Pediatric and Adolescent Nephrology Facing the Future: Diagnostic Advances and Prognostic Biomarkers in Everyday Practice

Pediatric and Adolescent Nephrology Facing the Future: Diagnostic Advances and Prognostic Biomarkers in Everyday Practice

Editors

Katarzyna Taranta-Janusz
Kinga Musiał

MDPI • Basel • Beijing • Wuhan • Barcelona • Belgrade • Manchester • Tokyo • Cluj • Tianjin

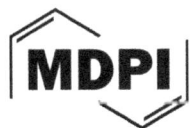

Editors
Katarzyna Taranta-Janusz
Medical University of
Bialystok
Poland

Kinga Musiał
Wroclaw Medical University
Poland

Editorial Office
MDPI
St. Alban-Anlage 66
4052 Basel, Switzerland

This is a reprint of articles from the Special Issue published online in the open access journal *Journal of Clinical Medicine* (ISSN 2077-0383) (available at: https://www.mdpi.com/journal/jcm/special_issues/Nephrology_Diagnostic_Prognostic_Biomarkers).

For citation purposes, cite each article independently as indicated on the article page online and as indicated below:

LastName, A.A.; LastName, B.B.; LastName, C.C. Article Title. *Journal Name* **Year**, *Volume Number*, Page Range.

ISBN 978-3-0365-5973-5 (Hbk)
ISBN 978-3-0365-5974-2 (PDF)

© 2022 by the authors. Articles in this book are Open Access and distributed under the Creative Commons Attribution (CC BY) license, which allows users to download, copy and build upon published articles, as long as the author and publisher are properly credited, which ensures maximum dissemination and a wider impact of our publications.

The book as a whole is distributed by MDPI under the terms and conditions of the Creative Commons license CC BY-NC-ND.

Contents

Kinga Musiał
Biomarkers in Pediatric Nephrology—From Bedside to Bench and Back Again
Reprinted from: *J. Clin. Med.* **2022**, *11*, 5919, doi:10.3390/jcm11195919 1

Małgorzata Mizerska-Wasiak, Emilia Płatos, Karolina Cichoń-Kawa, Urszula Demkow and Małgorzata Pańczyk-Tomaszewska
The Usefulness of Vanin-1 and Periostin as Markers of an Active Autoimmune Process or Renal Fibrosis in Children with IgA Nephropathy and IgA Vasculitis with Nephritis—A Pilot Study
Reprinted from: *J. Clin. Med.* **2022**, *11*, 1265, doi:10.3390/jcm11051265 5

Natalia Kopiczko, Aleksandra Dzik-Sawczuk, Karolina Szwarc, Anna Czyż and Anna Wasilewska
Analysis of Indications for Voiding Cystography in Children
Reprinted from: *J. Clin. Med.* **2021**, *10*, 5809, doi:10.3390/jcm10245809 17

Eryk Latoch, Katarzyna Konończuk, Katarzyna Taranta-Janusz, Katarzyna Muszyńska-Rosłan, Magdalena Sawicka, Anna Wasilewska and Maryna Krawczuk-Rybak
Urinary Beta-2-Microglobulin and Late Nephrotoxicity in Childhood Cancer Survivors
Reprinted from: *J. Clin. Med.* **2021**, *10*, 5279, doi:10.3390/jcm10225279 23

Katarzyna Werbel, Dorota Jankowska, Anna Wasilewska and Katarzyna Taranta-Janusz
Clinical and Epidemiological Analysis of Children's Urinary Tract Infections in Accordance with Antibiotic Resistance Patterns of Pathogens
Reprinted from: *J. Clin. Med.* **2021**, *10*, 5260, doi:10.3390/jcm10225260 35

Joanna Piechowicz, Andrzej Gamian, Danuta Zwolińska and Dorota Polak-Jonkisz
Adenine Nucleotide Metabolites in Uremic Erythrocytes as Metabolic Markers of Chronic Kidney Disease in Children
Reprinted from: *J. Clin. Med.* **2021**, *10*, 5208, doi:10.3390/jcm10215208 55

Karolina Nocuń-Wasilewska, Danuta Zwolińska, Agnieszka Zubkiewicz-Kucharska and Dorota Polak-Jonkisz
Evaluation of Vascular Endothelial Function in Children with Type 1 Diabetes Mellitus
Reprinted from: *J. Clin. Med.* **2021**, *10*, 5065, doi:10.3390/jcm10215065 67

Agnieszka Turczyn, Małgorzata Pańczyk-Tomaszewska, Grażyna Krzemień, Elżbieta Górska and Urszula Demkow
The Usefulness of Urinary Periostin, Cytokeratin-18, and Endoglin for Diagnosing Renal Fibrosis in Children with Congenital Obstructive Nephropathy
Reprinted from: *J. Clin. Med.* **2021**, *10*, 4899, doi:10.3390/jcm10214899 83

Kinga Musiał and Danuta Zwolińska
Bone Morphogenetic Proteins (BMPs), Extracellular Matrix Metalloproteinases Inducer (EMMPRIN), and Macrophage Migration Inhibitory Factor (MIF): Usefulness in the Assessment of Tubular Dysfunction Related to Chronic Kidney Disease (CKD)
Reprinted from: *J. Clin. Med.* **2021**, *10*, 4893, doi:10.3390/jcm10214893 99

Piotr Skrzypczyk, Magdalena Okarska-Napierała, Radosław Pietrzak, Katarzyna Pawlik, Katarzyna Waścińska, Bożena Werner and Małgorzata Pańczyk-Tomaszewska
NT-proBNP as a Potential Marker of Cardiovascular Damage in Children with Chronic Kidney Disease
Reprinted from: *J. Clin. Med.* **2021**, *10*, 4344, doi:10.3390/jcm10194344 109

Monika Kamianowska, Marek Szczepański, Anna Krukowska, Aleksandra Kamianowska and Anna Wasilewska
Urinary Levels of Cathepsin B in Preterm Newborns
Reprinted from: *J. Clin. Med.* **2021**, *10*, 4254, doi:10.3390/jcm10184254 . . . . **123**

Anna Medyńska, Joanna Chrzanowska, Katarzyna Kościelska-Kasprzak, Dorota Bartoszek, Marcelina Żabińska and Danuta Zwolińska
Alpha-1 Acid Glycoprotein and Podocin mRNA as Novel Biomarkers for Early Glomerular Injury in Obese Children
Reprinted from: *J. Clin. Med.* **2021**, *10*, 4129, doi:10.3390/jcm10184129 . . . . **133**

Katarzyna Maćkowiak-Lewandowicz, Danuta Ostalska-Nowicka, Jacek Zachwieja and Elżbieta Paszyńska
Differences between Obese and Non-Obese Children and Adolescents Regarding Their Oral Status and Blood Markers of Kidney Diseases
Reprinted from: *J. Clin. Med.* **2021**, *10*, 3723, doi:10.3390/jcm10163723 . . . . **143**

Piotr Skrzypczyk, Anna Ofiara, Michał Szyszka, Anna Stelmaszczyk-Emmel, Elżbieta Górska and Małgorzata Pańczyk-Tomaszewska
Serum Sclerostin Is Associated with Peripheral and Central Systolic Blood Pressure in Pediatric Patients with Primary Hypertension
Reprinted from: *J. Clin. Med.* **2021**, *10*, 3574, doi:10.3390/jcm10163574 . . . . **157**

Marcin Kołbuc, Beata Bieniaś, Sandra Habbig, Mateusz F. Kołek, Maria Szczepańska, Katarzyna Kiliś-Pstrusińska, Anna Wasilewska, Piotr Adamczyk, Rafał Motyka, Marcin Tkaczyk, Przemysław Sikora, Bodo B. Beck and Marcin Zaniew
Hyperuricemia Is an Early and Relatively Common Feature in Children with *HNF1B* Nephropathy but Its Utility as a Predictor of the Disease Is Limited
Reprinted from: *J. Clin. Med.* **2021**, *10*, 3265, doi:10.3390/jcm10153265 . . . . **171**

Agnieszka Pukajło-Marczyk and Danuta Zwolińska
Involvement of Hemopexin in the Pathogenesis of Proteinuria in Children with Idiopathic Nephrotic Syndrome
Reprinted from: *J. Clin. Med.* **2021**, *10*, 3160, doi:10.3390/jcm10143160 . . . . **185**

Joanna Bagińska, Edyta Sadowska and Agata Korzeniecka-Kozerska
An Examination of the Relationship between Urinary Neurotrophin Concentrations and Transcutaneous Electrical Nerve Stimulation (TENS) Used in Pediatric Overactive Bladder Therapy
Reprinted from: *J. Clin. Med.* **2021**, *10*, 3156, doi:10.3390/jcm10143156 . . . . **197**

Joanna Bagińska and Agata Korzeniecka-Kozerska
Are Tubular Injury Markers NGAL and KIM-1 Useful in Pediatric Neurogenic Bladder?
Reprinted from: *J. Clin. Med.* **2021**, *10*, 2353, doi:10.3390/jcm10112353 . . . . **209**

Michał Szyszka, Piotr Skrzypczyk, Anna Stelmaszczyk-Emmel and Małgorzata Pańczyk-Tomaszewska
Serum Periostin as a Potential Biomarker in Pediatric Patients with Primary Hypertension
Reprinted from: *J. Clin. Med.* **2021**, *10*, 2138, doi:10.3390/jcm10102138 . . . . **217**

Eryk Latoch, Katarzyna Konończuk, Anna Jander, Elżbieta Trembecka-Dubel, Anna Wasilewska and Katarzyna Taranta-Janusz
Galectin-3—A New Player of Kidney Damage or an Innocent Bystander in Children with a Single Kidney?
Reprinted from: *J. Clin. Med.* **2021**, *10*, 2012, doi:10.3390/jcm10092012 . . . . **231**

Monika Kamianowska, Marek Szczepański, Natalia Chomontowska, Justyna Trochim and Anna Wasilewska
Is Urinary Netrin-1 a Good Marker of Tubular Damage in Preterm Newborns?
Reprinted from: *J. Clin. Med.* **2021**, *10*, 847, doi:10.3390/jcm10040847 . . . . **243**

Hanna Nosek, Dorota Jankowska, Karolina Brzozowska, Katarzyna Kazberuk, Anna Wasilewska and Katarzyna Taranta-Janusz
Tumor Necrosis Factor-Like Weak Inducer of Apoptosis and Selected Cytokines—Potential Biomarkers in Children with Solitary Functioning Kidney
Reprinted from: *J. Clin. Med.* **2021**, *10*, 497, doi:10.3390/jcm10030497 . . . . **251**

Natalia Goździkiewicz, Danuta Zwolińska and Dorota Polak-Jonkisz
The Use of Artificial Intelligence Algorithms in the Diagnosis of Urinary Tract Infections—A Literature Review
Reprinted from: *J. Clin. Med.* **2022**, *11*, 2734, doi:10.3390/jcm11102734 . . . . **265**

Kinga Musiał
Current Concepts of Pediatric Acute Kidney Injury—Are We Ready to Translate Them into Everyday Practice?
Reprinted from: *J. Clin. Med.* **2021**, *10*, 3113, doi:10.3390/jcm10143113 . . . . **273**

Katarzyna Kilis-Pstrusinska, Artur Rogowski and Przemysław Bienkowski
Bacterial Colonization as a Possible Source of Overactive Bladder Symptoms in Pediatric Patients: A Literature Review
Reprinted from: *J. Clin. Med.* **2021**, *10*, 1645, doi:10.3390/jcm10081645 . . . . **285**

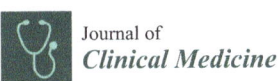

Editorial

Biomarkers in Pediatric Nephrology—From Bedside to Bench and Back Again

Kinga Musiał

Department of Pediatric Nephrology, Wrocław Medical University, Borowska 213, 50-556 Wrocław, Poland; kinga.musial@umw.edu.pl

The progress in biomarker research is characterized by the perpetual quest for parameters that fulfill the strict criteria of sensitivity, specificity, ease and speed in performance and cost-effectiveness. The expectations towards the range of functions the ideal index should deal with are increasing too. Lack of differentiation between biomarkers useful in the assessment of risk, prediction, prevention, diagnosis, progression or recovery raises the probability of functional overlap. Although unintentionally, such striving for perfection and versatility may lead to a dead end if there is no translation between sophisticated parameters and their use in clinical practice.

The example of acute kidney injury (AKI) clearly shows how difficult such implementation to the bedside can be. Despite years of research and subsequent recommendations, no internationally recognized definition of AKI has introduced any biomarker of damage so far [1]. Thus, only serum creatinine, estimated glomerular filtration rate, and urine output, condition clinical decisions regarding diagnosis, prognosis and treatment of AKI.

The problem seems even more serious in the pediatric field, where both physiological processes and pathological conditions largely depend on age and anthropometric data, extending presumed normal range values of biomarkers from prematures and neonates to adolescents [2]. Moreover, the profit advantage over the risk is always one of the priorities in the pediatric population, so noninvasive methods would overrate the invasive ones. Therefore, the evaluation of biomarkers in the urine would prioritize their assessment in the blood and the use of micro-methods would gain more attention than assays requiring excessive blood sampling [3,4]. The progress is also evident in bringing personalized medicine to everyday practice, where individual approach and adjustment of biomarkers to specific patients is the rule [5].

On the other hand, the assessment of biomarkers in specific panels seems superior to the evaluation of single parameters [4]. Last, but not least, the demands towards assessed parameters increase with time. Thus, today diagnostic indices are just the prelude, whereas prognostic markers or predictive models based on big data and built up with the tools of artificial intelligence are highly expected [6].

Pediatric nephrology seems to take on this challenge, tailoring parameters to various specific demands, including those of the neonatal period, rare diseases, inherited disorders or peritoneal dialysis [7–10].

However, with their specificity and multiplicity of topics, kidney diseases of childhood and adolescence don't make the search for ideal biomarkers easy. On the whole, understanding pediatric kidney meanders requires screening through the plethora of genetically conditioned, age-related, disease-specific and renal tissue-originating potential biomarkers. The pathology they illustrate is either restricted to clearly defined cells/milieu within the kidney, or to intrarenal interactions, or it triggers systemic engagement through interorgan crosslinks. Changes limited to the kidney are characteristic for the early phase of any renal pathology, then the systemic influence becomes the rule. However, it is usually challenging, because the dilemma whether the kidney is the culprit or the victim can remain unresolved.

Citation: Musiał, K. Biomarkers in Pediatric Nephrology—From Bedside to Bench and Back Again. *J. Clin. Med.* **2022**, *11*, 5919. https://doi.org/10.3390/jcm11195919

Received: 27 September 2022
Accepted: 5 October 2022
Published: 7 October 2022

Publisher's Note: MDPI stays neutral with regard to jurisdictional claims in published maps and institutional affiliations.

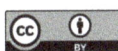

Copyright: © 2022 by the author. Licensee MDPI, Basel, Switzerland. This article is an open access article distributed under the terms and conditions of the Creative Commons Attribution (CC BY) license (https://creativecommons.org/licenses/by/4.0/).

Not unexpectedly, the kidney may also play both roles at the same time, as it occurs in the case of proteinuria in the course of chronic kidney disease.

Meanwhile, the examples of cardiorenal and hepatorenal syndromes unravel the truth of complex links between hemodynamic, metabolic, oxidative, inflammatory and neurohormonal conditions originating from distant organs [11,12]. They also highlight the role of holistic approaches as the optimal way of diagnosing and treating the patient as a whole, not just the disease itself. Additionally, functional links between various organs have created the possibility of universalization among markers, e.g., those reserved for cardiovascular comorbidities revealed their usefulness in chronic kidney disease [13].

The most recent example of a systemic approach towards the disease is the COVID-19-related pulmonary-renal crosstalk, placing the kidney as the second most frequently affected organ during SARS-CoV-2 infection. The existence of the lung-kidney axis has underlined the complexity and dynamism of interactions between the two organs and has given stimulus to new discoveries in the area of biomarkers predicting the development of complications and the patients' outcome [14,15].

In order to highlight the pathological background of a newly discovered disease, the molecular mechanisms of SARS-CoV-2 toxicity were analyzed within the clinical context. The first reports on the increased chemokine concentration, complement and coagulation overactivity stimulated a search for the molecular background of symptoms such as acute respiratory distress syndrome, thrombotic events or acute kidney injury [16,17]. Tracing the development of COVID-19 infection throughout various virus mutations enabled the acquisition of knowledge of SARS-CoV-2 structure, receptors, mechanisms of cell invasion and the way of systemic expansion with multiorgan affectation [14]. The invasion of SARS-CoV-2 was due to its entrance receptor, ACE-2, spreading all over the body and it was particularly abundant within the renal proximal tubules [18]. However, the direct viral toxicity was not sufficient and only its multiplication by overlapping innate immunity mechanisms, relied to the cascade activation of inflammation, necrosis, complement system, endothelial damage and thrombosis, could aggravate destructive mechanisms and lead to multiorgan failure [19]. The auto-amplification loops of several mechanisms, together with the interactions of circulating immune cells, gave way to the efficacious spread of stimulants such as chemokines or products released during cell damage [20]. Therefore, the subsequent stages of COVID-19-related research allowed for the definition of all clinical phenomena and connections between them, then the testing of the hypotheses explaining the molecular background of observed pathologies, and finally the introduction of innovative therapies based on recently acknowledged facts [21,22].

Thus, the turnover of candidate biomarkers, as well as their diagnostic/prognostic/therapeutic potentials during COVID-19 infection, were analyzed from bedside to bench and back again, and also in children [15]. Such attitudes should be implemented into pediatric biomarker research routinely.

The special issue entitled "Pediatric and adolescent nephrology facing the future: diagnostic advances and prognostic biomarkers in everyday practice" contains articles written in the era when COVID-19 had not yet been a major clinical problem in children. Now that we know its multifaceted clinical course, complications concerning the kidneys, and childhood-specific post-COVID pediatric inflammatory multisystem syndrome (PIMS), the value of diagnostic and prognostic biomarkers in the pediatric area should be appreciated, and their importance ought to increase [23].

The readers will have the opportunity to get acquainted with the spectrum of all major aspects of biomarker use in pediatric nephrology: from neonatal to adolescent perspectives, from rare genetic disorders to civilization diseases such as obesity, diabetes, and hypertension, from transient acute kidney injury to fibrosis and irreversible end-stage kidney disease, as well as from in situ sources to systemic manifestations.

The content should convince both the scientists and clinicians that re-shaping the attitude towards biomarkers is the only way to build up a de novo strategy, first based on in-depth analysis of the changeable clinical picture, then bridging clinical to molecular data, and coming back to the patient with molecular solutions to clinical challenges. No matter how far we reach, the patient remains in focus and gives the final answer to the question of the potential usefulness of tested biomarkers. Therefore, let these articles give us courage to come back to the bedside and start using biomarkers in everyday practice for the patients' good.

Funding: This research received no external funding.

Institutional Review Board Statement: Not applicable.

Informed Consent Statement: Not applicable.

Data Availability Statement: Not applicable.

Conflicts of Interest: The author declares no conflict of interest.

References

1. Ostermann, M.; Zarbock, A.; Goldstein, S.; Kashani, K.; Macedo, E.; Murugan, R.; Bell, M.; Forni, L.; Guizzi, L.; Joannidis, M.; et al. Recommendations on acute kidney injury biomarkers from the Acute Disease Quality Initiative consensus conference. A consensus statement. *JAMA Netw. Open* **2020**, *3*, e2019209. [CrossRef]
2. Bennett, M.R.; Nehus, E.; Haffner, C.; Ma, Q.; Devarajan, P. Pediatric reference ranges for acute kidney injury biomarkers. *Pediatr. Nephrol.* **2015**, *30*, 677–685. [CrossRef] [PubMed]
3. Valdimarsson, S.; Jodal, U.; Barregård, L.; Hansson, S. Urien neutrophil gelatinase-associated lipocalin and other biomarkers in infants with urinary tract infection and in febrile controls. *Pediatr. Nephrol.* **2017**, *32*, 2079–2087. [CrossRef]
4. Watson, D.; Yang, J.Y.C.; Sarwal, R.D.; Sigdel, T.K.; Liberto, J.M.; Damm, I.; Louie, V.; Sigdel, S.; Livingstone, D.; Soh, K.; et al. A novel multi-biomarker assay for non-invasive quantitative monitoring of kidney injury. *J. Clin. Med.* **2019**, *8*, 499. [CrossRef]
5. Cummins, T.D.; Korte, E.A.; Bhayana, S.; Merchant, M.L.; Barati, M.T.; Smoyer, W.E.; Klein, J.B. Advances in proteomic profiling of pediatric kidney diseases. *Pediatr. Nephrol.* **2022**, *37*, 2255–2265. [CrossRef]
6. Schena, F.P.; Magistroni, R.; Narducci, F.; Abbrescia, D.I.; Anelli, V.W.; Di Noia, T. Artificial intelligence in glomerular diseases. *Pediatr. Nephrol.* **2022**, *37*, 2533–2545. [CrossRef] [PubMed]
7. Coleman, C.; Perez, A.T.; Selewski, D.T.; Steflik, H.J. Neonatal acute kidney injury. *Front. Pediatr.* **2022**, *10*, 842544. [CrossRef]
8. Emma, F.; Montini, G.; Pennesi, M.; Peruzzi, L.; Verrina, E.; Goffredo, B.M.; Canalini, F.; Cassiman, D.; Rossi, S.; Levtchenko, E. Biomarkers in nephropatic cystinosis: Current and future perspectives. *Cells* **2022**, *11*, 1839. [CrossRef] [PubMed]
9. Sangeetha, G.; Babu, R. Comparing accuracy of urinary biomarkers in differentiation of ureteropelvic junction obstruction from nonobstructive dilatation in children. *Pediatr. Nephrol.* **2022**, *37*, 2277–2287. [CrossRef] [PubMed]
10. Trincianti, C.; Meleca, V.; La Porta, E.; Bruschi, M.; Candiano, G.; Garbarino, A.; Kajana, X.; Preda, A.; Lugani, F.; Ghiggeri, G.M.; et al. Proteomics and extracellular vesicles as novel biomarker sources in peritoneal dialysis in children. *Int. J. Mol. Sci.* **2022**, *23*, 5655. [CrossRef] [PubMed]
11. Liu, P.M.F.; de Carvalho, S.T.; Fradico, P.F.; Cazumbá, M.L.B.; Campos, R.G.B.; Simões e Silva, A.C. Hepatorenal syndrome in children: A review. *Pediatr. Nephrol.* **2021**, *36*, 2203–2215. [CrossRef] [PubMed]
12. Gembillo, G.; Visconti, L.; Giusti, M.A.; Siligato, R.; Gallo, A.; Santoro, D.; Mattina, A. Cardiorenal syndrome: New pathways and novel biomarkers. *Biomolecules* **2021**, *11*, 1581. [CrossRef]
13. Kula, A.; Bansal, N. Applications of cardiac biomarkers in chronic kidney disease. *Curr. Opin. Nephrol. Hypertens.* **2022**, *31*, 534–540. [CrossRef]
14. Perico, L.; Benigni, A.; Casiraghi, F.; Ng, L.F.P.; Renia, L.; Remuzzi, G. Immunity, endothelial injury and complement-induced coagulopathy in COVID-19. *Nat. Rev. Nephrol.* **2021**, *17*, 46–64. [CrossRef]
15. Önal, P.; Kilinç, A.A.; Aygün, F.D.; Aygün, F.; Durak, C.; Akkoç, G.; Ağbaş, A.; Elevli, M.; Çokuğraş, H. Diagnostic and prognostic biomarkers of coronavirus disease 2019 in children. *J. Trop. Pediatr.* **2022**, *68*, fmac003. [CrossRef]
16. Cabrera-Garcia, D.; Miltiades, A.; Yim, P.; Parsons, S.; Elisman, K.; Mansouri, M.T.; Wagener, G.; Harrison, N.L. Plasma biomarkers associated with survival and thrombosis in hospitalized COVID-19 patients. *Int. J. Hematol.* **2022**. [CrossRef]
17. Huber, S.; Massri, M.; Grasse, M.; Fleischer, V.; Kellnerová, S.; Harpf, V.; Knabl, L.; Knabl Sr, L.; Heiner, T.; Kummann, M.; et al. Systemic inflammation and complement activation parameters predict clinical outcome of severe SARS-CoV-2 infections. *Viruses* **2021**, *13*, 2376. [CrossRef]
18. Cruz, N.A.N.; de Oliveira, L.C.G.; Silva Junior, H.T.; Pestana, J.O.M.; Casarini, D.E. Angiotensin-converting enzyme 2 in the pathogenesis of renal abnormalities observed in COVID-19 patients. *Front. Physiol.* **2021**, *12*, 700220. [CrossRef]
19. Conway, E.M.; Mackman, N.; Warren, R.O.; Wolberg, A.S.; Mosnier, L.O.; Campbell, R.A.; Gralinski, L.E.; Rondina, M.T.; van de Veerdonk, F.L.; Hoffmeister, K.M.; et al. Understanding COVID-19-associated coagulopathy. *Nat. Rev. Immunol.* **2022**, *22*, 639–649. [CrossRef]
20. Lo, M.W.; Kemper, C.; Woodruff, T.M. COVID-19: Complement, coagulation, and collateral damage. *J. Immunol.* **2020**, *205*, 1488–1495. [CrossRef]

21. Vlaar, A.P.J.; Lim, E.H.T.; de Bruin, S.; Rückinger, S.; Pilz, K.; Brouwer, M.C.; Guo, R.-F.; Heunks, L.M.A.; Busch, M.H.; van Paassen, P.; et al. The anti-C5a antibody vilobelimab efficiently inhibits C5a in patients with severe COVID-19. *Clin. Transl. Sci.* **2022**, *15*, 854–858. [CrossRef] [PubMed]
22. Pitts, T.C. Soliris to stop immune-mediated death in COVID-19 (SOLID-C19)—A compassionate- use study of terminal complement blockade in critically ill patients with COVID-19-related adult respiratory distress syndrome. *Viruses* **2021**, *13*, 2429. [CrossRef] [PubMed]
23. Toraih, E.A.; Hussein, M.H.; Elshazli, R.M.; Kline, A.; Munshi, R.; Sultana, N.; Taghavi, S.; Killackey, M.; Duchesna, J.; Fawzy, M.S.; et al. Multisystem inflammatory syndrome in pediatric COVID-19 patients: A meta-analysis. *World J. Pediatr.* **2021**, *17*, 141–151. [CrossRef] [PubMed]

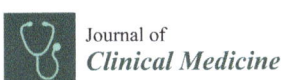

Article

The Usefulness of Vanin-1 and Periostin as Markers of an Active Autoimmune Process or Renal Fibrosis in Children with IgA Nephropathy and IgA Vasculitis with Nephritis—A Pilot Study

Małgorzata Mizerska-Wasiak [1,*,†], Emilia Płatos [2,†], Karolina Cichoń-Kawa [1], Urszula Demkow [3] and Małgorzata Pańczyk-Tomaszewska [1]

1. Department of Pediatrics and Nephrology, Medical University of Warsaw, 02-091 Warsaw, Poland; karolina.cichon@yahoo.com (K.C.-K.); mpanczyk1@wum.edu.pl (M.P.-T.)
2. Science Students' Association at the Department of Pediatrics and Nephrology, Medical University of Warsaw, 02-091 Warsaw, Poland; emiliaplatos@gmail.com
3. Department of Laboratory Diagnostics and Clinical Immunology of Developmental Age, Medical University of Warsaw, 02-091 Warsaw, Poland; urszula.demkow@wum.edu.pl
* Correspondence: mmizerska@wum.edu.pl
† These authors contributed equally to this work.

Abstract: This study aimed to evaluate the usefulness of vanin-1 and periostin in urine as markers of the autoimmune process in kidneys and renal fibrosis in IgA nephropathy (IgAN) and IgA vasculitis with nephritis (IgAVN). From a group of 194 patients from the Department of Pediatrics and Nephrology, who were included in the Polish Pediatric Registry of IgAN and IgAVN, we qualified 51 patients (20 with IgAN and 31 with IgAVN) between the ages of 3 and 17, diagnosed based on kidney biopsy, for inclusion in the study. All of the patients received glucocorticosteroids, immunosuppressive drugs, or renoprotective therapy. The control group consisted of 18 healthy individuals. The concentration of vanin was significantly higher in the IgAN and IgAVN groups than in the control group. The concentration of vanin/creatinine correlates positively with the level of IgA and negatively with the serum level of C3 at the end of the observation. Urinary vanin-1 concentration may be useful as a marker of the active autoimmune process in IgAN and IgAVN in children, but the study needs confirmation on a larger group of children, along with evaluation of the dynamics of this marker. Urinary periostin is not a good marker for children with IgAN and IgAVN, especially in stage 1 and 2 CKD.

Keywords: IgA nephropathy; IgA vasculitis with nephritis; vanin-1; periostin; biomarker; children

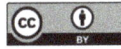

1. Introduction

IgA nephropathy (IgAN) is the most frequently diagnosed type of primary glomerulonephritis worldwide [1–3]. Its estimated incidence is 2.5/100,000/year; however, it varies across geographical locations. In Asia, the incidence rate is statistically higher than in Europe or the Americas [4,5]. Scientific research demonstrated an up to 8-fold higher increased frequency of occurrence of IgAN among Japanese children and teenagers than among American children [6,7].

IgA vasculitis (IgAV), previously known as Henoch–Schönlein purpura (HSP), is the most common cause of systemic childhood vasculitis [8–10]. Although its etiology remains vague, the strong predisposition among individuals with the HLA-DRB1*01 allele was revealed [8,9]. IgAV affects small vessels of the skin, gastrointestinal tract, and joints. Nonetheless, immunoglobulin A (IgA) vasculitis with nephritis (IgAVN) manifests in about one-third of IgAV patients [11].

Hallmarks of IgAN, a disease described by Burger and Hinglaise in 1968, are IgA-dominant deposits with co-dominant IgG and IgM deposits in mesangial glomeruli. Although complement C3 is almost always detected, C1q remains mostly absent [12,13]. The pathogenesis model is described as "multi-hit" and composed of a few stages: elevated galactose deficient IgA1 levels and the generation of anti-glycan antibodies, resulting in the formation of immune complexes out of themselves. Accumulation of those deposits leads to the activation of the alternative complement pathway and mesangial proliferation with inflammatory and fibrotic effects [12,14,15]. Acute kidney injury (AKI) occurs in up to 10% of IgAN patients and belongs to the risk factors for renal disease [16,17]. IgAN may lead to end-stage renal failure (ESRF) in up to 60% of cases [18].

The Oxford MEST-C Score facilitates the assessment of renal biopsy samples. It defines risk factors of kidney insufficiency and can be used in IgAVN patient samples [19,20].

IgAVN, despite different disease courses, has some common features with IgAN, which apply to a similar pathomechanism, linked to IgA complexes [21–23]. Although IgAN and IgAV are considered to be similar, they can be distinguished from each other with clinical manifestation or peak age ranges of diagnosis [24]. More recent evidence (Ozen et al., 2019) proposes SHARE recommendations for IgAV/IgAVN as a practical source of information. These recommendations underline the importance of renal and skin biopsy, eGFR, urinalysis, and ultrasound [25].

Vanin-1 has a crucial role in the recycling of pantothenic acid and is a precursor of CoA in the long term [26]. Since its discovery in 1945, coenzyme A has been known as a cofactor of lipid metabolic processes and energy production [27]. That explains its remarkable expression in tissues with CoA turnover, e.g., kidney, liver, or intestine [28]. Vnn1, which codes vanin-1, is involved in numerous metabolic pathways. For instance, in mice, it upregulates peroxisome proliferator-activated receptor alpha (PPAR-α)—liver's fasting regulator [29]. Proximal tubuli of the kidney are one of the places of vanin-1 expression [26]. Vanin-1 is a novel tissue sensor for oxidative stress and its level increases in AKI before the emergence of classic markers, e.g., N-acetyl-β-D-glucosaminidase (NAG), creatinine, or blood urea nitrogen (BUN) [30]. Vanin helps detect AKI, particularly kidney injuries triggered by nephrotoxic drugs and intoxication [31,32].

Novel studies have suggested its relevance to the prediction and evaluation of obstructive nephropathy (hydronephrosis) [32]. In addition, pantetheine, the substrate of vanin-1, may improve the vasculopathy observed in several inflammatory conditions. Enhanced levels of vanin-1 can be related to both positive and negative autoimmune disease prognoses [33,34].

Periostin is a protein expressed in multiple tissues during embryonal development; however, it is detected in collagen-rich tissues such as bone, dental tissues, and heart valves as well as in injured areas, e.g., kidneys [35–38]. It integrates an extracellular matrix (ECM) in physiological conditions; nonetheless, overexpression may lead to organ fibrosis [36,37]. AKI progression follows periostin expression and leads to renal fibrosis in response to hypoxia or ischemia [39]. That suggests its potentiality to become a novel CKD biomarker [35,37,40,41]. Patients with glomerulopathies might have increased periostin expression in the mesangium, tubular interstitium, and even areas of fibrosis according to biopsy findings. Interestingly, the external addition of TGF-β1 also leads to extreme periostin production [42]. De novo overexpression of periostin was found in several renal diseases such as lupus nephritis, diabetic nephropathy, IgA nephropathy, and focal-segmental glomerulosclerosis [42–45]. Moreover, complex periostin–human IgA1 in a ratio 1:1 might play a role in the pathomechanism of allergic diseases [46]. Although the trigger factors and mechanisms of periostin overexpression should still be elucidated, the interaction of periostin with ECM was extensively clarified [38].

This study aimed to evaluate the significance of vanin-1 and periostin in urine for the autoimmune inflammatory process in kidneys and renal fibrosis in IgAN and IgAVN.

2. Materials and Methods

We performed a prospective, cross-sectional study.

From the group of 194 patients hospitalized in the Department of Pediatrics and Nephrology with diagnosed IgAN or IgAVN, who were included in the Polish Pediatric

Registry of IgAN and IgAVN, we qualified 51 patients (20 with IgAN and 31 with IgAVN) between the ages of 3 and 17, diagnosed based on kidney biopsy, for inclusion in the study. The control group consisted of 18 healthy individuals after detailed physical examination without any symptoms of the diseases and any chronic illnesses in their past medical history. The patients included in the study fulfilled the following inclusion criteria: IgAN or IgAVN diagnosis based on renal biopsy with histological proof of predominant mesangial IgA immune deposits remained under the supervision of doctors in the clinic. All of the biopsy samples were screened by optical, immunofluorescence, and electron microscopy.

2.1. Clinical and Biological Features

The parameters assessed at the onset of the disease were age, weight, sex, protein in the 24 h urine collection, protein, and erythrocytes in the urinalysis, eGFR, creatinine, albumin, cholesterol, triglycerides, IgA, IgM, IgG, and complement components: C3 and C4. To diagnose the disease in all patients, we performed a histopathological examination of the material collected during the kidney biopsy. After treatment administration, we implemented follow-up measurements and tested the levels of vanin and periostin in the urine.

For each patient, their age, weight, and sex were determined by a nurse when the patient was admitted to the ward. General urine test samples, containing approximately 20 mL of midstream urine, were collected in plastic containers. Moreover, 50 mL of urine samples taken during the 24 h urine collection was transferred to plastic containers. Furthermore, 4 mL whole blood samples were collected in lithium heparin tubes aimed at the determination of creatinine, cholesterol, triglyceride levels, and complement components: C3 and C4 levels. To assess the level of albumin and immunoglobulins IgA, IgM, and IgG, 5 mL of whole blood was collected in test tubes with a separating gel. The material was stored at room temperature, centrifuged for 5 min at 4000 rpm, transferred to new tubes, and sent afterward to the hospital diagnostic laboratory.

A Human Vanin-1 (urine) ELISA Kit and Human Periostin ELISA Kit were used to test vanin and periostin levels. Ten mL urine samples were collected from each patient. The sensitivity of the Vanin-1 ELISA Kit was 9.6 pmol/L (=500 pg/mL) and the vanin concentration was converted according to the formula 1 pmol/L = 52.07 pg/mL (MW: 52.07 kDa). The sensitivity of the Periostin ELISA Kit was 20 pmol/L (=1800 pg/mL) and the periostin concentration was converted according to the formula 1 pmol/L = 91 pg/mL (MW: 91 kDa).

2.2. Renal Biopsy

After the detection of unexplained hematuria and proteinuria, the patients were qualified for renal biopsy. The diagnostic material was obtained from a large-needle percutaneous biopsy performed under ultrasound guidance. Three bioptates were evaluated under the light/electron microscope or in the immunofluorescence tests. A total of 25–50 serial 2–5 µm thick sections were analyzed. Direct immunofluorescence was performed with fluorescein-conjugated antibodies (FITC). A clear green fluorescence was assumed as a positive reaction, rated between 0 and +4. Immunomorphological diagnostics included the performance of reactions with antibodies against IgG, IgA, IgM, C3, C1q, fibrinogen, albumin, lambda, and kappa light chains. Findings were categorized according to the Oxford MEST-C score (M—mesangial hypercellularity: M0 > 50%, M1 < 50%; E—endocapillary hypercellularity: 0—absent, 1—present; S—segmental sclerosis/adhesion: 0—absent, 1—present; T—tubular atrophy/interstitial fibrosis: T0 0–25%, T1 26–50%, T2 > 50%; C—crescents: C0 0%, C1 0–25%, C2 > 25%. The overall score is calculated as the sum of M, E, S, T, and C).

2.3. Treatment

The patients received glucocorticosteroids (prednisone, deflazacort), immunosuppressive drugs (azathioprine, cyclophosphamide, cyclosporin A), renoprotective therapy (angiotensin-converting enzyme inhibitor (ACEI)/angiotensin receptor blocker (ARB): enalapril, amlodipine), and/or omega-3 fatty acid.

2.4. Monitoring and Follow-Up

Patients remain under the supervision of pediatric nephrologists at the Department of Pediatrics and Nephrology, Medical University of Warsaw. The development of their diseases is continuously monitored.

The study was approved by the Bioethics Committee at the Medical University of Warsaw (No. KB/147/2017).

The flow diagram of the study is shown in Figure 1.

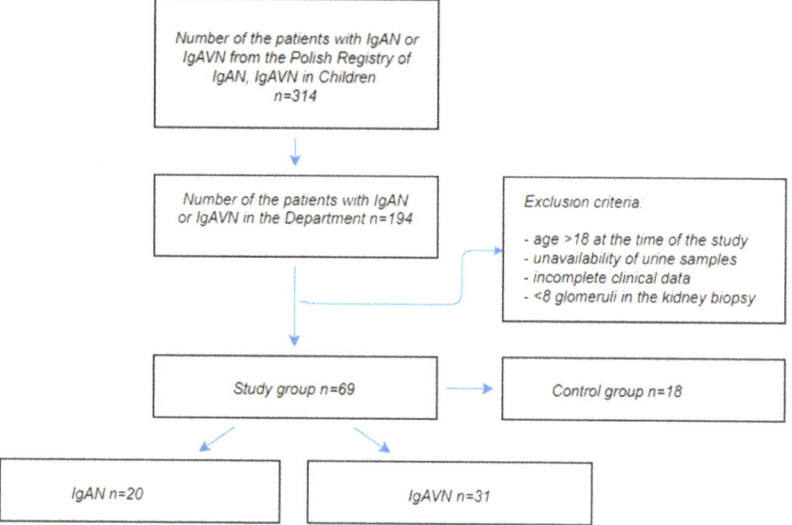

Figure 1. The flow diagram of the study.

Statistical analysis was performed with Statistica 13 (maintained by TIBCO Software, Inc., Palo Alto, CA, USA) using the Student's *t*-test for normally distributed variables: age, height, weight, and their values on growth charts, glomerular filtration rate (GFR), albumin, cholesterol, triglycerides, IgG, IgM, C3, C4, and the sum of the MEST-C score. For non-normally-distributed variables: proteinuria mg/kg/day, erythrocyturia, urea, creatinine, IgA, time to biopsy, vanin (pmol/L, pg/mg creatinine), and periostin (pg/mg creatinine), we used the Mann–Whitney test. The Kruskal–Wallis test was used to compare the values of vanin and periostin in the groups of IgAN and IgAVN patients with the control group (three groups). To evaluate differences between the baseline and follow-up values, the Student's *t*-test and the Wilcoxon test were used (for normally and non-normally distributed variables, respectively). Linear regression analysis and Spearman's rank correlation were also performed. The Mann–Whitney test was used to compare the individual components of MEST-C in the IgAN and IgAVN groups. The generalized GRM linear regression method helped us to find qualitative (group, gender) and quantitative variables that correlate with vanin, periostin, vanin/cr, and periostin/cr. Using the step-wise method, statistically, significant variables correlated with the above-mentioned variables were found.

Independently, the correlation between the variables was investigated using Spearman's rank method.

3. Results

The mean age at the diagnosis of IgAN/IgAVN was 8.84 ± 3.88 years. At baseline, the mean proteinuria was 28.8 (0–742) mg/kg/d; erythrocyturia was 80 (6–250) HPF; GFR was 108.89 ± 30.62 mL/min; IgA was 250.95 (57.8–1070); C3 was 109.65 ± 28.96; and C4 was 23.93 ± 7.89 mg/dL.

Renal biopsy was performed 1.0 (0–80.4) months after the onset of the disease.

The duration of follow-up was 3.31 ± 2.78 years. At the end of this period, proteinuria was 0 (0–180) mg/kg/d, erythrocyturia was 0 (0–200) HPF; GFR was 112.48 ± 17.71 mL/min; IgA was 192.1 (48.1–439) mg/dL; C3 was 93.62 ± 14.78 mg/dL; and C4 was 18.11 ± 6.9 mg/dL.

The clinical characteristics of the study patients divided into two groups, IgAN (group 1) and IgAVN (group 2), are shown in Table 1.

Table 1. Clinical characteristics of the IgAN and IgAVN patient groups.

Parameter	IgAN (n = 20)	IgAVN (n = 31)	p
Age at the disease onset (years)	11 ± 4.1	7.5 ± 3.1	0.001
Height (cm)	150.2 ± 26.6	129.2 ± 20.2	0.002
Weight (kg)	45.8 ± 20.8	31.8 ± 14.6	0.007
SDS to weight	0.6 ± 1.4	0.3 ± 0.9	NS
GFR (mL/min/1.73 m^2)	101.8 ± 30	113.5 ± 30.6	NS
Proteinuria at baseline (mg/kg/d)	19 (0–226)	34 (0–742)	NS
Erythrocyturia (RBC/HPF)	65.5 (0–250)	80 (0–250)	NS
Urea (mg/dL)	228 (18–43)	27 (15–159)	NS
Creatinine (mg/dL)	0.6 (0.3–1.3)	0.4 (0.3–2.1)	0.005
Albumin (g/dL)	3.7 ± 0.8	3.6 ± 0.7	NS
IgA (mg/dL)	302 (57.8–494)	213.4 (68.7–1070)	0.032
C3 (mg/dL)	106.6 ± 22.9	111.6 ± 32.5	NS
C4 (mg/dL)	24.8 ± 8	23.4 ± 7.9	NS
MEST-C score (sum)	2.2 ± 1.4	2.5 ± 1.2	NS
Time to biopsy (months)	3 (0–68.4)	1 (0–26)	0.03
Outcome (years)	2.9 ± 2.6	3.6 ± 2.9	NS
Age at FU (years)	14.1 ± 3.7	10.8 ± 3.6	0.004
Height at FU (cm)	154.4 ± 27.4	144.7 ± 18.6	NS
Weight at FU (kg)	53.6 ± 20.9	45.8 ± 19.8	NS
SDS to weight at FU	0 ± 1.5	0.7 ± 1.3	NS
GFR at FU (mL/min/1.73 m^2)	111 ± 14.6	113.4 ± 19.6	NS
Proteinuria at FU (mg/kg/d)	0 (0–76)	0 (0–190)	NS
Erythrocyturia at FU (RBC/HPF)	6 (0–200)	0 (0–35)	0.002
Creatinine at FU (mg/dL)	0.6 ± 0.2	0.6 ± 0.1	NS
Albumin at FU (g/dL)	4.2 ± 0.6	4.4 ± 0.2	NS
IgA at FU (mg/dL)	253 (51–439)	173.2 (49.1–396)	0.033
C3 at FU (mg/dL)	91.3 ± 13.6	95 ± 15.5	NS
C4 at FU (mg/dL)	18 ± 7.1	18.2 ± 6.9	NS

BMI = Body mass index; GFR = glomerular filtration rate; FU = follow up; MEST-C score = the Oxford classification of IgA nephropathy; SDS = standard deviation score; NS = not significant.

Subgroup analyses were also performed for the vanin and periostin in urine and further converted to creatinine, as shown in Table 2 and Figure 2.

The concentration of vanin was significantly higher in the IgAN and IgAVN groups than in the control group ($p < 0.05$). Furthermore, no significant differences were found in the concentration of vanin between the IgAN and IgAVN groups. In the study group, periostin concentration did not differ between the IgAN, IgAVN, and control groups (Figure 3).

Table 2. Vanin and periostin levels in the IgAV and IgAVN patient groups and the control group.

Parameter	Control Group (n = 18)	IgAN (n = 20)	IgAVN (n = 31)	p
Vanin (pmol/L)	61.1 (1–442.1)	203.4 (2.5–421.6)	190.4 (1.1–533)	0.016
Periostin (pmol/L)	21 (5–212.1)	16.7 (5–67.5)	22.8 (5–73.4)	NS
Vanin (pg/mg creatinine) *	0.5 (0.0–11.6)	1.8 (0.0–7.5)	1.8 (0–11.6)	NS
Perostin (pg/mg creatinine) *	0.2 (0.1–1.1)	0.2 (0.0–153.3)	0.4 (0.0–2.5)	NS

* pg/mg creatinine: We obtained the results in this parameter to adjust the results according to the gender of our patients and the different intensities of creatinine elimination; NS = not significant.

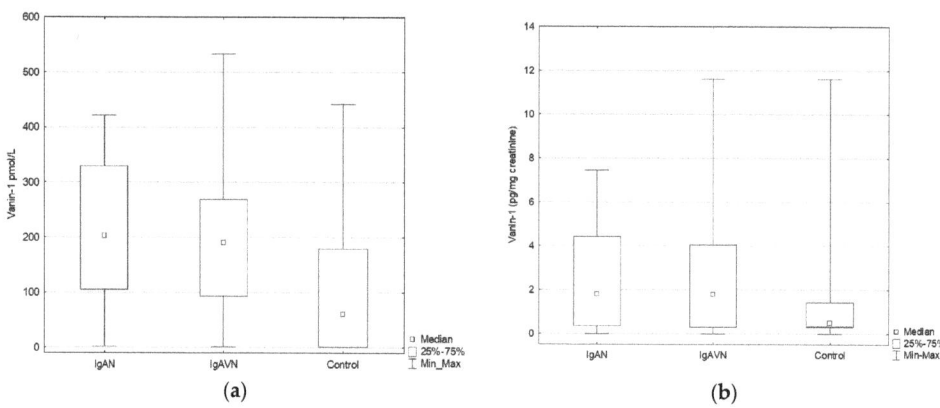

Figure 2. The concentration of vanin and vanin/creatinine in urine samples in children with IgAN, IgAVN, and in the control group. (a) The concentration of vanin in urine samples in IgAN, IgAVN and control group; (b) The concentration of vanin/creatinine in urine samples in IgAN, IgAVN and control group.

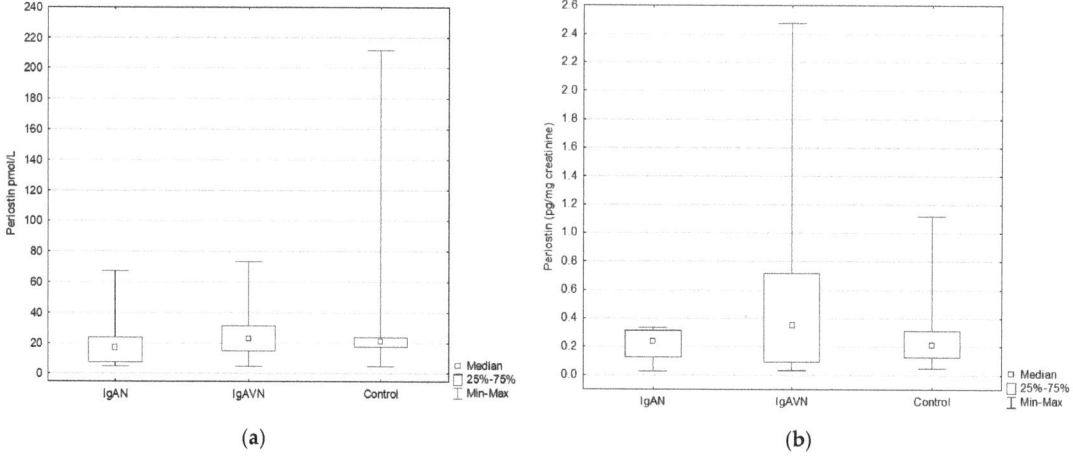

Figure 3. The concentration of periostin and periostin/creatinine in the urine samples in children with IgAN, IgAVN, and in the control group. (a) The concentration of periostin in urine samples in IgAN, IgAVN and control group; (b) The concentration of periostin/creatinine in urine samples in IgAN, IgAVN and control group.

A multivariate analysis of the concentration of vanin and periostin in urine was performed and the significant correlations were presented on a graph of linear correlations, as shown in Figures 4 and 5. The only statistically significant differences ($p < 0.05$) we observed were for the vanin-1 and vanin-1/creatinine concentration among patients with IgAVN and the whole study group (IgAVN and IgAN).

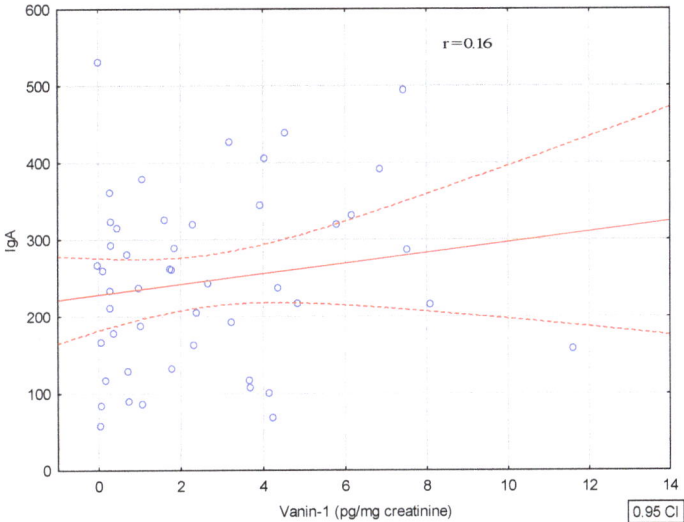

Figure 4. Correlation of vanin with serum IgA.

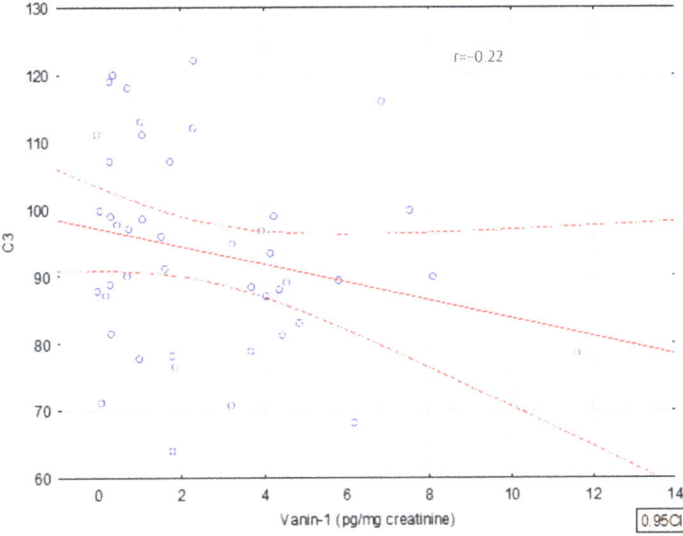

Figure 5. Correlation of urinary vanin with serum C3.

The concentration of vanin/cr correlates positively with the level of IgA and negatively with the serum level of C3 at the end of the observation.

The regression analysis confirmed a positive correlation of periostin and vanin (in pmol/l and ng/mg creatinine) in the IgAVN group and the whole study group.

In the multivariate GRM analysis (general regression model) of the dependence of vanin concentration, a weak negative correlation with C3 at the end of the observation and a positive correlation with the SDS of body weight was confirmed, as shown in Table 3.

Table 3. General regression model analysis results for vanin (pg/mg creatinine).

	Subgroup	Vanin (pg/mg Creatinine) Parameter Correlation	−95% CI	+95% CI	p
SDS to weight at FU		0.6757	−0.0755	1.2760	0.0285
GFR at FU		0.0075	−0.0416	0.0565	0.7582
C3 at FU		−0.0561	−0.1079	0.0047	0.0711
Group	IgAN	0.1450	−0.7856	1.0757	0.7533
Sex	F	−0.1197	−0.9952	0.7559	0.7827

FFU = foFFUFU = follow up; CI = confidence interval; SDS = standard deviation score; GFR = glomerular filtration rate.

GRM analysis did not confirm a correlation of periostin with the tested parameters.

We analyzed the results of kidney biopsy in the Oxford classification, and the levels of vanin and periostin in urine depending on the MEST-C score.

In the IgAN and IgAVN groups, no significant differences were found in the concentration of vanin or periostin in urine in E1, S1, T1-2, or C1-2 compared to E0, S0, T0, and C0 (M1 occurred in all IgAN patients).

The treatment analysis of children in the study group confirmed that 61% of all patients received immunosuppressive therapy, including 71% in the IgAVN group and 45% in the IgAN group, and therefore it should not influence the better or worse treatment of some groups of the patients.

4. Discussion

Vanin-1 had not been investigated among children nor adults with IgAN or IgAVN until now. Studies in the scope of periostin's role in IgAN include only adults and relate mostly to serum periostin levels. Thus, this study is a novelty and it was planned as a pilot study on a small group of patients.

The subgroups within the study group differed significantly only in the age of diagnosis and the time from diagnosis to a kidney biopsy, which results from the natural course of these diseases and the usually faster development of IgAVN.

In our study, we demonstrated the significant growth of urinary vanin-1 levels in children with IgAN or IgAVN diagnosis in comparison to the control group. Hosohata et al. were some of the first researchers who observed increased levels of urinary vanin-1 24 h after exposure to toxic solvents, and thus suggested vanin-1 to be a predictive biomarker of AKI [40]. GFR reduction at the onset of the disease was confirmed in nine patients (five with IgAN, four with IgAVN), whereas at the end of follow-up GFR < 90 mL/min had only two pediatric patients with IgAVN (GFR of 86 and 80 mL/min).

Although vanin-1 expression takes place in proximal tubuli, not in glomeruli, which would be remarkable for our findings, tubular atrophy is also recognized as one of the Oxford classifications (MEST-C). The MEST-C score enables stratification of the risks of IgAN nephropathy progression regarding, e.g., mesangial and endocapillary hypercellularity–proof of glomerular injury, or interstitial fibrosis/tubular atrophy–tubular compartment [20]. In our study, we did not observe significant differences between the levels of vanin in patients with T0 and T1-2.

The concentration of urinary vanin-1 correlates negatively with simultaneously measured serum C3 levels. However, in our study, we did not find the prognostic significance of the reduction of C3 in the serum of children with IgAN, which furthermore cannot confirm the prognostic significance of vanin [47].

The lack of significant differences, dependent on the Oxford-MEST-C score, might result from the time between kidney biopsy and vanin uptake and the influence of the implemented treatment on reversibility MEST-C classification elements.

There were no significant differences in the concentration of periostin in urine between the study group and the control group. Nevertheless, a relationship between periostin in the serum and the presence of fibrosis in the kidney tissue has been found in the studies performed so far. This relationship was shown in the study by Jia et al., especially for patients with severe CKD. Our group included children with CKD 1 and 2, and at the time of periostin uptake, only two patients presented CKD 2 [48].

Hwang et al. observed a positive correlation of periostin concentration in urine with interstitial fibrosis, interstitial inflammation, and glomerulosclerosis. Higher periostin levels in urine were linked to greater filtration failure in long-term observation, particularly with GFR < 60 mL/min. In our research, we have not confirmed this dependence, which might be associated with normal GFR in the long-term follow-up in 49 out of the 51 patients studied. Periostin levels were not tested during the renal biopsy, which may also play an important role [45].

Satirapoj et al. found that, in adults with diabetes mellitus type 2, urinary periostin correlates negatively with GFR and the severity of proteinuria; however, the investigated patients with an eGFR between 45.9 and 69.9 mL/min had a history of proteinuria. In our group, median proteinuria was 0, and mean GFR = 112.48 mL/min. It would be appropriate to investigate the level of microalbuminuria [44].

In Turczyn et al., in children with congenital obstructive nephropathy, a positive correlation of periostin with serum creatinine and cystatin C was found, with the presence of severe and moderate renal scars and borderline lesions in scintigraphy; in our study, periostin was measured after intensive treatment with positive effect for GFR and proteinuria [49].

Limitations

One of the limitations of our study is the lack of measurement of vanin and periostin concentration in the urine at the onset of the disease (at the time of the kidney biopsy); however, this is a pilot study.

5. Conclusions

Urinary vanin-1 concentration may be a biomarker of active inflammation in IgAN and IgAVN in children, but the study needs confirmation on a larger group of children, along with evaluation of the dynamics of this marker.

Urinary periostin is not a good marker for children with IgAN and IgAVN, especially in stage 1 and 2 CKD, but the study needs confirmation on a larger group and in higher stages of the disease progression.

Author Contributions: Conceptualization, M.M.-W. and E.P.; methodology, M.M.-W. and E.P.; software, K.C.-K.; validation, M.M.-W. and E.P.; formal analysis, M.M.-W. and E.P.; investigation, M.M.-W. and K.C.-K.; writing—original draft preparation, M.M.-W. and E.P.; writing—review and editing, M.M.-W., K.C.-K., and M.P.-T.; visualization, E.P. and M.M.-W.; supervision, M.P.-T. and U.D. All authors have read and agreed to the published version of the manuscript.

Funding: This research received no external funding.

Institutional Review Board Statement: The study was conducted according to the guidelines of the Declaration of Helsinki, and approved by the Bioethics Committee at the Medical University of Warsaw (No. KB/147/2017).

Informed Consent Statement: Informed consent for study participation was obtained from the legal guardians of the study participants.

Data Availability Statement: The data analyzed in this study are available from the corresponding author upon reasonable request.

Conflicts of Interest: The authors declare no conflict of interest.

References

1. Saha, M.K.; Julian, B.A.; Novak, J.; Rizk, D.V. Secondary IgA nephropathy. *Kidney Int.* **2018**, *94*, 674–681. [CrossRef] [PubMed]
2. Habib, R.; Murcia, I.; Beaufils, H.; Niaudet, P. Primary IgA nephropathies in children. *Biomed. Pharmacother.* **1990**, *44*, 159–162. [CrossRef]
3. Suzuki, H.; Yasutake, J.; Makita, Y.; Tanbo, Y.; Yamasaki, K.; Sofue, T.; Kano, T.; Suzuki, Y. IgA nephropathy and IgA vasculitis with nephritis have a shared feature involving galactose-deficient IgA1-oriented pathogenesis. *Kidney Int.* **2018**, *93*, 700–705. [CrossRef] [PubMed]
4. Kawasaki, Y.; Maeda, R.; Ohara, S.; Suyama, K.; Hosoya, M. Serum IgA/C3 and glomerular C3 staining predict severity of IgA nephropathy. *Pediatr. Int.* **2018**, *60*, 162–167. [CrossRef]
5. Schena, F.P.; Nistor, I. Epidemiology of IgA Nephropathy: A Global Perspective. *Semin. Nephrol.* **2018**, *38*, 435–442. [CrossRef]
6. Sehic, A.M.; Gaber, L.W.; Iii, S.R.; Miller, P.M.; Kritchevsky, S.B.; Wyatt, R. Increased recognition of IgA nephropathy in African-American children. *Pediatr. Nephrol.* **1997**, *11*, 435–437. [CrossRef]
7. Utsunomiya, Y.; Koda, T.; Kado, T.; Okada, S.; Hayashi, A.; Kanzaki, S.; Kasagi, T.; Hayashibara, H.; Okasora, T. Incidence of pediatric IgA nephropathy. *Pediatr. Nephrol.* **2003**, *18*, 511–515. [CrossRef]
8. Oni, L.; Sampath, S. Childhood IgA Vasculitis (Henoch Schonlein Purpura)—Advances and Knowledge Gaps. *Front. Pediatr.* **2019**, *7*, 257. [CrossRef]
9. Dyga, K.; Szczepanska, M. IgA vasculitis with nephritis in children. *Adv. Clin. Exp. Med.* **2020**, *29*, 513–519. [CrossRef]
10. González-Gay, M.A.; López-Mejias, R.; Pina, T.; Blanco, R.; Castañeda, S. IgA Vasculitis: Genetics and Clinical and Therapeutic Management. *Curr. Rheumatol. Rep.* **2018**, *20*, 24. [CrossRef]
11. Demir, S.; Kaplan, O.; Celebier, M.; Sag, E.; Bilginer, Y.; Lay, I.; Ozen, S. Predictive biomarkers of IgA vasculitis with nephritis by metabolomic analysis. *Semin. Arthritis Rheum.* **2020**, *50*, 1238–1244. [CrossRef] [PubMed]
12. Wyatt, R.J.; Julian, B.A. IgA nephropathy. *N. Engl. J. Med.* **2013**, *368*, 2402–2414. [CrossRef]
13. Novak, J.; Barratt, J.; Julian, B.A.; Renfrow, M.B. Aberrant Glycosylation of the IgA1 Molecule in IgA Nephropathy. *Semin. Nephrol.* **2018**, *38*, 461–476. [CrossRef] [PubMed]
14. Magistroni, R.; D'Agati, V.D.; Appel, G.B.; Kiryluk, K. New developments in the genetics, pathogenesis, and therapy of IgA nephropathy. *Kidney Int.* **2015**, *88*, 974–989. [CrossRef] [PubMed]
15. Rodrigues, J.C.; Haas, M.; Reich, H.N. Reich, IgA Nephropathy. *Clin. J. Am. Soc. Nephrol.* **2017**, *12*, 677–686. [CrossRef]
16. Zhang, L.; Li, J.; Yang, S.; Huang, N.; Zhou, Q.; Yang, Q.; Yu, X. Clinicopathological features and risk factors analysis of IgA nephropathy associated with acute kidney injury. *Ren. Fail.* **2016**, *38*, 799–805. [CrossRef]
17. Zhang, L.; Zhuang, X.; Liao, X. A proposed Oxford classification-based clinicopathological nomogram for predicting short-term renal outcomes in IgA nephropathy after acute kidney injury. *Eur. J. Intern. Med.* **2018**, *52*, 60–66. [CrossRef]
18. Coppo, R. Treatment of IgA nephropathy: Recent advances and prospects. *Nephrol. Ther.* **2018**, *14* (Suppl. S1), S13–S21. [CrossRef]
19. Trimarchi, H.; Barratt, J.; Cattran, D.C.; Cook, H.T.; Coppo, R.; Haas, M.; Liu, Z.-H.; Roberts, I.S.; Yuzawa, Y.; Zhang, H.; et al. Oxford Classification of IgA nephropathy 2016: An update from the IgA Nephropathy Classification Working Group. *Kidney Int.* **2017**, *91*, 1014–1021. [CrossRef]
20. Coppo, R.; Cattran, D.; Ian, S.D.R.; Troyanov, S.; Camilla, R.; Cook, T.; Feehally, J. The new Oxford Clinico-Pathological Classification of IgA nephropathy. *Prilozi* **2010**, *31*, 241–248.
21. Hetland, L.; Susrud, K.; Lindahl, K.; Bygum, A. Henoch-Schönlein Purpura: A Literature Review. *Acta Derm. Venereol.* **2017**, *97*, 1160–1166. [CrossRef] [PubMed]
22. Audemard-Verger, A.; Pillebout, E.; Guillevin, L.; Thervet, E.; Terrier, B. IgA vasculitis (Henoch–Shönlein purpura) in adults: Diagnostic and therapeutic aspects. *Autoimmun. Rev.* **2015**, *14*, 579–585. [CrossRef]
23. Chen, J.Y.; Mao, J.H. Henoch-Schönlein purpura nephritis in children: Incidence, pathogenesis and management. *World J. Pediatr.* **2015**, *11*, 29–34. [CrossRef]
24. Davin, J.C.; Ten Berge, I.J.; Weening, J.J. What is the difference between IgA nephropathy and Henoch-Schonlein purpura nephritis? *Kidney Int.* **2001**, *59*, 823–834. [CrossRef] [PubMed]
25. Ozen, S.; Marks, S.D.; Brogan, P.; Groot, N.; de Graeff, N.; Avcin, T.; Bader-Meunier, B.; Dolezalova, P.; Feldman, B.M.; Kone-Paut, I.; et al. European consensus-based recommendations for diagnosis and treatment of immunoglobulin A vasculitis—The SHARE initiative. *Rheumatology* **2019**, *58*, 1607–1616. [CrossRef] [PubMed]
26. Bartucci, R.; Salvati, A.; Olinga, P.; Boersma, Y.L. Vanin 1: Its Physiological Function and Role in Diseases. *Int. J. Mol. Sci.* **2019**, *20*, 3891. [CrossRef]
27. Theodoulou, F.L.; Sibon, O.C.; Jackowski, S.; Gout, I. Coenzyme A and its derivatives: Renaissance of a textbook classic. *Biochem. Soc. Trans.* **2014**, *42*, 1025–1032. [CrossRef]
28. Schalkwijk, J.; Jansen, P. Chemical biology tools to study pantetheinases of the vanin family. *Biochem. Soc. Trans.* **2014**, *42*, 1052–1055. [CrossRef]
29. Rommelaere, S.; Millet, V.; Gensollen, T.; Bourges, C.; Eeckhoute, J.; Hennuyer, N.; Baugé, E.; Chasson, L.; Cacciatore, I.; Staels, B.; et al. PPARalpha regulates the production of serum Vanin-1 by liver. *FEBS Lett.* **2013**, *587*, 3742–3748. [CrossRef]

30. Hosohata, K.; Matsuoka, H.; Kumagai, E. Association of urinary vanin-1 with kidney function decline in hypertensive patients. *J. Clin. Hypertens.* **2021**, *23*, 1316–1321. [CrossRef]
31. Hosohata, K.; Ando, H.; Fujimura, A. Urinary Vanin-1 As a Novel Biomarker for Early Detection of Drug-Induced Acute Kidney Injury. *J. Pharmacol. Exp. Ther.* **2012**, *341*, 656–662. [CrossRef]
32. Washino, S.; Hosohata, K.; Oshima, M.; Okochi, T.; Konishi, T.; Nakamura, Y.; Saito, K.; Miyagawa, T. A Novel Biomarker for Acute Kidney Injury, Vanin-1, for Obstructive Nephropathy: A Prospective Cohort Pilot Study. *Int. J. Mol. Sci.* **2019**, *20*, 899. [CrossRef] [PubMed]
33. Roisin-Bouffay, C.; Castellano, R.; Valéro, R.; Chasson, L.; Galland, F.; Naquet, P. Mouse vanin-1 is cytoprotective for islet beta cells and regulates the development of type 1 diabetes. *Diabetologia* **2008**, *51*, 1192–1201. [CrossRef] [PubMed]
34. Kavian, N.; Mehlal, S.; Marut, W.; Servettaz, A.; Giessner, C.; Bourges, C.; Nicco, C.; Chéreau, C.; Lemaréchal, H.; Dutilh, M.-F.; et al. Imbalance of the Vanin-1 Pathway in Systemic Sclerosis. *J. Immunol.* **2016**, *197*, 3326–3335. [CrossRef] [PubMed]
35. Kii, I. Practical Application of Periostin as a Biomarker for Pathological Conditions. *Single Mol. Single Cell Seq.* **2019**, *1132*, 195–204.
36. Guerrot, D.; Dussaule, J.-C.; Mael-Ainin, M.; Xu-Dubois, Y.-C.; Rondeau, E.; Chatziantoniou, C.; Placier, S. Identification of Periostin as a Critical Marker of Progression/Reversal of Hypertensive Nephropathy. *PLoS ONE* **2012**, *7*, e31974. [CrossRef]
37. Wallace, D.P. Periostin in the Kidney. *Adv. Exp. Med. Biol.* **2019**, *1132*, 99–112.
38. Prakoura, N.; Chatziantoniou, C. Periostin in kidney diseases. *Cell. Mol. Life Sci.* **2017**, *74*, 4315–4320. [CrossRef]
39. An, J.N.; Yang, S.H.; Kim, Y.C.; Hwang, J.H.; Park, J.Y.; Kim, D.K.; Kim, J.H.; Kim, D.W.; Hur, D.G.; Oh, Y.K.; et al. Periostin induces kidney fibrosis after acute kidney injury via the p38 MAPK pathway. *Am. J. Physiol. Physiol.* **2019**, *316*, F426–F437. [CrossRef]
40. François, H.; Chatziantoniou, C. Renal fibrosis: Recent translational aspects. *Matrix Biol.* **2018**, *68-69*, 318–332. [CrossRef]
41. Hwang, J.H.; Yang, S.H.; Kim, Y.C.; Kim, J.H.; An, J.N.; Moon, K.C.; Oh, Y.K.; Park, J.Y.; Kim, D.K.; Kim, Y.S.; et al. Experimental Inhibition of Periostin Attenuates Kidney Fibrosis. *Am. J. Nephrol.* **2017**, *46*, 501–517. [CrossRef] [PubMed]
42. Sen, K.; Lindenmeyer, M.T.; Gaspert, A.; Eichinger, F.; Neusser, M.A.; Kretzler, M.; Segerer, S.; Cohen, C.D. Periostin is induced in glomerular injury and expressed de novo in interstitial renal fibrosis. *Am. J. Pathol.* **2011**, *179*, 1756–1767. [CrossRef] [PubMed]
43. Wantanasiri, P.; Satirapoj, B.; Charoenpitakchai, M.; Aramwit, P. Periostin: A novel tissue biomarker correlates with chronicity index and renal function in lupus nephritis patients. *Lupus* **2015**, *24*, 835–845. [CrossRef] [PubMed]
44. Satirapoj, B.; Tassanasorn, S.; Charoenpitakchai, M.; Supasyndh, O. Periostin as a Tissue and Urinary Biomarker of Renal Injury in Type 2 Diabetes Mellitus. *PLoS ONE* **2015**, *10*, e0124055. [CrossRef] [PubMed]
45. Hwang, J.H.; Lee, J.P.; Kim, C.T.; Yang, S.H.; Kim, J.H.; An, J.N.; Moon, K.C.; Lee, H.; Oh, Y.K.; Joo, K.W.; et al. Urinary Periostin Excretion Predicts Renal Outcome in IgA Nephropathy. *Am. J. Nephrol.* **2016**, *44*, 481–492. [CrossRef]
46. Ono, J.; Takai, M.; Kamei, A.; Nunomura, S.; Nanri, Y.; Yoshihara, T.; Ohta, S.; Yasuda, K.; Conway, S.J.; Yokosaki, Y.; et al. Periostin forms a functional complex with IgA in human serum. *Allergol. Int.* **2020**, *69*, 111–120. [CrossRef]
47. Mizerska-Wasiak, M.; Such-Gruchot, A.; Cichoń-Kawa, K.; Turczyn, A.; Małdyk, J.; Miklaszewska, M.; Drożdż, D.; Firszt-Adamczyk, A.; Stankiewicz, R.; Rybi-Szumińska, A.; et al. The Role of Complement Component C3 Activation in the Clinical Presentation and Prognosis of IgA Nephropathy—A National Study in Children. *J. Clin. Med.* **2021**, *10*, 4405. [CrossRef]
48. Jia, Y.Y.; Yu, Y.; Li, H.J. The research status and prospect of Periostin in chronic kidney disease. *Ren. Fail.* **2020**, *42*, 1166–1172. [CrossRef]
49. Turczyn, A.; Pańczyk-Tomaszewska, M.; Krzemień, G.; Górska, E.; Demkow, U. The Usefulness of Urinary Periostin, Cytokeratin-18, and Endoglin for Diagnosing Renal Fibrosis in Children with Congenital Obstructive Nephropathy. *J. Clin. Med.* **2021**, *10*, 4899. [CrossRef]

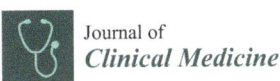

Article

Analysis of Indications for Voiding Cystography in Children

Natalia Kopiczko *, Aleksandra Dzik-Sawczuk, Karolina Szwarc, Anna Czyż and Anna Wasilewska

Department of Pediatrics and Nephrology, Medical University of Bialystok, ul. Waszyngtona 17, 15-274 Bialystok, Poland; aleksandradzik93@gmail.com (A.D.-S.); karolina.szwarc@interia.pl (K.S.); aczzz@wp.pl (A.C.); annwasil@interia.pl (A.W.)
* Correspondence: nwasilewska@interia.pl; Tel.: +48-788-880-352

Abstract: In this study, we report the experience of our center with the prognosis of vesicoureteral reflux, depending on the indications for voiding cystography, during a 12-year period. Retrospective analysis included 4302 children who were analyzed according to the indication for voiding cystography: (1) a febrile urinary tract infection, (2) urinary tract malformations on ultrasonography and (3) lower urinary tract dysfunction. Vesicoureteral reflux was found in 917 patients (21.32%; 24.1% of girls and 17.9% of boys). In group (1), reflux was found in 437/1849 cases (23.63%), group (2) in 324/1388 cases (23.34%) and group (3) in 156/1065 cases (14.65%). A significantly lower prevalence of reflux and its lower degree was found in children from group (3) when compared to other groups ($p < 0.01$). VURs were confirmed in over 20% of children with urinary tract malformations on ultrasonography or after a febrile urinary tract infection, suggesting the need for voiding cystography in these children. Indications for this examination in children with lower urinary tract dysfunction should be limited.

Keywords: voiding cystography; infection; urinary tract

Citation: Kopiczko, N.; Dzik-Sawczuk, A.; Szwarc, K.; Czyż, A.; Wasilewska, A. Analysis of Indications for Voiding Cystography in Children. *J. Clin. Med.* **2021**, *10*, 5809. https://doi.org/10.3390/jcm10245809

Academic Editors: Katarzyna Taranta-Janusz, Kinga Musiał and Emilio Sacco

Received: 2 November 2021
Accepted: 9 December 2021
Published: 11 December 2021

Publisher's Note: MDPI stays neutral with regard to jurisdictional claims in published maps and institutional affiliations.

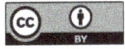

Copyright: © 2021 by the authors. Licensee MDPI, Basel, Switzerland. This article is an open access article distributed under the terms and conditions of the Creative Commons Attribution (CC BY) license (https://creativecommons.org/licenses/by/4.0/).

1. Introduction

Vesicoureteral reflux (VUR) is defined as a pathological retrograde flow of urine from the bladder to the upper parts of the urinary tract. The prevalence of VUR is still difficult to estimate. In an epidemiological study by Sargent, VUR was found in 0.4% to 1.8% of the general population of children and in over 30% of children after a febrile urinary tract infection (UTI) [1]. Similarly, other authors suggested VUR is a rather uncommon disorder that only affects a low percentage of all children [2]. However, the latest review article on VUR by Tullus, suggested the possibility of a much higher prevalence of VUR in the population (25%) [3]. This conclusion was based on large cohort studies, which reported vesicoureteral reflux in 65% of infants in the first 6 months of life [4]. Similarly, a Finnish group retrospectively diagnosed a large cohort of children who had undergone voiding cystography (VCUG) and confirmed reflux in 28% to 36% of cases, depending on the indication for this examination [5].

Although the percentage of children affected with VUR seems to be high, in recent years, there is a trend towards reducing the number of investigations for this abnormality. The guidelines from the UK National Institute for Health and Care Excellence and the American Academy of Pediatrics no longer recommend radiological investigations to detect vesicoureteral reflux in most children with an uncomplicated febrile UTI [6,7].

The indications for voiding cystography have been changed over time and usually include: a recent febrile urinary tract infection, especially in neonates and young children; abnormalities in renal and bladder ultrasonogram (RBUS) [6]; lower urinary tract dysfunction (LUTD), if they do not respond to standard therapy [8]. In the recent literature, the follow-up strategy for children after first-time acute pyelonephritis has been debated; however, no consensus has been achieved. It was shown that non-*E. coli* infections and elevated plasma creatinine are predictors of kidney scarring. Additionally, the authors showed that delayed clinical response time (>48 h), non-*E. coli* infection and an abnormal kidney US are significant predictors of an uneven differential kidney function [9]. That is why future work must focus on identifying further risk factors, new imaging modalities or specific urine or blood biomarkers, in order to minimize the number of investigations and identify those at risk for recurrent UTIs and loss of kidney function.

Diagnosis of a UTI in a febrile child requires both a positive urinalysis and urine culture. The method of obtaining a urine specimen is critical for accurate diagnosis. A urine specimen should be obtained either through sterile transurethral catheterization or suprapubic aspiration if a clean-catch specimen is not feasible. The diagnosis of UTI cannot be reliably established by a bagged specimen. [10]

In this study, we report the experience of our center with the prognosis of vesicoureteral reflux, depending on the indications for voiding cystography, during a 12-year period.

2. Materials and Methods

We performed a retrospective chart review of all children with VUR who were followed up at the Pediatric Nephrology Department, Medical University of Bialystok, Poland, between January 2003 and December 2014, as the recommendations for voiding cystography were quite wide during this period so we had a lot of patients for analysis. All children with VUR diagnosed with the use of VCUG were included in the study. They were graded using a 5-grade scale proposed by the International Reflux Study in Children [11].

During that time period, 4523 children had undergone voiding cystography (VCUG) in our center. Retrospective analysis included 4302 patients, whose medical charts allowed the determination of their indication for VCUG.

The inclusion criteria were patients aged 0–18 years who had undergone VCUG and whose medical charts were complete. Patients with a neurogenic bladder, myelomeningocele or posterior ureteral valves were excluded from the study. Reflux was also defined as passive (contrast solution is seen after filling the bladder) and active (during urination). The standard term 'reflux unit' was used to refer to reflux found on one side of the body. All patients had undergone ultrasonography of their urinary tract. The study group was divided into three subgroups based on their major indication for VCUG: (1) a febrile urinary tract infection (UTI), (2) urinary tract malformations on USG (UTM) and (3) lower urinary tract dysfunction (LUTD).

The definition of a febrile UTI was defined as: a UTI with a fever (above 38.5 °C) and increased inflammatory markers (leukocytosis, increased CRP and increased procalcitonin levels).

As recommendations changed during the analyzed period, the indications for VCUG were additionally assessed in two time intervals: (1) years 2003–2008 and (2) years 2009–2014.

The study had approval from the Local Bioethics Committee at the Medical University of Bialystok. Statistical analysis was performed using Statistica 10.0 software. The sample size was appropriate. The comparison between the groups was carried out with the Chi-square test for categorical variables. Statistical significance was set for $p < 0.05$.

3. Results

The median (IQR) age of patients included in the analysis was 4 years (0.8–9.0); 5 years (1.5–9.0) for girls and 3 years (0.5–8.0) for boys. Of the 4302 children who took part in our study, 2360 were females (55%) and 1942 were males (45%). Of the study population, 917 patients (21.3%) were positive for VUR (1266 reflux units). Girls were affected significantly more often than boys (569 vs. 348; $p < 0.01$). The discrepancy between the number of patients diagnosed with VUR and the number of reflux units is because 349 children (38.0%) had bilateral reflux. There were 533 (42.1%) active reflux cases and 733 (57.9%) passive reflux cases. The reflux units were found significantly more often on the left side (61.9%), when compared to the right side ($p < 0.01$). In children with a UTM, reflux was found on the affected side or on both sides—the affected side and additionally on the contralateral side. Out of all grades, the second one was most commonly found and made up 37.6% of the diagnosed reflux units (Table 1).

Table 1. Characteristics of examined children.

	N	Median Age (Q1–Q3)	Positive Reflux		Reflux Units	Positive Reflux (Unit)		Bilateral Reflux	Unilateral Reflux	
			N	%		Active	Passive		Right	Left
Total	4302	4 (0.8–9.0)	917	21.3	1266	533	733	349	210	358
Female	2360	5 (1.5–9.0)	569	24.1	790	318	472	221	122	226
Male	1942	3 (0.5–8.0)	348	17.9	476	215	261	128	88	132

The most frequent urinary tract malformation found on USG was hydronephrosis, with or without caliectasis, of a mild, moderate and severe degree, which was assessed according to the Society for Fetal Urology and anteroposterior diameter of the renal pelvis grading systems: grade 1 (urine in pelvis barely splits sinus), grade 2 (urine fills intrarenal pelvis ± major calyces dilated) and grade 3 (virtually all calyces are visualized), and grade 4 (similar to grade 3 plus parenchymal thinning) [12]. As we mentioned before, children with a neurogenic bladder, myelomeningocele or posterior ureteral valves were excluded from the study. In the group with a UTM and vesicoureteral reflux, hydronephrosis of grade 1 or 2 was found in 285/324 cases (88%), grade 3 in 33/324 cases (10%) and grade 4 in 6/324 cases (2%). Children who were diagnosed with reflux of grade 4 or 5, had grade 1 or 2 hydronephrosis in 66/114 cases (58%), grade 3 in 29/114 cases (25%) and grade 4 in 19/114 cases (17%). In the group with a UTM who were negative for reflux, most of children had hydronephrosis of grade 1 or 2, but still in about 9% of patients, it was grade 3 or 4.

Most of the children diagnosed with reflux from this group had grade 1 or grade 2 hydronephrosis, in 285/324 cases (88%). The rest of the children with reflux were classified as having grade 3 or grade 4 hydronephrosis.

The rate of VUR diagnosis was the highest in group (1), in children after a UTI (43.0%), lower with a UTM and the lowest with LUTD. The difference was statistically significant in group (3), when compared both to group (1) ($p < 0.01$) and group (2) ($p < 0.01$). No significant difference was observed between the incidence of positive VUR in group (1) and group (2) ($p > 0.05$).

A significantly higher incidence of moderate and severe reflux was found in group (1) and group (2), when compared to group (3) ($p < 0.01$ and $p < 0.01$, respectively). Children with LUTD had the highest incidence of reflux grade 1 and 2. The results are presented in Table 2.

Table 2. Grading of positive reflux, depending on indication for VCUG.

Grade (Total)	Urinary Tract Infection	Urinary Tract Malformations on USG	Lower Urinary Tract Dysfunction
1	134 (22%)	99 (23%)	76 (37.5%)
2	239 (39%)	146 (33%)	92 (44%)
3	132 (21%)	81 (18%)	34 (16%)
4	77 (12%)	60 (14%)	5 (2%)
5	36 (6%)	54 (12%)	1 (0.5%)

Further analysis included data in two time intervals. A significantly higher number of VCG were performed in the years 2003–2008, when compared to the years 2009–2014 ($p < 0.01$). Interestingly, the percentage of children diagnosed with VUR in the years 2009–2014 was higher (24.2%) than in 2003–2008 (19.2%) ($p < 0.01$). The rate of positive VUR was significantly higher in the years 2009–2014, in children from group (1) and group (3), than in the years 2003–2008 ($p < 0.01$ and $p < 0.05$, respectively). In the years 2003–2008, a UTM found on USG was the indication for VCUG significantly more often than the other two reasons ($p < 0.01$), while in 2009–2014, the most frequent sign was a febrile UTI (Table 3). When the patients had both indications (they had a UTI and additionally presented with a urinary tract malformation), the incidence of a positive examination for reflux was 31.55% and 44.92%, in both time intervals, respectively.

Table 3. Indications for VCG and positive reflux diagnosis in two time intervals (2003–2008 vs. 2009–2014).

	Years 2003–2008 (n = 2457)	Years 2009–2014 (n = 1845)	p Value
Urinary tract Infection	189/974 (19.4%)	248/874 (28.4%)	0.01
Urinary tract malformations on USG	197/814 (24.2%)	127/574 (22.1%)	0.37
Lower urinary tract dysfunction	85/669 (12.7%)	71/396 (17.9%)	0.02

4. Discussion

In this study, we evaluated the rate of detection of reflux in the population of children diagnosed in the Pediatric Nephrology Department, Medical University of Bialystok. In the entire study group, the prevalence of reflux was 21.3% and was almost as high as suggested by Tullus [3]. The prevalence of VUR in American children after a febrile UTI was almost twice as high as in our patients; however, this research only included children with a UTI and an age of less than 60 months [13]. Similar results were found in Swedish children with a UTI [14].

The incidence of VUR in children with a UTM on USG in our study was 23.3%, and this shared similarities with research by Brophy et al. [15]. In children with a febrile UTI or a UTM on USG, the incidence of moderate and severe reflux was significantly higher than in the group with LUTD. This may be explained because patients with higher grades of reflux are usually diagnosed earlier, because of symptomatic presentation (a UTI) or abnormal ultrasonography results. The frequency of VUR in children with LUTD in this study was only 14.6% and was similar to Iranian children [16] and much lower than in Japanese patients with enuresis [17]. Although Sillen et al. have indicated that patients who have both VUR and LUTD may have a worse final outcome after treatment, including an elevated risk of kidney damage, there is no indication for performing VCUG in all children with LUTD [18]. The results of the above study indicate that the coexistence of both conditions should be explored in any patient who has VUR, until the patient presents with symptoms suggestive of LUTD (urgency, wetting, constipation or holding maneuvers) and an extensive history, and has an examination, including voiding charts, uroflowmetry and residual urine determination. On the other hand, in LUTD, VUR is often low-grade and ultrasonography findings are often normal. It is recommended to ask all patients with LUTD if they have a history of febrile UTIs, in which case there is a greater possibility of finding VUR. Urodynamic study combined with VCUG is recommended in any child who fails standard therapy for LUTD.

On further analysis, we analyzed the results in two periods, as the recommendations for VCUG in these two periods changed. Previously, it was performed in most children after their first UTI. Similarly, increased pelvis size of the kidney was the indication for this diagnostic examination. Nowadays, we use the following approach, which avoids performing VCUG unnecessarily in most infants with fetal hydronephrosis. Voiding cystography is recommended if there is a bilateral antenatal hydronephrosis in a male or if the postnatal ultrasound shows persistent moderate or severe hydronephrosis (renal pelvic diameter >10 mm) and/or ureteral dilatation. Additionally, this examination should be considered if there is a family history of VUR. [19]. These recommendations are in line with the observation provided in this study. We found that reflux of a high grade (4 and 5) was found in only 114/1388 (8%) of all examined children with a UTM. In UTM group, high grade hydronephrosis was found in 12% of children who were positive for reflux, but also in 9% children who were negative for reflux.

Recently, routine imaging of infants with VCUG after the first UTI is no longer suggested, unless an ultrasonogram suggests selected renal abnormalities or obstruction, or a high-grade VUR. VCUG is usually indicated for children <2 years of age with a second well-documented UTI [7,20]. Starting from the year 2009, the number of VCUG decreased over time, from 2457 in the years 2003–2008 to 1845 in the years 2009–2014. What is even more important is that the accuracy of reflux diagnosis increased notably. This proves more accurate patient selection for this imaging study. Additional analysis showed that girls were diagnosed with VUR more often than boys. Low-grade reflux is often diagnosed during urological diagnostics. Significantly, a higher incidence of moderate and severe reflux was found in the group after a UTI and with a UTM, when compared to the group with LUTD. Analyzing two time intervals, the rate of positive VUR was less than 20% in the years 2003–2008 and increased to almost 25% in 2009–2014, which resulted from more accurate analysis of indications for VCUG.

The strength of this study is the long study period and large number of patients included in the study, analyzed in selected groups, reaching a power-calculated number of participants. Although our population reached a large number, our study still has its limitations. Primarily, it is a retrospective study and we assessed patients according to their major indication for VCUG, while in many children, the coexistence of two, or even three indications might be observed. The classification of a UTI was not always specified as atypical, recurrent or neither. This may influence evaluation of the classification of a UTI as a predictor for abnormal VCUG. A similar situation may apply to children with LUTD, as this diagnosis is sometimes difficult, especially in a retrospective study.

Starting from 2015, according to recommendations, we changed the indications for VCUG, and it is now only proposed for children with a recurrence of pyelonephritis or with significant abnormalities in an ultrasonogram. In the future, we will analyze the results of VCUG according the latest indications. It is in agreement with the results of RIVUR and CUTIE data, published in 2021, where the top-down approach (DMSA—as the first diagnostic study) was associated with a slightly higher recurrent UTI; however, compared to a bottom-up approach (VCUG as the first study), it significantly reduced the need of VCUG [21].

5. Conclusions

In our study, the incidence of positive reflux in the years 2003–2008 was the highest in children with abnormal USG, was lower with a febrile UTI and was the lowest with LUTD. However, after the recommendations changed in the years 2009–2014 the incidence of positive refluxes was the highest in UTI group. In conclusion, we would like to point out that the recommendations for voiding cystography in children is still a controversial area, but advances have been made towards less aggressive management than that applied traditionally. VCUG should be strongly considered in children after first-time acute pyelonephritis caused by non-*E. coli* infections, with elevated plasma creatinine, male with a bilateral antenatal hydronephrosis or if the postnatal ultrasound shows persistent moderate or severe hydronephrosis (renal pelvic diameter >10 mm), and/or ureteral dilatation, especially when there is a family history of VUR. Urodynamic study combined with VCUG is also recommended in any child who fails standard therapy for LUTD. The initial imaging approach for children with urinary tract infection, urinary tract malformations and disturbances is controversial, and further analysis is required to propose a strong recommendation in this field.

Author Contributions: N.K.: acquisition of data, analysis and interpretation of data, drafting of manuscript, critical revision; A.D.-S.: acquisition of data, critical revision; K.S.: acquisition of data, critical revision; A.C.: acquisition of data, critical revision; A.W.: study conception and design, critical revision. All authors have read and agreed to the published version of the manuscript.

Funding: The research was founded by Medical University of Bialystok.

Institutional Review Board Statement: The study was conducted according to the guidelines of the Declaration of Helsinki and approved by Ethics Committee of Medical University of Białystok (identification code: R-I-002/137/2018).

Informed Consent Statement: It was retrospective study performed many years ago we obtain an oral consent.

Conflicts of Interest: The authors declare no conflict of interest.

References

1. Sargent, M.A. What is the normal prevalence of vesicoureteral reflux? *Pediatr. Radiol.* **2000**, *30*, 587–593. [CrossRef] [PubMed]
2. Diamond, D.A.; Mattoo, T.K. Endoscopic treatment of primary vesicoureteral reflux. *N. Engl. J. Med.* **2012**, *366*, 1218–1226. [CrossRef] [PubMed]
3. Tullus, K. Vesicoureteric reflux in children. *Lancet* **2015**, *385*, 371–379. [CrossRef]
4. Köllermann, M.W.; Ludwig, H. On vesico-ureteral reflux in normal infants and children. *Z. für Kinderheilkd.* **1967**, *100*, 185–191. [CrossRef]
5. Venhola, M.; Hannula, A.; Huttunen, N.P.; Renko, M.; Pokka, T.; Uhari, M. Occurrence of vesicoureteral reflux in children. *Acta Paediatr.* **2010**, *99*, 1875–1878. [CrossRef]
6. Roberts, K.B.; Subcommittee on Urinary Tract Infection SeCoQIaM. Urinary tract infection: Clinical practice guideline for the diagnosis and management of the initial UTI in febrile infants and children 2 to 24 months. *Pediatrics* **2011**, *128*, 595–610. [CrossRef]
7. Mori, R.; Lakhanpaul, M.; Verrier-Jones, K. Diagnosis and management of urinary tract infection in children: Summary of NICE guidance. *BMJ* **2007**, *335*, 395–397. [CrossRef]
8. Tekgül, S.; Riedmiller, H.; Hoebeke, P.; Kočvara, R.; Nijman, R.J.; Radmayr, C.; Stein, R.; Dogan, H. SEAU guidelines on vesicoureteral reflux in children. *Eur. Urol.* **2012**, *62*, 534–542. [CrossRef]
9. Breinbjerg, A.; Jørgensen, C.S.; Frøkiær, J.; Tullus, K.; Kamperis, K.; Rittig, S. Risk factors for kidney scarring and vesicoureteral reflux in 421 children after their first acute pyelonephritis, and appraisal of international guidelines. *Pediatr. Nephrol.* **2021**, *36*, 2777. [CrossRef]
10. Roberts, K.B.; Wald, E.R. The diagnosis of UTI: Colony count criteria revisited. *Pediatrics* **2018**, *14*, e20173929. [CrossRef]
11. Lebowitz, R.L.; Olbing, H.; Parkkulainen, K.V.; Smellie, J.M.; Tamminen-Möbius, T.E. International system of radiographic grading of vesicoureteric reflux. *Pediatr. Radiol.* **1985**, *15*, 105–109. [CrossRef]
12. Nguyen, H.T.; Herndon, C.D.; Cooper, C.; Gatti, J.; Kirsch, A.; Kokorowski, P.; Lee, R.; Perez-Brayfield, M.; Metcalfe, P.; Yerkes, E.; et al. The Society for Fetal Urology consensus statement on the evaluation and management of antenatal hydronephrosis. *J. Pediatr. Urol.* **2010**, *6*, 212–231. [CrossRef]
13. Nelson, C.P.; Johnson, E.K.; Logvinenko, T.; Chow, J.S. Ultrasound as a screening test for genitourinary anomalies in children with UTI. *Pediatrics* **2014**, *133*, e394–e403. [CrossRef]
14. Swerkersson, S.; Jodal, U.; Sixt, R.; Stokland, E.; Hansson, S. Relationship among vesicoureteral reflux, urinary tract infection and renal damage in children. *J. Urol.* **2007**, *178*, 647–651. [CrossRef]
15. Brophy, M.M.; Austin, P.F.; Yan, Y.; Coplen, D.E. Vesicoureteral reflux and clinical outcomes in infants with prenatally detected hydronephrosis. *J. Urol.* **2002**, *168*, 1716–1719, discussion 9. [CrossRef]
16. Naseri, M. Association of nocturnal enuresis with vesicoureteral reflux and renal cortical damage. *Nephrourol. Mon.* **2012**, *4*, 448–453. [CrossRef]
17. Kawauchi, A.; Kitamori, T.; Imada, N.; Tanaka, Y.; Watanabe, H. Urological abnormalities in 1328 patients with nocturnal enuresis. *Eur. Urol.* **1996**, *29*, 231–234.
18. Sillén, U.; Brandström, P.; Jodal, U.; Holmdahl, G.; Sandin, A.; Sjöberg, I.; Hansson, S. The Swedish reflux trial in children: V. bladder dysfunction. *J. Urol.* **2010**, *184*, 298–304. [CrossRef]
19. Herthelius, M.; Axelsson, R.; Lidefelt, K.J. Antenatally detected urinary tract dilatation: A 12–15-year follow-up. *Pediatr. Nephrol.* **2020**, *35*, 2129. [CrossRef]
20. Żurowska, A.; Wasilewska, A.; Jung, A.; Kiliś-Pstrusińska, K.; Pańczyk-Tomaszewska, M.; Sikora, P.; Tkaczyk, M.; Zagożdżon, I. Zalecenia Polskiego Towarzystwa Nefrologii Dziecięcej (PTNFD) dotyczące postępowania z dzieckiem z zakażeniem układu moczowego. *Forum Med. Rodz.* **2016**, *10*, 159–178.
21. Scott Wang, H.H.; Cahill, D.; Panagides, J.; Logvinenko, T.; Nelson, C. Top-down versus bottom-up approach in children presenting with urinary tract infection: Comparative effectiveness analysis using RIVUR and CUTIE data. *J. Urol.* **2021**, *206*, 1284–1290. [CrossRef]

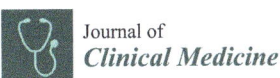

Article

Urinary Beta-2-Microglobulin and Late Nephrotoxicity in Childhood Cancer Survivors

Eryk Latoch [1,*], Katarzyna Konończuk [1], Katarzyna Taranta-Janusz [2], Katarzyna Muszyńska-Rosłan [1], Magdalena Sawicka [3], Anna Wasilewska [2] and Maryna Krawczuk-Rybak [1]

[1] Department of Pediatric Oncology and Hematology, Medical University of Bialystok, 15-274 Białystok, Poland; kononczukk@gmail.com (K.K.); kmroslan@post.pl (K.M.-R.); rybak@umb.edu.pl (M.K.-R.)
[2] Department of Pediatrics and Nephrology, Medical University of Bialystok, 15-274 Białystok, Poland; katarzyna.taranta@wp.pl (K.T.-J.); annwasil@interia.pl (A.W.)
[3] Department of Analysis and Bioanalysis of Medicines, Medical University of Bialystok, 15-089 Białystok, Poland; magdalena.sawicka@umb.edu.pl
* Correspondence: eryklatoch@gmail.com; Tel.: +48-85-745-0640

Abstract: The objectives of this study were to evaluate urinary beta-2-microglobulin (β2M) levels in long-term childhood cancer survivors and to establish its association with anticancer drug-induced nephrotoxicity. The study consisted of 165 childhood cancer survivors (CCS) who were in continuous complete remission. We reported that CCS had a significantly higher level of β2M ($p < 0.001$) and β2M/Cr. ratio ($p < 0.05$) than healthy peers. Among all participants, 24 (14.5%) had decreased eGFR (<90 mL/min/1.73 m^2). A significant positive correlation between β2M/Cr. ratio and body mass index (coef. 14.48, $p = 0.046$) was found. Furthermore, higher levels of urinary β2M were detected among CCS with a longer follow-up time (over 5 years) after treatment. Subjects with decreased eGFR showed statistically higher urinary β2M levels (20.06 ± 21.56 ng/mL vs. 8.55 ± 3.65 ng/mL, $p = 0.007$) compared with the healthy peers. Twelve survivors (7.2%) presented hyperfiltration and they had higher urinary β2M levels than CCS with normal glomerular filtration (46.33 ± 93.11 vs. 8.55 ± 3.65 ng/mL, $p = 0.029$). This study did not reveal an association between potential treatment-related risk factors such as chemotherapy, surgery, radiotherapy, and the urinary β2M level. The relationship between treatment with abdominal radiotherapy and reduced eGFR was confirmed ($p < 0.05$). We demonstrated that urinary beta-2-microglobulin may play a role in the subtle kidney injury in childhood cancer survivors; however, the treatment-related factors affecting the β2M level remain unknown. Further prospective studies with a longer follow-up time are needed to confirm the utility of urinary β2M and its role as a non-invasive biomarker of renal dysfunction.

Keywords: B2M; cancer; CCS; children; CKD; chronic kidney disease; nephropathies; renal toxicity

Citation: Latoch, E.; Konończuk, K.; Taranta-Janusz, K.; Muszyńska-Rosłan, K.; Sawicka, M.; Wasilewska, A.; Krawczuk-Rybak, M. Urinary Beta-2-Microglobulin and Late Nephrotoxicity in Childhood Cancer Survivors. *J. Clin. Med.* **2021**, *10*, 5279. https://doi.org/10.3390/jcm10225279

Academic Editor: Giacomo Garibotto

Received: 9 September 2021
Accepted: 11 November 2021
Published: 13 November 2021

Publisher's Note: MDPI stays neutral with regard to jurisdictional claims in published maps and institutional affiliations.

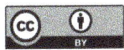

Copyright: © 2021 by the authors. Licensee MDPI, Basel, Switzerland. This article is an open access article distributed under the terms and conditions of the Creative Commons Attribution (CC BY) license (https:// creativecommons.org/licenses/by/ 4.0/).

1. Introduction

Improvements in the diagnosis and treatment of pediatric cancers have now resulted in significantly higher survival rates. However, childhood cancer survivors (CCS) are at greater risk of experiencing many treatment-related adverse effects that substantially affect later quality of life [1,2]. Nephrotoxicity is one of the most common late sequelae with prevalence ranging up to 80% based on the population studied [3]. There are many known causes of renal damage among CCS. These may result from the multimodal therapy (chemotherapy, radiotherapy, immunotherapy, and surgery), supportive treatment used (aminoglycoside antibiotics, diuretics, or antifungal agents), and the cancer itself—by tumor infiltration, disruption of glomerular and tubular development, acute tumor lysis syndrome, or urinary tract obstruction. The most nephrotoxic cytostatics include platinum-based drugs such as cisplatin and carboplatin, as well as ifosfamide, cyclophosphamide, and methotrexate. Overall, CCS have a nine-fold increased risk of developing chronic nephrotoxicity compared to their siblings, according to one of the largest studies available [4].

The extent of renal impairment can vary and depends on many factors. In some cases, the only sign of kidney damage is renal hypertension or Fanconi syndrome, while others develop chronic kidney disease (CKD) from mild damage to complete kidney failure at various ages in life. Based on available methods, it remains difficult to predict which patients will develop kidney disease after anticancer treatment. The primary parameter assessing renal function is estimated glomerular filtration rate (eGFR) based on creatinine level. However, there are many limitations affecting its level which include age, sex, race, muscle mass, diet, hydration status, physical activity, and medications taken regularly. New markers are being sought to identify individuals with early renal function impairment before it is clinically detectable by standard techniques. In recent years, there has been an increasing number of studies on the role of beta-2-microglobulin (β2M) in the development of acute kidney injury (AKI) and CKD. Some of them, but not all, reported its elevated levels following treatment with nephrotoxic drugs [5,6]. Still little is known about the association of β2M with late drug-induced nephrotoxicity in childhood cancer survivors.

Beta-2-microglobulin is a small protein (18 kDa) encoded by gen located on chromosome 15. In healthy subjects it is filtered by glomeruli and subsequently reabsorbed in the proximal tubule of the nephron, resulting in minimal urine concentration [7,8]. Tubular injury leads to increased urinary β2M levels due to impaired reabsorption. Furthermore, unlike creatinine, β2M levels do not depend on muscle mass, which makes it a potential candidate biomarker of kidney damage [9].

The aims of this study were to evaluate urinary beta-2-microglobulin levels in long-term childhood cancer survivors and determine its relationship with the type of anticancer treatment used.

2. Materials and Methods

The study included 165 childhood cancer survivors (80 males and 85 females) visiting the follow-up outpatients' clinic at the Department of Pediatric Oncology and Hematology, Medical University of Bialystok (Poland). All participants were in complete first continuous remission. Exclusion criteria included: congenital anomalies of kidney or urinary tract, current infection, relapse of cancer. All the children were treated according to the international protocols in line with the diagnosis, approved by the Polish Pediatric Leukemia and Lymphoma Group, and Polish Pediatric Solid Tumors Group. Written informed consent was obtained from the participants or their parents/guardians. The study was approved by the Ethical Committee of the Medical University of Bialystok in accordance with the Declaration of Helsinki (permission number: R-I-002/62/2018).

Clinical history, including demographic information, comorbidities, anticancer treatment used in each patient, especially cumulative dosage of nephrotoxic drugs (cyclophosphamide, ifosfamide, cisplatin, methotrexate), and abdominal radiotherapy was obtained from the CCS database. All the participants underwent a clinical examination and anthropometric measurements. Body mass index (BMI) was calculated as weight in kilograms divided by height in squared meters (kg/m^2). Blood pressure was measured using a standardized sphygmomanometer (performed three times at 1–2 min intervals); before the measurement, the participant rested peacefully for five minutes. Hypertension was defined as mean systolic blood pressure (SBP) and/or diastolic blood pressure (DBP) level $\geq$ 95th percentile adjusted for age, sex, and height [10]. The control group consisted of 50 healthy peers (27 female) without history of urinary tract infections, with a pair of normal kidneys, who were offspring of the departments' employees.

All participants had an abdominal ultrasound to assess the kidney and urinary tract performed by a qualified radiologist. After a 12 h night, fasting peripheral blood was collected from each participant for routine laboratory testing. Clean catch urine samples were stored at -80 °C for further analysis. The serum creatinine level was measured by enzymatic method, and the estimated glomerular filtration rate (mL/min/1.73 m^2) was calculated using the updated Schwartz formula: eGFR = 0.413 × (height in cm/serum cr. in mg/dL). Urinary beta-2-microglobulin level was measured using commercial immunoassays (R&D SYSTEMS a bio-techne brand, Quantikine® ELISA, Minneapolis, USA) according to the instructions for the ELISA kit. The tested urine biomarkers were calculated per milligram urine creatinine (cr.) in order to avoid the effect of urine dilution (β2M/cr. ratio). Urine albumin concentration was determined by Lowry's method. Subjects with a urinary albumin/creatinine ratio between 30 to 300 μg/mg were considered to have albuminuria. The stages of CKD were classified according to Kidney Disease: Improving Global Outcomes (KDIGO) guidelines, defined by structural or functional abnormalities of the kidney for ≥3 months, with or without decreased eGFR or eGFR < 60 mL/min/1.73 m^2 for ≥3 months, with or without kidney damage [11]. Glomerular hyperfiltration was define as eGFR higher than 175 mL/min/1.73 m^2 [12].

Statistical analysis. Normal distribution was tested by using the Shapiro–Wilk test. Mean and standard deviation (SD) or median (Me) and interquartile range (IQR) were used to presented data. The *t*-Student test or Mann–Whitney U test were applied to compare independent variables depending on normal distribution. Univariate analysis of variance was performed using ANOVA, and post hoc analysis using Tukey's test. The correlations between β2M and urine creatinine, blood pressure and cumulative dose of cytostatics used were calculated by Spearman or Pearson correlation coefficients. The STATA 12.1 version (StatCorp, College Station, TX, USA) was used to perform statistical analysis, and statistical significance was determined at 0.05.

3. Results

The clinical characteristics of the childhood cancer survivors (CCS) are presented in Table 1. The mean age at the time of diagnosis was 5.31 ± 4.16 years, while the mean time from treatment cessation to follow-up was 7.01 ± 5.28 years. The study group did not differ in age and sex from the control group.

Table 1. Clinical characteristics of the childhood cancer survivors (CCS).

	Total	Male	Female
Patients (*n*, %)	165 (100%)	80 (48.5%)	85 (51.5%)
Age at diagnosis (years)	5.31 ± 4.16 4.24 (2.66–7.20)	5.36 ± 4.16 3.82 (2.83–6.9)	5.9 ± 4.67 4.38 (2.34–7.57)
Age at study (years)	13.40 ± 5.96 14.21 (8.62–17.67)	12.25 ± 4.94 12.35 (8.09–16.21)	13.78 ± 5.94 14.5 (9.18–17.42)
Follow-up after treatment (years)	7.01 ± 5.28 6.55 (2.25–10.39)	6.22 ± 5.09 5.51 (2.03–9.25)	7.75 ± 5.27 7.45 (3.83–11.15)
Diagnosis:	165 (100%)		
Acute lymphoblastic leukemia	84 (50.9%)	41 (49%)	43 (51%)
Wilms tumor	17 (10.3%)	7 (41%)	10 (59%)
Sarcoma	14 (8.5%)	8 (57%)	6 (43%)
Non-Hodgkin lymphoma	13 (7.9%)	4 (31%)	9 (69%)
Hodgkin lymphoma	10 (6.1%)	4 (40%)	6 (10%)
Neuroblastoma	9 (5.5%)	3 (33%)	6 (64%)
Acute myeloid leukemia	8 (4.8%)	3 (37%)	5 (63%)
Hepatoblastoma	4 (2.4%)	2 (50%)	2 (50%)
Germ tumors	3 (1.8%)	2 (67%)	1 (33%)
Langerhans cell histiocytosis	3 (1.8%)	1 (33%)	2 (67%)

Table 1. Cont.

	Total	Male	Female
Chemotherapy:			
Methotrexate (cumulative dose in mg/m^2), $n = 100$ (60.6%)	13,373 ± 19,972 8000 (8000–10,000)	14,300 ± 20,059 8000 (8000–20,000)	12,409 ± 20,044 8000 (8000–8000) [b]
Cumulative corticosteroid [a] (dose in mg/m^2), $n = 109$ (66.1%)	1800 ± 791 1711 (1711–1711) [b]	1764 ± 763 1711 (1711–1711) [b]	1838 ± 825 1711 (1711–1748)
Cyclophosphamide (cumulative dose in mg/m^2), $n = 113$ (68.5%)	3893.36 ± 2448.33 3000 (3000–4000)	3868 ± 235 3000 (3000–3000) [b]	3919 ± 2557 3000 (3000–3000) [b]
Ifosfamide (cumulative dose in mg/m^2), $n = 14$ (8.5%)	74,857 ± 71,888 54,000 (36,000–84,000)	65,500 ± 40,242 54,000 (51,750–78,750)	87,333 ± 104,128 60,000 (18,500–139,500)
Cisplatin (cumulative dose in mg/m^2), $n = 16$ (9.7%)	430 ± 241.99 400 (240–480)	400 ± 153 400 (240–570)	460 ± 316 400 (240–480)
Radiotherapy (RT):	41 (24.8%)	19 (46%)	22 (54%)
Cranial radiotherapy (CRT) (cumulative dose in Gray), $n = 19$ (11.5%)	19.33 ± 14.04 12.0 (12–18)	21.2 ± 16.67 12.0 (12.0–34.2)	17.64 ± 11.85 12.0 (12.0–18.0)
Abdominal radiotherapy (cumulative dose in Gray), $n = 19$ (11.5%)	22.45 ± 10.26 21.0 (19.80–21)	21.98 ± 12.09 19.8 (13.95–21.0)	22.08 ± 9.32 21.0 (19.8–21)
Total body irradiation (TBI) (cumulative dose in Gray), $n = 5$ (3%)	12.0 ± 0.00 12.0 (12.0–12.0) [b]	12.0 ± 0.0 12.0 (12.0–12.0) [b]	12.0 ± 0.0 12.0 (12.0–12.0) [b]
No radiotherapy, $n = 124$ (75.2%)	124 (75.2%)		
Nephrectomy (unilateral)	16 (9.7%)	6 (37.5%)	10 (62.5%)
Hematopoietic stem cell transplantation (HSCT)	20 (12.1%)	9 (45%)	11 (55%)

Data are given as mean and standard deviation (SD) and median and interquartile range (IQR). There were no statistical differences between males and females; [a] calculated as prednisone equivalents; [b] most patients received the same dosage of anticancer agents or radiotherapy according to the treatment protocol; therefore, the first and third quartiles did not differ from the median.

Childhood cancer survivors revealed increased serum creatinine levels (0.60 ± 0.22 mg/dL vs. 0.52 ± 0.14 mg/dL, $p = 0.035$) as well as urine creatinine levels (131.24 ± 74.62 mg/L vs. 92.25 ± 45.97 mg/L, $p = 0.001$) than the healthy peers. However, we did not observe any difference in the eGFR (122.37 ± 34.93 mL/min/1.73 m^2 vs. 124.51 ± 38.49 mL/min/1.73 m^2, $p = 0.792$).

The study group presented a significantly higher concentration of β2M (33.64 ± 59.53 ng/mL vs. 8.55 ± 3.65 ng/mL, $p < 0.001$) and β2M/Cr. ratio (277.96 ± 405.67 ng/mg cr. vs. 140.98 ± 144.09 ng/mg cr., $p = 0.039$) compared to the control group (Figure 1). The summary of the biochemical parameters is shown in Table 2.

Table 2. Characteristics of biochemical parameters in childhood cancer survivors.

	Childhood Cancer Survivors $n = 165$	Control Group $n = 50$	p Value
Serum creatinine (mg/dL)	0.58 (0.43; 0.75)	0.50 (0.41; 0.63)	0.035
Urine creatinine (mg/L)	120.64 (73.67; 178.52)	89.40 (65.78; 116.44)	0.001
eGFR (mL/min/1.73 m^2)	117.47 (98.79; 139.87)	118.95 (103.25; 136.02)	0.792
β2M (ng/mL)	14.30 (8.62; 26.10)	8.67 (6.18; 11.48)	<0.001
β2M /cr. (ng/mg cr.)	139.87 (66.41; 305.48)	99.63 (55.34; 162.37)	0.039

eGFR: estimated glomerular filtration rate, β2M: beta-2-microglobulin, cr: creatinine. Data are given as median and interquartile range.

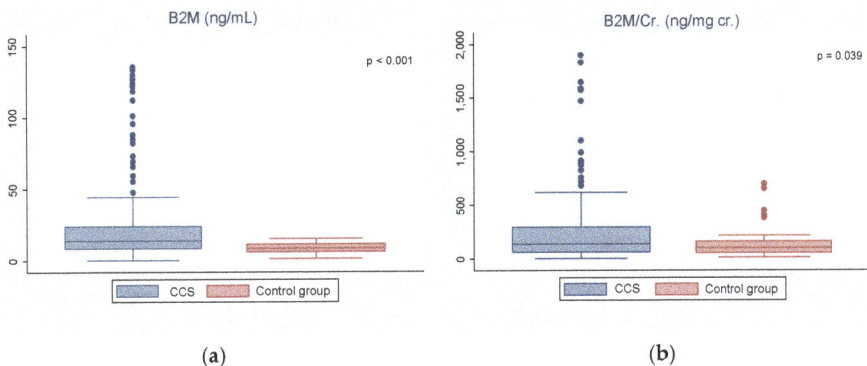

Figure 1. Comparison of (**a**) the urinary β2M (beta-2-microglobulin) and (**b**) the urinary β2M/Cr. ratio (beta-2-microglobulin/creatinine) between the childhood cancer survivors (CCS) and the control group.

We found no differences in β2M (33.43 ± 57.72 ng/mL vs. 33.86 ± 61.77 ng/mL, $p = 0.727$) and β2M/Cr. ratio (283.89 ± 438.08 ng/mg cr. vs. 271.65 ± 370.81 ng/mg cr., $p = 0.965$) concentrations according to sex. Both genders had significantly higher values of urine creatinine (female: 128.81 ± 71.87 mg/L vs. 96.76 ± 49.38 mg/L, $p = 0.045$; male: 133.82 ± 77.81 mg/L vs. 86.96 ± 42.08 mg/L, $p = 0.008$) and urinary β2M (female: 33.43 ± 57.72 ng/mL vs. 8.05 ± 3.64 ng/mL, $p < 0.001$; male: 33.86 ± 61.77 ng/mL vs. 9.13 ± 3.65 ng/mL, $p = 0.001$) when compared to the control group, but no gender differences were found within the study group. Of note, HSCT treatment had no effect on urinary β2M levels ($p < 0.05$).

Twenty-four of the study participants (14.5%) presented eGFR below 90 mL/min/1.7 m^2 of which only one had eGFR below 60 mL/min/1.73 m^2. Notably, before starting the treatment, eGFR was within normal range in all participants. The subgroup of subjects with reduced eGFR did not reveal any differences in β2M level and β2M/Cr. ratio in comparison to the normal eGFR subgroup. The analysis of patients with decreased eGFR compared with the healthy peers showed statistically higher β2M levels (20.06 ± 21.56 ng/mL vs. 8.55 ± 3.65 ng/mL, $p = 0.007$) in CCS, but no correlations between both the β2M level and β2M/Cr. ratio and eGFR were found. Among the whole study group, there were twelve individuals (7.2%) who presented hyperfiltration. Compared to those with normal glomerular filtration, they showed higher urinary creatinine (144.34 ± 75.35 mg/dL vs. 92.25 ± 45.97 mg/dL, $p = 0.009$) and β2M (46.33 ± 93.11 ng/mL vs. 8.55 ± 3.65 ng/mL, $p = 0.029$) levels.

We also investigated the association between the type of cytostatics used, abdominal radiotherapy, and the number of patients with reduced eGFR (<90 mL/min/1.73 m^2) in each group according to whether or not they were exposed to a particular nephrotoxic agent. Survivors who had radiation therapy in childhood were statistically more likely to have decreased eGFR at the time of the study compared to those who had never received RT (11% vs. 31%, $p = 0.024$).

Furthermore, we divided the study group according to the time of cessation of treatment. There were 101 subjects (61.2%) over 5 years after the end of treatment with significantly higher levels of sCr (0.68 ± 0.21 ng/mL vs. 0.48 ± 0.19 ng/mL, $p < 0.0001$), uCr (148.18 ± 79.62 mg/dL vs. 104.50 ± 56.98 mg/dL, $p < 0.001$), β2M (44.09 ± 71.76 ng/mL vs. 17.14 ± 24.50 ng/mL, $p = 0.0001$), β2M/Cr. ratio (306.17 ± 74.87 ng/mg cr. vs. 233.42 ± 363.09 ng/mg cr., $p = 0.049$), and lower eGFR (117.02 ± 28.68 mL/min/1.73 m^2 vs. 131.56 ± 42.37 mL/min/1.73 m^2, $p = 0.047$) than participants who were under 5 years from the end of treatment at follow-up (Table 3.).

Table 3. Characteristics of biochemical parameters according to the time after completion of treatment.

	<5 Years	>5 Years	p Value
	n = 64	n = 101	
Age at study (years)	6.90 (5.42; 11.67)	15.94 (12.99; 19.15)	<0.001
eGFR (mL/min/1.73 m^2)	127.00 (103.73; 151.96)	112.43 (98.01; 134.98)	0.047
β2M (ng/mL)	10.99 (5.31; 24.50)	16.59 (11.22; 39.82)	<0.0001
β2M /cr. (ng/mg cr.)	110.14 (41.00; 246.49)	151.56 (74.87; 328.48)	0.049

eGFR: estimated glomerular filtration rate, β2M: beta-2-microglobulin, cr: Creatinine. Data are given as median and interquartile range.

In the whole group, positive correlations between urine creatinine ($r = 0.25$, $p = 0.001$), systolic blood pressure ($r = 0.20$, $p = 0.015$), diastolic blood pressure ($r = 0.26$, $p = 0.001$), and β2M level were found; however, the strength of relationships was very weak ($r < 0.3$). Participants were also divided based on their initial diagnosis and treatment as follows: leukemia and non-Hodgkin lymphoma ($n = 105$), Hodgkin lymphoma ($n = 10$), and solid tumors ($n = 50$). No significant differences in eGFR ($p = 0.149$), β2M level ($p = 0.936$), and β2M/Cr. ratio ($p = 0.573$) were found between subgroups.

The β2M level and β2M/Cr. ratio were investigated depending on whether or not the patients received a specific cytostatic drug during the treatment (cyclophosphamide, ifosfamide, cisplatin, and methotrexate); however, no relationships were revealed ($p > 0.05$). Moreover, no correlations between the β2M level and β2M/Cr. ratio, and the cumulative dose of cyclophosphamide, ifosfamide, cisplatin, and methotrexate were found ($p > 0.05$).

Receiving operating curve (ROC) analyses were conducted to determine the diagnostic profile of β2M level and β2M/Cr. ratio in identifying participants with decreased eGFR (<90 mL/min/1.73 m^2). However, none of them showed any diagnostic value (the AUC for the β2M level was 0.46 and for the β2M/Cr. ratio was 0.43).

The univariable linear regression analysis showed significant correlation between β2M/Cr. ratio and BMI (coef. 14.48, $p = 0.046$, 95%CI 0.24–28.73). Other potential confounding factors such as abdominal radiotherapy, cumulative dose of nephrotoxic cytostatics, age at diagnosis, age at study, eGFR, albumin-to-creatinine ratio, and solitary functioning kidney did not affect the β2M level or β2M/Cr. ratio (Table 4).

Table 4. Univariable analysis of the beta-2-microglobulin/creatinine ratio (β2M/Cr. ratio) in childhood cancer survivors.

Variables	Coefficient	p
Ifosfamide (cumulative dose)	−17.6	0.120
Cyclophosphamide (cumulative dose)	0.02	0.368
Cisplatin (cumulative dose)	0.14	0.728
Methotrexate (cumulative dose)	−2.92	0.965
Abdominal radiotherapy (yes vs. no)	−89.6	0.368
Age at diagnosis (years)	6.43	0.372
Follow-up time (years)	−0.66	0.922
BMI (kg/m^2)	14.5	0.046
Hypertension (yes vs. no)	43.2	0.610
Nephrectomy (yes vs. no)	−10.7	0.361
HSCT (yes vs. no)	−45.4	0.642
Diagnosis (leukemia vs. lymphoma vs. solid tumors)	−29.2	0.401

BMI: body mass index, HSCT: hematopoietic stem cell transplantation.

4. Discussions

The exact etiology of late nephrotoxicity among childhood cancer survivors remains unclear. On the other hand, we know more about treatment-related factors leading to acute kidney injury. Some of these also increase the risk of chronic kidney disease later in life (the most common are described in the introduction). However, there is a population of CCS who had never experienced AKI but who developed CKD many years after treatment. In recent years, much effort has been concentrated on identifying those survivors who are at risk for developing kidney failure during adolescence and adulthood.

The available methods for accessing renal function have many limitations, and, thus, new biomarkers to access early kidney deterioration are needed. There are several urinary markers (highly sensitive and specific) for monitoring drug-induced kidney injury that have been approved in preclinical studies by the European Medicines Agency (EMA) and the Food and Drug Administration (FDA). The best candidates include β2-microglobulin (β2M), kidney injury molecule-1 (KIM-1), neutrophil gelatinase-associated lipocalin (NGAL), clusterin, and trefoil factor-3 (TFF-3) [13,14]. Most studies to date have focused specifically on AKI, and there are limited data on the utility of these biomarkers in late drug-induced nephrotoxicity [15]. In our previous studies on the association between urinary KIM-1 and NGAL levels and late renal toxicity, we showed that CCS had higher levels of both biomarkers, which was related to the cumulative dose of cisplatin and ifosfamide [16,17]. In this prospective cohort study, we focused on β-2-microglobulin and its applicability in accessing renal function in CCS.

In the overall group of CCS, subjects with reduced eGFR (<90 mL/min/1.73 m^2) accounted for 14.5% and this decreased in subsequent tests performed at least every 3 months. Our results are in accordance with one of the largest available studies conducted on a cohort of 1122 survivors, in which the probability of reduced eGFR among CCS treated with nephrotoxic agents was 6.6% by age 35 years compared to those who had never received such treatment, and eGFR continued to fall with time. The greater risk of nephrotoxicity was observed in survivors given ifosfamide and cisplatin, and with nephrectomy [18,19]. In the present study, no such relationship was noted. This may be explained by the fact that the mean age of our study group was two times lower than in the referred paper and the association is not yet noticeable.

Radiation-associated kidney injury can manifest as decreased eGFR, hypertension, or proteinuria. Dawson et al. reported that 46% of adults who were irradiated with a dose of 20 Gy developed nephropathy [20–22]. Similarly, our data showed a significantly higher number of individuals with reduced eGFR in the subset of CCS who were treated with abdominal radiotherapy compared to those who did not receive it, supporting the data on the damaging effects of RT on renal function.

Nowadays, it is increasingly discussed that the evaluation of decline in renal function only with eGFR has many limitations and may misidentify individuals in the early stages of kidney damage as healthy. Moreover, some authors emphasize that serum creatinine level increases when more than forty percent of renal tissue is damaged, which may underestimate the number of patients with early-onset renal injury as assessed by eGFR [23]. For this reason, there is a need for a new, preferably non-invasive biomarker to identify individuals with impaired renal function before it is detectable by standard methods.

The majority of studies conducted so far have looked at serum b2M rather than urine concentrations [5,18]. Most of them pointed to elevated β2M level in patients after chemotherapy with nephrotoxic agents and emphasized its high utility in detecting chemotherapy-induced acute kidney injury [14,24]. On the other hand, there are very limited data on the utility of urinary β2M in diagnosing the onset of CKD associated with anticancer treatment. In the present study, statistically higher level of β2M and β2M/Cr. ratio among CCS were reported. The association between urinary β2M and nephrotoxicity for the first time was described by Tiburcio et al. in a study of 41 CCS [25]. They reported in short-term survivors that urinary β2M level was significantly higher in the study group and was positively correlated with plasma creatinine concentration and negatively correlated with glomerular filtration rate. Similarly, our study confirmed a significantly higher level of urinary β2M in CCS but failed to confirm an association with creatinine level and eGFR value. Only in a small subset of patients with hyperfiltration (7%) was a significantly higher level of β2M found compared to subjects with normal and reduced filtration, which may indicate that increased filtration in the injured kidney enhances β2M excretion and, perhaps, may be a potential tool to assess impaired renal function. However, conclusions from this analysis should be drawn with caution due to the very small sample size. Another study carried out in children previously treated for central nervous system malignancy showed negative correlation between β2M level and eGFR [26]. However, we did not confirm this finding.

To our best knowledge, this is the first clinical study of the association of the urinary β2M among individuals previously treated for acute leukemia (61% of the study group), which has not been investigated so far. These individuals were analyzed separately but did not differ from CCS with other cancer types.

Higher levels of urinary β2M were observed in subjects with a follow-up time of more than 5 years. Interestingly, in the univariable linear regression analysis, significant positive correlations between β2M/Cr. ratio and BMI were observed. These results may suggest that urinary β2M level depends on age and body weight, as postulated by some authors; however, reference values are not available [27,28].

Reviewing the literature, there are many data reporting elevated serum β2M levels at the time of diagnosis in many types of cancer, as well as being a predictor of relapse in some of them [29–31]. It is important to note that all participants included in this study were in continuous first remission, and all were carefully screened for relapse and second malignancies.

Furthermore, there are many studies investigating the role of β2M in kidney diseases of different etiology. It has been demonstrated that β2M concentration is elevated among individuals with systemic lupus erythematosus, beta thalassemia major, type 1 diabetes, acute appendicitis, and congenital lower urinary tract obstruction, among others [32–36]. In addition, β2M levels are used as a tumor marker, primarily in monitoring the treatment of multiple myeloma, a cancer that occurs typically in advanced age [37].

Finally, there are several limitations that need to be considered. First, single-center studies may influence the occurrence of bias. Second, the heterogeneity of the study group in terms of different types of cancers made it unfeasible to analyze the effect of some specific treatment protocols (especially very rare tumors). For this reason, we targeted the impact of specific treatments modalities, such as cytostatic agents and radiotherapy. Third, we used the GFR estimated from creatinine level rather than measured by standard techniques such as plasma clearance of iohexol. Another limitation of the study is the non-inclusion of other markers for assessing renal function, such as cystatin C, which is considered to be more resistant to various confounding factors, such as body mass index. The authors did not use Gao's quadratic equation in addition to Schwartz's formula when glomerular hyperfiltration was suspected; however, the number of subjects with hyperfiltration was very limited [38].

The strengths of the study include the relatively large number of participants, long follow-up time, and ethnic homogeneity of the group.

Pooling all data, we demonstrated that 14.5% of childhood cancer survivors had reduced eGFR value, and the most adverse factor affecting renal function was abdominal radiotherapy used during the treatment. We also provided new data that this particular population has elevated urinary beta-2-microglobulin level regardless of initial diagnosis. Of the factors tested with potential effects on renal function, only a longer time of follow-up and high BMI were positively correlated with the level of urinary β2M. The results of this study do not explain what urinary β2M level depends on. None of the factors investigated, including type of cancer, cumulative dose of cytostatics used, radiotherapy, nephrectomy, or age at diagnosis significantly affected biomarker levels. It cannot be ruled out that genetic background is also relevant. Furthermore, in light of recent studies demonstrating premature aging of survivors, it is important to note that nephrotoxicity is a multifactorial process involving both environmental and genetic factors [39,40]. Since the process leading to elevated β2M concentration in CCS remains unclear, and its potential use as a biomarker in the assessment of deteriorating renal function is still unexplained, further longitudinal studies on urinary β2M concentration and its potential role as a tool in the assessment of declining renal function are needed.

Author Contributions: E.L. designed the study, wrote the manuscript, and performed statistical analysis, K.K. co-wrote the manuscript and performed statistical analysis, K.T.-J., K.M.-R. and A.W. contributed to the collection and interpretation of data, and assisted in the preparation of the manuscript. M.S. performed laboratory analysis and assisted in the preparation of the manuscript. M.K.-R. was comprehensively involved in the study. All authors have read and agreed to the published version of the manuscript.

Funding: This research received no external funding.

Institutional Review Board Statement: The study was conducted according to the guidelines of the Declaration of Helsinki and approved by the Institutional Review Board of the Medical University of Bialystok (R-I-002/62/2018).

Informed Consent Statement: Informed consent was obtained from all subjects involved in the study.

Data Availability Statement: The data presented in this study are available on request from the corresponding author.

Conflicts of Interest: The authors declare no conflict of interest.

References

1. Oeffinger, K.C.; Mertens, A.C.; Sklar, C.A.; Kawashima, T.; Hudson, M.M.; Meadows, A.T.; Friedman, D.L.; Marina, N.; Hobbie, W.; Kadan-Lottick, N.S.; et al. Childhood Cancer Survivors Study. Chronic Health Conditions in Adult Survivors of Childhood Cancer. *N. Engl. J. Med.* **2006**, *355*, 1572–1582. [CrossRef]
2. Krawczuk-Rybak, M.; Panasiuk, A.; Stachowicz-Stencel, T.; Zubowska, M.; Skalska-Sadowska, J.; Sęga-Pondel, D.; Czajńska-Deptuła, A.; Sławińska, D.; Badowska, W.; Kamieńska, E.; et al. Health Status of Polish Children and Adolescents after Cancer Treatment. *Eur. J. Pediatr.* **2018**, *177*, 437–447. [CrossRef]
3. Kooijmans, E.C.; Bökenkamp, A.; Tjahjadi, N.S.; Tettero, J.M.; van Dulmen-den Broeder, E.; van der Pal, H.J.; Veening, M.A. Early and Late Adverse Renal Effects after Potentially Nephrotoxic Treatment for Childhood Cancer. *Cochrane Database Syst. Rev.* **2019**, *3*, CD008944. [CrossRef] [PubMed]
4. Skinner, R. Late Renal Toxicity of Treatment for Childhood Malignancy: Risk Factors, Long-Term Outcomes, and Surveillance. *Pediatr. Nephrol.* **2018**, *33*, 215–225. [CrossRef]
5. Zubowska, M.; Wyka, K.; Fendler, W.; Młynarski, W.; Zalewska-Szewczyk, B. Interleukin 18 as a marker of chronic nephropathy in children after anticancer treatment. *Dis. Markers.* **2013**, *35*, 811–818. [CrossRef]
6. Sørensen, P.G.; Nissen, M.H.; Groth, S.; Rørth, M. Beta-2-microglobulin excretion: An indicator of long term nephrotoxicity during cis-platinum treatment? *Cancer Chemother. Pharmacol.* **1985**, *14*, 247–249. [CrossRef]
7. Argyropoulos, C.P.; Chen, S.S.; Ng, Y.H.; Roumelioti, M.E.; Shaffi, K.; Singh, P.P.; Tzamaloukas, A.H. Rediscovering Beta-2 Microglobulin As a Biomarker across the Spectrum of Kidney Diseases. *Front. Med.* **2017**, *4*, 73. [CrossRef] [PubMed]
8. Portman, R.J.; Kissane, J.M.; Robson, A.M. Use of beta 2 microglobulin to diagnose tubule-interstitial renal lesions in children. *Kidney Int.* **1986**, *30*, 91–98. [CrossRef]
9. Coca, S.G.; Parikh, C.R. Urinary biomarkers for acute kidney injury: Perspectives on translation. *Clin. J. Am. Soc. Nephrol.* **2008**, *3*, 481–490. [CrossRef] [PubMed]
10. Lurbe, E.; Agabiti-Rosei, E.; Cruickshank, J.K.; Dominiczak, A.; Erdine, S.; Hirth, A.; Invitti, C.; Litwin, M.; Mancia, G.; Pall, D.; et al. 2016 European Society of Hypertension guidelines for the management of high blood pressure in children and adolescents. *J. Hypertens.* **2016**, *34*, 1887–1920. [CrossRef] [PubMed]
11. Levin, A.; Stevens, P.E. Summary of KDIGO 2012 CKD Guideline: Behind the Scenes, Need for Guidance, and a Framework for Moving Forward. *Kidney Int.* **2014**, *85*, 49–61. [CrossRef] [PubMed]
12. Hjorth, L.; Wiebe, T.; Karpman, D. Hyperfiltration evaluated by glomerular filtration rate at diagnosis in children with cancer. *Pediatr. Blood Cancer* **2011**, *56*, 762–766. [CrossRef] [PubMed]
13. Griffin, B.R.; Faubel, S.; Edelstein, C.L. Biomarkers of Drug-Induced Kidney Toxicity. *Ther. Drug Monit.* **2019**, *41*, 213–226. [CrossRef]
14. George, B.; Joy, M.S.; Aleksunes, L.M. Urinary Protein Biomarkers of Kidney Injury in Patients Receiving Cisplatin Chemotherapy. *Exp. Biol. Med.* **2018**, *243*, 272–282. [CrossRef]
15. Finkel, K.W.; Foringer, J.R. Renal disease in patients with cancer. *Nat. Clin. Pract. Nephrol.* **2007**, *3*, 669–678. [CrossRef]

16. Latoch, E.; Konończuk, K.; Taranta-Janusz, K.; Muszyńska-Rosłan, K.; Szymczak, E.; Wasilewska, A.; Krawczuk-Rybak, M. Urine NGAL and KIM-1: Tubular Injury Markers in Acute Lymphoblastic Leukemia Survivors. *Cancer Chemother. Pharmacol.* **2020**, *86*, 741–749. [CrossRef]
17. Latoch, E.; Konończuk, K.; Muszyńska-Rosłan, K.; Taranta-Janusz, K.; Wasilewska, A.; Szymczak, E.; Trochim, J.; Krawczuk-Rybak, M. Urine NGAL and KIM-1-Tubular Injury Markers in Long-Term Survivors of Childhood Solid Tumors: A Cross-Sectional Study. *J. Clin. Med.* **2021**, *10*, 399. [CrossRef] [PubMed]
18. Ylinen, E.; Jahnukainen, K.; Saarinen-Pihkala, U.M.; Jahnukainen, T. Assessment of renal function during high-dose methotrexate treatment in children with acute lymphoblastic leukemia. *Pediatr. Blood Cancer* **2014**, *61*, 2199–2202. [CrossRef] [PubMed]
19. Mulder, R.L.; Knijnenburg, S.L.; Geskus, R.B.; van Dalen, E.C.; van der Pal, H.J.H.; Koning, C.C.E.; Bouts, A.H.; Caron, H.N.; Kremer, L.C.M. Glomerular Function Time Trends in Long-Term Survivors of Childhood Cancer: A Longitudinal Study. *Cancer Epidemiol. Biomarkers Prev.* **2013**, *22*, 1736–1746. [CrossRef]
20. Dawson, L.A.; Kavanagh, B.D.; Paulino, A.C.; Das, S.K.; Miften, M.; Li, X.A.; Pan, C.; Ten Haken, R.K.; Schultheiss, T.E. Radiation-associated kidney injury. *Int. J. Radiat. Oncol. Biol. Phys.* **2010**, *76*, S108–S115. [CrossRef]
21. Dekkers, I.A.; Blijdorp, K.; Cransberg, K.; Pluijm, S.M.; Pieters, R.; Neggers, S.J.; van den Heuvel-Eibrink, M.M. Long-term nephrotoxicity in adult survivors of childhood cancer. *Clin. J. Am. Soc. Nephrol.* **2013**, *8*, 922–929. [CrossRef]
22. Schiavetti, A.; Altavista, P.; De Luca, L.; Andreoli, G.; Megaro, G.; Versacci, P. Long-term renal function in unilateral non-syndromic renal tumor survivors treated according to International Society of Pediatric Oncology protocols. *Pediatr. Blood Cancer* **2015**, *62*, 1637–1644. [CrossRef] [PubMed]
23. Rysz, J.; Gluba-Brzózka, A.; Franczyk, B.; Jabłonowski, Z.; Ciałkowska-Rysz, A. Novel Biomarkers in the Diagnosis of Chronic Kidney Disease and the Prediction of Its Outcome. *Int. J. Mol. Sci.* **2017**, *18*, 1702. [CrossRef] [PubMed]
24. Puthiyottil, D.; Priyamvada, P.S.; Kumar, M.N.; Chellappan, A.; Zachariah, B.; Parameswaran, S. Role of Urinary Beta 2 Microglobulin and Kidney Injury Molecule-1 in Predicting Kidney Function at One Year Following Acute Kidney Injury. *Int. J. Nephrol. Renovasc. Dis.* **2021**, *14*, 225–234. [CrossRef] [PubMed]
25. Tibúrcio, F.R.; Rodrigues, K.; Belisário, A.R.; Simões-E-Silva, A.C. Glomerular hyperfiltration and β-2 microglobulin as biomarkers of incipient renal dysfunction in cancer survivors. *Future Sci. OA* **2018**, *4*, FSO333. [CrossRef]
26. Musiol, K.; Sobol-Milejska, G.; Nowotka, Ł.; Torba, K.; Kniażewska, M.; Wos, H. Renal function in children treated for central nervous system malignancies. *Childs Nerv. Syst.* **2016**, *32*, 1431–1440. [CrossRef]
27. Ikezumi, Y.; Uemura, O.; Nagai, T.; Ishikura, K.; Ito, S.; Hataya, H.; Fujita, N.; Akioka, Y.; Kaneko, T.; Iijima, K.; et al. Beta-2 microglobulin-based equation for estimating glomerular filtration rates in Japanese children and adolescents. *Clin. Exp. Nephrol.* **2015**, *19*, 450–457. [CrossRef]
28. Hibi, Y.; Uemura, O.; Nagai, T.; Yamakawa, S.; Yamasaki, Y.; Yamamoto, M.; Nakano, M.; Kasahara, K. The ratios of urinary β2-microglobulin and NAG to creatinine vary with age in children. *Pediatr. Int.* **2015**, *57*, 79–84. [CrossRef] [PubMed]
29. Prizment, A.E.; Linabery, A.M.; Lutsey, P.L.; Selvin, E.; Nelson, H.H.; Folsom, A.R.; Church, T.R.; Drake, C.G.; Platz, E.A.; Joshu, C. Circulating Beta-2 Microglobulin and Risk of Cancer: The Atherosclerosis Risk in Communities Study (ARIC). *Cancer Epidemiol. Biomark. Prev.* **2016**, *25*, 657–664. [CrossRef] [PubMed]
30. Wang, Q.; Qin, Y.; Zhou, S.; He, X.; Yang, J.; Kang, S.; Liu, P.; Yang, S.; Zhang, C.; Gui, L.; et al. Prognostic value of pretreatment serum beta-2 microglobulin level in advanced classical Hodgkin lymphoma treated in the modern era. *Oncotarget* **2016**, *7*, 72219–72228. [CrossRef] [PubMed]
31. Zhang, L.; Zhang, K.; Dong, W.; Li, R.; Huang, R.; Zhang, H.; Shi, W.; Liu, S.; Li, Z.; Chen, Y.; et al. Raised Plasma Levels of Asymmetric Dimethylarginine Are Associated with Pathological Type and Predict the Therapeutic Effect in Lupus Nephritis Patients Treated with Cyclophosphamide. *Kidney Dis.* **2020**, *6*, 355–363. [CrossRef] [PubMed]
32. Behairy, O.G.; Abd Almonaem, E.R.; Abed, N.T.; Abdel Haiea, O.M.; Zakaria, R.M.; AbdEllaty, R.I.; Asr, E.H.; Mansour, A.I.; Abdelrahman, A.M.; Elhady, H.A. Role of serum cystatin-C and beta-2 microglobulin as early markers of renal dysfunction in children with beta thalassemia major. *Int. J. Nephrol. Renovasc. Dis.* **2017**, *10*, 261–268. [CrossRef] [PubMed]
33. Monteiro, M.B.; Thieme, K.; Santos-Bezerra, D.P.; Queiroz, M.S.; Woronik, V.; Passarelli, M.; Machado, U.F.; Giannella-Neto, D.; Oliveira-Souza, M.; Corrêa-Giannella, M.L. Beta-2-microglobulin (B2M) expression in the urinary sediment correlates with clinical markers of kidney disease in patients with type 1 diabetes. *Metab. Clin. Exp.* **2016**, *65*, 816–824. [CrossRef] [PubMed]
34. Ugan, Y.; Korkmaz, H.; Dogru, A.; Koca, Y.S.; Balkarlı, A.; Aylak, F.; Tunc, S.E. The significance of urinary beta-2 microglobulin level for differential diagnosis of familial Mediterranean fever and acute appendicitis. *Clin. Rheumatol.* **2016**, *35*, 1669–1672. [CrossRef]
35. Katsoufis, C.P. Clinical predictors of chronic kidney disease in congenital lower urinary tract obstruction. *Pediatr. Nephrol.* **2020**, *35*, 1193–1201. [CrossRef] [PubMed]
36. Caro, J.; Al Hadidi, S.; Usmani, S.; Yee, A.J.; Raje, N.; Davies, F.E. How to Treat High-Risk Myeloma at Diagnosis and Relapse. *Am. Soc. Clin. Oncol. Educ. Book* **2021**, *41*, 291–309. [CrossRef]
37. Gao, A.; Cachat, F.; Faouzi, M.; Bardy, D.; Mosig, D.; Meyrat, B.J.; Girardin, E.; Chehade, H. Comparison of the glomerular filtration rate in children by the new revised Schwartz formula and a new generalized formula. *Kidney Int.* **2013**, *83*, 524–530. [CrossRef]

38. Kanemasa, Y.; Shimoyama, T.; Sasaki, Y.; Tamura, M.; Sawada, T.; Omuro, Y.; Hishima, T.; Maeda, Y. Beta-2 microglobulin as a significant prognostic factor and a new risk model for patients with diffuse large B-cell lymphoma. *Hematol. Oncol.* **2017**, *35*, 440–446. [CrossRef] [PubMed]
39. Krawczuk-Rybak, M.; Latoch, E. Risk Factors for Premature Aging in Childhood Cancer Survivors. *Dev. Period. Med.* **2019**, *23*, 97–103. [PubMed]
40. Ariffin, H.; Azanan, M.S.; Abd Ghafar, S.S.; Oh, L.; Lau, K.H.; Thirunavakarasu, T.; Sedan, A.; Ibrahim, K.; Chan, A.; Chin, T.F.; et al. Young Adult Survivors of Childhood Acute Lymphoblastic Leukemia Show Evidence of Chronic Inflammation and Cellular Aging. *Cancer* **2017**, *123*, 4207–4214. [CrossRef] [PubMed]

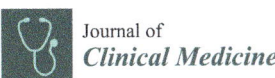

Article

Clinical and Epidemiological Analysis of Children's Urinary Tract Infections in Accordance with Antibiotic Resistance Patterns of Pathogens

Katarzyna Werbel [1], Dorota Jankowska [2], Anna Wasilewska [1] and Katarzyna Taranta-Janusz [1,*]

[1] Department of Pediatrics and Nephrology, Medical University of Białystok, 15-274 Białystok, Poland; katarzynawerbel@gmail.com (K.W.); annwasil@interia.pl (A.W.)
[2] Department of Statistics and Medical Informatics, Medical University of Białystok, 15-295 Białystok, Poland; dorota.jankowska@umb.edu.pl
* Correspondence: katarzyna.taranta@wp.pl; Tel.: +48-85-745-06-51; Fax: +48-85-742-18-38

Citation: Werbel, K.; Jankowska, D.; Wasilewska, A.; Taranta-Janusz, K. Clinical and Epidemiological Analysis of Children's Urinary Tract Infections in Accordance with Antibiotic Resistance Patterns of Pathogens. *J. Clin. Med.* **2021**, *10*, 5260. https://doi.org/10.3390/jcm10225260

Academic Editor: Bhaskar K. Somani

Received: 2 October 2021
Accepted: 10 November 2021
Published: 12 November 2021

Publisher's Note: MDPI stays neutral with regard to jurisdictional claims in published maps and institutional affiliations.

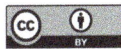

Copyright: © 2021 by the authors. Licensee MDPI, Basel, Switzerland. This article is an open access article distributed under the terms and conditions of the Creative Commons Attribution (CC BY) license (https://creativecommons.org/licenses/by/4.0/).

Abstract: The study was conducted to analyze urinary tract infections (UTI) in children by considering epidemiology and antibiotic resistance patterns of pathogens in accordance with inflammatory parameters. The research included 525 patients who demonstrated 627 episodes of UTI. The increasing resistance of bacteria was observed over the years covered by the study ($p < 0.001$). There was a significant increase of resistance to amoxicillin with clavulanic acid ($p = 0.001$), gentamicin ($p = 0.017$) and ceftazidime ($p = 0.0005$). According to the CART method, we managed to estimate C-reactive protein (CRP), procalcitonin (PCT) and white blood cell (WBC) values, in which antibiotic sensitivity was observed. In children with CRP > 97.91 mg/L, there was a high percentage of sensitive cases to amoxicillin with clavulanic acid (87.5%). Values of WBC above 14.45 K/μL were associated with *E. coli* more sensitivity to ampicillin. 100% of children with CRP > 0.42 mg/L and PCT ≤ 6.92 ng/mL had confirmed sensitivity to cefuroxime. Concerning sensitivity to gentamicin, the most optimal cut-off point of WBC was >7.80 K/μL, while in the case of nitrofurantoin, it was CRP value > 0.11 mg/L (which was presented in 98.50% of children). These results may guide us with antibiotic therapy and help to inhibit increasing antibiotic resistance.

Keywords: antibiotic resistance; *Escherichia coli*; inflammatory markers; urinary tract infection

1. Introduction

Urinary tract infections (UTI) are known as one of the most common bacterial diseases in children (after respiratory tract infections). Furthermore, they are often the cause of infant and toddler hospitalization [1]. Proper management of a UTI episode is a renal scarring prophylaxis, especially when associated with congenital anomalies of the urinary tract. Renal scarring may lead to complications in adulthood, including hypertension, proteinuria, renal damage and even chronic kidney disease. Therefore, it is important to initiate an effective antibiotic therapy early. Considering the numerous reports from the USA, Canada and Europe on the growing antibiotic resistance associated with often and inadequate use of antibacterial drugs, it is justified to regularly reassess the antibiotic sensitivity of bacterial strains responsible for UTI [2,3].

Due to conditions present in childhood age, such as short urethra, possibility of contamination with fecal bacteria, higher incidence of congenital defects and continuous development of human organ systems (including the immune system), the child's organism is more likely to develop UTI than an adult's. UTI occurs in 2–8% of children. Infections of this system affect 0.1–1% of full-term newborns [4], while in premature infants, this percentage rises to 25% [5].

In early infancy (especially <3 months old), the male sex is more predisposed to UTI due to higher incidence of CAKUT (congenital anomalies of kidney and urinary tract), whereas in adolescence, infections are more common in girls [6,7]. The incidence of UTI differs depending on race, which in white people is almost twice as high as in the African American population [8].

The most dominant etiological factor of UTI is *Escherichia coli*, which is responsible for about 90% of infections [2,9,10]. Proteus spp. is often found in urine cultures of young male infants because of its presence under the foreskin. Other bacteria known to be etiological factors of UTI are *Pseudomonas aeruginosa, Klebsiella pneumoniae* and *Enterobacter* spp. [11,12]. *Pseudomonas aeruginosa*, due to its properties, is a common cause of recurrent UTI.

Incidence of UTI is more frequent in groups of children with risk factors, including anomalies of urinary tract (including vesicoureteral reflux–VUR) and dysfunctional elimination syndrome [13,14].

The discovery of first antibiotic (penicillin) is one of the biggest achievements of medicine. Over the decades, it has helped to save millions of human lives. However, the common use of antibiotics reduced the effectiveness of this type of treatment. Klein et al. [15] analyzed global consumption of antibiotics from 2000 to 2015. The research showed that the highest DDD rates (daily defined dose) per 1000 habitants in 2015 were found in Turkey, Tunisia (~50 DDD), Spain, Greece, Algeria and Romania (~35–40 DDD). The biggest increase of DDD over the years covered by the study was observed in Turkey, Tunisia and Algeria.

It is known that the process of acquiring resistance is a natural example of evolution in response to usage of antibiotics. Unfortunately, irrational antibiotic therapy accelerates this trend. Tadesse et al. [16], conducted the research, in which they found out that multi–drug resistance of *Escherichia coli* is systematically increasing. The study showed the increase of resistance from 7.2% in the years from 1950–1959 to 63.6% in the years from 2000–2002.

Laboratory tests that can be helpful in making a diagnosis are markers of inflammation, e.g., elevated concentration of C-reactive protein–CRP. High CRP values are frequently found in patients with upper urinary tract infection and CRP testing has been shown to be useful in differentiating upper and lower UTI [17]. Raised CRP values may also be found in lower UTI in smaller children and as a result, there is a risk that antibiotics may be wrongly prescribed. For valid interpretations of inflammatory markers' results in patients with UTI, awareness of the range of values that can be expected when the infection is caused by antibiotic sensitive microorganisms would be useful.

The main aim of the study was to analyze antibiotic resistance trends over the years. We also assessed inflammatory parameters' association with patients' responsiveness to prescribed drugs and if it is possible to plan empiric therapy on the basis of inflammatory markers levels.

2. Materials and Methods

The retrospective study was conducted in 525 children hospitalized in the Department of Pediatrics and Nephrology (Children's Clinical University Hospital of Białystok, Poland) from 2010–2017, in which we observed 627 episodes of UTI. The inclusion criterion for the study group was a positive urine culture with accompanying clinical symptoms (a negative microbiological test result was acceptable in the case of use of outpatient antibiotic therapy before collecting urine for cultures in 33 cases; in these patients, UTI episodes were diagnosed and treatment had been started by general practitioner). The exclusion criteria were insignificant bacteriuria, leukocyturia with negative urine culture (except cases with administered outpatient antibiotic therapy). From among the performed microbiological tests, a significant growth of bacteria was obtained in 590 cases. Initially, 711 cases of UTI were included in the preliminary analysis. After excluding cases that did not meet the inclusion criteria or were not eligible for the study due to the exclusion criteria, the final analysis contained 627 episodes of UTI (398 in girls and 229 in boys). 318 episodes were febrile UTIs; patients without fever were hospitalized due to other symptoms, such as vomiting or severe abdominal pain. Twenty-nine of excluded cases were asymptomatic bacteriuria. Patients with history of recurrent UTIs and with VUR grade III–V were on chemoprohylaxis (110 girls and 51 boys). Renal scars and features of nephropathy were assessed in 51 cases by performing DMSA (as a feature of nephropathy (most often reflux nephropathy), a hypofunction of kidney determined as the split kidney function <30% shown on DMSA). Participants were aged between 7 days old and almost 18 years old (331 females and 194 males). The anthropometric measurements and laboratory tests were carried out at the time of admission to the hospital. In every patient, blood laboratory tests were performed, which included white blood count (WBC), C-reactive protein and procalcitonin (PCT). Blood count was examined from K-EDTA blood (Sysmex XT-4000i, Sysmex Europe GMBH, Bornbarch, Germany), however CRP and PCT concentrations were measured in serum with a clot activator (Cobas 6000 c501, Roche Diagnostics International Ltd., Rotkreuz, Switzerland). Urine samples for urinalysis and urine culture were collected by clean–catch of midstream urine or catheterization, also in infants (the method of clean–catch of midstream urine was used in cases when parents refused to consent catheterization). The use of a urine bag was only permitted for urinalysis. After bacteria growth in the urine culture, the antibiograms were marked in order to assess sensitivity of microbes to commonly used antibiotics (ampicillin, amoxicillin with clavulanic acid, cefuroxime, ceftazidime, gentamicin, cotrimoxazole and nitrofurantoin).

The research results were statistically analyzed using the Statistica 13.3 computer program (StatSoft, Tulsa, OK, USA). In the analyzes and tests, the significance level of $p < 0.05$ was used. For the analyzed numerical features, in each of the estimated group, the normality of the distribution was assessed using the Shapiro-Wilk test. Due to the lack of normal distribution the studied groups were compared with the non-parametric Mann-Whitney U test. Additionally, the non-parametric Pearson's Chi-square test of independence was used to assess the relationship between categorical features. The method of classification and regression trees (CART) was used to establish the optimal cut–off point for inflammatory markers, which allow to classify cases as sensitive or resistant to analyzed antibiotics.

The study was carried out after agreement of the Bioethics Committee of the Medical University of Bialystok (R-I-002/104/2018).

3. Results

The study included a total of 525 children hospitalized in the Department of Pediatrics and Nephrology (Children's Clinical University Hospital of Białystok, Poland) due to UTI in years 2010–2017. Girls constituted 63.1% (331) of children covered by the study, while boys—36.9% (194). Demographic and clinical parameters of participants are shown in Table 1.

The youngest patient developed UTI in the first week of life, while the oldest patient was 17 years and 11 months old. The median age was 2.08 years old. The age of patients with UTI differ significantly between males and females ($p < 0.001$). The analysis showed that girls have greater body weight than boys ($p < 0.001$), but there was no significant difference in BMI values ($p = 0.12$). Comparisons of concentrations of inflammatory markers showed significantly higher values of WBC in males ($p = 0.009$). Values of CRP and PCT did not differ significantly ($p > 0.05$). The diagram in Figure 1 shows the variability of UTI episodes depending on age and sex of patients. In boys, UTI was diagnosed mainly in the first year of life (with the prevalence of infections <6 months old). In girls, the distribution of UTI incidents was much more regular, with predomination of infections diagnosed after the second year of life.

Table 1. Demographic, anthropometric and biochemical parameters in patients; comparisons between males and females.

		n	Median	Q1	Q3	p-Value
Age (years)	all	627	2.08	0.5	8.67	
	male	229	0.58	0.25	4.75	<0.001
	female	398	3.88	0.92	10.42	
Body weight (kg)	all	600	12.00	7.40	26.00	
	male	219	8.70	6.20	15.00	<0.001
	female	381	16.40	9.10	31.00	
BMI (kg/m^2)	all	264	17.09	15.09	19.96	
	male	50	16.50	14.89	18.27	NS
	female	214	17.17	15.09	20.66	
CRP (mg/L)	all	622	14.93	1.56	66.38	
	male	229	14.95	1.78	62.90	NS
	female	393	14.90	1.52	70.00	
PCT (ng/mL)	all	228	0.65	0.15	4.16	
	male	95	0.75	0.11	6.70	NS
	female	133	0.60	0.16	3.46	
WBC (K/μL)	all	624	12.60	9.10	17.70	
	male	229	13.59	9.90	18.70	<0.01
	female	395	11.90	8.80	17.20	

Q1—lower quartile; Q3—upper quartile; NS—not significant.

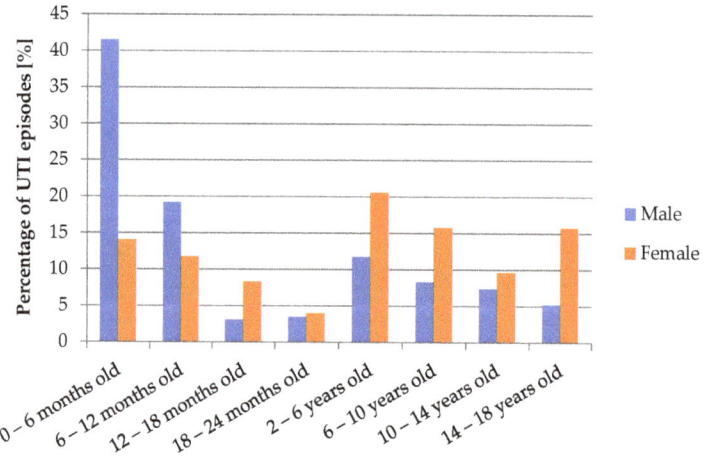

Figure 1. Number of UTI episodes depending on age and gender of patients.

In the study group, 147 patients had a history of recurrent UTIs—girls constituted 69.4% (102) and boys—30.6% (45). The recurrent UTIs were observed in 30.8% of girls and in 23.2% of boys. There was no significant dependence of sex on recurrent UTIs incidence ($p = 0.06$).

One of the risk factors of UTI is the presence of anatomical and functional abnormalities of the urinary tract. In the study group, 171 children were diagnosed with the urinary tract defect (Table 2) in which VUR was by far the most common diagnosis (92 patients).

Table 2. Anatomical defects of urinary tract depending on gender of patients.

Type of Anatomical Defect [1]		Male (n = 194)	Female (n = 331)	Total (n = 525)
Duplex collecting system	n	8	12	20
	[%]	4.12%	3.63%	3.81%
Ureteropelvic junction obstruction	n	6	8	14
	[%]	3.09%	2.42%	2.67%
Ureterovesical junction obstruction	n	5	4	9
	[%]	2.58%	1.21%	1.71%
Vesicoureteral reflux	n	31	61	92
	[%]	15.98%	18.43%	17.52%
Urethral valves	n	18	-	-
	[%]	9.28%	-	-

[1] Some patients had more than 1 type of anatomical defect.

In Table 3, the number of children with VUR depending on sex is shown. The conducted analysis showed that the gender of patient had a statistically significant dependence on the grade of VUR ($p = 0.013$). In boys, a high-grade VUR was observed more often (48.4%) than in girls (24.6%).

Table 3. Number of children with VUR depending on gender.

VUR		Male	Female	Total	
VUR I–III	n	16	47	63	
	[%]	51.6%	75.4%	68.5%	
VUR IV–V	n	15	14	29	$p = 0.013$
	[%]	48.4%	24.6%	31.5%	
Total	n	61	31	9	

Renal scintigraphy (DMSA) was performed in 51 patients to assess kidney function. In 31.4% of cases features of nephropathy were found, while in 19.6%, there were renal scars.

The diagram in Figure 2 presents the percentages of urine samples with or without leukocyturia. Leukocyturia was demonstrated in 78.8% of analyzed samples. The outpatient antibiotic therapy was administered in 34 cases out of 133 urine samples with no leukocyturia.

In Figure 3, there are shown percentages of microbes from urine cultures covered by the study. The most dominant bacteria in samples was *Escherichia coli* (72.7%). Other microbes found in the study were *Pseudomonas aeruginosa* (5.8%), *Proteus mirabilis* (5.8%) and *Klebsiella pneumonia* (3.9%); each of the rest of bacteria represented less than 2% of the total.

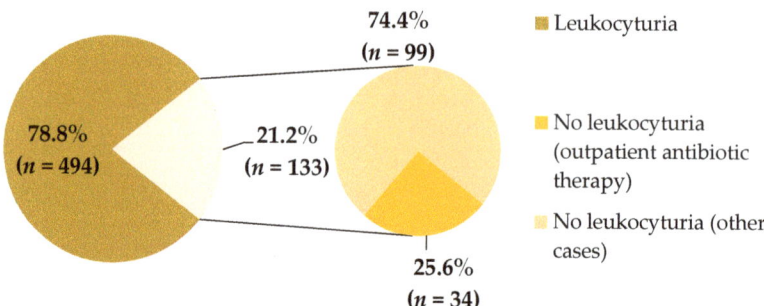

Figure 2. Percentage of leukocyturia in studied urine samples.

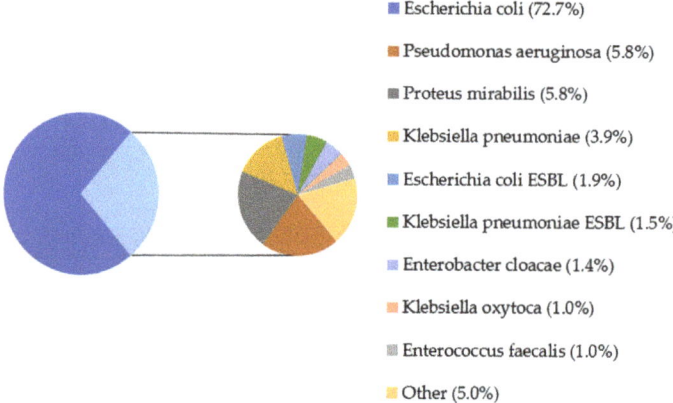

Figure 3. Percentage of bacterial strains in the urine cultures of patients; ESBL—extended-spectrum beta-lactamases. Other: *Proteus vulgaris* (0.68%), *Citrobacter freundii* (0.52%), *Citrobacter koseri*, *Staphylococcus saprophyticus* MSCNS, *Staphylococcus saprophyticus*, *Acinetobacter baumanii* (each 0.35%), *Enterococcus gallinarum*, *Escherichia coli* AMPc, *Staphylococcus epidermidis* MRSE, *Enterococcus faecalis* HLAR, *Providencia rettgeri*, *Streptococcus agalactiae*, *Streptococcus mitis*, *Morganellamorgani*, *Staphylococcus aureus*, *Enterobacter aerogenes*, *Staphylococcus simulans*, *Micrococcus* spp., *Staphylococcus epidermidis* MSCNS MLSB, *Staphylococcus epidermidis* (each 0.171%).

In the performed analysis, there was a lower percentage of urine samples with *Escherichia coli* in boys than in girls (64.8% vs. 77.3% in whole examined group), similar to the ESBL strain of this bacteria (1.4% vs. 2.2% in whole examined group). Other microbes accounted for a greater percentage in males than females (Figure 4).

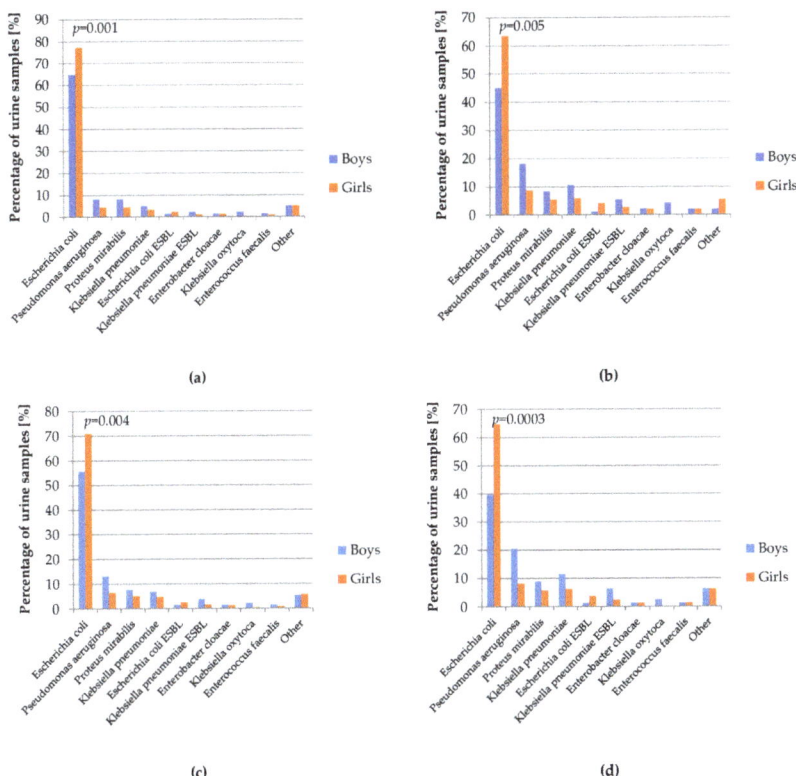

Figure 4. Percentage of bacterial strains in the urine cultures depending on gender of patients: (**a**) total; (**b**) patients with urinary tract defect; (**c**) patients on chemoprophylaxis; (**d**) patients with recurrent UTI.

The diagram in Figure 5 shows the variability of bacterial strains isolated from urine samples over the years covered by the study.

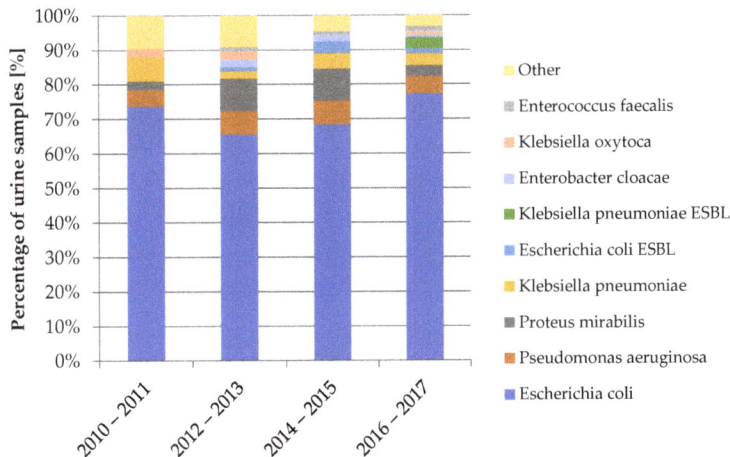

Figure 5. Variability of bacterial strains in the urine cultures from 2010–2017.

The increasing resistance of bacteria was observed in antibiograms of the urine cultures, shown in Figure 6. Dependency was statistically significant ($p < 0.001$).

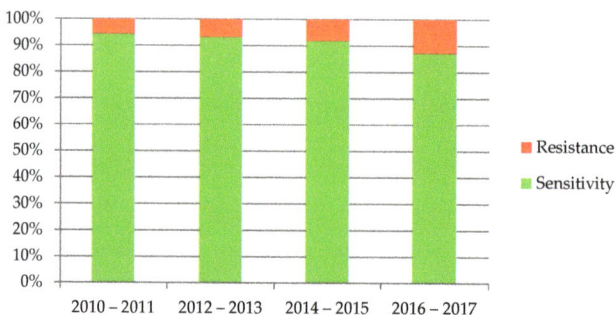

Figure 6. Sensitivity and resistance of bacteria to antibiotics from 2010–2017.

The diagrams in Figure 7 show the variability over time in antibiotic resistance of the most common bacteria. Statistical significance was found in the case of *E. coli* ($p = 0.0002$), *K. pneumoniae* ($p = 0.004$) and *P. mirabilis* ($p = 0.006$).

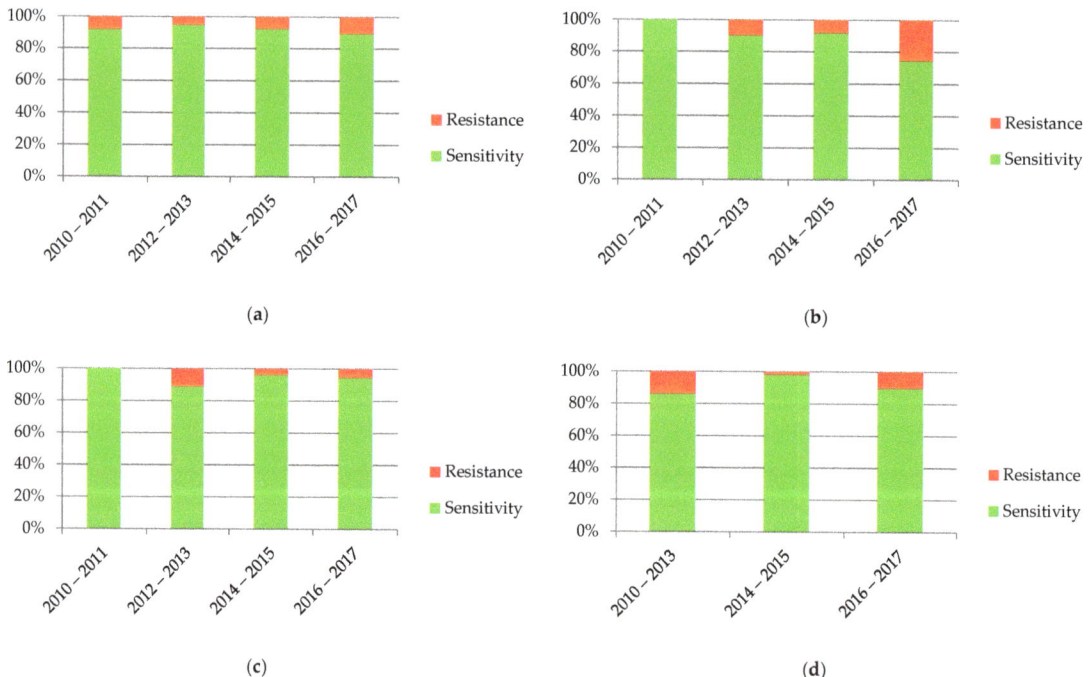

Figure 7. Sensitivity and resistance of bacteria to antibiotics from 2010–2017: (**a**) *Escherichia coli*; (**b**) *Pseudomonas aeruginosa*; (**c**) *Klebsiella pneumonia*; (**d**) *Proteus mirabilis*.

Comparisons of sensitivity of the most dominant bacteria to antibiotics are presented in Figure 8. In the case of *Escherichia coli*, the highest percentage of resistance was found in ampicillin (47.2%) and amoxicillin with clavulanic acid (24.8%). *Pseudomonas aeruginosa* was characterized by a high percentage of resistance to ticarcillin with clavulanic acid (42.9%). It is necessary to mention that sensitivity to this antibiotic was estimated on the basis of only seven antibiograms. *Klebsiella pneumoniae* was most resistant to amoxicillin with clavulanic acid (69.2%); however, *Proteus mirabilis* was most resistant to cotrimoxazole (33.3%).

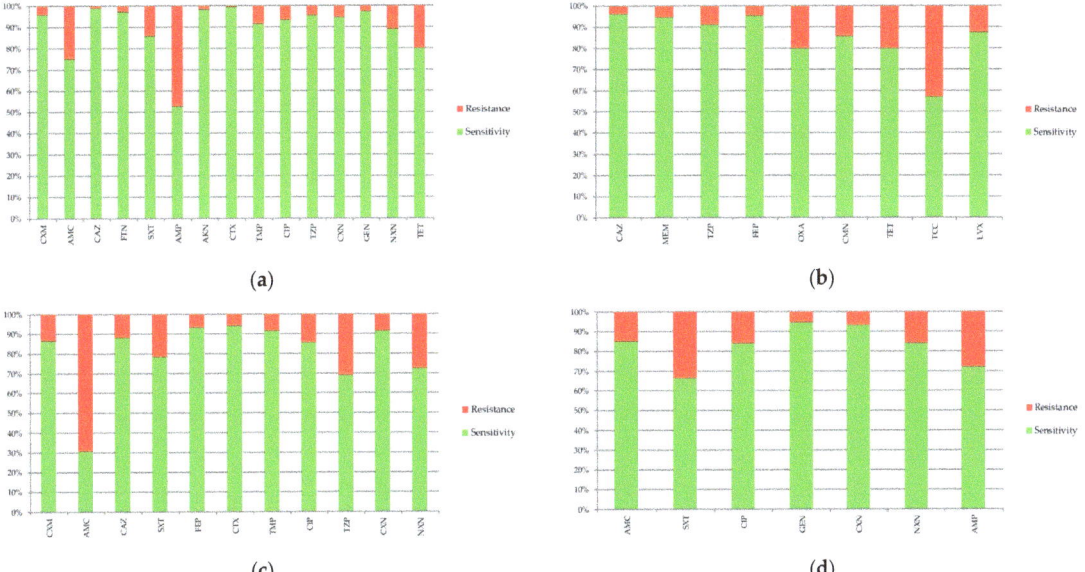

Figure 8. Sensitivity and resistance of bacteria to antibiotics: (**a**) *Escherichia coli*; (**b**) *Pseudomonas aeruginosa*; (**c**) *Klebsiella pneumonia*; (**d**) *Proteus mirabilis*. AKN—amikacin, AMC—amoxicillin with clavulanic acid, AMP—ampicillin, CAZ—ceftazidime, CFM—cefixime, CIP—ciprofloxacin, CMN—clindamycin, CTX—cefotaxime, CXM—cefuroxime, CXN—cephalexin, FEP—cefepime, FTN—nitrofurantoin, GEN—gentamicin, LVX—levofloxacin, MEM—meropenem, NXN—norfloxacin, OXA—oxacillin, SXT—cotrimoxazole, TCC—ticarcillin with clavulanic acid, TET—tetracycline, TMP—trimethoprim TZP—piperacillin with tazobactam.

Considering risk factors of UTI, such as VUR and recurrence of infections, the association between the presence of them and antibiotic resistance was assessed (Figure 9). Only episodes of UTI caused by *E. coli* were analyzed. Other etiological factors were not assessed due to the insufficient number of cases, which did not allow for obtaining reliable results. The percentage of antibiotic resistance were higher in UTI episodes in children with VUR ($p = 0.002$). Antibiotic resistance was observed a little more often in cases of recurrent UTI (9.93%) than in non-recurrent UTI (9.04%), but there was no statistical significance ($p = 0.37$). Additionally, assessment of antibiotic resistance in children on chemoprophylaxis was performed. Resistant *E. coli* was observed more often in children on chemoprophylaxis ($p < 0.001$).

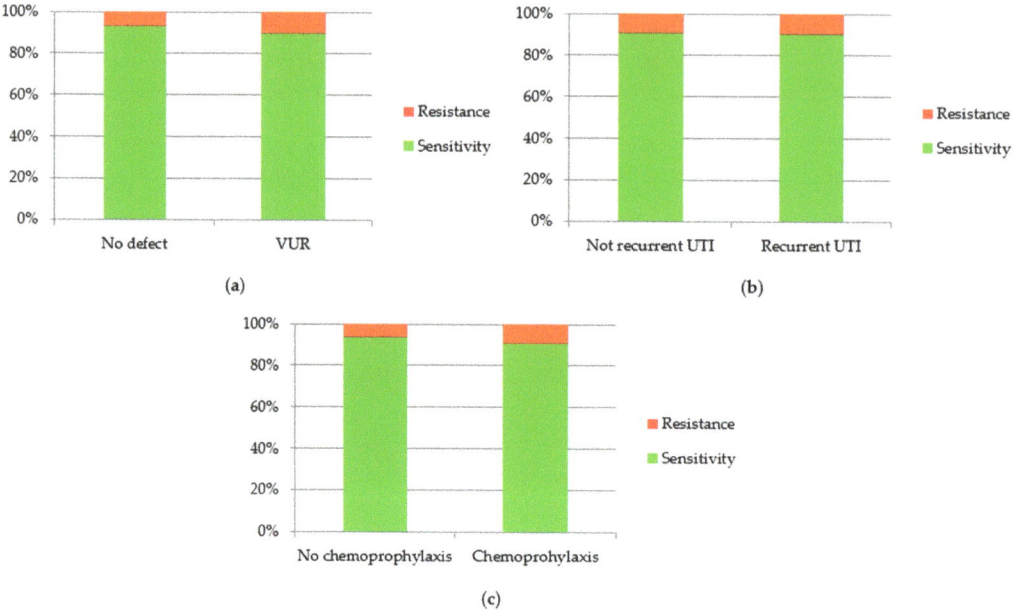

Figure 9. Sensitivity and resistance of *Escherichia coli* to antibiotics in children with: (**a**) VUR; (**b**) recurrent UTI; (**c**) chemoprophylaxis.

The diagrams in Figure 10 present the variability of sensitivity to most commonly used antibiotics. There was a significant increase of resistance to amoxicillin with clavulanic acid ($p = 0.001$), gentamicin ($p = 0.017$) and ceftazidime ($p = 0.0005$). The only drug where decreasing resistance was observed was nitrofurantoin ($p = 0.032$).

Further tests were carried out to identify differences in values of inflammatory markers between resistant and sensitive *Escherichia coli* to commonly used antibiotics. In the analysis, there were found to be significantly lower values of WBC in patients with *Escherichia coli* resistant to ampicillin ($p = 0.04$), cefuroxime ($p = 0.007$) and nitrofurantoin ($p = 0.0045$) beside sensitive ones. In the case of CRP, higher concentrations were observed in participants with *E. coli* sensitive to cefuroxime ($p = 0.045$) and nitrofurantoin ($p = 0.02$). There was no significant difference in analyzed values of PCT in the case of any antibiotic. It was not possible to evaluate statistical significance of PCT difference for nitrofurantoin because of no PCT test in patients with *E. coli* resistance to this antibiotic. However, for ceftazidime, too few resistant samples to carry out the analysis were observed.

Taking into consideration resistance to amoxicillin with clavulanic acid, the CART tree showed differences in CRP and PCT concentrations (Figure 11). In children with CRP value > 97.91 mg/L, there was great percentage of sensitive cases (87.5%), while CRP ≤ 97.91 mg/L was associated with higher risk of smaller sensitivity (72.54%). However, in cases with CRP ≤ 97.91 mg/L and PCT ≤ 2.14 ng/mL there was greater chance to have sensitivity to amoxicillin with clavulanic acid (81.97% of children) than in the case of PCT > 2.14 ng/mL.

Figure 12 shows that the most optimal cut–off point of WBC in case of ampicillin in the first node of the CART was 14.45 K/μL. Children with values of WBC above 14.45 K/μL were classified as patients with *E. coli* expected to be more sensitive to ampicillin. On the other hand, CRP in the CART was also taken into consideration. In participants with WBC > 14.45 K/μL, patients with CRP in the range of 43.91–123.47 mg/L were classified as patients with higher risk of resistance to ampicillin than children with CRP > 123.47 mg/L. Considering PCT concentration in this tree, children with WBC below or equal 14.45 K/μl and with PCT ≤ 0.08 ng/mL were at high risk of resistance to ampicillin (75.0% of samples). However, it is important to notice that there were only eight cases in this tree node. A similar situation took place in children with CRP values between 43.91 mg/L and 123.47 mg/L; patients with a concentration of PCT ≤ 0.28 ng/mL were at higher risk of resistance to ampicillin (85.71% of children). However, this tree node was also presented with small number of cases.

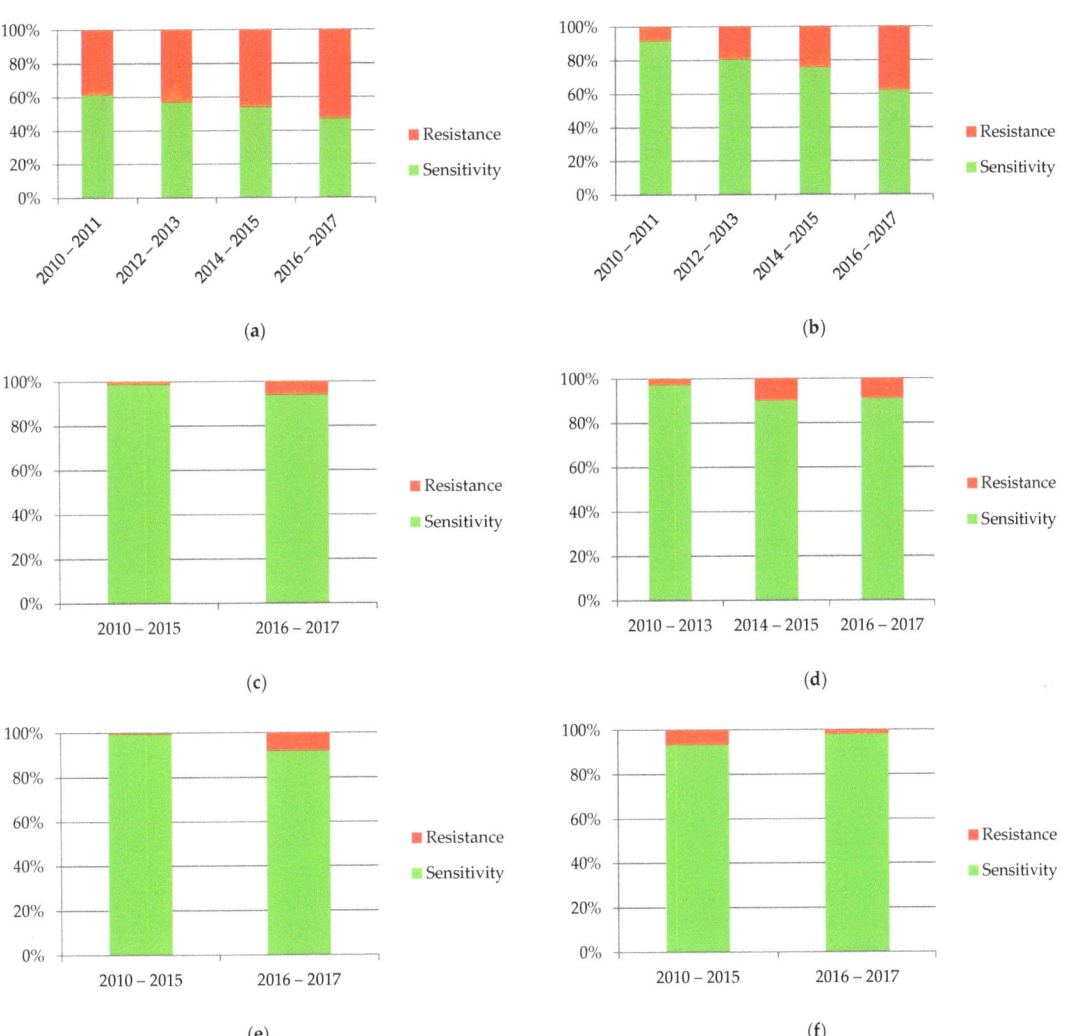

Figure 10. *Cont.*

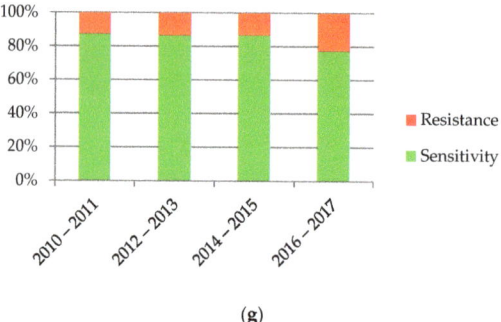

(g)

Figure 10. Sensitivity and resistance of bacteria to antibiotics from 2010–2017: (**a**) ampicillin; (**b**) amoxicillin with clavulanic acid; (**c**) gentamicin; (**d**) cefuroxime; (**e**) ceftazidime; (**f**) nitrofurantoin; (**g**) cotrimoxazole.

Further, in case of cefuroxime, there were optimal cut–off points of CRP and PCT values in estimating risk of resistance of *E. coli*. 100% of children with CRP > 0.42 mg/l and PCT ≤ 6.92 ng/mL had confirmed sensitivity to cefuroxime in antibiograms (Figure 13).

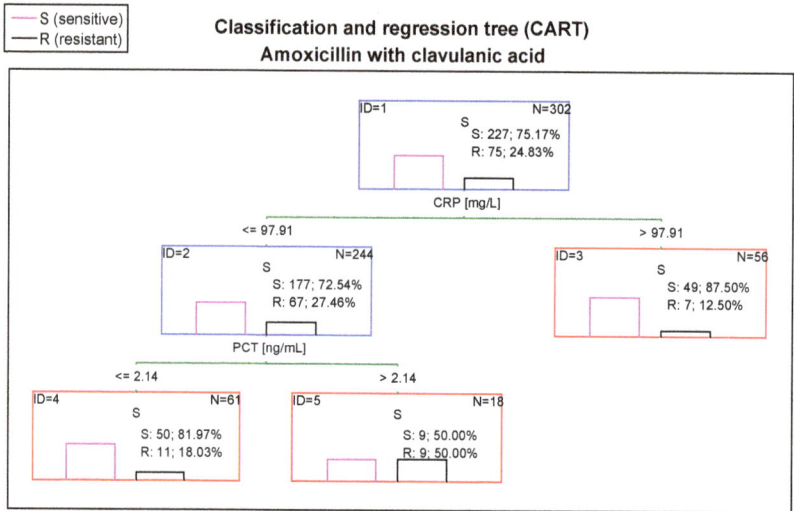

Figure 11. Classification and regression tree (CART) for resistance of *Escherichia coli* to amoxicillin with clavulanic acid created on basis of inflammatory markers.

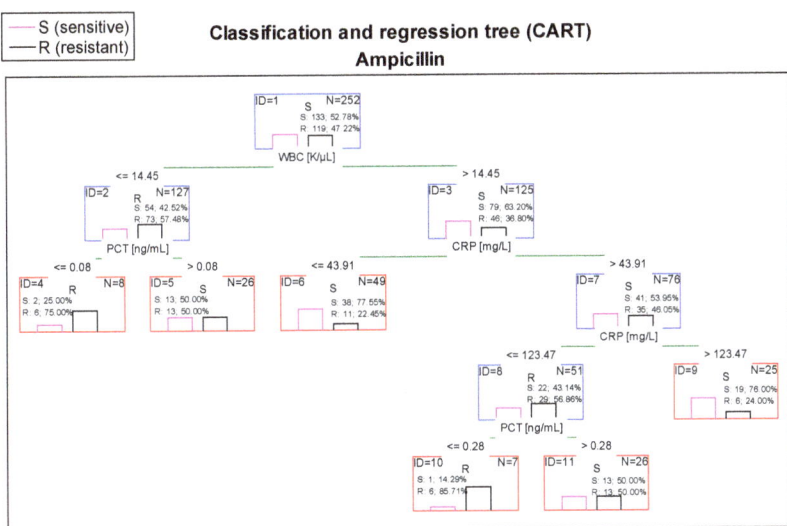

Figure 12. Classification and regression tree (CART) for resistance of *Escherichia coli* to ampicillin created on the basis of inflammatory markers.

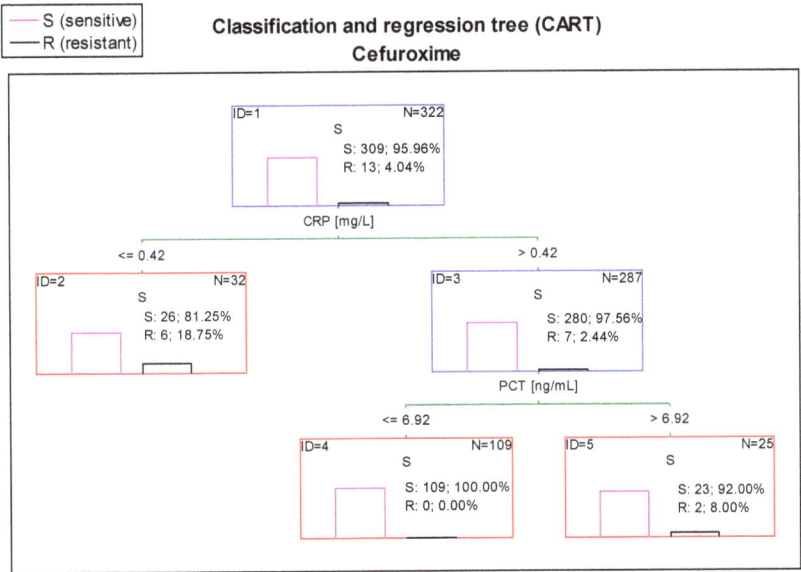

Figure 13. Classification and regression tree (CART) for resistance of *Escherichia coli* to cefuroxime created on the basis of inflammatory markers.

The CART tree in Figure 14, concerning sensitivity to gentamicin, sets the most optimal cut-off point of WBC at the level of 7.80 K/µL. Additionally, 100% of *E. coli* isolated from urine samples of patients with WBC > 7.80 K/µL and PCT concentration > 0.49 ng/mL were sensitive to this drug.

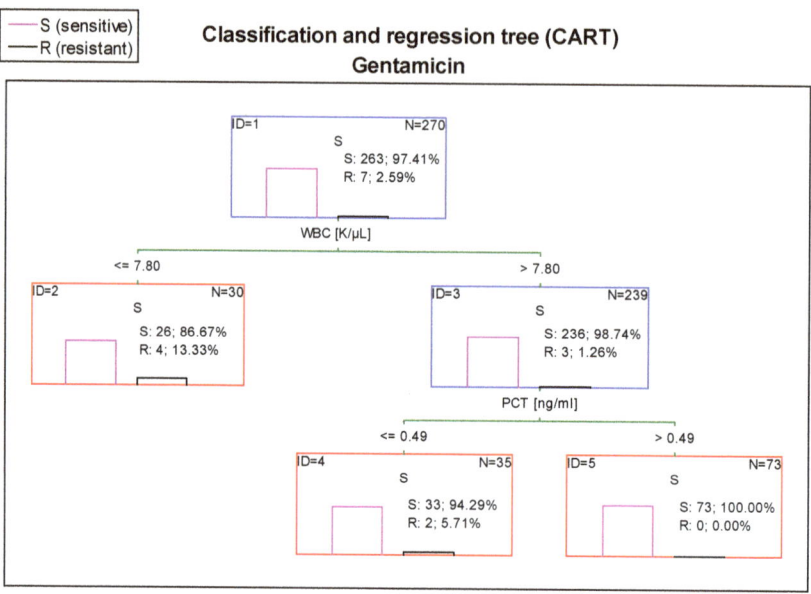

Figure 14. Classification and regression tree (CART) for resistance of *Escherichia coli* to gentamicin created on the basis of inflammatory markers.

The diagram in Figure 15 shows that 100% of patients who had UTI caused by *E. coli* sensitive to nitrofurantoin had CRP > 0.11 mg/L and WBC value higher than 12.18 K/μL.

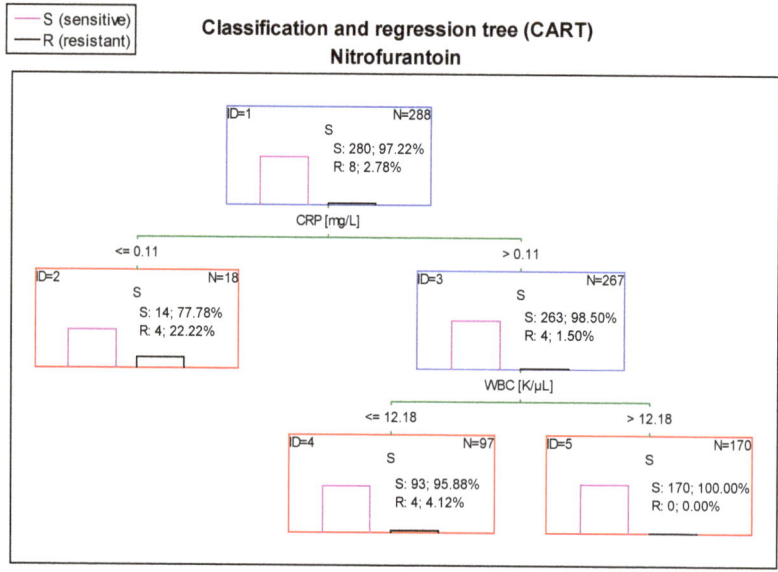

Figure 15. Classification and regression tree (CART) for resistance of *Escherichia coli* to nitrofurantoin created on the basis of inflammatory markers.

4. Discussion

Infections of the urinary tract in children are of great importance in epidemiology and clinical practice. They account for a large percentage of bacterial infections in the pediatric population. The proper diagnosis and treatment reduce the frequency of observed complications, such as chronic kidney disease or hypertension. Moreover, rationally conducted antibiotic therapy helps to inhibit the growing resistance of bacteria to drugs.

In the present study, we undertook the assessment of epidemiology and antibiotic resistance patterns of pathogens in accordance with inflammatory parameters. Research included 525 children aged between 1 week and 18 years old, in which there were observed 627 episodes of UTI. In prior research studies conducted in pediatric patients, more than 75% of children under 5 years old with febrile UTI showed features of pyelonephritis in renal scintigraphy [18,19], which in 27–64% led to kidney scarring [20,21]. Winberg et al. [22] estimated that up to the beginning of puberty, UTI was diagnosed in 1% of boys and 3% of girls, while a study by Stark [23], conducted in 1997 showed a higher percentage of UTI in prepubertal girls (8%). According to NICE (National Institute for Health and Care Excellence), 1/10 females and 1/30 males will have developed a UTI by the age of 16 [24]. In the study by Milas et al. [25], on the group of 1200 newborns, UTI was diagnosed in 4.5% of patients. Data from literature shows the highest percentage of infections among children < 1 year old [26,27]. According to the research work of Hanna–Wakim et al. [28], the median age of diagnosis of UTI was 16 months. Numerous prior studies about dependence of gender on UTI incidence unanimously indicate the superiority of diagnoses in boys in the first 2–3 months of life and the increase of incidence of UTI in females after the first year of life [29–33]. In our study, only children hospitalized at the Department of Pediatrics and Nephrology were assessed; therefore, it was impossible to estimate the overall incidence of UTI in the pediatric population. Our research showed that 38.6% of UTI episodes occurred in patients < 1 year old and infections in children < 2 years old accounted for 48.8% of all cases. The median age of UTI onset (25 months) was slightly higher than in Wakim's et al. research [28]. In the analysis, a significant relationship between gender and age of patients was found, confirming a prevalence of UTI episodes in boys < 6 months old and an increase of UTI incidence in girls after the second year of life.

Initially, we analyzed individual parameters of patients, including risk factors. One of them is a history of infections. In our study, we found that about one third of girls have a history of recurrent UTIs, while in boys this percentage was about 23%. Literature data shows that recurrent UTIs are observed in 13–33% of children with a predominance of females [22,34–37]. Herein, obtained results are consistent with prior studies.

The other risk factors, which were included in our analysis, were anatomical and functional disorders of the urinary tract. The most common abnormality is VUR. In our study, VUR was diagnosed in 18.4% of girls and in 16% of boys. There was a correlation between grade of VUR and gender of patients–boys were statistically more likely to have high-grade VUR than girls ($p < 0.05$). In the study by Orellana et al. [38], among 269 pediatric patients diagnosed with ≥1 UTI episodes, 55.8% of children had VUR (within 234 renal units); in the case of 101 renal units, it was a high-grade VUR. This defect was more common in children < 1 year old ($p = 0.001$) and, contrary to our results, in boys. In the research study by Swerkersson et al. [39], VUR were observed in 22% of boys and in 31% of girls. Interestingly, the high–grade VUR was found significantly more often in boys ($p < 0.01$), what was also obtained in our study.

The next step in our study was to assess the variability of bacterial strains in urine cultures and their susceptibility to antibiotics. Due to actual guidelines, the positive urine culture (with significant bacteriuria) and the presence of leukocyturia in urinalysis are necessary to reach a UTI diagnosis. In our analysis, pyuria was found in 78.8% of urine samples. In the remaining 21.2% of samples, in 34 cases there was outpatient antibiotic therapy administered (5.4% of all). In most of the remaining cases, lack of leukocyturia was concerned in infants and children < 2 years old who hadyet to complete toilet training. Therefore, urine is not kept in the bladder long enough to detect pyuria in the urinalysis in children at this age. Kim et al. [40] conducted the study to find out if absence of leukocyturia can exclude UTI in febrile children < 24 months of age. They observed that percentage of features of pyelonephritis in renal scintigraphy in both groups (patients with fulfilled diagnostic criteria of UTI and patients with clinical, even nonspecific, symptoms of UTI) were comparable (47.8% vs. 50.0%). Moreover, Shaikh et al. [41], estimated that about 12 children with UTI without pyuria were being overlooked to protect one patient with asymptomatic bacteriuria from antibiotic administration. Due to these studies and our analysis, it seems to be reasonable to diagnose UTI by considering all the components of clinical picture.

In recent years, the variability of microorganisms detected in urine cultures has increased. Considering the prior studies, the most dominant bacterial strain is still *Escherichia coli*, which varies between 53% and 87% [10,42–45]. The other microbes found in urine cultures were *Klebsiella pneumoniae* (7–36.2%), *Proteus mirabilis* (3.0–3.49%) and *Pseudomonas aeruginosa* (2.3–7.57%). Our study also identified *E. coli* as the most dominant UTI etiological factor (72.7%). Contrary to presented studies, we observed the lower percentage in UTIs caused by *K. pneumoniae* (3.9%) and greater number of cases with *P. mirabilis* etiology (5.8%), which may be correlated with no tradition of boys' circumcising in Poland and consequently with the presence of foreskin. The same studies took into consideration variability of antibiotic susceptibility. The antibiotic with the greatest percentage of resistance was ampicillin (83–87%). High-grade resistance was also found in ceftriaxone (40–62%), cotrimoxazole (40–93%) and amoxicillin with clavulanic acid (30–83%) [10,42–45]. Another Polish center (The Department of Medical Microbiology, Medical University of Silesia, Poland) carried out a research study on 710 urine samples, which showed high sensitivity of *E. coli* to gentamicin (97.7%) or amikacin (96.0%) and high resistance to ampicillin (70%) [46]. Another study was conducted in Granada (Spain) among <2-year-old patients, where Sorlózano-Puerto et al. [47], found that *E. coli* was resistant to amoxicillin with clavulanic acid and cotrimoxazole in about 20–30% of samples (depend on age group). These results showed similarity with our outcomes.

In our research, the percentage of resistance to commonly used antibiotics was lower than in prior studies, although we observed significantly decreasing susceptibility of bacteria. In the case of *E. coli*, the highest resistance was found against ampicillin (47.2%) and amoxicillin with clavulanic acid (24.8%). Moreover, our results were interesting with regard to obtained statistical significance in increasing antibiotics resistance to amoxicillin with clavulanic acid ($p < 0.01$), gentamicin ($p < 0.05$) and ceftazidime ($p < 0.01$). Interestingly, the increasing sensitivity to nitrofurantoin was observed ($p < 0.05$). Prior studies and our results confirmed an unwanted trend in increasing antibiotic resistance. In addition, this phenomenon is observed in relation to drugs used in severe infections, such as meningitis, which makes it even more alarming. On the other hand, an increasing sensitivity to nitrofurantoin may indicate more frequent use of antibiotics instead of chemotherapeutics in mild infections. Furthermore, the decreasing susceptibility to commonly used antibiotics, such as amoxicillin with clavulanic acid, is worth mentioning due to its misuse (e.g., in viral infections).

Finally, we tried to assess whether the inflammatory markers are associated with susceptibility of microbes to used antibiotics. In the available literature, we did not find any information about research studies related to this topic. Unfortunately, we were unabl to estimate precise values of CRP, PCT or WBC at which the antibiotic resistance can be ascertained. However, by using the CART trees method, we were able to slightly determine inflammatory markers' values to which we can suspect that bacteria are predisposed to be resistant to antibacterial drugs.

In summary, we made an attempt to evaluate cut-off points of inflammatory markers' values in case of amoxicillin with clavulanic acid, ampicillin, cefuroxime, gentamicin and nitrofurantoin (despite increasing antibiotic resistance, ampicillin and amoxicillin with clavulanic acid are still widely used). Considering amoxicillin with clavulanic acid, this point was determined at the value of CRP of 97.91 mg/L, above which there were observed higher percentages of sensitive cases. The high risk of resistance to ampicillin was found in children with WBC below or equal 14.45 K/µL and PCT ≤ 0.08 ng/mL. In the case of WBC > 14.45 K/µL, the resistance's risk was greater if CRP was in the range of 43.91–123.47 mg/L and PCT was ≤0.28 ng/mL. The most important results concerning cefuroxime revealed that all patients with values of CRP > 0.42 mg/L and PCT ≤ 6.92 ng/mL had confirmed susceptibility. Moreover, our results were interesting with regard to estimate the cut-off point for gentamicin—100% of *E. coli* isolated from children with WBC above 7.80 K/µL and PCT value > 0.49 ng/mL were sensitive. In case of nitrofurantoin, we found that values of CRP above 0.11 mg/L and WBC above 12.18 K/µL were associated with susceptibility to this drug (100% of cases). Results of our study seem to be useful due to the fact that urine culture is a time consuming method. There is a chance to initially assess whether the bacterium will be sensitive to used antibiotics and predict empiric antimicrobial treatment if we know the values of inflammatory markers, until urine cultures become available.

There were some limitations to this study, including that it was small, single–center and contained regional data. We have also focused on the one specific infection that could have had an impact on the calculated sensitivity of the inflammatory markers, which should therefore be interpreted with caution. Furthermore, there could have been clinical signs of severity in some patients that were not captured in our study and that would justify the use of antibiotics. Finally, we described the added value of markers of inflammation testing to guide antibiotic prescription without considering patient–related factors, such as the uptake of prescribed antibiotics and acceptance of a non–antibiotic management strategy by the patient. Not all clinical variables that may affect inflammatory markers, such as anaemia, were included in the evaluation.

Reached results indicate that increasing antibiotic resistance is a significant ongoing problem. Due to high percentage of resistance to amoxicillin with clavulanic acid, it is reasonable not to use this antibiotic empirically in our region. However, cefuroxime seems to be a promising choice as a first-line treatment. Our initial study results show that there are potential factors such as specific CRP and WBC levels, which can help in making decisions of first-line empiric antibiotic therapy. However, more studies on a larger group of patients are needed do confirm these data.

Author Contributions: K.W. and K.T.-J. designed the study, collected and interpreted data and wrote the manuscript. A.W. assisted in the preparation of the manuscript. D.J. performed statistical analysis and assisted in the preparation of the manuscript. All authors have read and agreed to the published version of the manuscript.

Funding: This research received no external funding.

Institutional Review Board Statement: The study was conducted according to the guidelines of Helsinki and approved by the Institutional Review Board of the Medical University of Białystok, Poland (R-I-002/104/2018).

Informed Consent Statement: The requirement for informed consent was waived by the approving authority due to the retrospective nature of the study.

Data Availability Statement: The datasets used and/or analyzed during the current study are available from the corresponding author on reasonable request.

Conflicts of Interest: The authors declare no conflict of interest.

References

1. Shaikh, N.; Morone, N.E.; Bost, J.E.; Farrell, M.H. Prevalence of urinary tract infection in childhood: A meta-analysis. *Pediatr. Infect. Dis. J.* **2008**, *27*, 302–308. [CrossRef]
2. Boczek, L.A.; Rice, E.W.; Johnston, B.; Johnson, J.R. Occurrence of antibiotic-resistant uropathogenic *Escherichia coli* clonal group A in wastewater effluents. *Appl. Environ. Microbiol.* **2007**, *73*, 4180–4184. [CrossRef] [PubMed]
3. Bean, D.C.; Krahe, D.; Wareham, D.W. Antimicrobial resistance on community and nosocomial *Escherichia coli* urianry tract isolates. *Ann. Clin. Microbiol. Antimicrob.* **2008**, *7*, 13. [CrossRef]
4. Szczapa, J. *Podstawy Neonatologii*, 1st ed.; PZWL: Warsaw, Poland, 2008; pp. 297–298.

5. Zies, L.; Ramirez, J.; Jannach, J.R. Incidence of bacteriuria in the premature infant as determined by suprapubic aspiration. *J. Fla. Med. Assoc.* **1968**, *55*, 452–454. [PubMed]
6. Goldman, M.; Lahat, E.; Strauss, S.; Reisler, G.; Livne, A.; Gordin, L.; Aladjem, M. Imaging after urinary tract infections in male neonates. *Pediatrics* **2000**, *105*, 1232–1235. [CrossRef]
7. Ismaili, K.; Lolin, K.; Damry, N.; Alexander, M.; Lepage, P.; Hall, M. Febrile Urinary Tract Infections in 0- to 3-Month-Old Infants: A prospective Follow-Up Study. *J. Pediatr.* **2011**, *158*, 91–94. [CrossRef] [PubMed]
8. Keeton, J.E.; Hillis, R.S. Urinary tract infections in black female children. *Urology* **1975**, *6*, 39–42. [CrossRef]
9. Akram, M.; Shahid, M.; Khan, A.U. Etiology and antibiotic resistance patterns of community acquired urinary tract infections in JNMC Hospital Aligarh, India. *Ann. Clin. Microbiol. Antimicrob.* **2007**, *6*, 4. [CrossRef] [PubMed]
10. Lutter, S.A.; Currie, M.L.; Mitz, L.B.; Greenbaum, L.A. Antibiotic resistance patterns in children hospitalized for urinary tract infections. *Arch. Pediatr. Adolesc. Med.* **2005**, *159*, 924–928. [CrossRef]
11. Dzierżanowska, D.; Kamińska, W.; Wieczyńska, J. Zakażenia układu moczowego w urologii–zapobieganie. *Przegl. Urol.* **2001**, *1*, 32–35.
12. Grzesiowski, P. Szpitalne zakażenia układu moczowego u pacjentów cewnikowanych. *Przegl Urolog.* **2003**, *3*, 79–85.
13. Jacobson, S.H.; Hansson, S.; Jakobsson, B. Vesicouretericreflux: Occurrence and long-term risks. *Acta Paediatr. Scand. Suppl.* **1999**, *431*, 22–30. [CrossRef] [PubMed]
14. Zaffanello, M.; Banzato, C.; Piacentini, G. Management of constipation in preventing urinary tract infections in children: A concise review. *Eur. Res. J.* **2019**, *5*, 236–243. [CrossRef]
15. Klein, E.Y.; Van Boeckel, T.P.; Martinez, E.; Pant, S.; Gandra, S.; Levin, S.A.; Goossens, H.; Laxminarayan, R. Global increase and geographic convergence in antibiotic consumption between 2000 and 2015. *Proc. Natl. Acad. Sci. USA* **2018**, *115*, 3463–3470. [CrossRef]
16. Tadesse, D.A.; Zhao, S.; Tong, E.; Ayers, S.; Singh, A.; Bartholomew, M.J.; McDermott, P.F. Antimicrobial Drug Resistance in *Escherichia coli* from Humans and Food Animals, United States, 1950–2002. *Emerg. Infect. Dis.* **2012**, *18*, 741–749. [CrossRef]
17. Xu, R.-Y.; Liu, H.-W.; Liu, J.-L.; Dong, J.-H. Procalcitonin and C-reactive protein in urinary tract infection diagnosis. *BMC Urol.* **2014**, *14*, 45. [CrossRef]
18. Benador, D.; Benador, N.; Slosman, D.O.; Nusslé, D.; Mermillod, B.; Girardin, E. Cortical scintigraphy in the evaluation of renal parenchymal changes in children with pyelonephritis. *J. Pediatr.* **1994**, *124*, 17–20. [CrossRef]
19. Bjorgvinsson, E.; Majd, M.; Eggli, K.D. Diagnosis of acute pyelonephritis in children: Comparison of sonography and 99mTc-DMSA scintigraphy. *AJR Am. J. Roentgenol.* **1991**, *157*, 539–543. [CrossRef] [PubMed]
20. Berg, U.B. Long-term follow-up of renal morphology and function in children with recurrent pyelonephritis. *J. Urol.* **1992**, *148*, 1715–1720. [CrossRef]
21. Rushton, H.G.; Majd, M.; Jantausch, B.; Wiedermann, B.L.; Belman, A.B. Renal scarring following reflux and nonreflux pyelonephritis in children: Evaluation with 99 mtechnetium-dimercaptosuccinic acid scintigraphy. *J. Urol.* **1992**, *147*, 1327–1332. [CrossRef]
22. Winberg, J.; Bergström, T.; Jacobsson, B. Morbidity, age and sex distribution, recurrences and renal scarring in symptomatic urinary tract infection in childhood. *Kidney Int. Suppl.* **1975**, *4*, 101–106.
23. Stark, H. Urinary tract infections in girls: The cost-effectiveness of currently recommended investigative routines. *Pediatr. Nephrol.* **1997**, *11*, 174–177. [CrossRef] [PubMed]
24. National Collaborating Centre for Women's and Children's Health (UK). Urinary tract infection in children: Diagnosis, treatment and long-term management. In *NICE Clinical Guidelines*; No. 54; RCOG Press: London, UK, 2007.
25. Milas, V.; Puseljić, S.; Stimac, M.; Dobrić, H.; Lukić, G. Urinary tract infection (UTI) in newborns: Risk factors, identification and prevention of consequences. *Coll. Antropol.* **2013**, *37*, 871–876. [PubMed]
26. Ladomenou, F.; Bitsori, M.; Galanakis, E. Incidence and morbidity of urinary tract infection in a prospective cohort of children. *Acta Paediatr.* **2015**, *104*, 324–329. [CrossRef]
27. Winberg, J.; Andersen, H.J.; Bergström, T.; Jacobsson, B.; Larson, H.; Lincoln, K. Epidemiology of symptomatic urinary tract infection in childhood. *Acta Paediatr.* **1964**, *63*, 1–20. [CrossRef]
28. Hanna-Wakim, R.H.; Ghanem, S.T.; El Helou, M.W.; Khafaja, S.A.; Shaker, R.A.; Hassan, S.A.; Saad, R.K.; Hedari, C.P.; Khinkarly, R.W.; Dbaibo, G.S. Epidemiology and characteristics of urinary tract infections in children and adolescents. *Front. Cell Infect. Microbiol.* **2015**, *5*, 45. [CrossRef]
29. Wettergren, B.; Jodal, U.; Jonasson, G. Epidemiology of bacteriuria during the first year life. *Acta Paediatr. Scan.* **1985**, *74*, 925. [CrossRef]
30. Zorc, J.J.; Levine, D.A.; Platt, S.L.; Dayan, P.S.; Macias, C.G.; Krief, W.; Schor, J.; Bank, D.; Shaw, K.N.; Kuppermann, N. Clinical and demographic factors associated with urinary tract infection in young febrile infants. *Pediatrics* **2005**, *116*, 644–648. [CrossRef]
31. Shaw, K.N.; Gorelick, M.; McGowan, K.L.; Yakscoe, N.M.; Schwartz, J.S. Prevalence of Urinary Tract Infection in Febrile Young Children in the Emergency Department. *Pediatrics* **1998**, *102*, e16. [CrossRef]
32. Dar-Shong, L.; Shing-Huey, H.; Chun-Chun, L.; Tung, Y.; Huang, T.-T.; Chiu, N.-C.; Koa, H.-A.; Hung, H.-Y.; Hsu, C.-H.; Hsieh, W.-S.; et al. Urinary Tract Infection in Febrile Infants Younger Than Eight Weeks of Age. *Pediatrics* **2000**, *105*, e20.
33. Ginsburg, C.M.; McCracken, G.H., Jr. Urinary tract infections in young infants. *Pediatrics* **1982**, *69*, 409–412. [CrossRef]

34. Nuutinen, M.; Uhari, M. Recurrence and follow-up after urinary tract infection under the age of 1 year. *Pediatr. Nephrol.* **2001**, *16*, 69–72. [CrossRef]
35. Panaretto, K.; Craig, J.; Knight, J.; Howman-Giles, R.; Sureshkumar, P.; Roy, L. Risk factors for recurrent urinary tract infection in preschool children. *J. Paediatr. Child. Health* **1999**, *35*, 454–459. [CrossRef]
36. Jakobsson, B.; Berg, U.; Svensson, L. Renal damage after acute pyelonephritis. *Arch. Dis. Child.* **1994**, *70*, 111–115. [CrossRef]
37. Conway, P.H.; Cnaan, A.; Zaoutis, T.; Henry, B.V.; Grundmeier, R.W.; Keren, R. Recurrent Urinary Tract Infections in Children: Risk Factors and Association with Prophylactic Antimicrobials. *JAMA* **2007**, *298*, 179–186. [CrossRef]
38. Orellana, P.; Baquedano, P.; Rangarajan, V.; Zhao, J.H.; Eng ND, C.; Fettich, J.; Chaiwatanarat, T.; Sonmezoglu, K.; Kumar, D.; Padhy, A.K.; et al. Relationship beteween acute pyelonephritis, renal scarring and vesicoureteral reflux. *Pediatr. Nephrol.* **2004**, *19*, 1122–1126. [CrossRef]
39. Swerkersson, S.; Jodal, U.; Sixt, R.; Stokland, E.; Hansson, S. Relationship among vesicoureteral reflux, urinary tract infection and renal damage in children. *J. Urol.* **2007**, *178*, 647. [CrossRef] [PubMed]
40. Kim, S.H.; Lyu, S.Y.; Kim, H.Y.; Park, S.E.; Kim, S.Y. Can absence of pyuria exclude urinary tract infection in febrile infants? About 2011 AAP guidelines on UTI. *Pediatr. Int.* **2016**, *58*, 472–475. [CrossRef]
41. Shaikh, N.; Osio, V.A.; Wessel, C.B.; Jeong, J.H. Prevalence of Asymptomatic Bacteriuria in Children: A Meta-Analysis. *J. Pediatr.* **2020**, *217*, 110–117. [CrossRef] [PubMed]
42. Chander, J.; Singla, N. Changing Etiology and Antibiogram od Urinary Tract Isolates from Pediatric Age Group. *Libyan J. Med.* **2008**, *3*, 122–123. [CrossRef] [PubMed]
43. Mirsoleymani, S.R.; Salimi, M.; Brojeni, M.S.; Ranjbar, M.; Mehtarpoor, M. Bacterial Pathogens and Antimicrobial Resistance Patterns in Pediatric Urinary Tract Infections: A Four-Year Surveillance Study (2009–2012). *Int. J. Pediatr.* **2014**, *2014*, 1–6. [CrossRef]
44. Jackowska, T.; Pawlik, K.; Załeska-Ponganis, J.; Kłyszewska, M. Etiology of urinary tract infections and antimicrobial susceptibility: A study conducted on a population of children hospitalized in the Department of Pediatrics at Warsaw Bielany Hospital; 2004–2006. *Med. Wieku Rozw.* **2008**, *12 Pt 2*, 705–712.
45. Shrestha, L.B.; Baral, R.; Poudel, P.; Khanal, B. Clinical, etiological and antimicrobial suscebility profile of pediatric urinary tract infections in a tertiary care hospital of Nepal. *BMC Pediatr.* **2019**, *19*, 36. [CrossRef]
46. Nowakowska, M.; Rogala-Zawada, D.; Wiechuła, B.; Rudy, M.; Radosz-Komoniewska, H.; Zientara, M. Czynniki etiologiczne zakażeń układu moczowego u dzieci i ich wrażliwość na antybiotyki. *Wiad Lek.* **2004**, *57*, 438–443. [PubMed]
47. Sorlózano-Puerto, A.; Gómez-Luque, J.M.; Luna-del-Castillo, J.D.D.; Navarro-Marí, J.M.; Gutiérrez-Fernández, J. Etiological and Resistance Profile of Bacteria Involved in Urinary Tract Infections in Young Children. *BioMed Res. Int.* **2017**, *2017*, 4909452. [CrossRef] [PubMed]

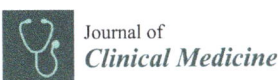

Article

Adenine Nucleotide Metabolites in Uremic Erythrocytes as Metabolic Markers of Chronic Kidney Disease in Children

Joanna Piechowicz [1], Andrzej Gamian [2], Danuta Zwolińska [3] and Dorota Polak-Jonkisz [3],*

1. Department of Medical Biochemistry, Wroclaw Medical University, 50-556 Wroclaw, Poland; joanna.piechowicz@onet.pl
2. Hirszfeld Institute of Immunology and Experimental Therapy, Polish Academy of Sciences, 50-556 Wroclaw, Poland; andrzej.gamian@hirszfeld.pl
3. Department of Pediatric Nephrology, Wroclaw Medical University, 50-556 Wroclaw, Poland; danuta.zwolinska@umed.wroc.pl
* Correspondence: dorota.polak-jonkisz@umed.wroc.pl

Abstract: Chronic kidney disease (CKD) is associated with multifaceted pathophysiological lesions including metabolic pathways in red blood cells (RBC). The aim of the study was to determine the concentration of adenine nucleotide metabolites, i.e., nicotinamide adenine dinucleotide (NAD)-oxidized form, nicotinamide adenine dinucleotide hydrate (NADH)-reduced form, nicotinic acid mononucleotide (NAMN), β-nicotinamide mononucleotide (NMN), nicotinic acid adenine dinucleotide (NAAD), nicotinic acid (NA) and nicotinamide (NAM) in RBC and to determine a relationship between NAD metabolites and CKD progression. Forty-eight CKD children and 33 age-matched controls were examined. Patients were divided into groups depending on the CKD stages (Group II-stage II, Group III- stage III, Group IV- stage IV and Group RRT children on dialysis). To determine the above-mentioned metabolites concentrations in RBC liquid chromatography-mass spectrometry was used. Results: the only difference between the groups was shown concerning NAD in RBC, although the values did not differ significantly from controls. The lowest NAD values were found in Group II (188.6 ± 124.49 nmol/mL, the highest in group IV (324.94 ± 63.06 nmol/mL. Between Groups II and IV, as well as III and IV, the differences were statistically significant ($p < 0.032$, $p < 0.046$ respectively). Conclusions. CKD children do not have evident abnormalities of RBC metabolism with respect to adenine nucleotide metabolites. The significant differences in erythrocyte NAD concentrations between CKD stages may suggest the activation of adaptive defense mechanisms aimed at erythrocyte metabolic stabilization. It seems that the implementation of RRT has a positive impact on RBC NAD metabolism, but further research performed on a larger population is needed to confirm it.

Keywords: adenine nucleotide metabolites; chronic renal failure; children

Citation: Piechowicz, J.; Gamian, A.; Zwolińska, D.; Polak-Jonkisz, D. Adenine Nucleotide Metabolites in Uremic Erythrocytes as Metabolic Markers of Chronic Kidney Disease in Children. *J. Clin. Med.* **2021**, *10*, 5208. https://doi.org/10.3390/jcm10215208

Academic Editor: Katarzyna Taranta-Janusz

Received: 7 October 2021
Accepted: 3 November 2021
Published: 8 November 2021

Publisher's Note: MDPI stays neutral with regard to jurisdictional claims in published maps and institutional affiliations.

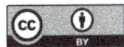

Copyright: © 2021 by the authors. Licensee MDPI, Basel, Switzerland. This article is an open access article distributed under the terms and conditions of the Creative Commons Attribution (CC BY) license (https://creativecommons.org/licenses/by/4.0/).

1. Introduction

Chronic kidney disease (CKD), along with cardiovascular diseases, obesity or diabetes, belongs to diseases of affluence. CKD is a challenge for the medical world in the 21st century not only due to the increase in the number of cases, overburdens incurred by prevention measures concerning the development of the disease and its accompanying complications, but also due to the search for methods of its early diagnosis [1].

The origin of CKD is associated with multifaceted pathophysiological lesions including i.a. arginine-creatine metabolic pathways, arginine methylation, urea cycle or glycolytic pathways. Such metabolic pathway disorders are co-responsible for changes in the concentration of various metabolites determined e.g., in patients' blood, also important for the diagnosis of disease processes [2–5]. Therefore, according to Cisek et al., Markers identified by 'omics' research technologies (metabolomics, proteomics, transcriptomics) can improve not only the prediction of the development of various diseases (including CKD) but will even allow the development of personalized therapy [6].

Although CKD is a global health problem, little information is available concerning metabolomics in the pediatric patient population. For pediatrics and neonatology, according to Mussap et al., metabolomics offers new perspectives in the treatment of sick children, allows for early diagnosis of metabolic profiles associated with the development of the disease, as well as provides personalised therapy for this population [7]. This is of great importance for children because all chronic diseases lead to the inhibition of the body's growth along with irreversible processes of hormonal imbalance, bone or cardiovascular lesions and the development of hypertension. Currently, the mechanism of CKD development at the molecular level is still not fully understood.

Thus, NAD plays a key role in biological processes related to the response to cellular or genotoxic stress and participates in the metabolism of carbohydrates and fats through SIRT1 activity [8–12]. In the human body, NAD can be synthesized de novo or by a 'salvage pathway' ('recovery process'). The energy metabolism of the red blood cell is mainly based on glycolysis.

Reduced concentrations of NAM and NMN can be explained by an impaired *"recovery process"* in erythrocytes or weakened NAM incorporation due to cell membrane deformation when deficiency of ATP leads to dehydration of cells and their spiky shape [4,13–15].

The debate on pathophysiology and biochemistry of processes accompanying kidney damage during CKD development remains open. The identification and validation of the analytes of the ongoing processes will contribute significantly to the understanding of CKD pathomechanisms, the development of accurate prevention principles and the implementation of innovative, effective therapies.

The aim of the study was to determine the concentration of adenine nucleotide metabolites, i.e., nicotinamide adenine dinucleotide (NAD)-oxidized form, nicotinamide adenine dinucleotide hydrate (NADH)-reduced form, nicotinic acid mononucleotide (NAMN), β-nicotinamide mononucleotide (NMN), nicotinic acid adenine dinucleotide (NAAD), nicotinic acid (NA) and nicotinamide (NAM) in erythrocytes of children with chronic kidney disease and to establish a relationship between the concentrations of these NAD metabolites and the development of CKD.

2. Materials

2.1. The Study Group

The study included 48 patients with chronic kidney disease (16 girls and 32 boys) aged 3–18 years (mean age 11.00 ± 4.72 years) treated in the Department of Pediatric Nephrology and Dialysis Station of the University Hospital.

All the respondents met the inclusion criteria which were:

- Age of 3–18 years,
- Diagnosed CKD of varying degrees of progression
- And written consent to participate in the study.

Patients meeting the exclusion criteria, i.e., failure to meet the inclusion criteria, such as recognition of another acute/chronic inflammatory disease, lack of cooperation and/or abnormalities that may affect the course of the research procedure, were not eligible for the study.

Taking GFR (glomerular filtration rate) values into account (estimated on the basis of Schwartz formula: eGFR (mL/min per 1.73 m^2) = 0.413 * [height (cm)/serum creatinine (mg/dL)]), groups corresponding to a given stage of disease progression have been distinguished among CKD patients [16,17].

The size of groups in each stage of CKD is as follows:

Group II—15 patients with stage II CKD; including 11 boys, 4 girls;
Group III—16 patients with stage III CKD; including 10 boys, 6 girls;
Group IV—8 patients with stage IV CKD; including 4 boys, 4 girls;

Group of children undergoing renal replacement therapy (RRT)—9 patients undergoing RRT (hemodialysis, peritoneal dialysis); including 7 boys, 2 girls.

The cause of chronic kidney disease (CKD) in the studied population of patients was glomerulonephritis (18), pyelonephritis (20), and congenital defects of the urinary tracts (10). The hemodialysis [3–4 sessions per week (3–3.5 h)] was applied in 4 children using polysulfone membranes, $NaHCO_3$-buffered dialysate, Ca^{+2} content—1.25 or 1.5 mmol/L. Peritoneal dialysis applied in 5 children includes NIPD—nocturnal intermittent peritoneal dialysis and CCPD—continuous cycling peritoneal dialysis with Baxter's Home Choice using 1.36% or 2.27% Physioneal. The duration of renal replacement therapy (RRT) is 2.02 ± 0.51 years.

In pediatric population with CKD, depending on the clinical condition and the results of laboratory tests, as well as the type of treatment of RRT in pharmacotherapy, the following drugs (in individual doses), were used: antihypertensive drugs (e.g., calcium channel blockers, angiotensin-converting enzyme inhibitors—ACE inhibitors, β-blockers), vitamins: D_3, C, B, folic acid, proton pump blockers, erythropoietin, calcium carbonate, iron preparations.

Control group (Group I)—Thirty-three healthy children (14 boys, 19 girls) with normal kidney function. These children were hospitalized in the Department of Pediatric Nephrology of the University Hospital due to suspected dysfunctions of the lower urinary tract (mainly nocturnal enuresis). On the basis of diagnostic tests carried out at that time, the above-mentioned abnormalities were excluded. None of these patients were diagnosed with a chronic disease nor were they treated with specialist pharmacotherapy.

The biochemical parameters in the CKD children and control group are presented in Table 1.

Table 1. The biochemical characteristics of the blood of studied population of patients.

Material	Studied Parameter	Study Group/Patient Group		Control Group		Significance Level p-Value
		N	Mean ± SD	N	Mean ± SD	
blood	GFR (mL/min/1.73 m^2)	48	45.96 ± 26.81	33	103.15 ± 10.88	0.0001
	creatinine (mg/dL)	48	2.25 ± 1.99	33	0.56 ± 0.11	0.0001
	inorganic phosphorus (mg/dL)	44	4.94 ± 0.84	33	5.36 ± 1.17	0.194 (NS)
	calcium (mg/dL)	43	9.80 ± 0.68	32	10.04 ± 0.47	0.020
	sodium (mg/dL)	48	139.46 ± 3.35	33	138.94 ± 2.73	0.381 (NS)
	potassium (mg/dL)	48	4.47 ± 0.46	32	4.42 ± 0.39	0.643 (NS)
	urea (mg/dL)	47	60.85 ± 38,91	32	26.16 ± 15.86	0.0001
	Hb (g/dL)	48	11.7 ± 1.51	34	14.4 ± 1.74	0.0001
	Ht (%)	48	34.33 ± 4.15	34	41.38 ± 4.88	0.0001
	RBC (*10^6/μL)	48	4.14 ± 0.71	34	4.85 ± 0.55	0.0001

Legend: NS—not significant; SD—standard deviation.

2.2. Ethical Issues

The research project has been approved by the Bioethics Committee of the Wrocław Medical University, issue KB-369/2017 of 6 June 2017.

All procedures involving human participants were in accordance with the highest ethical standards of the institutional research committee and were performed according to the Declaration of Helsinki on the treatment of human subjects and its later amendments. Both the children of all groups participating in the study (≥16 years) and their parents were informed about the aims, principles, benefits and informed consent was obtained.

3. Methods

3.1. Collection of Test Material Samples

Blood samples from selected pediatric patients were collected in the morning in the sitting position, from the ulnar vein, during the planned diagnostic and therapeutic procedures. In dialysis patients, blood was collected between hemodialysis sessions. The material was collected from fasting patients in two ways: whole blood collected into test tubes with EDTA-K and into test tubes with citrate as an anticoagulant. Samples were prepared according to the procedure described in Section 3.3 for the determination of nucleotide metabolites. The samples were stored in a freezer at −80 °C until the liquid chromatography-mass spectrometry (LC-MS/MS) analysis was performed.

3.2. Reagents

Water, acetonitrile and methanol (Merck); NAMN, NMN, NAAD, NA, BCl and PCA (perchloric acid) (Sigma, Saint Louis, MA, USA); NAM, NAD and NADH (Koch Light Laboratory GmbH) were used in the research. The research was carried out in the Chair and Department of Medical Biochemistry of the Medical University and in the Mass Spectrometry Laboratory of the Technology Park (WTP) [18].

3.3. Preparation of Samples for the Determination of Nucleotide-Related Metabolites

The analysis of samples taken for the determination of adenine nucleotide-related metabolites (NAD, NADH, NA, NAM, NMN, NAMN, NAAD) was carried out on red blood cells obtained from whole blood collected on EDTA. Procedure for patient samples: 400 μL of whole blood (1000× g, 5 min, 4 °C) was centrifuged. Plasma and buffy coat were discarded, blood cells were flushed twice with 0.9% NaCl and counted (applied dilution of blood cells; 1:1 trypan blue stain). As much as 50 μL of erythrocytes were added to 400 μL of 0.5 N perchloric acid (PCA), shaken (5 min, 800 g) and centrifuged (15,000× g, 10 min, 4 °C). Samples were kept on ice for 30 min at −20 °C. In the next step, 300 μL of supernatant was removed. Before measurements, 100 μL of supernatant was diluted in 0.1% formic acid (FA) solution in water. In the case of standards, 400 μL of 0.5 N PCA was added to 100 μL of the standard solution. Subsequently, the samples were shaken (5 min, 800 g), centrifuged (15,000× g, 10 min, 4 °C) and then placed on ice for 30 min at −20 °C. As much as 100 μL of 0.1% FA solution in water was added to 100 μL of the supernatant obtained.

3.4. Method of Analysis for Nucleotide Metabolites

In order to analyze metabolites in the sample at the same time, it was necessary to develop a method for their determination. The analysis time for an individual sample was 13 min and the volume of the sample for analysis was only 50 μL of erythrocytes. By using the appropriate concentration and elution time of the mobile phase during the chromatographic separation (Table 2), it was possible to separate individual nucleotide metabolites.

Table 2. Percentage gradient distribution of mobile phases during chromatographic separation of LC-MS/MS for nucleotide-related metabolites (phase A—10 mM of ammonium acetate with 0.1% FA in water, phase B—10 mM ammonium acetate with 0.1% FA in methanol).

Time [min]	Phase A [%]	Phase B [%]
0	99	1
2.7	0	100
5.7	0	100
5.71	99	1
13	99	1

The chromatographic separation of adenine nucleotide-related metabolite samples was performed with Acquity UHPLC liquid chromatograph with a cooled autosampler and Acquity HSS T3 column (50 m × 1.0 mm, 1.75 μm), coupled with Xevo G2 Q-TOF mass spectrometer (Waters). The separation time of a single injection of 2 μL was 13 min and the mobile phase flow was 95 μL/min. For gradient elution (Table 2), 10 mM ammonium acetate with 0.1% FA in water was used as phase A and 10 mM ammonium acetate with 0.1% FA in methanol was used as phase B. In the spectrometer, the ion source was of electrospray ionization (ES) type, operating in positive ion mode. The samples were ionized using the ESI. The source parameters were optimized to obtain the highest sensitivity for the tested compounds. The electrode voltage was 4500 V. The other parameters of the ion source were set as follows: ion source temperature: 110 °C; desolvation temperature: 350 °C. Nitrogen was used as a nebulizing and drying gas. Quanlynx software (Waters) was applied to collect and process the data. The following ions were used for quantitative analysis: 123.0553 *m/z (mass-to-charge ratio)* for NAM; 124.0393 *m/z* for NA; 664.1169 *m/z* for NAD; 666.1169 *m/z* for NADH; 335.0644 *m/z* for NMN; 336.0484 *m/z* for NAMN; 665.1010 *m/z* for NAAD.

The chromatograms of NAD metabolites of sample from representative patient are shown in Figure 1.

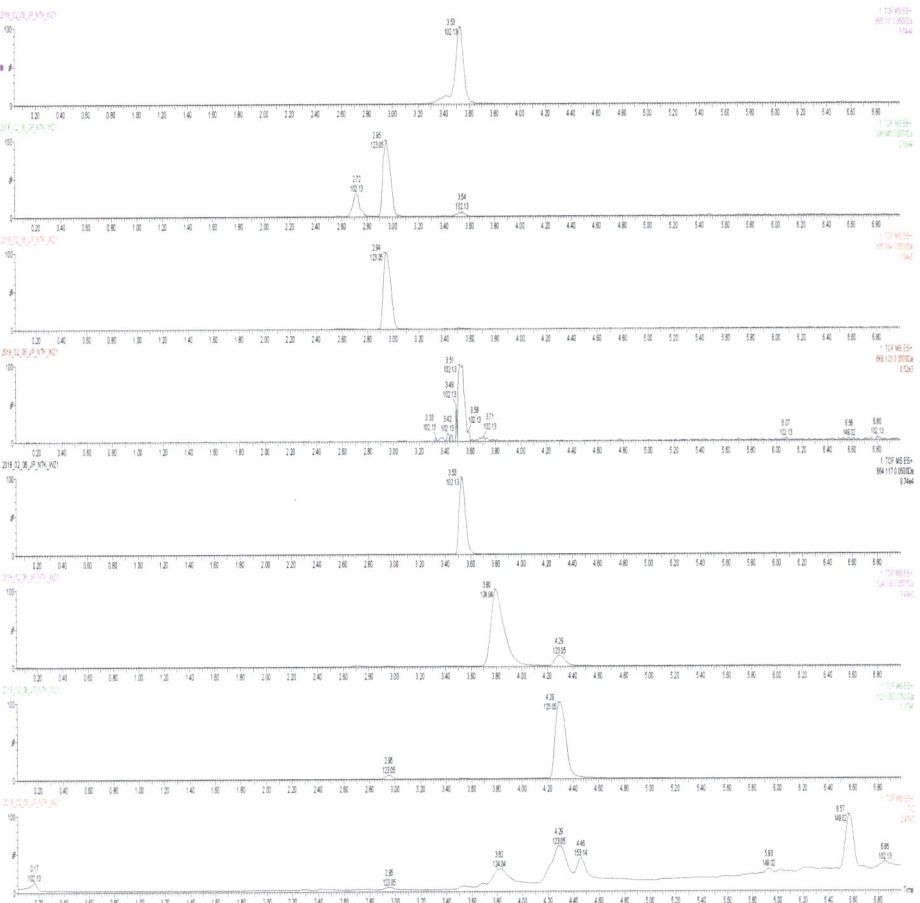

Figure 1. Total ionic current (TIC) chromatogram for patient exemplified sample. Data represent single ion current chromatograms for particular metabolites (NAAD, NAMN, NMN, NADH, NAD, NA and NAM, from the top) from with their retention times on horizontal axis and total ion current on the bottom chromatogram for patient sample.

The peak area ratio of the tested compound in relation to the peak area of the corresponding standard was used to perform linear regression analysis. A linear regression coefficient (r^2) was calculated for each standard. For nucleotide metabolites $r^2 > 0.956$.

3.5. Statistical Analysis

The results of the analyses were presented as mean (x), standard deviations (SD), median (M), lower and upper quartiles (25–75 Q). The equality of means in independent groups was tested with ANOVA analysis of variance. A nonparametric Mann–Whitney U test and the Kruskal–Wallis test were performed. Spearman's correlation coefficient was used to analyze the relationships between the tested parameters. Statistically significant differences at $p < 0.05$ level were assumed. A statistical analysis was performed using STATISTICA 8 software (StatSoft).

4. Results

4.1. Comparison of the Results of Determinations between the CKD Children and Control Group

The results of all statistical analyses for the determination of nucleotide metabolites in erythrocytes are presented in relevant tables. A detailed representation of the mean, standard deviation and median for each parameter is shown in Table 3.

Table 3. Comparison of test results for both study and control group (N = 81).

Material	Studied Parameter	Study Group/Patient Group			Control Group			Significance Level p-Value
		N	Mean ± SD	Median (Q25 Q75)	N	Mean ± SD	Median (Q25 Q75)	
erythrocytes	NAD	48	216.98 ± 117.87 [N]	222.48 (119.84–317.8)	33	233.30 ± 113.11	256.08 (177,60–289.12)	0.269 (NS)
	NA	47	8.69 ± 5.08 [N]	7.84 (5.44–10.24)	33	9.04 ± 4.66	8.00 (6.40–11.52)	0.756 (NS)
	NAM	46	298.56 ± 238.78	171.04 (132.16–510.72)	33	242.39 ± 204.04	150.64 (139.6–183.52)	0.183 (NS)
	NAAD	47	119.29 ± 73.45 [N]	121.92 (49.04–188.00)	33	136.40 ± 69.60	156.00 (86.40–172.24)	0.350 (NS)
	NAMN	47	40.00 ± 8.61	38.56 (33.28–44.40)	33	41.28 ± 10.30	38.00 (33.76–46.48)	0.809 (NS)
	NMN	47	40.90 ± 9.75	40.08 (33.52–48.16)	33	43.53 ± 10.68	41.44 (34.80–49.84)	0.350 (NS)
	NADH	47	92.38 ± 53.66 [N]	106.64 (32.64–129.44)	33	105.61 ± 59.30	101.84 (62.72–146.72)	0.273 (NS)

Legends: NS—non-significant; the index [N] means that the studied parameter has the normal distribution; SD—standard deviation.

The higher concentrations (although not statistically significant) of nucleotide were observed in the control group for NAD, NA, NAAD, NADH, NAMN, NMN in relation to CKD children. Only in the case of NAM, lower concentrations of this compound (without statistical significance) were found in the group of healthy children (mean 242.39 ± 204.04 nmol/mL), whereas the mean in CKD patients was 298.56 ± 238.78 nmol/mL.

4.2. Comparison of the Content of Nucleotide-Related Metabolites with the CKD Severity

Differences between individual stages of CKD are only for NAD. NAD concentrations reached the lowest values in Group II patients.

Statistically significant differences in NAD concentrations were observed between CKD patients with stages II–IV and III–IV.

On the other hand, in CKD patients, the highest NAD concentrations were observed in Group IV (mean 324.94 ± 63.06), which was statistically significantly different in relation to Group II ($p = 0.032$) and Group III ($p = 0.045$).

Table 4 shows average NAD concentration values of erythrocytes for individual stages of CKD and control (nmol/mL).

Table 4. Differences between stages of CKD severity for NAD.

Variable		NAD	Multiple Comparisons p Values (with a Bonferroni Adjustment)				
Stages of CKD	N	Median (Q25 Q75)	Control	II	III	IV	RRT
Control	33	256.08 (177.6–289.12)		1.000	1.000	0.148	1.000
II	15	201.6 (78.64–303.28)	1.000		1.000	0.032	1.000
III	16	221.12 (144.84–261.84)	1.000	1.000		0.046	1.000
IV	8	340.52 (315.88–353.28)	0.148	0.032	0.046		0.194
RRT	9	252.00 (23.44–304.88)	1.000	1.000	1.000	0.194	

Legends: RRT—renal replacement therapy; C (I)—control; II, III, IV—stage of CKD.

Similar correlations are also found for other nucleotides, i.e., higher concentrations (although not statistically significant) were observed in the control group for NA, NAAD, NADH, NAMN, NMN in relation to CKD children. Only in the case of NAM, were lower concentrations of this compound (without statistical significance) found in the group of healthy children (mean 242.39 ± 204.04 nmol/mL), whereas the mean in CKD patients was 298.56 ± 238.78 nmol/mL.

Table 5 shows the average values of NA, NAM, NAAD, NAMN and NMN concentration in erythrocytes for individual stages of CKD and control group (nmol/mL).

Table 5. Median of NA, NAM, NAAD, NAMN, NMN and NADH concentration values for individual stages of CKD and control group (nmol/mL).

Variables	NA		NAM		NAAD		NAMN		NMN		NADH	
Stages of CKD	N	Median (Q25 Q75)	N	Median (Q25 Q75)	N	Median (Q25 Q75)	N	Median (Q25 Q75)	N	Median (Q25 Q75)	N	Median (Q25 Q75)
Control	33	8.00 (6.40–11.52)	33	150,64 (139.6–183.52)	33	156.00 (86.40–172.24)	33	38.00 (33.76–46.48)	33	41.44 (34.8–49.84)	33	101.84 (62.72–146.72)
II	14	8.08 (5.44–9.76)	14	202.52 (147.52–566.88)	14	117.60 (44.08–178.16)	14	38.88 (34.56–45.92)	14	40.44 (34.32–49.36)	14	97.36 (27.20–121.52)
III	16	7.72 (5.40–10.44)	15	136.56 (128.88–510.72)	16	120.64 (61.72–152.76)	16	37.28 (33.24–42.84)	16	40.24 (33.56–47.52)	16	74.56 (39.16–110.92)
IV	8	8.76 (6.44–15.60)	8	177.48 (151.64–362.32)	8	192.88 (66.40–212.00)	8	38.64 (31.64–45.16)	8	40.52 (32.00–50.80)	8	125.88 (116.56–181.04)
RRT	9	6.32 (3.36–8.72)	9	159.52 (138.64–184.4)	9	141.76 (16.24–188.00)	9	42.24 (33.92–47.84)	9	38.56 (31.28–48.08)	9	97.92 (26.00–126.56)

Legends: RRT—renal replacement therapy; C (I)—control; II, III, IV—stage of CKD. (The Kruskal-Wallis H test with a Bonferroni adjustment showed no statistically significant differences between the various stages of CKD).

4.3. Assessment of Dependence in the Groups of Children with CKD

The test results showed the following correlations in the groups of children with CKD: Positive correlations of statistical significance between:

- NAD and NAAD (r = 0.852, p = 0.001),
  and NAMN (r = 0.564, p = 0.001),
  and NMN (r = 0.641, p = 0.001),
  and with NADH (r = 0.850; p = 0.001).
- NAAD and NAMN (r = 0.677, p = 0.001),

and NMN (r = 0.742, p = 0.001)
and with NADH (r = 0.765, p = 0.001).
- NAMN and NMN (r = 0.874, p = 0.001)
and with NADH (r = 0.542, p = 0.001)
- NMN correlated positively with NADH (r = 0.585, p = 0.001)

NAD did not show any correlation with NAM in any study group.

5. Discussion

Maintaining an adequate physiological concentration of ATP/nucleotides in RBC affects cell life expectancy [19]. These processes are undoubtedly intensified during metabolic diseases, chronic inflammation, and in the case of chronic kidney disease, they are co-responsible for eryptosis.

Our observations revealed that in CDK children there are no obvious red blood cell metabolism disorders regarding the metabolites of adenine nucleotides. In contrast, erythrocytic NAD concentration shows significant differences between stage II and IV as well as stage III and IV of the disease. This indicates the activation of the defence mechanisms, leading to metabolic/energy stabilization of the erythrocyte.

NAD plays a fundamental role in energy reactions, but also in other basic processes of cell signaling, gene expression or DNA repair [20–22]. According to many researchers, the level of adenosine triphosphate (ATP) in red blood cells depends on the proper course of glycolysis, and thus on the appropriate concentration of NAD [20–23].

Hikosaka et al. additionally showed that the blockade of the glycolytic pathway in red blood cells (RBC) occurred at the stage of glyceraldehyde-3-phosphate dehydrogenase (GAPDH) due to lack of NAD coenzyme [4]. These observations revealed the unexpected role of Nmnat3 in maintaining the appropriate NAD concentration in erythrocytes and related regulation of RBC lifespan [4].

A number of studies have been undertaken on the occurrence of abnormalities in the metabolism of compounds involved in glycolysis, and thus in the basic physiological processes. In 6-phosphate dehydrogenase (G6PD) deficiency, decreased NADPH regeneration in the pentose phosphate pathway and diminished levels of reduced glutathione cause insufficient antioxidant defenses, increased sensitivity of red blood cells to oxidative stress and acute hemolysis after exposure to pro-oxidants and inflammation [4,24].

In mammals, NAD is synthesized from various sources. Its main precursors include tryptophan (Trp), nicotinic acid (NA), nicotinamide riboside (NR), nicotinamide mononucleotide (NMN) and nicotinamide (NAM). Based on the bioavailability of these precursors, there are three pathways for the synthesis of NAD in cells: from Trp through the de novo biosynthesis pathway or the kynurenine pathway; from NA in the Preiss–Handler path; and with NAM, NR and NMN in the rescue path [25]. Maintaining NAD homeostasis as a response to environmental factors or stimuli highlights NAD activities in coordinating metabolic reprogramming and maintaining physiological cell biology. Hence, NAD and its metabolites serve as a metabolic center in both physiological and pathophysiological processes. They may also represent future therapeutic potential in NAD modulation in the treatment of metabolic diseases, neurodegenerative and oncological diseases.

In turn, NAAD and NAD initially show in stage III of the disease a downward trend in concentrations (without statistical significance) and already in stage III–IV an increase is observed in their cellular level. In the case of uremic red blood cells, NAD fluctuations are statistically significant in stages II to IV of the disease. Although the studied nucleotide NAM does not show statistically significant changes in uremic blood cell levels, it nevertheless has an interesting (and thought-provoking) "course" of concentrations in the progression of CKD. The trend of these changes is different in relation to the remaining metabolites of adenine nucleotides analyzed. In stage II of the disease, it shows the highest value among the other stages of CKD, reaching the lowest concentration value in stage III. Taking into account the rescue pathway of the NAD cellular synthesis, we can consider that the observed growth fluctuation in stage III of NAD disease results from, among others, the use of NAM as a substrate. In CKD patients, increased activation of enzymes affecting NAM metabolism, including poly(ADP-ribose) polymerase, is also possible. The cytoprotective properties of NAM are associated with the inhibition of poly(ADP-ribose) polymerase activity.

An interesting phenomenon was noted by us regarding the statistically insignificant fluctuation tendency of concentration of metabolites NA, NAM, NAAD, NAMN and NMN for stage III CKD. All mentioned parameters had either the lowest or one of the lower cellular levels in the uremic RBC. Patients with stage IV CKD had higher concentrations of NAD than patients in stage II and III, however, no difference was noted in comparison to control group and between other groups. Given relatively small sample sizes of subgroups, it is possible that type II error has occurred. Further studies are needed to establish the relationship between NAD levels CKD stages and RRT. In the course of chronic kidney disease progression, each stage of the disease has more or less expressed "newly" attached metabolic disorders. In the pediatric population, the body maintains homeostasis for a relatively long time, through a variety of repair processes. Such stabilization takes place especially in the first two stages of CKD. From a practical point of view, stage III is a clear beginning of the clinical manifestation of multifaceted metabolic disorders of the body, including the first symptoms of uremic anemia, which are the result of a shortened period of life of the red blood cell. Hikosaka's team published a study linking NAD and NADH metabolism insufficiency in erythrocytes with splenomegaly and hemolytic anemia in mice [4].

These concentrations were significantly reduced compared to those of the control group. For other NAD-associated metabolites, these authors recorded slight decreases for NAM and NMN in erythrocytes in mice with hemolytic anemia. Hikosaka and coworkers believe that the reduced concentration of NAM and NMN may be caused by an impairment of the "recovery process" in erythrocytes [4]. On the basis of results, we are inclined to agree with this conclusion.

The pre-dialysis stage of the disease (i.e., stage IV CKD) at the cellular level is characterized by the highest concentrations for NAM, NAAD, and NAD and NADH. Only for NAD concentration are the values statistically significant compared to those of stage II and III of the disease. At the same time, for NA, NAMN, NMN, cellular concentrations remain at a level similar to those of the physiological erythrocytes of the control group. Stage IV CKD is the culmination of the biochemical repair processes taking place in the cell undergoing increasing uremic toxemia.

Red blood cell red-ox homeostasis requires a continuous supply of energy, i.e., maintaining a sufficiently high concentration of erythrocytic adenosine triphosphate (ATP_e), and energy potential (energy charge) inside the cell. The level of cytoplasmic ATP_e and the "energy charge" values of erythrocytes are determined not only by the rate of synthesis in the process of anaerobic glycolysis and the process of reutilization of adenyl nucleotides. In our 2012 study also conducted on CKD children, we observed a gradual increase in ATP_e concentration from stage I-III CKD [26]. In the pre-dialysis stage, however, there was a large decrease in the concentration of erythrocytic ATP_e. The reason for such a change in ATP concentration is probably a decrease in the activity of lactate dehydrogenase (LDH) as well as the "redirection" of glucose catabolism towards the pentose-phosphate pathway. Such a direction in erythrocytic metabolic disorders is confirmed by our subsequent research also presented in the aforementioned publication. In the process of the erythrocyte anaerobic glycolysis, a special role plays LDH, whose activity and direction of action is decisive for the rate of glycolysis and the associated energy consequences and red-ox of the cell. In the studied population of CKD children, we initially had a gradual increase in LDH activity to stage III of CKD. In the pre-dialysis period, however, there was a significant decrease in LDH activity in relation to the examined patients and in relation to the control group. The accompanying CKD hypoxia is also of importance; greater transport of lactates and ion H^+ ions inside the cell as a result of, among others, inactivation of LDH [26].

Stressors such as ischemia induce enzymes consuming NAD such as poly-ADP-ribose polymerases (PARPs), and the induction of these enzymes lowers cellular NAD [27]. The above observations on the onset of metabolic disorders at the cell level are reflected in the clinical state of the CKD patient.

In the group of children treated with renal replacement for NA and NMN, the lowest cellular concentrations in the course of the disease were found, but without signs of statistical significance. The other metabolites NAM, NAAD, NAMN and NAD present concentrations similar to those found in a healthy population. Such a metabolic state of red blood cells allows us to suppose that renal replacement treatment brings the cells closer to biological physiology. However, the question remains of the duration of dialysis therapy and its secondary metabolic complications.

Although the results obtained in the current publication did not identify clearly statistically significant disturbances in the erythrocytic concentrations of adenine nucleotide metabolites besides NAD, the observations made seem to be helpful in better understanding the relationship between the metabolism of individual parameters involved in different biochemical cycles, and above all its energy level. In addition, they shed more light on the complex pathomechanism of metabolic profiles of chronic kidney disease. Maintaining physiological (low levels) oxidative stress, also referred to as oxidative eustress, is critical in regulating biological processes and physiological functions, including the RBC cell cycle [28,29]. From a clinical point of view, according to Na Xie's team, it is important that the new NAD red-ox regulation through sirtin -3 (SIRT3) dependent deacetylation in response to oxidative stress, improve resistance to the harmful effects of oxidative damage [23].

On the basis of the performed experiments in this paper, we agree with the opinion of Benito and co-workers that a multivariate analysis of data on plasma concentration of metabolites of the urea cycle, arginine methylation and metabolic pathways of arginine and creatinine in pediatrics makes it possible to "classify" a child to a specific stage of the disease with 74% accuracy with currently up to 90% of the diagnoses performed by doctors (one stage above or below) regarding the advancement of CKD being erroneous [2,3]. Therefore, further metabolomic studies are necessary and will undoubtedly contribute to the identification of disorders and later therapeutic implications.

Considering the overall design of our observation, it should be emphasized that this is the first study of CKD children regarding adenine nucleotide metabolites. However, this study has limitations. We are aware that it would be necessary to analyze more patients. It would also be useful to expand the study group to include children who have had a kidney transplant. Investigation of the correlations of NAD metabolites concentrations with other erythrocyte characteristics such as size and hemoglobin content should be also performed.

6. Conclusions

1. CKD children do not have evident abnormalities of RBC metabolism with respect to adenine nucleotide metabolites.
2. The significant differences in erythrocyte NAD concentrations between CKD stages may suggest the activation of adaptive defense mechanisms aimed at erythrocyte metabolic stabilization.
3. It seems that the implementation of RRT has a positive impact on RBC NAD metabolism, but further research performed on a larger population is needed to confirm it.

Author Contributions: J.P.: conceptualization, methodology, investigation, and writing. A.G.: conceptualization, funding acquisition, review and editing. D.Z.: project administration, review and editing. D.P.-J.: conceptualization, supervision, writing-original draft preparation, review, and editing. All authors have read and agreed to the published version of the manuscript.

Funding: This research received no external funding except statutory funds of Wroclaw Medical University and by the Institute of Immunology and Experimental Therapy grant 501-15.

Institutional Review Board Statement: The study was conducted according to the guidelines of the Declaration of Helsinki, and approved by the Ethics Committee of Wroclaw Medical University (protocol KB-369/2017 dated 06.06.2017).

Informed Consent Statement: Informed consent was obtained from all subjects involved in the study.

Conflicts of Interest: The authors declare no conflict of interest.

References

1. Chen, T.; Knicely, D.H.; Grams, M.E. Chronic Kidney Disease Diagnosis and Management. *JAMA* **2019**, *322*, 1294–1304. [CrossRef]
2. Benito, S.; Sanchez-Ortega, A.; Unceta, N.; Andrade, F.; Aldámiz-Echevarria, L.; Goicolea, M.A.; Barrio, R.J. LC-QTOF-MS-based targeted metabolomics of arginine-creatine metabolic pathway-related compounds in plasma: Application to identify potential biomarkers in pediatric chronic kidney disease. *Anal. Bioanal. Chem.* **2016**, *408*, 747–760. [CrossRef]
3. Benito, S.; Sánchez-Ortega, A.; Unceta, N.; Jansen, J.; Postma, G.; Andrade, F.; Aldámiz-Echevarria, L.; Kupdens, K.L.M.; Goicolea, M.A.; Barrio, R.J. Plasma biomarker discovery for early chronic kidney disease diagnosis based on chemometric approaches using LC-QTOF targeted metabolomics data. *J. Pharm Biomed. Anal.* **2018**, *149*, 46–56. [CrossRef]
4. Hikosaka, K.; Ikutani, M.; Shito, M.; Kazuma, K.; Gulshan, M.; Nagai, J.; Takatsu, K.; Konno, K.; Tobe, K.; Kanno, H.; et al. Deficiency of nicotinamide mononucleotide adenylyltransferase 3 (nmnat3) causes hemolytic anemia by altering the glycolytic flow in mature erythrocytes. *J. Biol. Chem.* **2014**, *289*, 14796–14811. [CrossRef]
5. Slee, A.D. Exploring metabolic dysfunction in chronic kidney disease. *Nutr. Metab.* **2012**, *9*, 36. [CrossRef]
6. Cisek, K.; Krochmal, M.; Klein, J.; Mischak, H. The application of multi-omics and systems biology to identify therapeutic targets in chronic kidney disease. *Nephrol. Dial. Transplant.* **2016**, *31*, 2003–2011. [CrossRef]
7. Mussap, M.; Antonucci, R.; Noto, A.; Fanos, V. The role of metabolomics in neonatal and pediatric laboratory medicine. *Clin. Chim. Acta* **2013**, *426*, 127–138. [CrossRef]
8. Imai, S.; Guarente, L. NAD$^+$ and sirtuins in aging and disease. *Trends Cell Biol.* **2014**, *25*, 464–471. [CrossRef]
9. Chiarugi, A.; Dölle, C.; Felici, R.; Ziegler, M. The NAD metabolome: A key determinant of cancer cell biology. *Nat. Rev. Cancer.* **2012**, *12*, 741–752. [CrossRef]
10. Houtkooper, R.H.; Canto, C.; Wanders, R.J.; Auwerx, J. The secret life of NAD: An old metabolite controlling new metabolic signaling pathways. *Endocr. Rev.* **2010**, *31*, 194–223. [CrossRef]
11. Picard, F.; Kurtev, M.; Chung, N.; Topark-Ngarm, A.; Senawong, T.; De Oliveira, R.M.; Leid, M.; McBurney, M.W.; Guarente, L. Sirt1 promotes fat mobilization in white adipocytes by repressing PPAR-gamma. *Nature* **2004**, *6993*, 771–776. [CrossRef]
12. Rodgers, J.T.; Lerin, C.; Haas, W.; Gygi, P.; Spiegelman, B.M.; Puigserver, P. Nutrient control of glucose homeostasis through a complex of PGC-1alpha and SIRT1. *Nature* **2005**, *7029*, 113–118. [CrossRef]
13. Liu, J.; Mohandas, N.; An, X. Membrane assembly during erythropoiesis. *Curr. Opin. Hematol.* **2011**, *18*, 133–138. [CrossRef]
14. Liu, R.; Orgel, L.E. Enzymatic synthesis of polymers containing nicotinamide mononucleotide. *Nucleic Acids Res.* **1995**, *23*, 3742–3749. [CrossRef]
15. Yamada, K.; Hara, N.; Shibata, T.; Osago, H.; Tsuchiya, M. The simultaneous measurement of nicotinamide adenine dinucleotide and related compounds by liquid chromatography/electrospray ionization tandem mass spectrometry. *Anal. Biochem.* **2006**, *352*, 282–285. [CrossRef]
16. Schwartz, G.J.; Muñoz, A.; Schneider, M.F.; Mak, R.H.; Kaskel, F.; Furthet, S.L. New equations to estimate GFR in children with CKD. *J. Am. Soc. Nephrol.* **2009**, *20*, 629–637. [CrossRef]
17. Graves, J.W. Diagnosis and management of chronic kidney disease. *Mayo Clin. Proc.* **2008**, *83*, 1064–1069. [CrossRef]
18. Piechowicz, J.; Gajewska-Naryniecka, A.; Kukula, M.; Wiśniewski, J.; Gamian, A. Mass Spectrometry in Clinical Diagnostics. *Med. Sci. Technol.* **2017**, *58*, 98–110. [CrossRef]
19. Cho, J.; Seo, J.; Lim, C. Mitochondrial ATP transporter Ant2 depletion impairs erythropoiesis and B lymphopoiesis. *Cell Death Differ.* **2015**, *22*, 1437–1450. [CrossRef]
20. Rose, I.A. Regulation of human red cell glycolysis: A review. *Exp. Eye Res.* **1971**, *11*, 264–272. [CrossRef]
21. Szołkiewicz, A. Purine Nucleotide Metabolism in Erythrocytes in Children with Cancer. Dissertation, Medical University of Gdańsk, Gdansk, Poland, 2013; pp. 50–63.
22. Alexandrovich, Y.G.; Kosenko, E.A.; Sinauridze, E.I.; Obydennyi, S.I.; Kiree, I.I.; Ataullakhanov, F.I.; Kaminsky, Y.G. Rapid Elimination of Blood Alcohol Using Erythrocytes: Mathematical Modeling and In Vitro Study. *BioMed Res. Int.* **2017**, *2017*, 5849593. [CrossRef]
23. Xie, N.; Zhang, L.; Gao, W.; Huang, C.; Huber, P.E.; Zhou, X.; Li, H.; Shen, G.; Zou, B. NAD$^+$ metabolism: Pathophysiologic mechanisms and therapeutic potential. *Signal Transduct. Target. Ther.* **2020**, *5*, 227. [CrossRef]
24. Reisz, J.A.; Tzounakas, V.L.; Nemkov, T. Metabolic Linkage and Correlations to Storage Capacity in Erythrocytes from Glucose 6-Phosphate Dehydrogenase-Deficient Donors. *Front. Med.* **2018**, *4*, 248. [CrossRef]
25. Pericom, L.; Benigni, A. The iNADequacy of renal cell metabolism: Modulating NAD$^+$ biosynthetic pathways to forestall kidney diseases. *Kidney Int.* **2019**, *96*, 264–267. [CrossRef]
26. Polak-Jonkisz, D.; Purzyc, L.; Szczepańska, M.; Makulska, I. Erythrocyte caspase-3 levels in children with chronic kidney disease. *Clin. Biochem.* **2012**, *46*, 11–14. [CrossRef]

27. Parikh, S.M. Metabolic Stress Resistance in AKI: Evidence for a PGC1α-NAD+ Pathway. *Nephron* **2019**, *143*, 184–187. [CrossRef]
28. Ralto, K.M.; Rhee, E.P.; Parikh, S.M. NAD$^+$ homeostasis in renal health and disease. *Nat. Rev. Nephrol.* **2020**, *16*, 99–111. [CrossRef]
29. Mehr, A.P.; Tran, M.T.; Ralto, K.M.; Leaf, D.E.; Washco, V.; Messmer, J.; Lerner, A.; Kher, A.; Kim, S.H.; Khoury, C.C.; et al. De novo NAD+ biosynthetic impairment in acute kidney injury in humans. *Nat. Med.* **2018**, *24*, 1351–1359. [CrossRef]

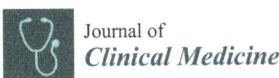

Article

Evaluation of Vascular Endothelial Function in Children with Type 1 Diabetes Mellitus

Karolina Nocuń-Wasilewska [1], Danuta Zwolińska [1], Agnieszka Zubkiewicz-Kucharska [2] and Dorota Polak-Jonkisz [1,*]

[1] Department of Pediatric Nephrology, Wroclaw Medical Univeristy, 50-367 Wrocław, Poland; nocun-wasilewska@wp.pl (K.N.-W.); danuta.zwolinska@umed.wroc.pl (D.Z.)

[2] Department of Pediatric Endocrinology and Diabetology, Wroclaw Medical University, 50-367 Wrocław, Poland; agnieszka.zubkiewicz-kucharska@umed.wroc.pl

* Correspondence: dorota.polak-jonkisz@umed.wroc.pl; Tel.: +48-717364400; Fax: +48-717364409

Abstract: Diabetic kidney disease belongs to the major complications of diabetes mellitus. Here, hyperglycaemia is a key metabolic factor that causes endothelial dysfunction and vascular changes within the renal glomerulus. The aim of the present study was to assess the function of the vascular endothelium in children with type 1 diabetes mellitus (type 1 diabetes) by measuring selected endothelial lesion markers in blood serum. The selected markers of endothelial lesions (sVCAM-1, sICAM-1, sE-SELECTIN, PAI-1, ADMA and RAGE) were assayed by the immunoenzymatic ELISA method. The study involved 66 patients (age: 5–18 years) with type 1 diabetes and 21 healthy controls (age: 5–16 years). In the type 1 diabetes patients, significantly higher concentrations of all of the assayed markers were observed compared to the healthy controls ($p < 0.001$). All of the evaluated markers positively correlated with the disease duration, the age, and BMI of the patients, while only PAI-1 and sE-SELECTIN were characteristic of linear correlations with the estimated glomerular filtration rate (eGFR). It can be concluded that endothelial inflammatory disease occurs in the early stages of type 1 diabetes mellitus in children. The correlations between PAI-1, sE-SELECTIN, and eGFR suggest an advantage of these markers over other markers of endothelial dysfunction as prognostic factors for kidney dysfunction in children with type 1 diabetes.

Keywords: diabetic kidney disease; vascular endothelial markers; children; eGFR

1. Introduction

Diabetes is a significant health problem in children, including children who are very young. Since the year 2006, it diabetes has been considered to be one of the main health conditions with the potential of endangering public health around the world [1]. Chronic hyperglycaemia results in the enhanced production of toxic oxygen derivatives that, together with their impaired elimination by the antioxidative systems of the body, cause a specific status to emerge called "oxidative stress" [2–4]. This entails modifications in the structures of proteins, lipids, carbohydrates, or nucleic acids, resulting in degenerative changes to tissues, mainly those in the vascular area. Diabetic nephropathy, one of the most serious complications of diabetes mellitus, as a clinical picture of renal microangiopathy, results from metabolic disturbances (the "glucotoxicity" effect) and coexisting inflammation. Pathomorphologic changes in the renal structure may be present at the time of diabetes diagnosis, resulting in initial hypertrophy and hyperfunction at the early stages and throughout albuminuria, eventually leading to end-stage renal failure.

An enhanced, non-enzymatic glycation of the basal lamina has been observed from both the glomeruli and the mesangial matrix and shows the formation of advanced glycation products that contribute to the loss of the negative charge of the filtration membrane, increased intraglomerular pressure, and glomerular hyperfiltration [5]. At present, albuminuria is considered the marker of generalised vascular endothelium damage [6]. However, the increased concentrations of inflammation indices can already be found during the early period where changes occur in the kidneys, which occur long before glomerulosclerosis and which may disappear after the metabolic balance of the disease is regained. The risk of the occurrence and progression of chronic complications principally depend on the effective metabolic control of diabetes mellitus; therefore, people with well-controlled disease are much less likely to be endangered by chronic complications. In addition, extraglycaemic risk factors of sclerosis, such as hypertension, hyperlipidemia, and obesity, also influence the progression of vascular changes [7–9].

The vascular endothelium is the largest endothelial structure in the body and produces numerous substances that maintain vascular homeostasis. Endothelial products, depending on their functions, are divided into three categories. These include vasomotor substances (e.g., asymmetric dimethylarginine-ADMA), substances affecting coagulation and fibrinolysis (e.g., plasminogen activator inhibitor-PAI-1), and substances regulating vascular permeability and inflammatory processes (e.g., E-selectin, vascular adhesion molecule-VCAM-1, intercellular adhesion molecule-ICAM-1). These markers, together with circulating serum receptors for advanced glycation end-products-RAGE, are considered as new biomarkers for endothelial damage and atherosclerosis development. This is because their high concentrations have been observed in cardiovascular diseases and because they have been shown to correlate with the presence of cardiovascular risk factors. What is more, their baseline value decreases after statin therapy [10]. The very fact that their expression is increased by inflammatory mediators such as IL-1, TNF, and LPS is certainly not without significance [11,12].

Taking into account the finding that chronic hyperglycemia is the most significant, unfavourable factor and that it affects the endothelial cells in particular, the identification of reliable markers of progressive endothelium dysfunction seems to be a primary objective. The existing knowledge gap as to whether biomarkers of inflammation and endothelial dysfunction are associated with prognosis in type 1 diabetes needs to be filled. [9].

The Aim of the Study

The aim of this study was to assess the vascular endothelium function in children with type 1 diabetes mellitus (type 1 diabetes, DM1) based on selected markers of endothelial lesions such as sVCAM-1, sICAM-1, sE-SELECTIN, PAI-1, ADMA, and RAGE. The tests performed in the present research were supplemented with an analysis of the effects of type 1 diabetes duration, the degree of its metabolic balance, as well as of the effects of the patient's age, sex, and BMI on the extent of endothelial damage.

2. Materials and Methods

The prospective observational study involved sixty-six (66) children (36 boys and 30 girls) with diagnosed type 1 diabetes who were being treated at the Department of Pediatric Endocrinology and Diabetology at the University Hospital. The presence of other chronic diseases that could have been either inflammatory or influential for the selected parameters were excluded.

The control group included twenty-one (21) healthy children (10 boys and 11 girls). The control children were hospitalized at the Department of Pediatric Nephrology at the University Hospital due to suspected urinary tract abnormalities or bedwetting. On the basis of the diagnostic examinations performed at that time, the above-mentioned abnormalities were excluded.

Anthropometric measurements were conducted in both the group of children with type 1 diabetes (the study group) and the control group and included body height and weight with body mass index (BMI) estimation measurements as per the BMI centile charts developed by the WHO (see the WHO Child Growth Standards). The study patients were qualified to four (4) groups depending on their nutrition status: UN—undernourished children (BMI < 15 centiles), N—properly nourished children (BMI < 15–85 centiles), OV—children with overweight (BMI 85–90 centiles), and O—obese children (BMI ≥ 90 centiles).

Blood and urine from the patients were used as the research material. Blood was collected in the morning from the veins of the elbow fossa into tubes without anticoagulant (the so-called "clot") a minimum of 12 h after the patient had last ingested food or fluids. Then, the blood samples were centrifuged for 15 min at +4 °C at 1000× g. The obtained serum, which was necessary for the determination of the vascular endothelial damage markers (sVCAM-1, sICAM-1, sE-SELECTIN, ADMA, PAI-1, RAGE), was stored in Eppendorf tubes in the amount of approx. 400 µL and at a temperature −70 °C until the planned determinations were made.

Albuminuria was assessed by the immunoturbidimetric method, having collected a 24 h urine sample.

All of the studied endothelial inflammation markers were assayed by means of the immunoenzymatic ELISA test and by its variant, i.e., the so-called "sandwich" ELISA (a double-binding test) in particular, where the antigen is bound between two layers of antibodies [13,14]. The assays were conducted using the following sets: R&D Systems (sICAM-1, sVCAM-1, sE-SELECTIN, PAI-1) and Wuhan EIAab Science (RAGE, ADMA), according to the manufacturer's instructions. The degree of metabolic DM control was evaluated using the HbA1c concentration measured with high-performance liquid chromatography (HPLC). The eGFR value was assessed on the basis of serum creatinine concentration and was assayed by the Jaffe method and the Schwartz formula.

k-factor: 0.33—low birth weight infants; 0.45—normal birth weight infants; 0.55—children 2–12 years; 0.55—girls 13 years and older; 0.70—boys 13 years and older [15,16]. The results were related to age- and sex-specific norms for children.

Ethical Issues

A statistical analysis was conducted by means of the Statistica software (TIBCO Software Inc. (2017). Statistica (data analysis software system), version 13. http://statistica.io (accessed on 25 August 2021)). A single-factor analysis of variance (ANOVA) was applied for the statistical material analysis using Tukey's post hoc test or the Mann–Whitney nonparametric test. The correlation among continuous features was also determined using the Spearman correlation coefficient. The studied continuous features were characterised by their distribution parameters, i.e., the mean value, the standard deviation (SD), and the sample size (N).

Two-sided p-values less than 0.05 were considered significant. Calculated p-values were not adjusted for multiple testing. Standard boxplots with bold lines indicating median value were made, with the upper and lower edges of the box showing the first quantile and third quantile results. Black dots are individual data points.

3. Results

The clinical characteristics of the study groups are present Table 1. Compared to the control group, the DM1 group had significantly higher age, BMI, CRP, and percentage of males (see Table 1).

The children with type 1 diabetes demonstrated significantly higher concentrations of all of the studied markers of vascular endothelial damage, i.e., sICAM-1, sVCAM-1, sE-SELECTIN, ADMA, PAI-1 and RAGE, when compared to the corresponding values in the control group (see Table 1).

For all of the studied biomarkers, the minimal values in the DM1 group were higher than the maximal values in the control group: the sICAM-1 ranged from 102.55 to 117.8 in control group vs. from 162.41 to 425.35; sVCAM-1 ranged from 313.86 to 357.27 in the control group vs. from 400.20 to 762.65; sE-SELECTIN ranged from 29.12 to 35.38 in the control group vs. from 41.94 to 79.95; ADMA ranged from 68.49 to 75.81 in the control group vs. from 104.71 to 693.67; PAI-1 ranged from 6.02 to 6.82 in the control group vs. from 12.82 to 19.38; and RAGE ranged from 80.10 to 88.12 in the control group vs. from 114.47 to 796.66. Thus, it was possible to predict DM1 based on each biomarker with 100% accuracy.

Table 1. Baseline data in diabetic patients (studied group) and in control group.

Parameter	Studied Group n = 66		Control Group n = 21		p Value
	Mean ± SD	Median Value	Mean ± SD	Median Value	
Sex (female, n (%))	31 (46.97%)		16 (76.19%)		0.0367
Age (years)	12.69 ± 3.6	13.5	9.26 ± 2.9	9	<0.001
BMI (kg/m^2)	19.45 ± 3.9	19.02	17.47 ± 2.7	17	0.024
Duration of diabetes (years)	3.8 ± 4.2	2			
HbA1c (%)	10.47 ± 3.07	9			
Haemoglobin (g/dL)	13.21 ± 0.89	13.6	13.21 ± 0.89	13.21	1
Leukocytes (thousand/μL)	6.74 ± 1.81	6.9	6.83 ± 1.71	6.83	0.837
PLT [thousand/μL]	260.66 ± 76.07	261	305.2 ± 75.74	286	0.096
Sodium (mmol/L)	138 ± 3.15	138	138.5 ± 1.36	139	0.402
Potassium (mmol/L)	4.18 ± 0.45	4.2	4.19 ± 0.24	4.19	0.262
CRP [mg/L]	3.54 ± 6.0	0.67	0.77 ± 1.2	0.3	0.011
AspAT	26.33 ± 13.24	24	27.93 ± 5.80	28	0.566
AlAT	17.38 ± 8.53	16	15.73 ± 4.27	14.5	0.273
TSH	2.43 ± 1.45	2.06	2.22 ± 0.85	2.06	0.154
Cholesterol	165.52 ± 32.49	161	172.67 ± 11.67	175	0.104
Triglycerides	98.30 ± 41.53	92	83.5 ± 21.99	83.5	0.089
Urea (mg/dL)	21.13 ± 9.40	22.5	23.55 ± 5.71	23.55	0.353
Creatinine (mg/dL)	0.58 ± 0.14	0.56	0.66 ± 0.09	0.65	0.013
eGFR (mL/min/1.73 m^2)	166.04 ± 32.86	160.26	114.11 ± 11.00	114.81	<0.001
sICAM-1 (ng/mL)	267.15 ± 111.89	229.2	110.48 ± 4.53	110	<0.001
sVCAM-1 (ng/mL)	554.01 ± 132.11	522.48	337.33 ± 11.73	337.45	<0.001
sE-SELECTIN (ng/mL)	57.74 ± 14.19	52.49	32.64 ± 1.27	32.56	<0.001
ADMA (ng/mL)	325.03 ± 233.39	227.75	71.91 ± 2.31	71.01	<0.001
PAI-1 (ng/mL)	16.03 ± 2.41	16.12	6.51 ± 0.21	6.53	<0.001
RAGE (pg/mL)	380.20 ± 282.90	265.52	84.94 ± 2.27	85.48	<0.001

Legends: SD—standard deviation.

A positive, linear correlation was observed in the study group between the concentrations of the assayed endothelial damage markers and the disease duration. A significant increase in the concentrations of those markers was found already at very early stages of the disease, i.e., from the moment of its diagnosis, while the levels of C-reactive protein (CRP), the inflammation marker in the body, did not differ statistically significantly in relation to the control group (0.8 ± 1.2 vs. 2.97 ± 4.53 mg/L; $p = 0.161$) (see Figure 1a–g).

Table 2 lists the data based on DM1 duration (Group I, II, III) and the control group (Control).

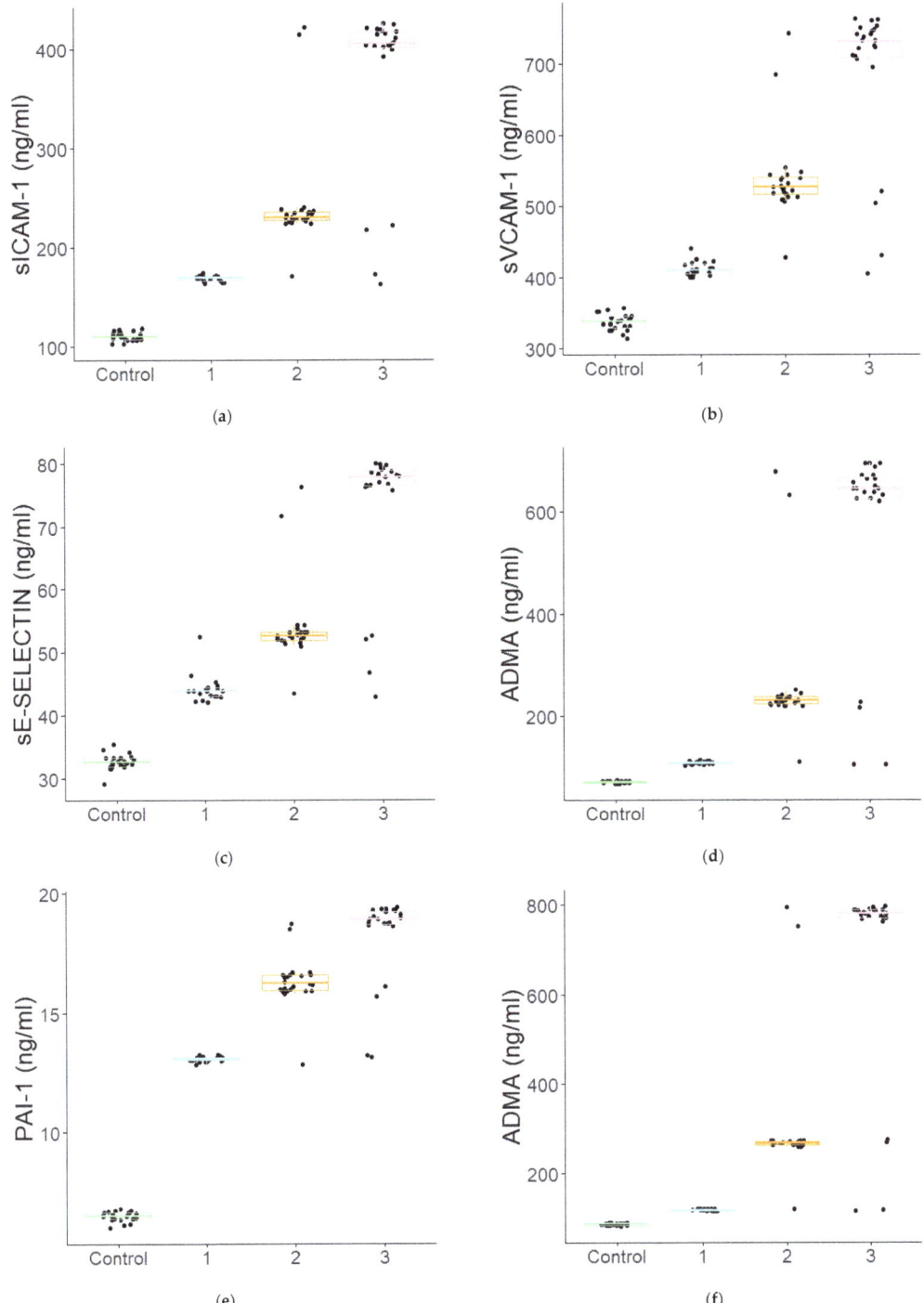

Figure 1. *Cont.*

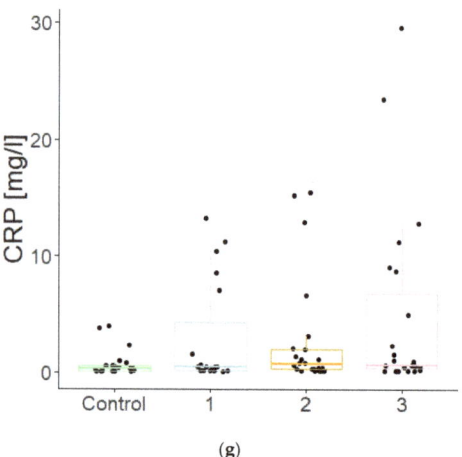

(g)

Figure 1. (**a**–**g**). A comparison of the distribution of selected parameters vs. DM1 duration. Boxplot of values for each subgroup. ((**a**)—the mean sICAM-1 values: 110.48 ± 4.53 vs. 168.47 ± 3.05 vs. 243.97 ± 55.18 vs. 372.85 ± 85.31 ng/mL; (**b**)—the mean sVCAM-1 values: 337.33 ± 11.73 vs. 412.56 ± 10.29 vs. 538.29 ± 59.77 vs. 687.26 ± 107.84 ng/mL; (**c**)—the mean sE-SELECTIN values: 5.43 ± 0.21 vs. 44.17 ± 2.27 vs. 54.01 ± 6.5 vs. 72.84 ± 11.56 ng/mL; (**d**)—the mean ADMA values: 71.91 ± 2.31 vs. 109.32 ± 2.38 vs. 261.05 ± 124.20 vs. 569.99 ± 193.44 ng/mL; (**e**)—the mean PAI-1 values: 6.51 ± 0.21 vs. 13.07 ± 0.11 vs. 16.29 ± 1.04 vs. 18.21 ± 1.84 ng/mL; (**f**)—the mean RAGE values: 84.94 ± 2.27 vs. 116.78 ± 1.53 vs. 301.95 ± 148.48 vs. 679.45 ± 230.59 pg/mL; and (**g**)—the mean CRP values: 0.8 ± 1.2 vs. 2.97 ± 4.53 vs. 2.78 ± 4.77 vs. 4.82 ± 7.92 mg/L). Legends: Control—control group; 1—the patients with newly diagnosed diabetes mellitus (DM1 duration < 1 year), n = 19; 2—the patients with DM1 duration of 1–5 years, n = 24; 3—the patients with DM1 duration of at least 5 years, n = 23.

Table 2. Demographic, clinical, and biochemical data of the groups depending on DM1 duration Legends: Control—control group; Group 1—the patients with newly diagnosed diabetes mellitus (DM1 duration < 1 year), n = 19; Group 2—the patients with DM1 duration of 1–5 years, n = 24; Group 3—the patients with DM1 duration of at least 5 years, n = 23. [a]: difference between group I and II is significant ($p < 0.05$), [b]: difference between Group II and III is significant ($p < 0.05$), [c]: difference between Group I and III is significant ($p < 0.05$), [d]: difference between Control group and Group I is significant ($p < 0.05$), [e]: difference between Control group and Group II is significant ($p < 0.05$), [f]: difference between Control group and Group III is significant ($p < 0.05$).

Variables.	Control	Group 1	Group 2	Group 3
Age (years)	(9.3 ± 2.9) [e,f]	(11.2 ± 3.4) [c]	(11.9 ± 3.8) [b,e]	(14.8 ± 2.5) [b,c,f]
BMI (kg/m^2)	(17.5 ± 2.7) [f]	(17.3 ± 3.0) [c]	19.8 ± 4.5	(20.9 ± 3.1) [c,f]
HbA1c (%)		(12.2 ± 3.2) [a]	(9.2 ± 2.5) [a]	10.3 ± 2.9
eGFR mL/min/1.73 m^2	(114.1 ± 1) [d,e,f]	(175.5 ± 28.0) [c,d]	(165.6 ± 33.6) [e]	(158.4 ± 35.2) [c,f]
S-creatinine (mg/dL)	(0.6 ± 0.1) [d,e]	(0.5 ± 0.1) [c,d]	(0.6 ± 0.1) [b,e]	(0.6 ± 0.1) [b,c]
Albuminuria (mg/24 h)		15.2 ± 10.8	14.4 ± 14.2	21.5 ± 19.5
sICAM-1 (ng/mL)	(110.5 ± 4.5) [d,e,f]	(168.5 ± 3.0) [a,c,d]	(244.0 ± 55.2) [a,b,e]	(372.8 ± 85.3) [b,c,f]
sVCAM-1 (ng/mL)	(337.3 ± 11.7) [d,e,f]	(412.6 ± 10.3) [a,c,d]	(538.3 ± 59.8) [a,b,e]	(687.3 ± 107.8) [b,c,f]
sE-SELECTIN (ng/mL)	(5.4 ± 0.2) [d,e,f]	(44.2 ± 2.3) [a,c,d]	(54.0 ± 6.5) [a,b,e]	(72.8 ± 11.6) [b,c,f]
ADMA (ng/mL)	(71.9 ± 2.3) [d,e,f]	(109.3 ± 2.4) [a,c,d]	(261.1 ± 124.2) [a,b,e]	(570.0 ± 193.4) [b,c,f]
PAI-1 (ng/mL)	(6.5 ± 0.2) [d,e,f]	(13.1 ± 0.1) [a,c,d]	(16.3 ± 1.0) [a,b,e]	(18.2 ± 1.8) [b,c,f]
RAGE (pg/mL)	(84.9 ± 2.3) [d,e,f]	(116.8 ± 1.5) [a,c,d]	(301.9 ± 148.5) [a,b,e]	(679.5 ± 230.6) [b,c,f]
CRP (mg/L)	(0.8 ± 1.2) [e,f]	3.0 ± 4.5	(2.8 ± 4.8) [e]	(4.8 ± 7.9) [f]

A positive correlation was also proven between all of the studied endothelial damage markers and the age of the patients; however, statistically significant differences were observed in the youngest children when compared to the patients in the intermediate age group, a finding that specifically concerned ADMA concentrations (196.99 ± 135.66 vs. 331.71 ± 246.17 ng/mL; $p \leq 0.01$) (see Figure 2).

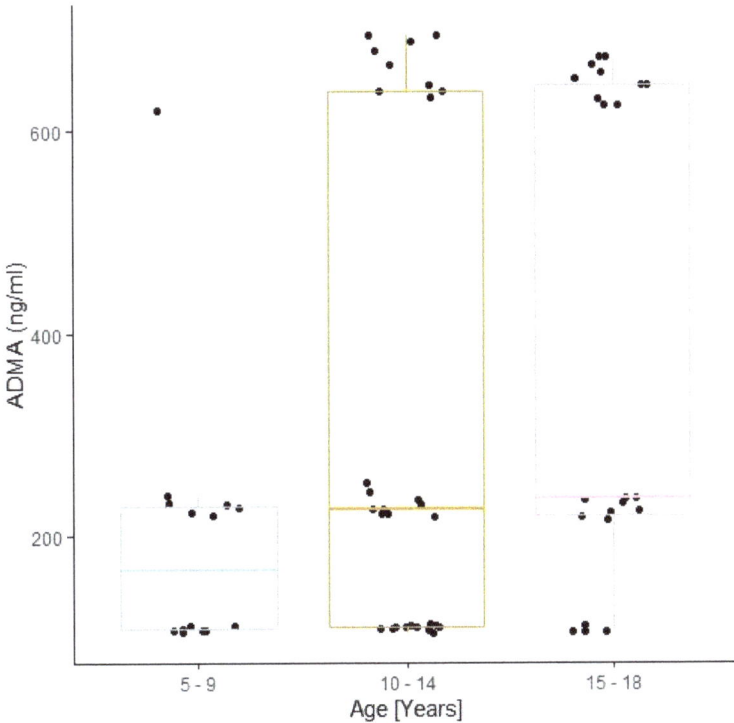

Figure 2. A comparison of the ADMA values depending on the patient's age (196.99 ± 135.66 vs. 331.71 ± 246.17 vs. 397.40 ± 238.84 ng/mL). Boxplot of values for each subgroup. Legends: patients aged 5–9-years-old, n = 14; patients aged 10–14-years-old, n = 30; patients aged 15–18-years-old, n = 22.

In addition, a linear correlation was identified between the concentrations of all of the assayed endothelial dysfunction markers and the BMI values of the patients. The children with diabetes mellitus and who were underweight (the "U" subgroup) presented statistically significant concentrations of sICAM (209.94 ± 70.31 vs. 279.44 ± 108.54 ng/mL; $p \leq 0.05$), sVCAM-1 (481.18 ± 99.39 vs. 568.94 ± 141.01 ng/mL; $p \leq 0.05$), and RAGE (231.46 ± 198.32 vs. 414.20 ± 298.22 pg/mL; $p \leq 0.05$) when compared to the children with a normal body weight (the "N" subgroup), while the patients who were overweight (the "O" subgroup) demonstrated much higher albuminuria vs. the normal-weight patients (23.67 ± 16.08 vs. 15.81 ± 14.41 mg/day; $p \leq 0.05$); however, there was no linear correlation between those parameters (see Figure 3a–d).

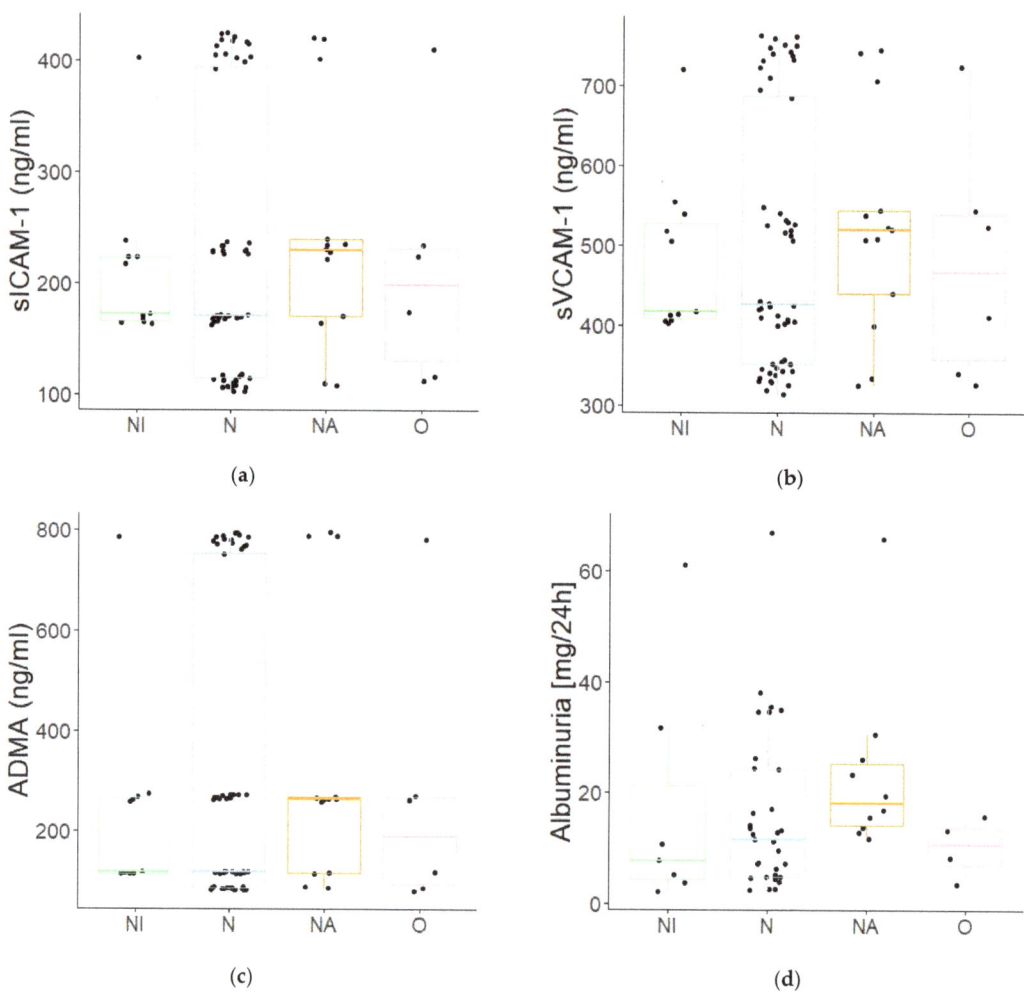

Figure 3. (**a–d**). A comparison of selected parameters depending on BMI ((**a**)—the mean sICAM-1 values: 209.94 ± 70.31 vs. 279.44 ± 108.54 vs. 269.65 ± 96.13 vs. 261.02 ± 103.28 ng/mL; (**b**)—the mean sVCAM-1 values: 481.18 ± 99.39 vs. 568.94 ± 141.01 vs. 560.93 ± 117.07 vs. 550.41 ± 129.89 ng/mL; (**c**)—the mean RAGE values: 231.46 ± 198.32 vs. 414.20 ± 298.22 vs. 380.62 ± 269.90 vs. 357.74 ± 291.02 pg/mL; (**d**)—the mean albuminuria values: 17.51 ± 21.68 vs. 15.81 ± 14.41 vs. 23.67 ± 16.08 vs. 10.23 ± 5.41 mg/24 h). Boxplot of values for each subgroup. Legends: NI—the patients underweight patients, $n = 11$; N—the patients with normal body weight, $n = 39$; NA—the overweight patients, $n = 11$; O—the patients with obesity, $n = 4$.

Taking into account the degree of metabolic control of diabetes mellitus, the highest concentrations of the studied endothelial damage markers were observed in the children with the lowest HbA1c values, i.e., between 6.5 and 8.9%, while the lowest ones were observed in the children with the worst glycaemic control (HbA1c $\geq$ 14%) (see Figure 4a–f). In case of sVCAM-1 and PAI-1, there was a negative correlation between those two markers and HbA1c concentration levels.

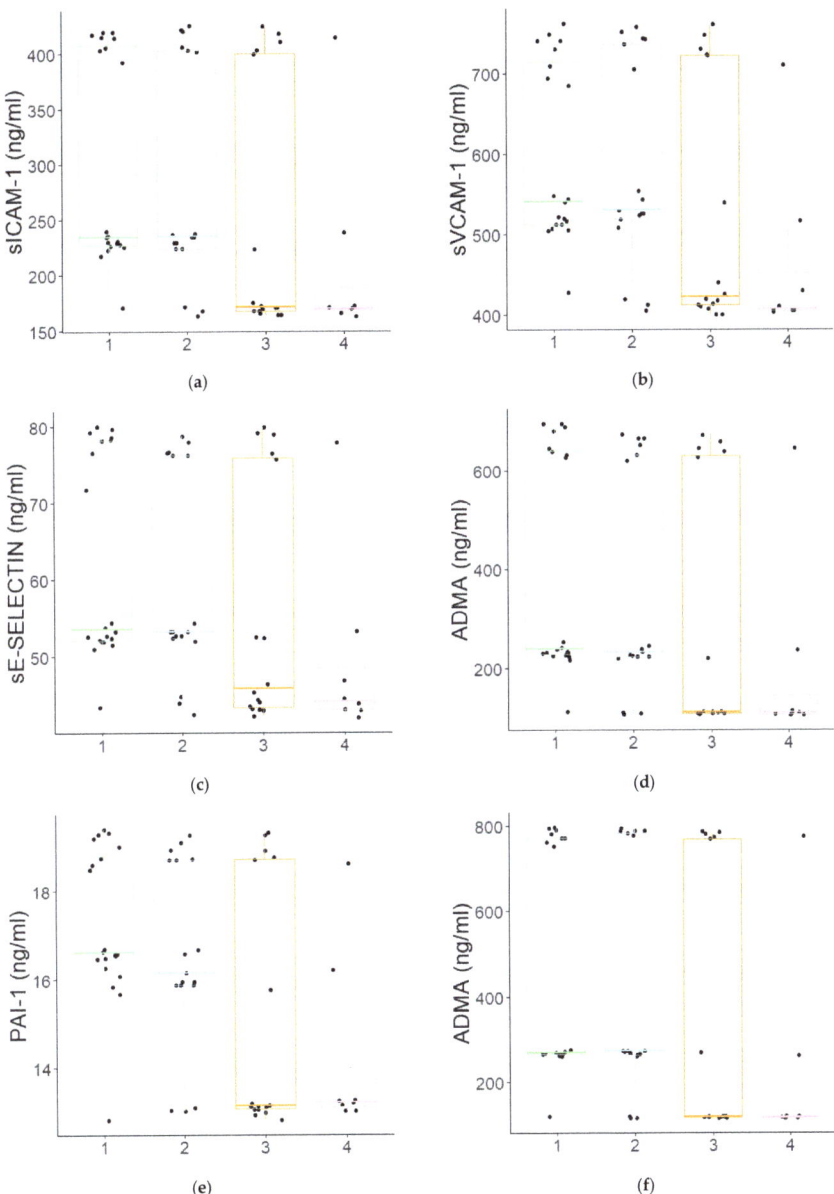

Figure 4. (**a**–**f**). A comparison of endothelial damage markers depending on the degree of metabolic (non)balancing of type 1 diabetes ((**a**)—the mean sICAM-1 values: 298.69 ± 95.06 vs. 284.13 ± 101.18 vs. 247.87 ± 114.65 vs. 207.70 ± 86.90 ng/mL; (**b**)—the mean sVCAM-1 values: 598.80 ± 111.06 vs. 583.04 ± 127.85 vs. 523.53 ± 152.63 vs. 461.07 ± 108.22 ng/mL; (**c**)—the mean sE-SELECTIN values: 62.13 ± 13.35 vs. 59.81 ± 13.58 vs. 55.57 ± 15.92 vs. 49.24 ± 12.07 ng/mL; (**d**)—the mean ADMA values: 397.44 ± 223.47 vs. 356.19 ± 228.50 vs. 284.21 ± 254.30 vs. 191.14 ± 188.38 ng/mL; (**e**)—the mean PAI-1 values: 17.23 ± 1.70 vs. 16.56 ± 2.12 vs. 15.08 ± 2.80 vs. 4.22 ± 2.07 ng/mL; (**f**)—the mean RAGE values: 462.95 ± 265.67 vs. 424.01 ± 281.86 vs. 333.59 ± 312.73 vs. 216.76 ± 231.39 pg/mL). Boxplot of values for each subgroup. Legends: 1—the patients with HbA1c: 6.5–8.9%, n = 20; 2—the patients with HbA1c: 9–11.4%, n = 17; 3—the patients with HbA1c: 11.5–13.9%, n = 16; 4—the patients with HbA1c: $\geq$14%, n = 8.

Urine albumin concentration measurements were available for 55 DM1 patients. The median concentration of urine albumin was 12.9 mg/24 h, with an interquartile range 5.25 mg/24 h–23.85 mg/24 h. In 10 patients (18.18%), the urine albumin concentration exceeded 30 mg/24 h. There were not any statistically significant differences in the levels of the biomarkers between the groups with and without albuminuria.

In turn, while comparing the results of the patients with reference to their sex, it was found that the boys were characterised by statistically significantly higher glomerular filtration rates vs. the studied girls. Otherwise, no statistically significant differences were demonstrated between the boys and the girls regarding the endothelial damage markers.

All of the studied vascular endothelial dysfunction markers correlated with one another (see Figure 5).

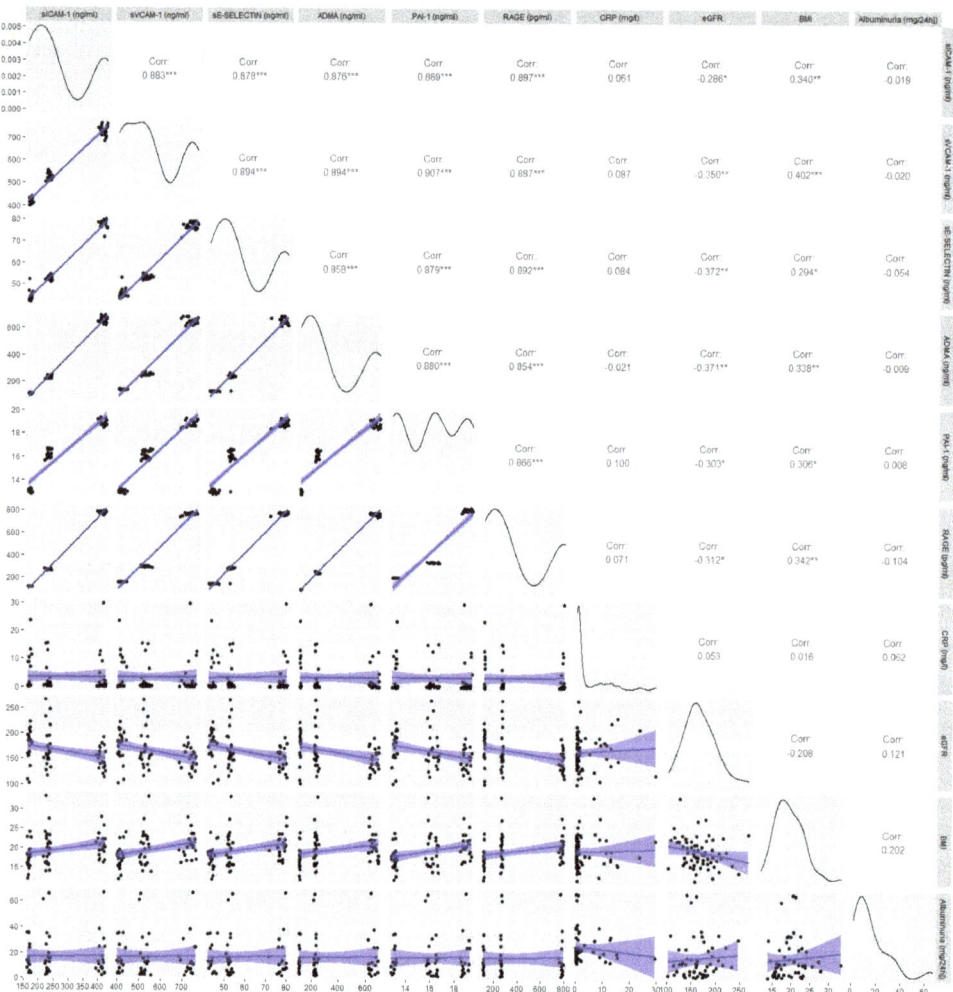

Figure 5. The indices of correlation among selected diagnostic features. Correlogram shows scatterplots for each pair variables in the bottom left part, and Spearman's correlation coefficient is shown in the upper right part. Distribution of variables is shown diagonally. Legend: *—p-value < 0.05; **—p-value < 0.01; ***—p-value < 0.001.

Simple linear regression was performed to predict eGFR based on each one of studied biomarkers. Among them, sE-SELECTIN had the highest R2 = 0.09 and had a regression coefficient = −0.75, SE = 0.28, and intercept = 209.28, p = 0.0088. In the multiple linear regression analysis, sE-SELECTIN was proven to be an independent predictor (p = 0.033) of eGFR. The model was adjusted for age, gender, and duration of DM1.

4. Discussion

Although many insights and knowledge about diabetes mellitus have been developed over the last 5000 years, there are many still unanswered questions [17,18]. It is not known what underlies the destruction of pancreatic β-cells. It has, however, been demonstrated that persistent hyperglycaemia leads to progressive vascular endothelial dysfunction which, in turn, underpins the development of diabetic micro- and macroangiopathy [19,20]. Since the early diagnosis of the disease is so important for the prevention of these dangerous complications, the identification of reliable endothelial dysfunction markers should become our priority. In this study, we used the serum from patients to determine the biochemical substances produced by the endothelium, such as vascular cell adhesion molecules (VCAM-1), intercellular adhesion molecules (sICAM-1), selectin E (sE-Selektin), asymmetric dimethylarginine (ADMA), plasminogen activator inhibitor 1 (PAI-1), and receptors for advanced glycation end products (AGEs), because their concentrations increase rapidly in states of cellular stress.

In the analysed material, the children with type 1 diabetes demonstrated significantly higher concentrations of all six studied endothelial damage markers (sICAM-1, sVCAM-1, sE-SELECTIN, PAI-1, ADMA, RAGE) when compared to the healthy controls. A significant increase in the concentrations of the markers was already found in the patients with newly diagnosed diabetes mellitus, i.e., at a very early stage of the disease, while the systemic inflammation index (CRP) was normal. The longer the disease duration was, the more distinctive the increase in the concentrations of the above-mentioned inflammation markers was. This was confirmed by the high positive correlation values between the concentrations of the studied markers and the disease duration. Moreover, the markers grew linearly against one another. This observation confirms earlier reports that diabetes duration is an important risk factor for the development of chronic diabetes complications, which are characterized by chronic subclinical endothelial inflammation [21,22].

Taking into account the degree of metabolic balance in diabetes mellitus, the highest concentrations of the studied endothelial damage markers were observed in the children with the lowest HbA1c values, while the lowest ones were observed in the children with the worst glycaemic control. In addition, in the case of sVCAM-1 and PAI-1, there was a negative correlation between those two markers and HbA1c concentration levels. Since poor glycaemic control is a significant risk factor for complications in diabetes mellitus, an inverse relation could have been expected. However, it should be noted that the diabetic patients with the best glycaemic control were also characterised by the lowest glomerular filtration rates and had been suffering from diabetes mellitus longer than those with the statistically significantly lower concentrations of endothelial damage markers. In fact, there was a strong positive correlation between the studied endothelial damage markers and the duration of diabetes mellitus, while the marker levels decreased linearly with the growing glomerular filtration rate. Observations from other authors regarding the issues have been divided: the same researchers, while evaluating the concentrations of various endothelial inflammation markers, simultaneously obtained positive and negative correlations with glomerular filtration rates [20,23]. Moreover, the correlation between the levels of the markers and diabetes mellitus duration was often not indicated at all, even showing other factors, such as the metabolic control of DM or the patient's age [24,25]. Moreover, it should be underlined that it is not only hyperglycemia that has a damaging effect on the endothelium; hypoglycemia also induces inflammation [26–28]. Therefore, increased risk of chronic complications resulting from endothelial inflammation is a consequence of all glycemic fluctuations (so called glycemic variability) should be considered in diabetes, as these fluctuations undoubtedly have a negative impact on the endothelium [29–31]. This may explain the inverse relationship between HbA1c and the concentration of the investigated markers of inflammation. Frequent episodes of hypoglycaemia lower the level of HbA1c, but at the same time, hypoglycaemia also negatively affects endothelial condition. Furthermore, in our cohort, the majority of children with the highest HbA1c level were the newly diagnosed patients. Such disproportion might have biased the result, as in those patients, the levels of studied parameters were the lowest, indicating the inverse correlation of who had had the disease for longer.

In our study, we also examined the impact of the patient's age on the status of the vascular endothelium. Similar to other studies, that correlation proved to be an important factor for the progress of vascular changes, indicating a positive, linear correlation with all of the studied markers of endothelial damage as well as a positive correlation with the Y variable, which corresponds to the endothelial inflammation intensity [24,32]. Although the concentrations of all of those indices demonstrated the lowest values in the subgroup with the youngest patients, statistically significant differences were only found for ADMA. This result proves the suitability and usability of the asymmetric dimethylarginine concentration assay for the prognosis of early changes in the endothelium, especially in younger patients. Other significant differences that were analysed with regard to the patient's age concerned disease duration, the metabolic degree to which the patient's diabetes mellitus was balanced, and albuminuria. This implies that the oldest children would have been suffering from the disease for the longest period of time, and they were characterised by the worst glycaemic control and the highest albuminuria. Such results should certainly not come as a surprise. They once again confirm the mutual correlation of the above-mentioned parameters, as both poor glycaemic control and DM duration are the risk factors of diabetic kidney disease and consequently contribute to enhanced albuminuria [32,33].

In turn, while comparing the results of the patients with reference to their sex, it was only found that the boys had been characterised by statistically significantly higher glomerular filtration rates vs. those of the studied girls. That result was in line with the expectations since eGFR, when taking into account the parameters of the maturing body (the patient's height, age and sex) as calculated by the Schwartz method, requires higher values [15]. On the other hand, no statistically significant differences were demonstrated between the boys and the girls regarding either the endothelial damage markers or the other evaluated parameters.

In addition, the in-house research results have allowed us to determine that children with diabetes mellitus and who are underweight present statistically significantly lower concentrations of sICAM, sVCAM-1, and RAGE when compared to children with a normal body weight. What is more, a linear correlation has been confirmed between the BMI values of the patients and the concentrations of these and other markers of endothelial dysfunction. Many publications also confirm such correlations [34–39]. On the other hand, the children who are overweight demonstrated significantly higher albuminuria vs. normal weight children, who had no linear correlation between the parameters. Moreover, positive correlations with BMI were found, both in terms of the patient's age and the duration of the patient's diabetes mellitus. Increased concentrations of endothelial dysfunction markers accompanied by increased BMI values may indicate the inflammatory state of the endothelium in the course of the developing metabolic syndrome (obesity as the risk factor of sclerosis). It could also be the case that the concomitance of these two conditions increases the risk of angiopathic complications, including diabetic kidney disease.

In contrast, while analysing the correlations between those markers and the other parameters, based on the assays in all of the patients (i.e., both in the study group and the control group), our attention was driven by the positive correlations between both PAI-1 and eGFR and between sE-SELECTIN and eGFR. While all of the studied markers revealed positive correlations with the risk factors for vascular complications (BMI, the patient's age, disease duration), only the two above-mentioned factors demonstrated linear correlations with the kidney damage factor (eGFR), and they thus seem to be more suitable in the prognoses and detection of early unfavourable changes in the kidneys.

Musial and Zwolinska reported that the concentrations of matrix metalloproteinases (MMPs) and their tissue inhibitors (TIMPs) correlate not only with the markers of inflammation, e.g., e selectin, but also with eGFR, thus indicating increased inflammation and endothelial dysfunction in patients with renal failure [40]. Similar findings were reported by Gheissari et al. and Meamar et al. [41,42]. As such, it may be assumed that markers of inflammation, i.e., e-selectin, may act not only as the predictors of cardiovascular complications in chronic kidney disease but also to predict late diabetes complications, including nephropathy.

To sum up, the assayed endothelial dysfunction markers proved the presence of inflammatory condition in the endothelium, which was already at the very early stages of the disease, i.e., from the time of its diagnosis, when the inflammation marker (CRP) was not yet elevated. The enhanced inflammation of the endothelium depended on the already well-known risk factors for vascular complications, namely disease duration, the patient's age, or his/her BMI. What is more, all of the studied markers demonstrated positive linear correlations between one another, while their increasing concentrations reflected progressive endothelial inflammation. Therefore, the essential issue is whether the evaluated markers are sensitive and specific enough to be used for the assessment of vascular endothelial inflammation and thereby for the estimation of the risk of vascular complications in diabetes mellitus. Such studies should be conducted in children in future to fully determine this. When looking at this issue in the context of nephrological complications, attention should be given to the linear correlations between PAI-1 and eGFR as well as to those between sE-SELECTIN and eGFR, as such results may suggest a certain advantage of PAI-1 and sE-SELECTIN over the other endothelial dysfunction markers, especially regarding the identification of early changes in the kidneys.

5. Conclusions

1. In the patients with type 1 diabetes, statistically significantly higher concentrations were demonstrated for all the assayed markers when compared to the corresponding values in the control group.
2. A significant increase in the concentrations of those markers was already observed at the early stages of the disease.
3. All of the evaluated endothelial dysfunction markers were positively correlated with the disease duration, the age of the patients, and their BMI, while only PAI-1 and sE-SELECTIN were characteristic of linear correlations with the estimated glomerular filtration rate (eGFR).

Author Contributions: Conceptualization, K.N.-W., D.Z.; Data curation, D.P.-J.; Formal analysis, D.Z.; Investigation, A.Z.-K.; Methodology, K.N.-W., D.Z., A.Z.-K. and D.P.-J.; Project administration, D.Z.; Resources, K.N.-W.; Supervision, D.Z., A.Z.-K.; Validation, A.Z.-K.; Writing—original draft, K.N.-W.; Writing—review & editing, D.P.-J. All authors have read and agreed to the published version of the manuscript.

Funding: This work was supported by the Wrocław Medical University grant ST. 942.

Institutional Review Board Statement: The study was conducted according to the guidelines of the Declaration of Helsinki, and approved by the Bioethical Commission at the Wrocław Piastów Śląskich Medical University in Wrocław (ethical approval no. 184/2017).

Informed Consent Statement: Both the children in all of the participating groups ($\geq$16 years) and their parents were informed about the aims, principles, and benefits of the current research, and informed consent was obtained from all of the participants and their legal guardians.

Data Availability Statement: The datasets generated and/or analyzed during the current study available from the corresponding author on reasonable request.

Conflicts of Interest: The authors declare that they have no competing interest.

References

1. Guariguata, L.; Whiting, D.; Hambleton, I.; Beagley, J.; Linnenkamp, U.; Shaw, J. Global estimates of diabetes prevalence for 2013 and projections for 2035. *Diabetes Res. Clin. Pract.* **2014**, *103*, 137–149. [CrossRef] [PubMed]
2. Knapik-Kordecka, M.; Piwowar, A.; Warwas, M. Oxidative-antioxidant imbalances and risk factors for atherosclerosis and vascular complications in patients with type 2 diabetes. *Med. News* **2007**, *40*, 7–8.
3. Giugliano, D.; Ceriello, A.; Paolisso, G. Oxidative stress and diabetic vascular complications. *Diabetes Care* **1996**, *19*, 257–267. [CrossRef]
4. Lipinski, B. Pathophysiology of oxidative stress in diabetes mellitus. *J. Diabetes Its Complicat.* **2001**, *15*, 203–210. [CrossRef]
5. Mogensen, C.E.; Christensen, C.K.; Vittinghus, E. The stages in diabetic renal disease: With emphasis on the stage of incipient diabetic nephropathy. *Diabetes* **1983**, *32*, 64–78. [CrossRef]
6. Deckert, T.; Feldt-Rasmussen, B.; Borch-Johnsen, K.; Jensen, T.; Kofoed-Enevoldsen, A. Albuminuria reflects widespread vascular damage. *Diabetologia* **1989**, *32*, 219–226. [CrossRef]
7. Krol, G.L.; Kunisaki, M.; Nishio, T.; Inoguchi, T.; Shiba, P. Biochemical and molecular mechanisms in the development of diabetic vascular complications. *Diabetes* **1996**, *45*, S105–S108.
8. Tatoń, J.; Czech, A.; Łaz, R. *Angiotoxic Effects of Increased Oxidative Stress in Diabetes. Diabetic Heart Disease*; Wydawnictwo Medyczne via Medica: Gdańsk, Poland, 2005; pp. 93–99.
9. Astrup, A.S.; Tarnow, L.; Pietraszek, L.; Schalkwijk, C.G.; Stehouwer, C.D.; Parving, H.H.; Rossing, P. Markers of endothelial dysfunction and inflammation in type 1 diabetic patients with or without diabetic nephropathy followed for 10 years: Association with mortality and decline of glomerular filtration rate. *Diabetes Care* **2008**, *31*, 1170–1176. [CrossRef]
10. Polek, A.; Sobiczewski, W.; Matowicka-Karna, J. P-selektyna i jej rola w niektórych chorobach P-selectin and its role in some diseases. *Postepy Hig. Med. Dosw.* **2009**, *63*, 465–470.
11. Chase, S.D.; Magnani, J.L.; Simon, S.I. E-selectin ligands as mechanosensitive receptors on neutrophils in health and disease. *Ann. Biomed. Eng.* **2012**, *40*, 849–859. [CrossRef]
12. Abbassi, O.M.I.D.; Kishimoto, T.K.; McIntire, L.V.; Anderson, D.C.; Smith, C.W. E-selectin supports neutrophil rolling in vitro under conditions of flow. *J. Clin. Investig.* **1993**, *92*, 2719. [CrossRef]
13. Lequin, R.M. Enzyme immunoassay (EIA)/enzyme-linked immunosorbent assay (ELISA). *Clin. Chem.* **2005**, *51*, 2415–2418. [CrossRef]
14. Fossceco, S.L. Exploring Enzyme-Linked Immunosorbent Assay (ELISA) Data with the SAS®. *Anal. Appl.* 1999. Available online: https://stats.idre.ucla.edu/wpcontent/uploads/2016/02/analystelisa.pdf (accessed on 11 June 2018).
15. Schwartz, G.J.; Haycock, G.B.; Edelmann, C.M.; Spitzer, A. A simple estimate of glomerular filtration rate in children derived from body length and plasma creatinine. *Pediatrics* **1976**, *582*, 259–263.
16. Miklaszewska, M. Laboratory Indicators of Renal Function-Determination Method and Clinical Value. Available online: https://www.mp.pl/pediatria/praktyka-kliniczna/badania-laboratoryjne/176082,laboratoryjne-wskazniki-czynnosci-nerek (accessed on 11 June 2018).
17. Korzeniowska, K.; Jabłecka, A. Diabetes (Part I). *Farm. Współ.* **2008**, *1*, 231–235. Available online: http://www.akademiamedycyny.pl/wp-content/uploads/2016/05/200804_Farmacja_003.pdf (accessed on 25 August 2021).
18. Schalkwijk, C.G.; Stehouwer, C.D. Vascular complications in diabetes mellitus: The role of endothelial dysfunction. *Clin. Sci.* **2005**, *109*, 143–159. [CrossRef] [PubMed]
19. Wierusz-Wysocka, B. Pathogenetic relationships between diabetic micro- and macroangiopathy Part I. Diabetic microangiopathy-what's new. *Clin. Diabetol.* **2009**, *10*, 151–156.
20. Araszkiewicz, A.; Mackiewicz-Wysocka, M.; Wierusz-Wysocka, B. Skin dysfunction in diabetes. Part 2—Microcirculation and peripheral nerve function. *Clin. Diabetol.* **2014**, *3*, 117–124.
21. Romero, P.; Salvat, M.; Fernandez, J.; Baget, M.; Martinez, I. Renal and retinal microangiopathy after 15 years of follow-up study in a sample of type 1 diabetes mellitus patients. *J. Diabetes Its Complicat.* **2007**, *21*, 93–100. [CrossRef]
22. Karamanos, B.; Porta, M.; Songini, M.; Metelko, Z.; Kerenyi, Z.; Tamas, G.; Fuller, J.H. Different risk factors of microangiopathy in patients with type I diabetes mellitus of short versus long duration. The EURODIAB IDDM Complications Study. *Diabetologia* **2000**, *43*, 348–355. [CrossRef] [PubMed]
23. Karimi, Z.; Kahe, F.; Jamil, A.; Marszalek, J.; Ghanbari, A.; Afarideh, M.; Chi, G. Intercellular adhesion molecule-1 in diabetic patients with and without microalbuminuria. *Diabetes Metab. Syndrome* **2018**, *12*, 365–368. [CrossRef]
24. Liu, J.J.; Yeoh, L.Y.; Sum, C.F.; Tavintharan, S.; Ng, X.W.; Liu, S.; Lim, S.C. Vascular cell adhesion molecule-1, but not intercellular adhesion molecule-1, is associated with diabetic kidney disease in Asians with type 2 diabetes. *J. Diabetes Its Complicat.* **2015**, *29*, 707–712. [CrossRef] [PubMed]
25. Lee, S.W.; Song, K.E.; Shin, D.S.; Ahn, S.M.; Ha, E.S.; Kim, D.J.; Lee, K.W. Alterations in peripheral blood levels of TIMP-1, MMP-2, and MMP-9 in patients with type-2 diabetes. *Diabetes Res. Clin. Pract.* **2005**, *69*, 175–179. [CrossRef] [PubMed]
26. Marfella, R.; Esposito, K.; Giunta, A.; Coppola, G.; De Angelis, L.; Farzati, B.; Giugliano, D. Circulating adhesion molecules in humans: Role of hyperglycemia and hyperinsulinemia. *Circulation* **2000**, *101*, 2247–2251. [CrossRef]
27. El Amine, M.; Sohawon, S.; Lagneau, L.; Gaham, N.; Noordally, S. Plasma levels of icam-1 and circulating endothelial cells are elevated in unstable types 1 and 2 diabetes. *Endocr. Regul.* **2010**, *44*, 17–24. [CrossRef]

28. Joy, N.G.; Hedrington, M.S.; Briscoe, V.J.; Tate, D.B.; Ertl, A.C.; Davis, S.N. Effects of acute hypoglycemia on inflammatory and pro-atherothrombotic biomarkers in individuals with type 1 diabetes and healthy individuals. *Diabetes Care* **2010**, *33*, 1529–1535.
29. Kilpatrick, E.S.; Rigby, A.S.; Atkin, S.L. For debate. Glucose variability and diabetes complication risk: We need to know the answer. *Diabet. Med.* **2010**, *27*, 868–871. [CrossRef]
30. Ceriello, A.; Ihnat, M.A. 'Glycaemic variability': A new therapeutic challenge in diabetes and the critical care setting. *Diabet. Med.* **2010**, *27*, 862–867. [CrossRef] [PubMed]
31. Lachin, J.M.; Bebu, I.; Bergenstal, R.M.; Pop-Busui, R.; Service, F.J.; Zinman, B.; Nathan, D.M. DCCT/EDIC Research Group. Association of Glycemic Variability in Type 1 Diabetes with Progression of Microvascular Outcomes in the Diabetes Control and Complications Trial. *Diabetes Care* **2017**, *40*, 777–783. [CrossRef]
32. Auwerx, J.; Bouillon, R.; Collen, D.; Geboers, J. Tissue-type plasminogen activator antigen and plasminogen activator inhibitor in diabetes mellitus. *Arterioscler. Thromb. Vasc. Biol.* **1988**, *8*, 68–72. [CrossRef]
33. Yarmolinsky, J.; Bordin Barbieri, N.; Weinmann, T. Plasminogen activator inhibitor-1 and type 2 diabetes: A systematic review and meta-analysis of observational studies. *Sci. Rep.* **2016**, *6*, 17714. [CrossRef]
34. Xiong, Y.; Lei, M.; Fu, S.; Fu, Y. Effect of diabetic duration on serum concentrations of endogenous inhibitor of nitric oxide synthase in patients and rats with diabetes. *Life Sci.* **2005**, *77*, 149–159. [CrossRef]
35. Bogdanović, R. Diabetic nephropathy in children and adolescents. *Pediatric Nephrol.* **2008**, *23*, 507–525. [CrossRef]
36. Głowińska, B.; Urban, M.; Peczyńska, J.; Florys, B. Soluble adhesion molecules (sICAM-1, sVCAM-1) and selectins (sE selectin, sP selectin, sL selectin) levels in children and adolescents with obesity, hypertension, and diabetes. *Metabolism* **2005**, *54*, 1020–1026. [CrossRef] [PubMed]
37. Juhan-Vague, I.; Roul, C.; Alessi, M.C.; Ardissone, J.P.; Heim, M. Increased plasminogen activator inhibitor activity in non insulin dependent diabetic patients-relationship with plasma insulin. *Thromb. Haemost.* **1989**, *61*, 370–373. [CrossRef]
38. Juhan-Vague, I.; Alessi, M.C.; Vague, P. Increased plasma plasminogen activator inhibitor 1 levels. A possible link between insulin resistance and atherothrombosis. *Diabetologia* **1991**, *34*, 457–462. [CrossRef]
39. Henry, M.; Tregouet, D.A.; Alessi, M.C.; Aillaud, M.F.; Visvikis, S.; Siest, G.; Tiret, L.; Juhan-Vague, I. Metabolic determinants are much more important than genetic polymorphisms in determining the PAI-1 activity and antigen plasma concentrations: A family study with part of the Stanislas Cohort. *Arterioscler. Thromb. Vasc. Biol.* **1988**, *18*, 84–91. [CrossRef]
40. Musiał, K.; Zwolińska, D. Matrix metalloproteinases (MMP-2, 9) and their tissue inhibitors (TIMP-1, 2) as novel markers of stress response and atherogenesis in children with chronic kidney disease (CKD) on conservative treatment. *Cell Stress Chaperones* **2011**, *16*, 97–103. [CrossRef]
41. Gheissari, A.; Meamar, R.; Abedini, A.; Roomizadeh, P.; Shafiei, M.; Samaninobandegani, Z.; Najafi, T.E. Association of matrix metalloproteinase-2 and matrix metalloproteinase-9 with endothelial dysfunction, cardiovascular disease risk factors and thrombotic events in children with end-stage renal disease. *Iran. J. Kidney Dis.* **2018**, *12*, 169–177. [PubMed]
42. Meamar, R.; Shafiei, M.; Abedini, A.; Ghazvini MR, A.; Roomizadeh, P.; Taheri, S.; Gheissari, A. Association of E-selectin with hematological, hormonal levels and plasma proteins in children with end stage renal disease. *Adv. Biomed. Res.* **2016**, *5*, 118. [PubMed]

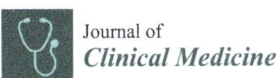

Article

The Usefulness of Urinary Periostin, Cytokeratin-18, and Endoglin for Diagnosing Renal Fibrosis in Children with Congenital Obstructive Nephropathy

Agnieszka Turczyn [1,*], Małgorzata Pańczyk-Tomaszewska [1], Grażyna Krzemień [1], Elżbieta Górska [2] and Urszula Demkow [2]

1. Department of Pediatrics and Nephrology, Medical University of Warsaw, 02-091 Warsaw, Poland; mpanczyk1@wum.edu.pl (M.P.-T.); grazyna.krzemien@wum.edu.pl (G.K.)
2. Department of Laboratory Diagnostics and Clinical Immunology of Developmental Age, Medical University of Warsaw, 02-091 Warsaw, Poland; elzbieta.gorska@uckwum.pl (E.G.); urszula.demkow@wum.edu.pl (U.D.)
* Correspondence: agnieszka.turczyn@wum.edu.pl; Tel.: +48-22-317-96-53; Fax: +48-22-317-99-54

Abstract: Congenital obstructive nephropathy (CON) leads to renal fibrosis and chronic kidney disease. The aim of the study was to investigate the predictive value of urinary endoglin, periostin, cytokeratin-18, and transforming growth factor-β1 (TGF-β1) for assessing the severity of renal fibrosis in 81 children with CON and 60 controls. Children were divided into three subgroups: severe, moderate scars, and borderline lesions based on 99mTc-ethylenedicysteine scintigraphy results. Periostin, periostin/Cr, and cytokeratin-18 levels were significantly higher in the study group compared to the controls. Children with severe scars had significantly higher urinary periostin/Cr levels than those with borderline lesions. In multivariate analysis, only periostin and cytokeratin-18 were independently related to the presence of severe and moderate scars, and periostin was independently related to borderline lesions. However, periostin did not differentiate advanced scars from borderline lesions. In ROC analysis, periostin and periostin/Cr demonstrated better diagnostic profiles for detection of advanced scars than TGF-β1 and cytokeratin-18 (AUC 0.849; 0.810 vs. 0.630; 0.611, respectively) and periostin for detecting borderline lesions than endoglin and periostin/Cr (AUC 0.777 vs. 0.661; 0.658, respectively). In conclusion, periostin seems to be a promising, non-invasive marker for assessing renal fibrosis in children with CON. CK-18 and TGF-β1 demonstrated low utility, and endoglin was not useful for diagnosing advanced scars.

Keywords: periostin; cytokeratin-18; endoglin; transforming growth factor-β1; renal fibrosis; congenital obstructive nephropathy; children

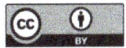

1. Introduction

Congenital anomalies of the kidneys and urinary tract (CAKUT) are the leading cause of chronic kidney disease (CKD) in children, and a large part of them is related to congenital obstructive nephropathy (CON) [1,2]. The pathogenesis of CON is complex and results from various functional and morphological changes associated with impaired urinary outflow. Obstruction in the urine flow causes an increase in the pressure in the urinary tract and leads to tubular dilatation. Renal response to mechanical compression involves angiotensin (Ang)-dependent renal vasoconstriction, ischemia, hypoxia, and accumulation of reactive oxygen species (ROS) [3]. These are mediated by altered expression of growth factors, cytokines, including transforming growth factor-β1 (TGF-β1) and adhesion molecules [3–5]. Functional lesions lead to cell apoptosis, interstitial macrophage recruitment, epithelial–mesenchymal transition (EMT), fibroblast–myofibroblast transformation, and accumulation of extracellular matrix (ECM) proteins. Morphological changes are responsible for interstitial fibrosis, tubular and vascular atrophy, and glomerular sclerosis.

CON leads to the reduction of functioning nephrons. It causes glomerular hyperfiltration and consequent glomerular sclerosis of the remaining nephrons and is responsible for the occurrence of CKD in childhood or adulthood [2,6].

Widely used imaging studies such as ultrasonography (US) and scintigraphy and currently available laboratory indices of the kidney injury such as serum creatinine (Cr), cystatin C, estimated glomerular filtration rate (GFR), and urinary albumin excretion do not provide information about the early stage of renal fibrosis and are poor predictors of the future course of CON [2,7]. Therefore, unfavorable prognosis in children with CON mandates a search for non-invasive fibrotic markers, which would enable early diagnosis of the fibrosis process, assessment of the severity of fibrosis, and early intervention in children at risk of renal injury progression.

TGF-β1 is a 25 kDA well-known cytokine that plays a pivotal role in renal fibrosis. It is secreted by epithelial cells, macrophages, and fibroblasts as an inactive latent complex [5,8]. After activation, TGF-β1 binds to its type II receptor (TβRII), which recruits two types I receptors (TβRI)—Activin like kinase 1 (ALK1) and ALK5. Depending on the TβRI recruited, different kinds of Smad proteins become phosphorylated for cellular response to TGF-β1. The complex composed of TβRII and ALK1 leads to Smad1/5/8 phosphorylation, and the complex composed of TβRII and ALK5 leads to Smad2/3 phosphorylation. Smad cascade is one of the most essential and well-known pathways in progressive renal fibrosis [9–11]. TGF-β1 promotes fibrosis by cell apoptosis, increasing macrophage infiltration, EMT, and myofibroblast transformation [3]. Overexpression of TGF-β1 mRNA and protein was demonstrated in multiple models of renal fibrosis [5,12,13]. Increased urinary TGF-β1 levels were found in CKD [14] and various types of nephropathies, including glomerular (GN), diabetic (DN), and obstructive nephropathy [8,15–17].

Endoglin is a 180 kDa homodimeric protein consisting of extracellular, transmembrane, and intracellular domain. Endoglin expression was identified in endothelial, smooth muscle and mesangial cells, macrophages, and fibroblasts [9,18,19]. Ang II and TGF-β1 are the most important stimulators of endoglin expression [18,20]. Endoglin acts as a TGF-β1 co-receptor known as TβRIII and binds to TGF-β1 by ALK1 and ALK5 receptors [18]. It modulates cellular responses to TGF-β1, mainly related to myofibroblast transformation and ECM accumulation [11,20]. Cytoplasmatic domain differentiates two endoglin isoforms, named large (L-Eng) and short (S-Eng), according to the length of their cytoplasmatic tails. Upregulation of L-Eng leads to Smad1 and Smad2/3 phosphorylation and promotes fibrosis, while upregulation of S-Eng acts oppositely [9,19]. Overexpression of endoglin was shown in renal fibrosis models [21–23] and in various human diseases, including CKD and DN [11,24].

Periostin is a 90 kDa matricellular protein with a multi-domain structure [25–27]. It is induced during organogenesis and found only in small amounts in a healthy kidney. Periostin was expressed de novo during the chronic disease of several organs [26,28,29]. In the kidney, periostin is released from fibroblasts and myofibroblasts in response to many factors, including Ang II and TGF-β1, which stimulate periostin expression by Smad phosphorylation and through Smad independent pathways [25,30]. It is expressed mainly in the location of tissue damage in ECM areas and directly interacts with multiple ECM proteins such as integrin, fibronectin, collagens, tenascin C, and bone morphogenic protein-1 (BMP-1) [27,28]. After binding to integrin, periostin induces fibrosis by increasing inflammatory cell infiltration, ECM remodeling, and TGF-β1 pathway upregulation [29,31]. Overexpression of periostin was reported in numerous experimental and clinical studies of renal fibrosis [25,32]. Increased urinary periostin levels were described in CKD, polycystic kidney disease (PKD), and various types of nephropathies, including IgA nephropathy (IgAN) [29,32,33].

Cytokeratin-18 (CK-18) is a 45 kDA cytoskeletal protein consisting of three domains [34,35]. It is a family member of intermediate filament proteins and represents about 5% of total cell proteins in most epithelial and parenchymal cells [36,37]. CK-18 is involved in maintaining cell shape and integrity, mechanical stability, intracellular organization, and cell signaling, transport, and differentiation [35,38,39]. In addition, it protects cells from mechanical and non-mechanical stress [35,40]. In response to various stress situations, CK-18 undergoes phosphorylation that modifies its solubility, filaments organization, prevents interaction with other molecules, and protects from proteolysis and degradation [35,39]. Overexpression of CK-18 was found in models of renal fibrosis and in humans with diabetic and lupus nephropathy [39]. High urinary CK-18 levels were reported in acute kidney injury (AKI) and CKD [37,39].

To the best of our knowledge, there are no studies in the available literature investigating the usefulness of urinary endoglin, periostin, and CK-18 in children with CON. Therefore, the aim of our study was to investigate the predictive value of urinary endoglin, periostin, CK-18, and TGF-β1 for assessing the severity of renal fibrosis in children with congenital obstructive nephropathy.

2. Materials and Methods

2.1. Study Group

This single-center cross-sectional study included 81 children with congenital obstructive nephropathy who were diagnosed at the Department of Pediatrics and Nephrology of the Medical University of Warsaw, Poland. The study was performed from July 2016 to April 2019. The inclusion criteria were age from 6 months to 18 years and presence of obstructive nephropathy: ureteropelvic junction obstruction (UPJO), ureterovesical junction obstruction (UVJO), and posterior urethral valves (PUV). The exclusion criteria were occurrence of another CAKUT history of urinary tract infection (UTI) during the last 6 months, surgery in the last 12 months, fibrotic disease of other organs, and acute infections (temporary exclusion). Sixty healthy children were included in the control group. The study design is displayed on the flow diagram in Figure 1. A sample size of the study and control groups was estimated based on the available literature on renal biomarkers with a statistical power of 0.8 and statistical significance $p = 0.05$.

2.2. Ethical Issues

The study was approved by the local Bioethics Committee for Human Research (No. KB/152/2016) before the initiation. The clinical investigation was conducted in accordance ethical standards of the institutional research committee and with the guidelines of the 2013 Declaration of Helsinki. Informed consent was obtained from all participant representatives and participants (≥ 16 years) prior to study inclusion.

2.3. Clinical Parameters

In all participants, the following clinical data were evaluated: age (years), sex, body height (cm), body weight (kg), and blood pressure measurement.

2.4. Biochemical Parameters

In all participants, the following laboratory data were evaluated: serum Cr (mg/dL), serum cystatin C (ng/L), urinary albumin (mg/L), and urinary Cr (mg/dL). Urinalysis and urine culture were performed to rule out urinary tract infection (UTI). Estimated GFR (mL/min/1.73 m^2), according to the revised 2009 Schwartz formula [41], and urinary albumin to urinary Cr ratio (ACR) were calculated. Biochemical parameters were measured using VITROS 5600 Integrated System (Ortho Clinical Diagnostics) except cystatin C (IMMAGE 800 Beckman Coulter Company, Koto, Tokyo). In line with local recommendations, normal serum Cr (depending on age 0.2–0.7 mg/dL), serum cystatin C (depending on age 0.51–1.15 mg/L), and ACR (<30 mg/g Cr) were derived from the manufacturers' reference values.

2.5. Urinary Biomarkers

Urine samples were taken on fasting in the morning, immediately centrifuged according to the manufacturers' instructions, frozen, and stored at $-80\ °C$ until further assays were performed. All biomarkers were measured using enzyme-linked immunosorbent assays (ELISA) kits from Reagent Genie, Dublin, Ireland: TGF-β1-Cat. No. HUFI 00248, Human TGF-β1/TGF-beta-1; endoglin-Cat. No. HUFI 00064, Human CD105/Endoglin; periostin-Cat. No. HUDLO 0236 Human Periostin (POSTN); cytokeratin-18-Cat. No. HUFI 02320, Human CK-18/KRT18/Cytokeratin-18. The urinary TGF-β1, endoglin, periostin and CK-18 levels were normalized to the urinary Cr levels, measured from the same urine samples, and expressed as ng/mg Cr.

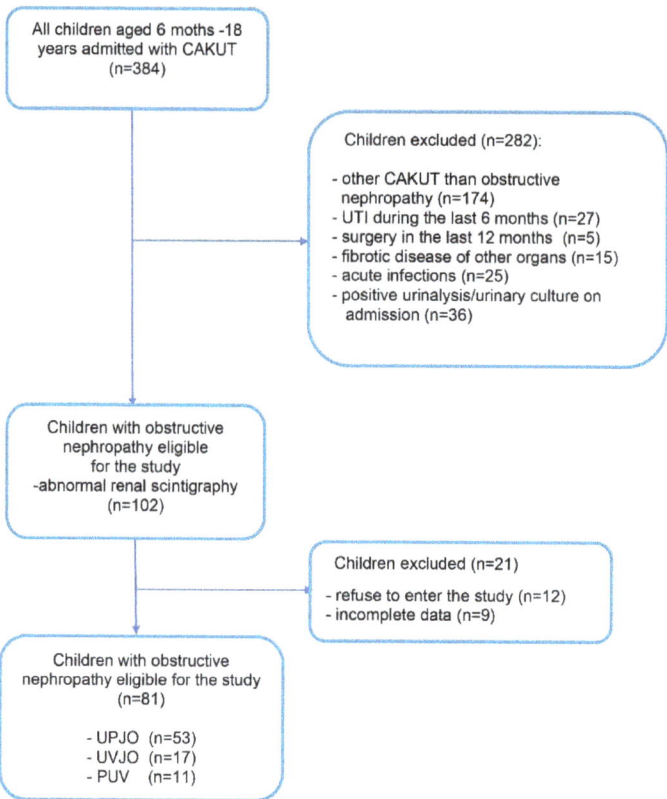

Figure 1. Study flow diagram. CAKUT—congenital anomalies of the kidney and urinary tract; UTI—urinary tract infection; UPJO—ureteropelvic junction obstruction; UVJO—ureterovesical junction obstruction; PUV—posterior urethral valves.

2.6. Imaging Data

In all patients, abdominal ultrasonography and 99mTechnetium-ethylenedicysteine (99mTc-EC) scintigraphy were evaluated at the study entry. US was performed using Philips Epiq 5G device (Royal Philips, Amsterdam, The Netherlands) in B-mode. Pelvic dilatation was classified based on the anterior–posterior diameter (mm) (APD) as follows: severe APD—>20 mm, moderate APD—10–20 mm, and mild APD—<10 mm [42,43].

99mTc-EC was conducted to evaluate renal scarring and relative renal function (RRF). Children were injected with an adequate dose of 99mTc-EC for the child's age and body weight. Two experienced nuclear medicine specialists evaluated radionuclide scans. Renal scars were diagnosed as an abnormal parenchymal layer, irregular renal contour, disorders of tracer placement and uptake [44]. RRF of affected kidney ≥45% was considered normal, and RRF of <45% or >55% was considered abnormal. Renal scars were classified as follows: severe—narrowed parenchymal layer, focal or diffuse tracers placement disorders, and renal radionuclide uptake below 45%; moderate—narrowed parenchymal layer or abnormal kidney outline, focal or diffuse tracers placement disorder, and renal radionuclide uptake above or equal to 45%; borderline lesions—normal parenchymal layer, discreet tracers placement disorder and renal radionuclide uptake above or equal to 45%.

Voiding cystourethrography (VCUG) was evaluated at the moment of CON diagnosis. Children with VUR were excluded from the study, except those with secondary VUR as a consequence of PUV.

2.7. Statistical Analysis

Statistical analysis was performed using Statistica 13.3 PL software (StatSoft, Tulsa, OK, USA). The results were presented as the mean ± standard deviation or the median, interquartile ranges based on the Shapiro–Wilk and the Lilliefors normality test results. The Student's t-test or the Mann–Whitney U-test was used to compare two groups of variables. ANOVA test or Kruskal–Wallis test and post hoc test were performed to analyze differences between three subgroups. The relationship between variables was evaluated using the Pearson or the Spearman's rank correlation. Odds ratio (OR), including 95% confidence interval (CI), were calculated by univariate and multivariate logistic regression analysis to identify variables associated with the presence of renal scars. Variables associated with renal scars in the univariate analysis were included in the multivariate model. Variables that correlated with each other with $r > 0.600$ were excluded from the regression model to avoid collinearity. Receiver operating curve (ROC) analysis was used to calculate the area under the curves (AUC) for laboratory variables and to find the best cut-off values (including 95% CI), sensitivity, and specificity in the detection of renal scarring for each variable. p values less than 0.05 were considered statistically significant for all tests.

3. Results

3.1. Clinical and Laboratory Parameters

Clinical and laboratory data in the study group and in the control group are shown in Table 1. We evaluated 81 children with CON and 60 healthy children. CON was diagnosed due to UPJO in 53 (65%) of children, UVJO in 17 (21%) of children, and PUV in 11 (14%) of children. US at the moment of study entry found severe dilatation of pelvis in 23% of children, moderate dilatation in 63% of children, and mild in 14% of children.

Children with CON had significantly higher levels of cystatin C and ACR, significantly lower GFR, and significantly higher urinary periostin, CK-18, and periostin/Cr compared to the controls. Groups did not differ in terms of age, sex, serum Cr and other urinary biomarkers. The levels of serum Cr were slightly elevated in 6 (7.4%) children, cystatin C in 15 (18.5%) children, and ACR in 15 (18.5%) children. Arterial hypertension was diagnosed in four children who were treated with calcium channel blocker (three children) and angiotensin-converting enzyme inhibitor (one child). Fourteen (17%) children were treated surgically because of a significant obstruction in urine outflow.

3.2. Renal Scintigraphy

Comparison of laboratory variables with the results of renal scintigraphy in the study group is shown in Table 2. According to the 99mTc-EC results, children with CON were divided into three subgroups: group 1 (n = 32, 39.5%)—severe renal scars, group 2 (n = 31, 38.3%)—moderate renal scars, and group 3 (n = 18, 22.2%)—borderline lesions. Children with severe scars had a significantly higher periostin/Cr ratio than those with borderline results. No other differences in laboratory indices of kidney injury and urinary biomarkers were found between children with severe, moderate scars, and borderline lesions. The group of borderline lesions demonstrated significantly higher levels of cystatin C and urinary periostin compared to the control group (0.92 ± 0.21 vs. 0.81 ± 0.15, $p = 0.012$; 0.102 (0.034; 0.149) vs. 0.028 (0.013; 0.053) $p = 0.001$, respectively) and significantly lower levels of GFR compared to the control group (106.18 ± 19.11 vs. 121.60 ± 26.09, $p = 0.018$).

The groups did not differ in terms of other laboratory indices of kidney injury and urinary biomarkers (data not shown).

Table 1. Clinical and laboratory data in the study group and in the control group.

Variables	Study Group (n = 81)	Control Group (n = 60)	p
Demographic data			
Sex, male, n (%)	58 (71.6)	39 (65.0)	0.223
Age at the diagnosis (years)	0.40 (0.10; 4.98)		-
Age at the study entry (years)	3.92 (0.67; 9.17)	4.08 (1.83; 10.08)	0.247
Obstructive uropathy, n (%)			
UPJO	53 (65)		
UVJO	17 (21)		
PUV	11 (14)		
Ultrasonography			
Dilatation of renal pelvis, n (%)			
Severe (APD > 20 mm)	19 (23)		
Moderate (APD 10–20 mm)	51 (63)		
Mild (APD < 10 mm)	11 (14)		
Laboratory data			
Serum Cr (mg/dL)	0.40 (0.30; 0.50)	0.40 (0.30; 0.50)	0.603
Cystatin C (mg/L)	0.91 ± 0.22	0.81 ± 0.15	0.005
GFR (mL/min/1.73 m^2)	106.90 ± 18.57	121.60 ± 26.09	<0.001
ACR (mg/g)	16.87 (7.04; 26.12)	11.67 (4.85; 18.83)	0.024
Urinary biomarkers			
TGF-β1 (ng/mL)	0.038 ± 0.021	0.046 ± 0.027	0.069
Endoglin (ng/mL)	8.82 ± 3.68	9.85 ± 4.86	0.090
Periostin (ng/mL)	0.092 (0.062; 0.160)	0.028 (0.013; 0.053)	<0.001
Cytokeratin-18 (ng/mL)	0.383 ± 0.152	0.320 ± 0.162	0.012
TGF-β1/Cr (ng/mg)	0.088 (0.028; 0.261)	0.103 (0.040; 0.281)	0.450
Endoglin/Cr (ng/mg)	21.39 (6.55; 57.04)	22.47 (9.82; 55.55)	0.580
Periostea/Cr (ng/mg)	0.258 (0.131; 0.508)	0.081 (0.024; 0.164)	<0.001
Cytokeratin-18/Cr (ng/mg)	0.838 (0.310; 1.984)	0.562 (0.293; 1.580)	0.260

UPJO—ureteropelvic junction obstruction; UVJO—ureterovesical junction obstruction; PUV—posterior urethral valves; APD—anterior-posterior diameter; Cr—creatinine; GFR—estimated glomerular filtration rate; ACR—urinary albumin/creatinine ratio; TGF-β1—transforming growth factor- β1.

Table 2. Comparison of laboratory variables with the results of renal scintigraphy in the study group.

Variables	Severe Scars (1)	Moderate Scars (2)	Borderline Lesions (3)
No. patients (%)	32 (39.5%)	31 (38.3%)	18 (22.2%)
Laboratory data			
Serum Cr (mg/dL)	0.35 (0.3; 0.5)	0.3 (0.3; 0.5)	0.5 (0.33; 0.6)
Cystatin C (mg/L)	0.90 ± 0.22	0.91 ± 0.23	0.92 ± 0.21
GFR (mL/min/1.73 m^2)	107.47 ± 21.37	106.70 ± 15.5	106.18 ± 19.11
ACR (mg/g)	17.22 (7.31; 25.00)	19.2 (9.06; 26.74)	9.45 (4.09; 24.28)
Urinary biomarkers			
TGF-β1 (ng/mL)	0.039 ± 0.018	0.036 ± 0.020	0.040 ± 0.026
Endoglin (ng/mL)	9.07 ± 4.57	9.22 ± 3.25	7.70 ± 2.31
Periostin (ng/mL)	0.098 (0.073; 0.208)	0.080 (0.063; 0.125)	0.102 (0.034; 0.149)
Cytokeratin-18 (ng/mL)	0.370 ± 0.142	0.391 ± 0.153	0.394 ± 0.174
TGF-β1/Cr (ng/mg)	0.095 (0.034; 0.286)	0.088 (0.026; 0.238)	0.038 (0.014; 0.228)
Endoglin/Cr (ng/mg)	22.16 (8.30; 60.55)	25.16 (8.65; 62.36)	9.73 (4.48; 44.45)
Periostin/Cr (ng/mg)	0.342 (0.161; 0.616) *	0.269 (0.172; 0.473)	0.110 (0.070; 0.250)
Cytokeratin-18/Cr (ng/mg)	0.976 (0.355; 2.188)	0.961 (0.530; 1.774)	0.442 (0.268; 1.530)

Cr—creatinine; GFR—estimated glomerular filtration rate; ACR—urinary albumin/creatinine ratio; TGF-β1—transforming growth factor-β1. * p—0.010 versus borderline lesions.

Normal RRF (45–55%) demonstrated 49 (60.5%) of children and decreased RRF < 45% 32 (39.5%) of children. RRF less than 10% was found in 2 (2.5%) of children, RRF 10–19% in 4 (5%) of children, 20–39% in 13 (16%) of children, and 40–44% in 13 (16%) of children. Correlations of urinary biomarkers with RRF in the scintigraphy in the study group are shown in Table 3. No correlation between urinary biomarkers and RRF was found.

Table 3. Correlations between urinary biomarkers and %RRF in the study group.

Variables	%RRF	
	r	p
TGF-β1	0.04	0.708
Endoglin	0.10	0.386
Periostin	−0.15	0.190
Cytokeratin-18	−0.01	0.921
TGF-β1/Cr	0.03	0.785
Endoglin/Cr	0.07	0.560
Periostin/Cr	−0.12	0.293
Cytokeratin-18/Cr	0.02	0.868

%RRF—relative renal function Cr—creatinine; TGF-β1—transforming growth factor-β1.

3.3. Correlation of Laboratory Parameters

Correlations between urinary biomarkers and widely used laboratory indices of kidney injury in the studied children are shown in Table 4. All standardized to Cr biomarkers correlated with cystatin C and ACR. There was a negative correlation between biomarkers and serum Cr. None of the biomarkers correlated with GFR except endoglin/Cr.

Table 4. Correlations between urinary biomarkers and laboratory indices of kidney injury in the studied children.

Variables	Serum Cr		Cystatin C		GFR		ACR	
	r	p	r	p	r	p	r	p
TGF-β1/Cr	−0.45	<0.001	0.27	<0.001	0.14	0.104	0.35	<0.001
Endoglin/Cr	−0.54	<0.001	0.24	0.004	0.18	0.037	0.44	<0.001
Periostin/Cr	−0.48	<0.001	0.26	0.002	0.11	0.210	0.49	<0.001
Cytokeratin-18/Cr	−0.57	<0.001	0.27	<0.001	0.06	0.448	0.47	<0.001

Cr—creatinine; GFR—estimated glomerular filtration rate; ACR—urinary albumin/creatinine ratio; TGF-β1—transforming growth factor-β1.

Inter-correlations of normalized urinary biomarkers in the studied children are shown in Table 5. A strong positive correlation was found between TGF-β1/Cr and endoglin/Cr, TGF-β1/Cr, and CK-18/Cr, as well between endoglin/Cr and CK-18/Cr. A weaker correlation was revealed between periostin/Cr and other biomarkers.

Table 5. Inter-correlations of normalized urinary biomarkers in the studied children.

Variables	TGF-β1/Cr		Periostin/Cr		Cytokeratin-18/Cr	
	r	p	r	p	r	p
TGF-β1/Cr	-	-	0.37	<0.001	0.71	<0.001
Endoglin/Cr	0.72	<0.001	0.53	<0.001	0.73	<0.001
Periostin/Cr	0.39	<0.001	-	-	0.54	<0.001

TGF-β1—transforming growth factor-β1.

3.4. Relation between Laboratory Parameters and Renal Scars

Univariate and multivariate logistic regression analysis of laboratory variables related to the presence of severe and moderate scars are shown in Table 6a, and related to the presence of borderline lesions are shown in Table 6b. In univariate logistic regression analysis, cystatin C, GFR ACR, and urinary biomarkers—TGF-β1, CK-18, periostin, and periostin/Cr were associated with the presence of severe and moderate renal scars. Multivariate analysis demonstrated that GFR, TGF-β1, and periostin were independently related to the presence of severe and moderate scars. Urinary periostin/Cr was excluded from the multivariate model due to collinearity.

Table 6. Univariate and multivariate logistic regression analysis of laboratory variables related to the presence of severe, moderate renal scars and borderline lesions in the scintigraphy. **a.** Univariate and multivariate logistic regression analysis of laboratory variables related to the presence of severe and moderate renal scars in the scintigraphy (n = 63). **b.** Univariate and multivariate logistic regression analysis of laboratory variables related to the presence of borderline lesions in the scintigraphy (n = 18).

	Variables	Univariate Regression Analysis		Multivariate Regression Analysis	
		OR (95% CI)	p	OR (95% CI)	p
a					
	Laboratory data				
	Serum Cr (mg/dL)	1.23 (0.15–9.90)	0.841	-	-
	Cystatin C (mg/L)	12.58 (1.62–97.58)	0.014	7.09 (0.61–82.54)	0.114
	GFR (mL/min/1.73 m^2)	0.97 (0.95–0.99)	0.001	0.96 (0.94–0.98)	<0.001
	ACR (mg/g)	1.03 (1.00–1.06)	0.027	1.04 (1.00–1.07)	0.053
	Urinary biomarkers				
	TGF-β1 (ng/mL)	0.85 (0.72–0.99)	0.036	0.89 (0.73–1.08)	0.225
	Endoglin (ng/mL)	0.96 (0.89–1.05)	0.374	-	-
	Periostin (ng/mL)	1.28 (1.15–1.43)	<0.001	1.26 (1.12–1.40)	<0.001
	Cytokeratin-18 (ng/mL)	12.93 (1.13–148.19)	0.038	25.99 (1.25–539.35)	0.033
	TGF-β1/Cr (ng/mg)	0.99 (0.98–1.01)	0.441	-	-
	Endoglin/Cr (ng/mg)	0.90 (0.65–1.24)	0.512	-	-
	Periostin/Cr (ng/mg) *	1.05 (1.03–1.07)	<0.001	-	-
	Cytokeratin-18/Cr (ng/mg)	1.13 (0.92–1.39)	0.229	-	-
b					
	Laboratory data				
	Serum Cr (mg/dL)	14.23 (0.75–269.34)	0.072	-	-
	Cystatin C (mg/L)	35.80 (1.45–885.94)	0.026	62.83 (1.65–2397.05)	0.023
	GFR (mL/min/1.73 m^2)	0.97 (0.94–1.00)	0.027	1.00 (0.96–1.04)	0.055
	ACR (mg/g)	1.00 (0.96–1.04)	0.906	-	-
	Urinary biomarkers				
	TGF-β1 (ng/mL)	0.91 (0.75–1.11)	0.343	-	-
	Endoglin (ng/mL)	0.89 (0.78–1.01)	0.077	-	-
	Periostin (ng/mL)	1.20 (1.08–1.33)	0.001	1.17 (1.05–1.31)	0.005
	Cytokeratin-18 (ng/mL)	14.48 (0.55–384.17)	0.104	-	-
	TGF-β1/Cr (ng/mg)	1.00 (0.98–1.02)	0.939	-	-
	Endoglin/Cr (ng/mg) **	0.61 (0.38–0.98)	0.038	-	-
	Periostin/Cr (ng/mg)	1.01 (0.99–1.04)	0.288	-	-
	Cytokeratin–18/Cr (ng/mg)	0.95 (0.66–1.38)	0.805	-	-

Cr—creatinine; GFR—estimated glomerular filtration rate; ACR—urinary albumin/creatinine ratio; TGF-β1—transforming growth factor-β1. * Periostin/Cr excluded from multivariate model due to collinearity. ** Endoglin/Cr excluded from multivariate model due to collinearity.

Cystatin C, GFR, periostin, and endoglin/Cr were related to the presence of borderline lesions in univariate analysis, whereas in multivariate analysis, cystatin C and periostin were independently related to borderline lesions. Endoglin/Cr was excluded from multivariate analysis due to collinearity.

Diagnostic usefulness of laboratory variables for diagnosing severe and moderate renal scars in the scintigraphy is shown in Table 7a, and for diagnosing borderline lesions, in the scintigraphy in Table 7b. ROC analysis demonstrated that periostin and periostin/Cr had higher AUC for detection of severe and moderate scars than cystatin C, GFR, ACR, TGF-β1, and CK-18 (Table 7a), and periostin had higher AUC than cystatin C, GFR, endoglin, and periostin/Cr for diagnosing borderline lesions (Table 7b).

Table 7. Diagnostic usefulness of laboratory variables for diagnosing severe, moderate renal scars and borderline lesions.
a. Diagnostic usefulness of laboratory variables for diagnosing severe and moderate renal scars in the scintigraphy (n = 63).
b. Diagnostic usefulness of laboratory variables for diagnosing renal borderline lesions in the scintigraphy (n = 18).

	Variables	AUC (95%CI)	p	Cut-Off	Sensitivity (%)	Specificity (%)
a						
	Laboratory data					
	Serum Cr (mg/dL)	0.503 (0.400–0.606)	0.958	0.40	55.0	52.4
	Cystatin C (mg/L)	0.624 (0.525–0.723)	0.014	0.92	47.6	74.6
	GFR (mL/min/1.73 m^2)	0.678 (0.583–0.772)	<0.001	104.90	75.0	55.6
	ACR (mg/g)	0.647 (0.550–0.744)	0.003	16.40	56.5	68.3
	Urinary biomarkers					
	TGF-β1 (ng/mL)	0.630 (0.526–0.733)	0.014	0.052	53.3	79.4
	Endoglin (ng/mL)	0.579 (0.475–0.684)	0.136	11.825	38.3	87.3
	Periostin (ng/mL)	0.849 (0.780–0.918)	<0.001	0.053	84.1	75.0
	Cytokeratin-18 (ng/mL)	0.611 (0.511–0.712)	0.030	0.292	74.6	50.0
	TGF-β1/Cr (ng/mg)	0.514 (0.410–0.618)	0.791	0.092	60.0	50.8
	Endoglin/Cr (ng/mg)	0.527 (0.423–0.632)	0.606	6.794	87.5	23.8
	Periostin/Cr (ng/mg)	0.810 (0.731–0.888)	<0.001	0.131	84.1	70.0
	Cytokeratin-18/Cr (ng/mg)	0.580 (0.479–0.682)	0.121	0.758	60.3	58.3
b						
	Laboratory data					
	Serum Cr (mg/dL)	0.625 (0.473–0.778)	0.108	0.50	55.6	66.7
	Cystatin C (mg/L)	0.645 (0.502–0.789)	0.047	0.80	83.3	49.2
	GFR (mL/min/1.73 m^2)	0.669 (0.533–0.804)	0.015	118.40	50.0	83.3
	ACR (mg/g)	0.508 (0.341–0.676)	0.922	4.51	81.7	33.3
	Urinary biomarkers					
	TGF-β1 (ng/mL)	0.566 (0.426–0.706)	0.358	0.055	46.7	72.2
	Endoglin (ng/mL)	0.661 (0.544–0.779)	0.007	10.444	48.3	94.4
	Periostin (ng/mL)	0.777 (0.642–0.911)	<0.001	0.086	66.7	86.0
	Cytokeratin-18 (ng/mL)	0.626 (0.480–0.771)	0.090	0.397	61.1	70.0
	TGF-β1/Cr (ng/mg)	0.553 (0.396–0.710)	0.506	0.043	73.3	55.6
	Endoglin/Cr (ng/mg)	0.655 (0.491–0.818)	0.064	5.496	92.9	44.4
	Periostin/Cr (ng/mg)	0.658 (0.530–0.785)	0.015	0.046	94.4	38.3
	Cytokeratin-18/Cr (ng/mg)	0.532 (0.377–0.688)	0.682	0.493	56.7	61.1

Cr—creatinine; GFR—estimated glomerular filtration rate; ACR—urinary albumin/creatinine ratio; TGF-β1—transforming growth factor-β1.

4. Discussion

Our cross-sectional single-center study investigated the predictive value of new biomarkers, such as endoglin, periostin, and CK-18, for assessing the severity of renal scarring in children with CON. We also evaluated TGF-β1, the most recognized fibrotic factor, which served as our reference ("gold standard"). Here, we report that urinary periostin, periostin/Cr, and CK-18 were significantly higher in children with CON compared to the healthy controls. In addition, children with severe scars had significantly higher urinary periostin/Cr levels than those with borderline lesions. Thus, periostin and periostin/Cr demonstrated a better diagnostic profile for diagnosing renal scars than other evaluated biomarkers. However, both periostin and periostin/Cr did not differentiate severe and moderate scars from borderline lesions. Endoglin showed moderate usefulness for diagnosing borderline lesions, and CK-18 and TGF-β1 revealed low utility for diagnosing severe and moderate scars.

Multiple clinical studies confirmed the usefulness of urinary TGF-β1 for the diagnosis of urinary tract obstruction and tubulointerstitial fibrosis. Children with obstructive uropathy demonstrated significantly higher TGF-β1 levels than those with non-obstructive hydronephrosis and healthy controls [4,45,46]. A significant decrease in elevated TGF-β1 levels was observed after pyeloplasty [47]. Patients who improved renal function after nephrostomy (i.e., those in whom GFR increased) had significantly lower TGF-β1 levels at presentation compared to those who did not [48]. Elevated urinary TGF-β1 demonstrated 82% accuracy for differentiation reversible obstruction from irreversible [48] and 90.8% accuracy for long-term follow-up after pyeloplasty [47]. The ESCAPE trial revealed markedly higher urinary TGF-β1 levels in children with mild to moderate CKD and CON compared to those with CKD and other kidney diseases [14].

In contrast, our study found no differences in urinary TGF-β1 and TGF-β1/Cr levels between children with CON and healthy controls. Palmer et al. reported elevated TGF-β1 levels only in the pelvis of the obstructed kidney but not in the bladder urine [49]. Some authors suppose that the production of TGF-β1 is increased in the early phase of tissue damage and reduced in the terminal stage of tissue degeneration [14,17]. We did not find any differences in TGF-β1 and TGF-β1/Cr levels between subgroups with severe, moderate scars and borderline lesions. Despite this, urinary TGF-β1 was associated with the presence of advanced scars. However, its diagnostic potential for detecting scars was low. In our study, 17% of children were at least one year after surgery of urinary tract obstruction, which could reduce their TGF-β1 level. A slight increase in serum Cr was found in 7.4% of children and in cystatin C in 18.5% of children. RRF in scintigraphy less than 10% demonstrated in 2.5% of patients. It could also have had an impact on the results obtained.

The importance of endoglin in renal fibrosis was documented in several animal models of renal fibrosis. For example, the model of tubulointerstitial fibrosis induced by unilateral ureteral obstruction (UUO) demonstrated an increase in endoglin mRNA and protein expression in the obstructed kidney [9,19,50]. Model of renal ischemia–reperfusion (I-R) injury showed coincidence endoglin expression with increased TGF-β1 mRNA expression. In this study, haploinsufficient mice of endoglin (Eng+/−) were protected for renal I-R injury compared to their wild type (WT) littermates (Eng+/+) [20]. Roy-Chaudhury et al. described an association of interstitial endoglin expression and chronic histological damage in biopsies from patients with progressive CKD [24]. A recent study by Gerrits et al. revealed an increase in interstitial endoglin expression in autopsy samples obtained from diabetic patients with DN compared to those without DN. Renal endoglin expression correlated with the degree of interstitial fibrosis and increased serum Cr, reduced GFR, and hypertension in DN [11].

In our cohort of pediatric patients, we demonstrated no differences in urinary endoglin and endoglin/Cr levels between children with CON and the controls, as well as between subgroups with severe, moderate scars, and borderline lesions. Only endoglin/Cr was related to the presence of borderline lesions. In ROC analysis, endoglin showed moderate utility as a biomarker for diagnosing borderline lesions. However, its specificity was very high. We did not evaluate L-Eng and S-Eng isoforms. Therefore, we do not know if an association of endoglin with borderline lesions is due to the upregulation of pro-fibrotic L-Eng or anti-fibrotic S-Eng, especially in children with borderline lesions.

Recent studies have identified periostin as a novel key factor in the progression of kidney disease. Overexpression of periostin following renal injury was described in different models of renal fibrosis, such as UUO, 5/6 nephrectomy, hypertensive renal injury, and renal I-R injury [31,51,52]. High expression of periostin was associated with acceleration of cyst growth and fibrosis in PKD [33,53]. Periostin overexpression was observed in patients with different types of progressive nephropathies, including lupus nephropathy and chronic allograft nephropathy (CAN) [7,32,54]. Patients with high levels of urinary periostin at the time of AKI episode were more likely to progress to CKD [52]. In the study by Hwang et al., higher urinary periostin/Cr levels at the time of renal biopsy were associated with tissue periostin overexpression, a higher degree of fibrosis, a greater decline in GFR, and poor renal outcome in IgAN patients [29]. Some studies demonstrated a protective effect of periostin suppression for CKD progression. Periostin-null mice showed a decrease in apoptosis compared to the WT mice [25,52].

In the present study, we demonstrated significantly higher urinary periostin and periostin/Cr levels in children with CON compared to the controls and significantly higher periostin/Cr levels in children with severe scars compared to those with borderline lesions. Both periostin and periostin/Cr demonstrated relatively high utility for diagnosing scars and moderate utility for diagnosing borderline lesions. However, based on diagnostic profile and cut-off in ROC analysis, periostin did not allow for differentiation of severe and moderate scars from borderline lesions.

It is difficult to explain why periostin was of no use to differentiate scars from borderline lesions, especially that we showed significantly higher levels of periostin/Cr in children with severe scars compared to those with borderline lesions. Although we confirmed that periostin is strongly related to renal fibrosis, we still know too little about the regulation of periostin expression and its signaling pathways [33]. Recent evidence suggests that periostin might be a tissue repair molecule that stimulates signaling pathways involved in tissue regeneration [33,55,56]. Korman et al. revealed a protective effect of periostin in the model of AKI induced by renal I-R injury. They demonstrated that periostin overexpression was associated with lower expression of pro-inflammatory cytokines, less epithelial damage, increased proliferation of pro-regenerative macrophage phenotypes, and less severe injury than the periostin-null mouse. In the authors' opinion, periostin may play a protective role in AKI and a detrimental role in CKD [56]. In our study, we followed patients with chronic renal fibrosis. Therefore, periostin overexpression could not be related to renal tissue regeneration.

CK-18 is a cell-protective and stress-responsive protein that seems to be a novel sensitive marker of renal tubular cell stress and tubular injury. Experimental studies demonstrated an increase in CK-18 expression in different models of renal injury. In the model of UUO, upregulation of CK-18 occurred very early after UUO induction and increased with renal injury progression. Additionally, the model of progressive GN with secondary tubulointerstitial injury and fibrosis showed only slight CK-18 expression in the early stage of disease and significantly higher expression in the late stage. Overexpression of CK-18 in renal biopsy was reported in the majority of renal tubules in the cast, diabetic, and lupus nephropathy, as well in the Bowman capsule in crescentic necrotic GN [39].

In this study, we found significantly higher urinary CK-18 levels in children with CON compared to the controls, but no differences were observed in terms of CK-18 and CK-18/Cr between the three subgroups. Urinary CK-18 was associated with the presence of scars, but its diagnostic value was low. In the study by Djudjaj et al., elevated urinary CK-18 levels were found in animals with adenine nephropathy and Alport syndrome and in patients with AKI [39]. Roth et al. reported significantly higher urinary CK-18 levels in CKD stage 5 compared to the healthy controls [37]. During cell degeneration, CK-18 is released in two forms depending on the type of cell death. In cells apoptosis, caspase cleaved CK-18 fragments are produced, while in cell necrosis, CK-18 is liberated without caspase-mediated modifications [57]. In CKD, cell loss results mainly from cell necrosis, while in the obstructed kidney, cell death is most susceptible to apoptosis [3,58]. Choi et al. confirmed a progressive increase in tubular and interstitial cell apoptosis during the duration of renal obstruction [59]. We did not assess caspase cleaved CK-18. However, we can speculate that our patients could have high levels of CK-18 fragments due to apoptosis followed by urinary tract obstruction.

It is not known whether urinary fibrotic biomarkers are associated with clinical and laboratory indices of kidney injury. In the ESCAPE trial, GFR inversely correlated with urinary TGF-β1 [14]. Similarly, a negative correlation was reported with urinary periostin in IgAN [29] and chronic allograft nephropathy (CAN) [7] and urinary CK-18 in CKD [37]. Some studies reported positive correlations of TGF-β1 with proteinuria and urinary α1-microglobulin in CON [4], urinary periostin with proteinuria in CAN [7], and CK-18 with proteinuria and albuminuria in CKD stage 5 [37]. In contrast, other authors did not show any correlations of urinary TGF-β1 with serum Cr, GFR, ACR, proteinuria, and degree of tubulointerstitial fibrosis [4,17].

We found positive correlations of the normalized biomarkers with cystatin C and ACR, negative correlations with serum Cr, and no relation with GFR except endoglin/Cr.

These negative correlations with serum Cr were probably related to our study's relatively large number of young children. In infants and young children, low serum Cr levels, due to small muscle mass in this age, and greater Cr tubular reabsorption lead to low urinary Cr excretion [2]. It results in higher values of normalized biomarkers and is responsible for a negative correlation with serum Cr. Due to the heterogenicity of children's age in our study, we assessed biomarkers with and without normalization.

In our study, we also evaluated the association of widely used laboratory indices of kidney injury with the presence of renal scars and borderline lesions. We found that only ACR was able to differentiate children with scars from those with borderline lesions. However, its diagnostic value was relatively low. The ESCAPE trial also demonstrated inter-correlation of urinary TGF-β1 with other biomarkers that participated in the progression of tissue injury in CKD [14]. In line with this study, we found an inter-correlation of all normalized biomarkers. These results are not unexpected. It is well-known that TGF-β1 is the major stimulator of endoglin and periostin expression, periostin creates a feedback loop with TGF-β1, and CK18 was identified as an important factor in renal fibrosis [9,10,27,32,33,39].

Some studies evaluated the correlation of the intensity of renal fibrosis and urinary biomarkers with RRF of obstructed kidney in a nuclear renal scan. Zhang demonstrated a correlation between the intensity of renal fibrosis in renal biopsy performed during pyeloplasty and RRF of affected kidney [60]. In contrast, other authors did not show any correlation between urinary TGF-β1 and RRF [4,47]. In the present study, 99mTc-EC scintigraphy was used for renal scars assessment, which is an alternative to 99mTc-dimercaptosuccinic acid (DMSA) scintigraphy, with high sensitivity (98.75%) and specificity (99.15%) for detection of scars in normally positioned kidneys but with lower radiation dose [61]. We demonstrated that approximately half of our children with advanced scars demonstrated tracer uptake higher than 45%. We also did not find a correlation between urinary biomarkers and RRF in children with CON.

Urinary tract obstruction leads to a reduction in functioning nephrons and to the compensatory adaptation of the remaining. Therefore, it may affect RRF results [2]. In addition, in hydronephrosis, tracer accumulation in the obstructed kidney, as well as an increase in blood flow caused by altered renal hemodynamics, may cause falsely high RRF [62,63]. Men-Meir et al. demonstrated that "supranormal" RRF in the obstructed kidney is not always a favorable sign and may even be a warning sign of impending decompensation. Therefore, a measure of RRT has a low predictive value for renal fibrosis in children with CON.

Our study has some limitations. This single-center research may be associated with the bias occurrence. The cross-sectional design of the study prevents from drawing definitive and causative conclusions. The number of analyzed patients in subgroups was relatively low. Heterogenicity of patients' ages, various causes of obstructive nephropathy, and different patient follow-up may impact the results. In addition, we have not analyzed the fibrosis markers in other groups of patients, e.g., in glomerulopathies.

5. Conclusions

To the best of our knowledge, this study, for the first time, demonstrates that periostin, endoglin, and CK-18 are associated with renal fibrosis in children with congenital obstructive nephropathy. Periostin showed a higher diagnostic profile for diagnosing renal scars than other evaluated biomarkers. However, periostin did not differentiate advanced scars from borderline lesions. CK-18 and TGF-β1 demonstrated low utility, and endoglin was not useful for diagnosing advanced scars. In our opinion, periostin seems to be a promising, non-invasive marker for the assessment of renal fibrosis in children with CON. However, future studies on more patients are needed to confirm our results.

Author Contributions: Conceptualization, A.T. and M.P.-T.; methodology, A.T., M.P.-T., G.K., E.G. and U.D.; validation, A.T., M.P.-T. and G.K.; formal analysis, A.T. and G.K.; investigation, A.T., E.G. and U.D.; resources, M.P.-T.; data curation, A.T.; writing—original draft preparation, A.T. and G.K.; writing—review and editing, M.P.-T.; visualization, A.T.; supervision, M.P.-T.; project administration, A.T. and M.P.-T.; funding acquisition, M.P.-T. All authors have read and agreed to the published version of the manuscript.

Funding: This research was funded from the statutory funds of the Department of Pediatrics and Nephrology, Medical University of Warsaw.

Institutional Review Board Statement: The study was conducted according to the guidelines of the Declaration of Helsinki and approved by the Local Bioethics Committee of the Medical University of Warsaw (approval No. KB/152/2016).

Informed Consent Statement: Informed consent was obtained from all subjects ($\geq$16 years) and their representatives involved in the study.

Data Availability Statement: The data analyzed in this study are available from the corresponding author on reasonable request.

Conflicts of Interest: The authors declare no conflict of interest.

References

1. Harambat, J.; van Stralen, K.J.; Kim, J.J.; Tizard, E.J. Epidemiology of chronic kidney disease in children. *Pediatr. Nephrol.* **2012**, *27*, 363–373. [CrossRef]
2. Chevalier, R.L. Prognostic factors and biomarkers of congenital obstructive nephropathy. *Pediatr. Nephrol.* **2015**, *31*, 1411–1420. [CrossRef]
3. Chevalier, R.L.; Thornhill, B.A.; Forbes, M.S.; Kiley, S.C. Mechanisms of renal injury and progression of renal disease in congenital obstructive nephropathy. *Pediatr. Nephrol.* **2009**, *25*, 687–697. [CrossRef]
4. Zieg, J.; Blahova, K.; Seeman, T.; Bronsky, J.; Dvorakova, H.; Pechova, M.; Janda, J.; Matousovic, K. Urinary transforming growth factor-β1 in children with obstructive uropathy. *Nephrology* **2011**, *16*, 595–598. [CrossRef]
5. Misseri, R.; Rink, R.C.; Meldrum, D.R.; Meldrum, K.K. Inflammatory mediators and growth factors in obstructive renal injury. *J. Surg. Res.* **2004**, *119*, 149–159. [CrossRef]
6. Zhang, Z.; Quinlan, J.; Hoy, W.; Hughson, M.D.; Lemire, M.; Hudson, T.; Hueber, P.A.; Benjamin, A.; Roy, A.; Pascuet, E.; et al. A common RET variant is associated with reduced newborn kidney size and function. *J. Am. Soc. Nephrol.* **2008**, *19*, 2027–2034. [CrossRef] [PubMed]
7. Satirapoj, B.; Witoon, R.; Ruangkanchanasetr, P.; Wantanasiri, P.; Charoenpitakchai, M.; Choovichian, P. Urine Periostin as a Biomarker of Renal Injury in Chronic Allograft Nephropathy. *Transplant. Proc.* **2014**, *46*, 135–140. [CrossRef] [PubMed]
8. Goumenos, D.S.; Tsamandas, A.C.; Oldroyd, S.; Sotsiou, F.; Tsakas, S.; Petropoulou, C.; Bonikos, D.; El Nahas, A.M.; Vlachojannis, J.G. Transforming growth factor-beta(1) and myofibroblasts: A potential pathway towards renal scarring in human glomerular disease. *Nephron* **2001**, *87*, 240–248. [CrossRef]
9. Muñoz-Félix, J.M.; Pérez-Roque, L.; Núñez-Gómez, E.; Oujo, B.; Arévalo, M.; Ruiz-Remolina, L.; Cuesta, C.; Langa, C.; Pérez-Barriocanal, F.; Bernabeu, C.; et al. Overexpression of the short endoglin isoform reduces renal fibrosis and inflammation after unilateral ureteral obstruction. *Biochim. Biophys. Acta* **2016**, *1862*, 1801–1814. [CrossRef]
10. Meng, X.-M.; Nikolic-Paterson, D.J.; Lan, H.Y. TGF-β: The master regulator of fibrosis. *Nat. Rev. Nephrol.* **2016**, *12*, 325–338. [CrossRef] [PubMed]
11. Gerrits, T.; Zandbergen, M.; Wolterbeek, R.; Bruijn, J.A.; Baelde, H.J.; Scharpfenecker, M. Endoglin Promotes Myofibroblast Differentiation and Extracellular Matrix Production in Diabetic Nephropathy. *Int. J. Mol. Sci.* **2020**, *21*, 7713. [CrossRef]
12. Diamond, J.R.; Kees-Folts, D.; Ding, G.; Frye, J.E.; Restrepo, N.C. Macrophages, monocyte chemoattractant peptide-1, and TGF-beta 1 in experimental hydronephrosis. *Am. J. Physiol. Physiol.* **1994**, *266*, F926–F933. [CrossRef] [PubMed]
13. Fukuda, K.; Yoshitomi, K.; Yanagida, T.; Tokumoto, M.; Hirakata, H. Quantification of TGF-beta1 mRNA along rat nephron in obstructive nephropathy. *Am. J. Physiol. Renal Physiol.* **2001**, *281*, F513–F521. [CrossRef] [PubMed]
14. Grenda, R.; Wühl, E.; Litwin, M.; Janas, R.; Sladowska, J.; Arbeiter, K.; Berg, U.; Caldas-Afonso, A.; Fischbach, M.; Mehls, O.; et al. Urinary excretion of endothelin-1 (ET-1), transforming growth factor- beta1 (TGF-beta1) and vascular endothelial growth factor (VEGF165) in paediatric chronic kidney diseases: Results of the ESCAPE trial. *Nephrol. Dial. Transplant.* **2007**, *22*, 3487–3494. [CrossRef]
15. Goumenos, D.S.; Tsakas, S.; El Nahas, A.M.; Alexandri, S.; Oldroyd, S.; Kalliakmani, P.; Vlachojannis, J.G. Transforming growth factor-beta(1) in the kidney and urine of patients with glomerular disease and proteinuria. *Nephrol. Dial. Transplant.* **2002**, *17*, 2145–2152. [CrossRef] [PubMed]

16. Goumenos, D.S.; Kalliakmani, P.; Tsakas, S.; Sotsiou, F.; Vlachojannis, J.G. Urinary Transforming Growth Factor-beta 1 as a marker of response to immunosuppressive treatment, in patients with crescentic nephritis. *BMC Nephrol.* **2005**, *6*, 16. [CrossRef] [PubMed]
17. De Muro, P.; Faedda, R.; Fresu, P.; Masala, A.; Cigni, A.; Concas, G.; Mela, M.G.; Satta, A.; Carcassi, A.; Sanna, G.M.; et al. Urinary transforming growth factor-beta 1 in various types of nephropathy. *Pharmacol. Res.* **2004**, *49*, 293–298.
18. Muñoz-Felix, J.M.; Oujo, B.; Lopez-Novoa, J.M. The role of endoglin in kidney fibrosis. *Expert Rev. Mol. Med.* **2014**, *16*, e18. [CrossRef] [PubMed]
19. Oujo, B.; Muñoz-Félix, J.M.; Arevalo, M.; Nuñez-Gomez, E.; Perez-Roque, L.; Pericacho, M.; Gonzalez-Nunez, M.; Langa, C.; Martinez-Salgado, C.; Pérez-Barriocanal, F.; et al. L-Endoglin Overexpression Increases Renal Fibrosis after Unilateral Ureteral Obstruction. *PLoS ONE* **2014**, *9*, e110365. [CrossRef] [PubMed]
20. Docherty, N.; López-Novoa, J.M.; Arevalo, M.; Düwel, A.; Rodriguez-Peña, A.; Pérez-Barriocanal, F.; Bernabeu, C.; Eleno, N. Endoglin regulates renal ischaemia–reperfusion injury. *Nephrol. Dial. Transplant.* **2006**, *21*, 2106–2119. [CrossRef] [PubMed]
21. Scharpfenecker, M.; Floot, B.; Russell, N.S.; Stewart, F.A. The TGF-β co-receptor endoglin regulates macrophage infiltration and cytokine production in the irradiated mouse kidney. *Radiother. Oncol.* **2012**, *105*, 313–320. [CrossRef]
22. Rodríguez-Peña, A.; Prieto, M.; Duwel, A.; Rivas, J.V.; Eleno, N.; Pérez-Barriocanal, F.; Arévalo, M.; Smith, J.D.; Vary, C.P.; Bernabeu, C.; et al. Up-regulation of endoglin, a TGF-beta-binding protein, in rats with experimental renal fibrosis induced by renal mass reduction. *Nephrol. Dial. Transplant.* **2001**, *16* (Suppl. 1), 34–39. [CrossRef] [PubMed]
23. Rodríguez-Peña, A.; Eleno, N.; Düwell, A.; Arévalo, M.; Pérez-Barriocanal, F.; Flores, O.; Docherty, N.; Bernabeu, C.; Letarte, M.; Lopez-Novoa, J.M. Endoglin Upregulation During Experimental Renal Interstitial Fibrosis in Mice. *Hypertension* **2002**, *40*, 713–720. [CrossRef]
24. Roy-Chaudhury, P.; Simpson, J.G.; Power, D. Endoglin, a transforming growth factor-beta-binding protein, is upregulated in chronic progressive renal disease. *Exp. Nephrol.* **1997**, *5*, 55–60. [PubMed]
25. Hwang, J.H.; Yang, S.H.; Kim, Y.C.; Kim, J.H.; An, J.N.; Moon, K.C.; Oh, Y.K.; Park, J.Y.; Kim, D.K.; Kim, Y.S.; et al. Experimental Inhibition of Periostin Attenuates Kidney Fibrosis. *Am. J. Nephrol.* **2017**, *46*, 501–517. [CrossRef] [PubMed]
26. Conway, S.J.; Izuhara, K.; Kudo, Y.; Litvin, J.; Markwald, R.; Ouyang, G.; Arron, J.; Holweg, C.T.J.; Kudo, A. The role of periostin in tissue remodeling across health and disease. *Experientia* **2013**, *71*, 1279–1288. [CrossRef]
27. Kudo, A.; Kii, I. Periostin function in communication with extracellular matrices. *J. Cell Commun. Signal.* **2017**, *12*, 301–308. [CrossRef] [PubMed]
28. Kudo, A. Periostin in fibrillogenesis for tissue regeneration: Periostin actions inside and outside the cell. *Experientia* **2011**, *68*, 3201–3207. [CrossRef] [PubMed]
29. Hwang, J.H.; Lee, J.P.; Kim, C.T.; Yang, S.H.; Kim, J.H.; An, J.N.; Moon, K.C.; Lee, H.; Oh, Y.K.; Joo, K.W.; et al. Urinary Periostin Excretion Predicts Renal Outcome in IgA Nephropathy. *Am. J. Nephrol.* **2016**, *44*, 481–492. [CrossRef] [PubMed]
30. Prakoura, N.; Kavvadas, P.; Kormann, R.; Dussaule, J.C.; Chadjichristos, C.E.; Chatziantoniou, C. NFκB-Induced Periostin Activates Integrin-β3 Signaling to Promote Renal Injury in GN. *J. Am. Soc. Nephrol.* **2017**, *28*, 1475–1490.
31. Mael-Ainin, M.; Abed, A.; Conway, S.J.; Dussaule, J.C.; Chatziantoniou, C. Inhibition of Periostin Expression Protects against the Development of Renal Inflammation and Fibrosis. *J. Am. Soc. Nephrol.* **2014**, *25*, 1724–1736. [CrossRef] [PubMed]
32. Sen, K.; Lindenmeyer, M.T.; Gaspert, A.; Eichinger, F.; Neusser, M.A.; Kretzler, M.; Segerer, S.; Cohen, C.D. Periostin is induced in glomerular injury and expressed de novo in interstitial renal fibrosis. *Am. J. Pathol.* **2011**, *179*, 1756–1767.
33. Wallace, D.P. Periostin in the Kidney. *Single Mol. Single Cell Seq.* **2019**, *1132*, 99–112. [CrossRef]
34. Steinert, P.M.; Parry, D.A.; Racoosin, E.L.; Idler, W.W.; Steven, A.C.; Trus, B.L.; Roop, D.R. The complete cDNA and deduced amino acid sequence of a type II mouse epidermal keratin of 60,000 Da: Analysis of sequence differences between type I and type II keratins. *Proc. Natl. Acad. Sci. USA* **1984**, *81*, 5709–5713. [CrossRef]
35. Bragulla, H.H.; Homberger, D.G. Structure and functions of keratin proteins in simple, stratified, keratinized and cornified epithelia. *J. Anat.* **2009**, *214*, 516–559. [CrossRef] [PubMed]
36. Chu, P.G.; Weiss, L.M. Keratin expression in human tissues and neoplasms. *Histopathology* **2002**, *40*, 403–439. [CrossRef]
37. Roth, G.A.; Lebherz-Eichinger, D.; Ankersmit, H.J.; Hacker, S.; Hetz, H.; Vukovich, T.; Perne, A.; Reiter, T.; Farr, A.; Hörl, W.H.; et al. Increased total cytokeratin-18 serum and urine levels in chronic kidney disease. *Clin. Chim. Acta* **2011**, *412*, 713–717. [CrossRef] [PubMed]
38. Ku, N.-O.; Zhou, X.; Toivola, D.M.; Omary, M.B. The cytoskeleton of digestive epithelia in health and disease. *Am. J. Physiol. Liver Physiol.* **1999**, *277*, G1108–G1137. [CrossRef] [PubMed]
39. Djudjaj, S.; Papasotiriou, M.; Bülow, R.D.; Wagner, A.; Lindenmeyer, M.T.; Cohen, C.D.; Strnad, P.; Goumenos, D.S.; Floege, J.; Boor, P. Keratins are novel markers of renal epithelial cell injury. *Kidney Int.* **2016**, *89*, 792–808. [CrossRef] [PubMed]
40. Helenius, T.O.; Antman, C.A.; Asghar, M.N.; Nyström, J.H.; Toivola, D.M. Keratins Are Altered in Intestinal Disease-Related Stress Responses. *Cells* **2016**, *5*, 35. [CrossRef]
41. Schwartz, G.J.; Muñoz, A.; Schneider, M.F.; Mak, R.H.; Kaskel, F.; Warady, B.A.; Furth, S.L. New equations to estimate GFR in children with CKD. *J. Am. Soc. Nephrol.* **2009**, *20*, 629–637.
42. Dias, C.S.; Silva, J.M.; Pereira, A.K.; Marino, V.S.; Silva, L.A.; Coelho, A.M.; Costa, F.P.; Quirino, I.G.; Simões, E.S.A.C.; Oliveira, E.A. Diagnostic accuracy of renal pelvic dilatation for detecting surgically managed ureteropelvic junction obstruction. *J. Urol.* **2013**, *190*, 661–666. [CrossRef] [PubMed]

43. Swenson, D.W.; Darge, K.; Ziniel, S.I.; Chow, J.S. Characterizing upper urinary tract dilation on ultrasound: A survey of North American pediatric radiologists' practices. *Pediatr. Radiol.* **2014**, *45*, 686–694. [CrossRef]
44. Piepsz, A.; Colarinha, P.; Gordon, I.; Hahn, K.; Olivier, P.; Roca, I.; Sixt, R.; van Velzen, J. Guidelines for 99mTc-DMSA scintigraphy in children. *Eur. J. Nucl. Med.* **2001**, *28*, 37–41.
45. El-Sherbiny, M.T.; Mousa, O.M.; Shokeir, A.; Ghoneim, M. Role of urinary transforming growth factor-beta1 concentration in the diagnosis of upper urinary tract obstruction in children. *J. Urol.* **2002**, *168*. [CrossRef]
46. Furness, P.D.; Maizels, M.; Han, S.W.; Cohn, R.A.; Cheng, E.Y. Elevated bladder urine concentration of transforming growth factor-beta1 correlates with upper urinary tract obstruction in children. *J. Urol.* **1999**, *162*, 1033–1036.
47. Taha, M.A.; Shokeir, A.A.; Osman, H.G.; El-Aziz, A.A.; Farahat, S.E. Pelvi-ureteric junction obstruction in children: The role of urinary transforming growth factor-beta and epidermal growth factor. *BJU Int.* **2007**, *99*, 899–903. [CrossRef] [PubMed]
48. Chen, X.; Zhu, W.; Al-Hayek, S.; Yan, X.; Jiang, C.; Zheng, X.; Guo, H. Urinary TGF-1 has a supplementary value in predicting renal function recovery post unilateral ureteral obstruction. *Int. Urol. Nephrol.* **2014**, *47*, 33–37. [CrossRef] [PubMed]
49. Palmer, L.S.; Maizels, M.; Kaplan, W.E.; Firlit, C.F.; Cheng, E.Y. Urine levels of transforming growth factor-beta 1 in children with ureteropelvic junction obstruction. *Urology* **1997**, *50*, 769–773. [CrossRef]
50. Prieto, M.; Rodríguez-Peña, A.B.; Düwel, A.; Rivas, J.V.; Docherty, N.; Pérez-Barriocanal, F.; Arévalo, M.; Vary, C.P.; Bernabeu, C.; López-Novoa, J.M.; et al. Temporal changes in renal endoglin and TGF-beta1 expression following ureteral obstruction in rats. *J. Physiol. Biochem.* **2005**, *61*, 457–467. [CrossRef] [PubMed]
51. Satirapoj, B.; Wang, Y.; Chamberlin, M.P.; Dai, T.; LaPage, J.; Phillips, L.; Nast, C.C.; Adler, S.G. Periostin: Novel tissue and urinary biomarker of progressive renal injury induces a coordinated mesenchymal phenotype in tubular cells. *Nephrol. Dial. Transplant.* **2011**, *27*, 2702–2711. [CrossRef]
52. An, J.N.; Yang, S.H.; Kim, Y.C.; Hwang, J.H.; Park, J.Y.; Kim, D.K.; Kim, J.H.; Kim, D.W.; Hur, D.G.; Oh, Y.K.; et al. Periostin induces kidney fibrosis after acute kidney injury via the p38 MAPK pathway. *Am. J. Physiol. Physiol.* **2019**, *316*, F426–F437. [CrossRef] [PubMed]
53. Wallace, D.P.; White, C.; Savinkova, L.; Nivens, E.; Reif, G.A.; Pinto, C.S.; Raman, A.; Parnell, S.C.; Conway, S.J.; Fields, T.A. Periostin promotes renal cyst growth and interstitial fibrosis in polycystic kidney disease. *Kidney Int.* **2014**, *85*, 845–854. [CrossRef]
54. Wantanasiri, P.; Satirapoj, B.; Charoenpitakchai, M.; Aramwit, P. Periostin: A novel tissue biomarker correlates with chronicity index and renal function in lupus nephritis patients. *Lupus* **2015**, *24*, 835–845. [CrossRef]
55. Kühn, B.; Del Monte, F.; Hajjar, R.J.; Chang, Y.-S.; Lebeche, D.; Arab, S.; Keating, M.T. Periostin induces proliferation of differentiated cardiomyocytes and promotes cardiac repair. *Nat. Med.* **2007**, *13*, 962–969. [CrossRef]
56. Kormann, R.; Kavvadas, P.; Placier, S.; Vandermeersch, S.; Dorison, A.; Dussaule, J.-C.; Chadjichristos, C.E.; Prakoura, N.; Chatziantoniou, C. Periostin Promotes Cell Proliferation and Macrophage Polarization to Drive Repair after AKI. *J. Am. Soc. Nephrol.* **2019**, *31*, 85–100. [CrossRef] [PubMed]
57. Lebherz-Eichinger, D.; Krenn, C.G.; Roth, G.A. Keratin 18 and Heat-Shock Protein in Chronic Kidney Disease. *Adv. Clin. Chem.* **2013**, *62*, 123–149. [CrossRef] [PubMed]
58. Truong, L.D.; Sheikh-Hamad, D.; Chakraborty, S.; Suki, W.N. Cell apoptosis and proliferation in obstructive uropathy. *Semin. Nephrol.* **1998**, *18*.
59. Choi, Y.-J.; Baranowska-Daca, E.; Nguyen, V.; Koji, T.; Ballantyne, C.M.; Sheikh-Hamad, D.; Suki, W.N.; Truong, L.D. Mechanism of chronic obstructive uropathy: Increased expression of apoptosis-promoting molecules. *Kidney Int.* **2000**, *58*, 1481–1491. [CrossRef] [PubMed]
60. Zhang, P.L.; Peters, C.; Rosen, S. Ureteropelvic junction obstruction: Morphological and clinical studies. *Pediatr. Nephrol.* **2000**, *14*, 820–826. [CrossRef]
61. Pawar, S.U.; Dharmalingam, A.; Parelkar, S.V.; Shetye, S.S.; Ghorpade, M.K.; Tilve, G.H. Tc-99m ethylenedicysteine and Tc-99m dimercaptosuccinic acid scintigraphy-comparison of the two for detection of scarring and differential cortical function. *Indian J. Nucl. Med.* **2017**, *32*, 93–97. [CrossRef] [PubMed]
62. Piepsz, A. The predictive value of the renogram. *Eur. J. Nucl. Med. Mol. Imaging* **2009**, *36*, 1661–1664. [CrossRef] [PubMed]
63. Ben-Meir, D.; Hutson, J.M.; Donath, S.; Chiang, D.; Cook, D.J. The prognostic value of relative renal function greater than 51% in the pelvi-ureteric junction-obstructed kidney on 99mtechnetium mercaptoacetyltriglycine study. *J. Pediatr. Urol.* **2007**, *3*, 184–188. [CrossRef] [PubMed]

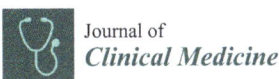

Article

Bone Morphogenetic Proteins (BMPs), Extracellular Matrix Metalloproteinases Inducer (EMMPRIN), and Macrophage Migration Inhibitory Factor (MIF): Usefulness in the Assessment of Tubular Dysfunction Related to Chronic Kidney Disease (CKD)

Kinga Musiał * and Danuta Zwolińska

Department of Pediatric Nephrology, Wrocław Medical University, Borowska 213, 50-556 Wrocław, Poland; danuta.zwolinska@umw.edu.pl
* Correspondence: kinga.musial@umw.edu.pl; Tel.: +48-71-736-44-70

Citation: Musiał, K.; Zwolińska, D. Bone Morphogenetic Proteins (BMPs), Extracellular Matrix Metalloproteinases Inducer (EMMPRIN), and Macrophage Migration Inhibitory Factor (MIF): Usefulness in the Assessment of Tubular Dysfunction Related to Chronic Kidney Disease (CKD). *J. Clin. Med.* **2021**, *10*, 4893. https://doi.org/10.3390/jcm10214893

Academic Editor: Giacomo Garibotto

Received: 5 September 2021
Accepted: 21 October 2021
Published: 23 October 2021

Publisher's Note: MDPI stays neutral with regard to jurisdictional claims in published maps and institutional affiliations.

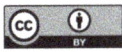

Copyright: © 2021 by the authors. Licensee MDPI, Basel, Switzerland. This article is an open access article distributed under the terms and conditions of the Creative Commons Attribution (CC BY) license (https://creativecommons.org/licenses/by/4.0/).

Abstract: Bone morphogenetic proteins (BMP), extracellular matrix metalloproteinases inducer (EMMPRIN), and macrophage migration inhibitory factor (MIF) are known to be closely connected to renal tubule damage by experimental data; however, this has not been analyzed in children with chronic kidney disease (CKD). The aim of this study was to determine their usefulness in the assessment of CKD-related tubular dysfunction. The study group consisted of 61 children with CKD stages 1–5 and 23 controls. The serum and urine concentrations of BMP-2, BMP-6, EMMPRIN, and MIF were assessed by ELISA and their fractional excretion (FE) was calculated. The serum and urine concentrations of BMP-2, BMP-6, EMMPRIN, and MIF were significantly elevated in children with CKD vs. controls. The FE of BMP-2, FE BMP-6, and EMMPRIN increased significantly in CKD stages 1–2, but exceeded 1% in CKD stages 3–5. FE MIF became higher than in controls no sooner than in CKD 3–5, but remained below 1%. The FE values for BMP-2, BMP-6, and EMMPRIN of <1% may result from the tubular adaptive mechanisms, whereas those surpassing 1% suggest irreversible tubular damage. The analysis of serum/urinary concentrations and fractional excretion of examined parameters may allow the assessment of CKD-related tubular dysfunction.

Keywords: bone morphogenetic protein (BMP)-2; bone morphogenetic protein (BMP)-6; extracellular matrix metalloproteinases inducer (EMMPRIN); macrophage migration inhibitory factor (MIF); tubular functional reserve; tubular damage

1. Introduction

Tubular damage is an early marker of kidney injury and a major determinant of renal outcome [1]. The regenerative potential of renal tubules is clearly seen in the course of acute tubular necrosis, when the increased fractional excretion of sodium results from the timely dysfunction of proximal tubules and allows sequential control until its normalization preceding recovery. The working hypothesis is that similar follow-up of tubular reabsorption capacity is available in the course of chronic kidney disease (CKD) and that it is possible to define a breakthrough point at which reversal of tubular dysfunction is no longer possible [2]. The breakthrough is usually preceded by compensatory mechanisms aimed at maintaining the status quo. One of the nephrological examples is glomerular functional reserve, which defines the ability of glomeruli to increase filtration under unfavorable conditions. Such a situation occurs in patients with CKD stage 1, who demonstrate normal or even increased values of estimated glomerular filtration rate (eGFR), even though the features of kidney damage, such as decreased nephron mass, are already present. Similarly, tubular functional reserve should identify the ability of tubules to respond to the increasing urinary net content of various molecules during the course of CKD. Previous attempts have focused on the tubular secretory response to creatinine load as a tool to detect the subclinical condition of reduced nephron mass [3,4]. A furosemide stress test gave way to a more clinical approach [5]. However, no standardized test to assess tubular reserve has yet been developed.

From a clinical perspective, it is essential to determine a turning point at which tubular reabsorption is no longer able to mitigate the increasing net content of various substances in the urine. To evaluate the process, both specific markers and an effective method of tubular function assessment are needed. Classical markers of tubular damage, such as kidney injury molecule (KIM)-1 or α1microglobulin, were promising in the assessment of subclinical kidney injury and the prediction of renal function deterioration in patients with normal kidney function, but failed in patients with chronic kidney injury [6,7]. Therefore, when screening for suitable parameters, molecules with regenerative potential towards renal tubules may serve as candidate markers of their adaptive abilities.

Bone morphogenetic proteins (BMPs) are the members of the transforming growth factor (TGF)-β superfamily, which is responsible for cell proliferation and regeneration [8]. Animal studies have demonstrated close relations between the decreased expression of BMP-6 and damage to renal tubular cells [9]. BMP-6 null mice present more extensive tubular epithelial necrosis than their wild-type littermates [9]. BMP-2 also appears to play an important role in the regeneration of tubular cells; increased BMP-2 expression in the course of acute kidney injury was shown to induce the myofibroblastic transition in renal progenitor cells [10].

Other potential markers of tubular function are the molecules localized within the tubular structures, which will react directly to the in situ injury. Extracellular matrix metalloproteinases inducer (EMMPRIN) is expressed on the basolateral side of tubular epithelial cells. When these cells are injured in the course of AKI, EMMPRIN expression decreases as it is excreted in the urine [11]. Such a decrease has been also noted in advanced stages of fibrosis compared with the early phase [12]. Our previous studies in children with advanced CKD revealed increased serum and urinary concentrations of EMMPRIN [13,14]. Tubular macrophage migration inhibitory factor (MIF) has been characterized as an endogenous renoprotective factor, attenuating the progression of kidney damage [15]. Its activity is closely connected with the M1 subpopulation of macrophages, triggering inflammatory and regenerative responses, which lead to extracellular matrix deposition [16].

To assess the dynamic changes in tubular function, we decided to evaluate the fractional excretion of BMPs, EMMRIN, and MIF, taking into account the difference in proportion between their serum and urine pools in relation to corresponding creatinine concentrations. This compilation enables the interpretation of the behavior of a selected molecule under different CKD conditions, enriched by the context of glomerular (serum creatinine) and tubular (urinary creatinine) function. The abovementioned parameters have not previously been analyzed as markers of tubular damage in children with CKD. Moreover, nothing is known about the impact of tubular functional reserve, expressed as the values of urinary fractional excretion of the selected parameters, in CKD.

2. Aim of Study

Therefore, the aim of this study was to analyze the ability of renal tubules to adapt to changeable conditions, namely decreased eGFR, by assessing serum and urine concentrations of BMP-2, BMP-6, EMMPRIN, and MIF in the consecutive stages of CKD. We also assessed the fractional excretion (FE) values of BMP-2, BMP-6, EMMPRIN, and MIF in children with CKD and in controls, in order to evaluate their potential usefulness as markers of tubular dysfunction.

3. Methods

3.1. Study Design and Sampling

This was a single-center cross-sectional study concerning 61 children with CKD and 23 controls. Blood samples were drawn from peripheral veins after an overnight fast.

Samples were clotted for 30 min and centrifuged for 10 min. Then serum was stored at −20 °C until being assayed. Urine from the first morning sample was collected aseptically, centrifuged for 10 min, and then stored at −20 °C until being assayed.

3.2. Assay Characteristics

The serum and urine concentrations of BMP-2, BMP-6, EMMPRIN, and MIF were evaluated by commercially available ELISA kits: BMP-2 (Cloud-Clone Corp., Houston, TX, USA), reagent kit SEA013Hu; BMP-6 (Cloud-Clone Corp., Houston, TX, USA), reagent kit SEA646Hu; EMMPRIN (R&D Systems, Minneapolis, MN, USA), reagent kit DEMP00; MIF (R&D Systems, Minneapolis, MN, USA), reagent kit PDMF00B. Standards, serum and urine samples were transferred to 96-well microplates pre-coated with recombinant antibodies to human BMP-2, BMP-6, EMMPRIN, and MIF. Measurements were performed in according to the manufacturer's instructions, and results were calculated by reference to standard curves.

Serum and urine chemical parameters were measured using automated routine diagnostic tests. The serum and urine creatinine were assessed using the Creatinine OSR61204 reagent (Beckman Coulter, Aurora, OH, USA) on the Beckman Coulter AU2700 analyzer (Beckman Coulter, Aurora, OH, USA). Estimated glomerular filtration rate (eGFR) was calculated using the Schwartz formula [17]. All urinary concentrations of evaluated parameters were normalized to urinary creatinine values.

The fractional excretion (FE) of a parameter with urine was calculated according to the formula: FE [%] = ((urine parameter concentration) × (serum creatinine concentration)) ÷ ((serum parameter concentration) × (urine creatinine concentration)) × 100.

3.3. Statistical Analysis

The results were expressed as median values and interquartile ranges. The null hypothesis of normality of distribution was rejected by the Shapiro–Wilk test. Thus, the comparisons between variables were evaluated by using nonparametric tests (Kruskal–Wallis, Mann–Whitney U). Relations between parameters were defined by Spearman's correlation coefficient R. Statistical analysis was performed using the package Statistica ver. 13.3 (StatSoft Inc., Tulsa, OK, USA). A p value of <0.05 was considered significant.

4. Results

4.1. Patient Characteristics

Eighty-four patients were divided into three groups. The first group (CKD I) consisted of 20 children with CKD stages 1–2, the second group (CKD II) contained 41 patients with CKD stages 3–5, and the control group consisted of 23 children with monosymptomatic nocturnal enuresis and normal kidney function. The basic clinical data are presented in Table 1.

The major causative factors for CKD were congenital anomalies of the kidney and urinary tract (CAKUT) (45 children), including reflux nephropathy (19 cases), obstructive uropathy (14 patients), and hypo/dysplastic kidneys (12). Other underlying diseases were: chronic glomerulonephritis (10), polycystic kidney disease (4), and hemolytic uremic syndrome (2). CAKUT was the only cause of CKD in CKD I and the dominant cause in CKD II (Table 1).

Patients did not show clinical evidence of infection and did not smoke or take antibiotics or statins. They were also free of such co-morbidities as diabetes, malignancies, connective tissue diseases, cardiovascular disease, peripheral vascular disease, or obesity. Thirty-five children from the CKD group were normotensive based on the criteria of the European Society of Hypertension in children and adolescents [18]. Sixteen patients had clinically well-controlled blood pressure, using ACE inhibitors (8 children), calcium channel blockers (6 patients), and β-blockers (2 children); 10 patients required combined therapy. All patients with CKD stages 3–5 were supplemented with phosphate binders and vitamin D metabolites.

Table 1. Basic clinical characteristics of the patients.

Parameter	Median (Lower–Upper Quartile)		
	Control Group (n = 23)	CKD I (n = 20)	CKD II (n = 41)
Age (years)	10.5 (5.0–16.5)	9.5 (4.0–12.5)	11.0 (4.5–16.5)
Gender	13 girls, 10 boys	5 girls, 15 boys	17 girls, 24 boys
Primary cause of CKD	-	CAKUT/GN/other 20/0/0	CAKUT/GN/other 25/10/6
Serum creatinine [mg/dL]	0.6 (0.5–0.7)	1.1 (1.0–1.2) [a]	1.9 (1.3–3.7) [b]
Urine creatinine [mg/dL]	114 (100–126)	131 (118–140) [a]	76 (60–82) [b]
Proteinuria [g/L]	0.01 (0.0–0.1)	0.02 (0.02–0.2)	0.4 (0.03–0.6) [b]
eGFR [mL/min/1.73 m^2]	97.1 (92.3–115.0)	79.5 (65.7–97.4) [a]	26.2 (17.3–41.5) [b]

Mann–Whitney U test: [a] $p < 0.001$ CKD I vs. control gr.; [b] $p < 0.001$ CKD II vs. CKD I; CAKUT, congenital anomalies of the kidney and urinary tract; GN, glomerulonephritis.

4.2. Serum and Urine Concentrations of BMP-2, BMP-6, EMMPRIN, and MIF

The serum concentrations of all examined parameters in CKD patients were significantly higher than in controls, irrespective of the stage of the disease (Table 2). Serum BMP-2 and BMP-6 levels reached their maximum in early stages of CKD (CKD I) and then decreased significantly throughout advanced CKD (CKD II), although remained elevated vs. controls. In contrast, serum EMMPRIN and MIF values continued to increase as CKD progressed (Table 2).

Table 2. Serum concentrations of examined parameters in children with CKD and in the control group.

Parameters in Serum	Median Value (Lower–Upper Quartile)		
	Control Group (n = 23)	CKD I (n = 20)	CKD II (n = 41)
sBMP-2 [pg/mL]	523.8 (513.8–538.9)	1574.1 (1540.1–1645.1) [a]	1527.6 (1495.9–1570.5) [b]
sBMP-6 [ng/mL]	33.3 (31.8–34.7)	96.6 (95.9–97.7) [a]	92.5 (90.6–96.3) [b]
sEMMPRIN [pg/mL]	871.9 (854.9–906.1)	1114.4 (1085.1–1137.8) [a]	1175 (1150.6–1199.4) [b]
sMIF [ng/mL]	20.1 (19.4–21.4)	61.9 (61.7–62.4) [a]	66.5 (62.4–68.5) [b]

Mann–Whitney U test: [a] $p < 0.0001$ CKD I vs. control gr.; [b] $p < 0.001$ CKD II vs. CKD I.

The urine concentrations of BMP-2, BMP-6, and EMMPRIN were higher in children with CKD compared with the controls and gradually increased with CKD progression (Table 3). The MIF values increased in CKD I vs. the control and then reached a plateau phase between mild (CKD I) and advanced (CKD II) CKD (Table 3). Urine creatinine concentrations were elevated in patients with CKD I in comparison with the controls, but in the CKD II group they were lower than in the CKD I and control group (Table 1).

Table 3. Urine concentrations of examined parameters in children with CKD and in the control group.

Parameters in Urine	Median Value (Lower–Upper Quartile)		
	Control Group (n = 23)	CKD I (n = 20)	CKD II (n = 41)
uBMP-2 [pg/mg creatinine]	160.3 (146.2–198.1)	571.8 (516.7–611.7) [a]	900.7 (797.7–1172.4) [b]
uBMP-6 [ng/mg creatinine]	12.4 (11.4–14.7)	39.8 (37.2–44.3) [a]	62.2 (56.5–84.4) [b]
uEMMPRIN [pg/mg creatinine]	375 (313.3–402.4)	629.2 (572.2–690.1) [a]	1117.9 (962.1–1361.5) [b]
uMIF [ng/mg creatinine]	0.9 (0.8–1.1)	3.5 (3.2–3.7) [a]	3.8 (3.4–4.6) [b]

Mann–Whitney U test: [a] $p < 0.0001$ CKD I vs. control gr.; [b] $p < 0.01$ CKD II vs. CKD I.

4.3. Fractional Excretion of BMP-2, BMP-6, EMMPRIN, and MIF

The fractional excretion (FE) values of BMP-2, BMP-6, and EMMPRIN were significantly elevated in all children with CKD when compared with the control group, and increased with the progression of CKD (Table 4). However, FE BMP-2, FE BMP-6, and FE EMMPRIN in mild CKD remained below 1% and exceeded this threshold no sooner than in the CKD II group. The FE values of BMP-2, BMP-6, EMMPRIN, and MIF in the control group were all below 1%. FE MIF values remained unchanged in the CKD I group vs. the control group, and then increased significantly in the CKD II group, but did not exceed 1% (Table 4).

Table 4. Fractional excretion of examined parameters in children with CKD and in the control group.

Fractional Excretion of Parameters	Median Value (Lower–Upper Quartile)		
	Control Group ($n = 23$)	CKD I ($n = 20$)	CKD II ($n = 41$)
FE BMP-2 [%]	0.21 (0.19–0.24)	0.39 (0.35–0.45) [a]	0.74 (0.45–1.42) [b]
FE BMP-6 [%]	0.27 (0.24–0.28)	0.45 (0.41–0.54) [a]	0.81 (0.54–1.78) [b]
FE EMMPRIN [%]	0.30 (0.28–0.31)	0.62 (0.57–0.72) [a]	1.12 (0.73–2.13) [b]
FE MIF [%]	0.03 (0.02–0.04)	0.03 (0.02–0.04) [a]	0.06 (0.04–0.14) [b]

Mann–Whitney U test: [a] $p < 0.0001$ CKD I vs. the control group; [b] $p < 0.00001$ CKD II vs. CKD I.

4.4. Correlations

The BMP-2, BMP-6, EMMPRIN, and MIF serum concentrations were significantly correlated with each other, with eGFR, and with the corresponding urine values (Table 5).

Table 5. Selected correlations between serum (s) and urine (u) parameters in children with CKD assessed by Spearman's correlation coefficient (R).

Examined Parameters	sBMP-2	sBMP-6	sEMMPRIN	sMIF	eGFR	Urine Corresponding Values
sBMP-2	-	$R = 0.49$, $p < 0.0001$	$R = -0.35$, $p < 0.01$	$R = -0.29$, $p < 0.01$	$R = 0.34$, $p < 0.01$	uBMP-2 $R = 0.02$, $p = 0.8$
sBMP-6	$R = 0.49$, $p < 0.0001$	-	$R = -0.61$, $p < 0.00001$	$R = -0.66$, $p < 0.00001$	$R = 0.63$, $p < 0.00001$	uBMP-6 $R = -0.55$, $p < 0.0001$
sEMMPRIN	$R = -0.35$, $p < 0.01$	$R = -0.61$, $p < 0.00001$	-	$R = 0.57$, $p < 0.00001$	$R = -0.62$, $p < 0.00001$	uEMMPRIN $R = 0.48$, $p < 0.0001$
sMIF	$R = -0.29$, $p < 0.01$	$R = -0.66$, $p < 0.00001$	$R = 0.57$, $p < 0.00001$	-	$R = -0.53$, $p < 0.0001$	uMIF $R = 0.78$, $p < 0.000001$

The urine concentrations of all the analyzed parameters were also correlated with each other, and the strength of these correlations was more significant than for the serum values ($-0.54 \leq R \leq -0.49$; $p < 0.0001$). The urine concentrations of BMP-2, BMP-6, EMMPRIN, and MIF were negatively correlated with eGFR ($-0.59 \leq R \leq -0.55$; $p < 0.0001$).

5. Discussion

Our investigation revealed changes in the serum and urine concentrations of BMP-2, BMP-6, EMMPRIN, and MIF, as well as adaptive changes in the FE values, in children with CKD when compared with the controls. The kinetics of these changes were dependent upon the analyzed molecule.

5.1. Bone Morphogenetic Proteins

The serum concentrations of BMP-2 and BMP-6 followed similar patterns to each other, but were different to those of other examined molecules. An early rise in CKD stages 1–2 was followed by a statistically significant, although not large, decrease in CKD stages 3–5.

However, the concentrations remained higher than those in the controls. The serum values of BMPs were positively correlated with eGFR, which could explain the decrease in their concentration as CKD progressed. The progressively increasing urinary concentrations of BMP-2 and BMP-6 were strongly dependent on the eGFR values. Moreover, BMPs are low-molecular-weight proteins, so they can be freely filtered into urine. Thus, the decrease in serum BMPs during the late stages of CKD can be partially explained by the excretion of molecules in the urine. Meanwhile, the FE BMP-2 and BMP-6 values, which increased with the progression of CKD, but did not exceed the 1% threshold in CKD stages 1–2, could act as surrogate markers for the enhanced tubular activity. Experimental studies suggest that the change in creatinine tubular secretion, triggered, e.g., by protein meal, may serve as a marker of tubular functional reserve [19]. Indeed, such overactivity was seen in our study, where children with CKD I demonstrated increased creatinine urine concentrations compared with the controls. This may be indirect proof of aggravated tubular activity. Such mobilization of the tubular functional reserve would aid the reabsorption of excessive urinary BMPs in order to prevent the loss of filtered proteins. Crossing the borderline of 1% in advanced CKD indicates that the renal tubules are unable to cope with the urinary protein overload. Indeed, this exhaustion of renal tubule function was clearly shown by the urine creatinine values, decreasing to the level below that of the control group owing to the impaired secretory abilities of the tubules. Thus, the simultaneous analysis of serum/urine/fractional excretion values broadens the horizon of dynamic adaptive changes that the tubules may undergo during CKD progression.

5.2. EMMPRIN

The decrease in EMMPRIN expression has been demonstrated in human kidney allografts, along with the progression of fibrosis and tubular atrophy [12]. Increased plasma and urinary EMMPRIN levels have been reported in patients with tubular atrophy/interstitial fibrosis in the course of IgA nephropathy and diabetic kidney disease [20]. Moreover, the strong correlation of both plasma and urinary EMMPRIN with eGFR has been noted [20]. Therefore, EMMPRIN has been identified as a marker that can accurately reflect disease activity and tubular damage. In our study, EMMPRIN serum and urinary concentrations, as well as FE values, also increased systematically and significantly with CKD progression. Likewise, both serum and urine EMMPRIN values were correlated negatively with eGFR. Thus, the gradual increase in serum can be explained by both the accumulation and overproduction during disease progression, whereas the increase in EMMPRIN in urine can be explained by the cumulative effects of molecule leakage and release by damaged tubular cells into urine. Consequently, this would justify the rise in FE values from the earliest stages of CKD and the surpassing of the 1% borderline, indicating the adaptive ability of tubular function in early CKD, as well as the irreversible tubular damage in advanced CKD and an inability to acquire the increased net content of EMMPRIN in the urine.

5.3. MIF

MIF is an anti-inflammatory cytokine that inhibits migration of macrophages and triggers their adhesion and accumulation at the sites of inflammation and phagocytosis. Increased serum concentrations of MIF have been reported in adults with uremic cardiomyopathy [21]. Therefore, the MIF systemic pool appears to represent destructive mechanisms in the course of CKD. The gradual increase in serum MIF in our patients was concordant with previous results and could indicate the accumulation of the molecule. An additional argument for this explanation is the negative correlation with eGFR. In contrast, owing to its low molecular weight, MIF could be freely filtered through a glomerular filtration barrier. Thus, the MIF overproduction in the systemic pool due to the chronic inflammatory process, which is characteristic for CKD, was also likely. Moreover, the increase in serum MIF concentration was noticeable, despite the undisturbed elimination of the molecule in urine; thus, the cumulative effect of accumulation and overproduction was the most likely explanation.

The increased MIF in urine in the early stages of CKD was the most notable among all parameters, whereas urinary concentrations in advanced CKD remained stable despite the increasing serum values, unlike other markers. MIF activity in the kidney is strongly dependent on the presence of M1 macrophages, which are predominant in the early period of injury but give way to type M2 in advanced fibrosis [16]. Therefore, the abrupt early MIF increase in urine could indicate the cumulative effects of molecule leakage and its protective overactivity in situ. Meanwhile, the stable urinary values of MIF in CKD stages 3–5 vs. stages 1–2, as well as their negative correlation with eGFR, suggest a suppression of pro-inflammatory activity in response to the progression of fibrosis, which is characteristic of the advanced stages of CKD. They may also be an indirect marker of the switch from the pro-inflammatory M1 macrophage phenotype to M2. Tubular MIF also has been known for its regenerative potential during the course of AKI [22,23]. Therefore, the increase in urinary MIF may serve as proof of its regenerative activity in the course of early CKD, whereas the later plateau phase toward advanced CKD may illustrate that this activity is exhausted and the transition of active inflammatory process creates irreversible damage. Consequently, owing to the various stimuli that influence MIF concentrations, FE MIF values only increased to higher than the control group in CKD stages 3–5 and they did not exceed 1% in any of the analyzed groups.

5.4. The Role of Fractional Excretion

Collectively, the complex analysis of serum, urine, and fractional excretion values of BMPs and EMMPRIN enabled the differentiation between the mobilization of tubular functional reserve in the face of increased parameter urine load and the subsequent tubular damage during the progression of CKD. The value of the obtained results was strengthened by the fact that the critical period of tubular adaptive activity was analyzed in a group of children with CAKUT as a major reason for CKD development. This homogeneity allowed the exclusion of any potential glomerular interference from the background of dysfunction. The analyzed group became more heterogenous in advanced stages of CKD, when tubular damage is common to all underlying diseases leading to CKD.

Fractional excretion has been shown to be a useful tool in the assessment of CKD-related tubular dysfunction, provided that free filtration of the molecule was the major mechanism of its elimination in urine. Given that none of the FE values in the control group exceeded 1%, we could assume that none of the examined molecules were actively secreted by the tubules. However, when additional mechanisms were considered to contribute to the final serum and urine concentrations, such as inflammation or macrophage transition/fibrosis in the case of MIF, this analysis yielded inconclusive results.

We must also acknowledge the limitations of our study. First, the heterogeneity of factors influencing serum and urine concentrations of BMPs, EMMPRIN, and MIF, as well as a cross-sectional design, could create a bias and make the interpretation of their increased/decreased/stable concentrations a challenge. The narrow range in FE variation may also increase difficulties in the proper interpretation of obtained results. However, our main goal was to evaluate the proportion between the serum and urinary pools and identify a common pattern of tubular adaptive mechanisms, rather than analyze the selected molecules separately. Second, our hypothesis is new and this is the first attempt to use FE as a tool to assess tubular activity in chronic conditions, so our results cannot be compared with any previous data from experimental or physiology studies. We are also aware of the small number of patients, which limits the power of our conclusions and necessitates continued study of a larger group of patients.

6. Conclusions

The FE values of BMP-2, BMP-6, and EMMPRIN, which were below 1% in CKD stages 1–2, may result from adaptive tubular mechanisms, whereas FE values surpassing the 1% threshold in CKD stages 3–5 suggest irreversible tubular damage.

The complex analysis of serum/urinary concentrations and FE values of multiple parameters may demonstrate the features of CKD-related tubular dysfunction.

Author Contributions: Conceptualization, K.M.; investigation, K.M.; resources, D.Z.; formal analysis, K.M.; writing—original draft, K.M.; writing—review and editing, K.M. and D.Z.; visualization, K.M.; funding acquisition: D.Z. All authors have read and agreed to the published version of the manuscript.

Funding: The project was financed by the University funds (ST.841).

Institutional Review Board Statement: All procedures were performed in accordance with the 1964 Helsinki declaration and its further amendments. The research project was approved by the Wroclaw Medical University Ethics Committee (ethical approval no. 567/2016).

Informed Consent Statement: Written informed consent was obtained from all participants older than 16 years and from all parents prior to study.

Data Availability Statement: The datasets generated and analyzed during the current study are available from the corresponding author on reasonable request.

Conflicts of Interest: The authors declare no conflict of interest regarding the publication of this manuscript.

References

1. Takaori, K.; Nakamura, J.; Yamamoto, S.; Nakata, H.; Sato, Y.; Takase, M.; Nameta, M.; Yamamoto, T.; Economides, A.; Kohno, K.; et al. Severity and Frequency of Proximal Tubule Injury Determines Renal Prognosis. *J. Am. Soc. Nephrol.* **2015**, *27*, 2393–2406. [CrossRef] [PubMed]
2. Musiał, K. Current Concepts of Pediatric Acute Kidney Injury—Are We Ready to Translate Them into Everyday Practice? *J. Clin. Med.* **2021**, *10*, 3113. [CrossRef] [PubMed]
3. Herrera, J.; Rodriguez-Iturbe, B. Stimulation of tubular secretion of creatinine in health and in conditions associated with reduced nephron mass. Evidence for a tubular functional reserve. *Nephrol. Dial. Transplant.* **1998**, *13*, 623–629. [CrossRef]
4. Rodriguez-Iturbe, B.; Herrera, J.; Marin, C.; Manalich, R. Tubular stress test detects subclinical reduction in renal functioning mass. *Kidney Int.* **2001**, *59*, 1094–1102. [CrossRef]
5. Ronco, C.; Chawla, L.S. Glomerular and tubular kidney stress test: New tools for a deeper evaluation of kidney function. *Nephron* **2016**, *134*, 191–194. [CrossRef]
6. Fuhrman, D.Y.; Nguyen, L.; Hindes, M.; Kellum, J.A. Baseline tubular biomarkers in young adults with congenital heart disease as compared to healthy young adults: Detecting subclinical kidney injury. *Congenit. Hearth Dis.* **2019**, *14*, 963–967. [CrossRef]
7. Schulz, C.-A.; Engström, G.; Nilsson, J.; Almgren, P.; Petkovic, M.; Christensson, A.; Nilsson, P.M.; Melander, O.; Orho-Melander, M. Plasma kidney injury molecule-1 (p-KIM-1) levels and deterioration of kidney function over 16 years. *Nephrol. Dial. Transplant.* **2019**, *35*, 265–273. [CrossRef]
8. Yang, J.; Shi, P.; Tu, M.; Wang, Y.; Liu, M.; Fan, F.; Du, M. Bone morphogenetic proteins: Relationship between molecular structure and their osteogenic activity. *Food Sci. Hum. Wellness* **2014**, *3*, 127–135. [CrossRef]
9. Dendooven, A.; van Oostrom, O.; van der Giezen, D.M.; Leeuwis, J.W.; Snijckers, C.; Joles, J.A.; Robertson, E.J.; Verhaar, M.C.; Nguyen, T.Q.; Goldschmeding, R. Loss of endogenous bone morphogenetic protein-6 aggravates renal fibrosis. *Am. J. Pathol.* **2011**, *178*, 1069–1079. [CrossRef]
10. Simone, S.; Cosola, C.; Loverre, A.; Cariello, M.; Sallustio, F.; Rascio, F.; Gesualdo, L.; Schena, F.P.; Grandaliano, G.; Pertosa, G. BMP-2 induces a profibrotic phenotype in adult renal progenitor cells through Nox4 activation. *Am. J. Physiol. Renal Physiol.* **2012**, *303*, F23–F34. [CrossRef] [PubMed]
11. Kosugi, T.; Maeda, K.; Sato, W.; Maruyama, S.; Kadomatsu, K. CD147 (EMMPRIN/Basigin) in kidney diseases: From an inflammation and immune system viewpoint. *Nephrol. Dial. Transplant.* **2014**, *30*, 1097–1103. [CrossRef]
12. Kemmner, S.; Schulte, C.; Von Weyhern, C.H.; Schmidt, R.; Baumann, M.; Heemann, U.; Renders, L.; Schmaderer, C. EMMPRIN expression is involved in the development of interstitial fibrosis and tubular atrophy in human kidney allografts. *Clin. Transplant.* **2016**, *30*, 218–225. [CrossRef]
13. Musiał, K.; Bargenda, A.; Zwolińska, D. Urine matrix metalloproteinases and their extracellular inducer EMMPRIN in children with chronic kidney disease. *Ren. Fail.* **2015**, *37*, 980–984. [CrossRef]
14. Musial, K.; Bargenda, A.; Zwolinska, D. SP719 Fractional Excretion Ofsurvivin, Emmprin and MMP-7 in Children with Chronic Kidney Disease. *Nephrol. Dial. Transplant.* **2016**, *31*, i335–i336. [CrossRef]

15. Djudjaj, S.; Martin, I.V.; Buhl, E.M.; Nothofer, N.J.; Leng, L.; Piecychna, M.; Floege, J.; Bernhagen, J.; Bucala, R.; Boor, P. Macrophage migration inhibitory factor limits renal inflammation and fibrosis by counteracting tubular cell cycle arrest. *J. Am. Soc. Nephrol.* **2017**, *28*, 3590–3604. [CrossRef] [PubMed]
16. Lu, H.; Bai, Y.; Wu, L.; Hong, W.; Liang, Y.; Chen, B.; Bai, Y. Inhibition of macrophage migration inhibitory factor protects against inflammation and matrix deposition in kidney tissues after injury. *Mediat. Inflamm.* **2016**, *2016*, 2174682. [CrossRef]
17. Schwartz, G.J.; Munoz, A.; Schneider, M.F.; Mak, R.H.; Kaskel, F.; Warady, B.A.; Furth, S.L. New equations to estimate GFR in children with CKD. *J. Am. Soc. Nephrol.* **2009**, *20*, 629–637. [CrossRef] [PubMed]
18. Lurbe, E.; Agabiti-Rosei, E.; Cruickshank, J.K.; Dominiczak, A.; Erdine, S.; Hirth, A.; Invitti, C.; Litwin, M.; Mancia, G.; Pall, D.; et al. 2016 European Society of Hypertension guidelines for the management of high blood pressure in children and adolescents. *J. Hypertens.* **2016**, *34*, 1887–1920. [CrossRef] [PubMed]
19. Mittal, A.; Sethi, S.K. Functional Renal Reserve and Furosemide Stress Test. In *Advances in Critical Care Pediatric Nephrology*; Sethi, S.K., Raina, R., McCulloch, M., Bunchman, T.E., Eds.; Springer: Singapore, 2021; Chapter 18; pp. 177–189.
20. Mori, Y.; Masuda, T.; Kosugi, T.; Yoshioka, T.; Hori, M.; Nagaya, H.; Maeda, K.; Sato, Y.; Kojima, H.; Kato, N.; et al. The clinical relevance of plasma CD147/basigin in biopsy-proven kidney diseases. *Clin. Exp. Nephrol.* **2017**, *22*, 815–824. [CrossRef] [PubMed]
21. Hu, Z.; Liu, Y.; Zhang, X.; Liu, G.; Huang, J.; Pan, Y. Expressions of macrophage migration inhibitory factor in patients with chronic kidney disease. *Niger. J. Clin. Pract.* **2016**, *19*, 778. [CrossRef] [PubMed]
22. Ochi, A.; Chen, D.; Schulte, W.; Leng, L.; Moeckel, N.; Piecychna, M.; Averdunk, L.; Stoppe, C.; Bucala, R.; Moeckel, G. MIF-2/D-DT enhances proximal tubular cell regeneration through SLPI- and ATF4-dependent mechanisms. *Am. J. Physiol. Renal Physiol.* **2017**, *313*, F767–F780. [CrossRef] [PubMed]
23. Stoppe, C.; Averdunk, L.; Goetzenich, A.; Soppert, J.; Marlier, A.; Kraemer, S.; Vieten, J.; Coburn, M.; Kowark, A.; Kim, B.-S.; et al. The protective role of macrophage migration inhibitory factor in acute kidney injury after cardiac surgery. *Sci. Transl. Med.* **2018**, *10*, eaan4886. [CrossRef] [PubMed]

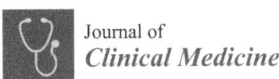

Article

NT-proBNP as a Potential Marker of Cardiovascular Damage in Children with Chronic Kidney Disease

Piotr Skrzypczyk [1,*], Magdalena Okarska-Napierała [1,2], Radosław Pietrzak [3], Katarzyna Pawlik [4], Katarzyna Waścińska [4], Bożena Werner [3] and Małgorzata Pańczyk-Tomaszewska [1]

1. Department of Pediatrics and Nephrology, Medical University of Warsaw, 02-091 Warsaw, Poland; magda.okarska@gmail.com (M.O.-N.); mpanczyk1@wum.edu.pl (M.P.-T.)
2. Department of Pediatrics with Clinical Assessment Unit, Medical University of Warsaw, 02-091 Warsaw, Poland
3. Department of Paediatric Cardiology and General Paediatrics, Medical University of Warsaw, 02-091 Warsaw, Poland; radoslaw.pietrzak@wum.edu.pl (R.P.); bozena.werner@wum.edu.pl (B.W.)
4. Student Scientific Group at the Department of Pediatrics and Nephrology, Medical University of Warsaw, 02-091 Warsaw, Poland; katarzynapawlik97@gmail.com (K.P.); s068819@student.wum.edu.pl (K.W.)
* Correspondence: pskrzypczyk@wum.edu.pl; Tel.: +48-22-317-96-53; Fax: +48-22-317-99-54

Abstract: Assessing cardiovascular disease (CVD) in children with chronic kidney disease (CKD) is difficult. Great expectations have been associated with biomarkers, including the N-terminal pro-brain natriuretic peptide (NT-proBNP). This study aimed to determine the correlation between NT-proBNP and cardiovascular complications in children with CKD. Serum NT-proBNP, arterial stiffness, common carotid artery intima-media thickness (cIMT), echocardiographic (ECHO) parameters (including tissue Doppler imaging), and biochemical and clinical data were analyzed in 38 pediatric patients with CKD (21 boys, 12.2 ± 4.2 years). Mean NT-proBNP in CKD patients was 1068.1 ± 4630 pg/mL. NT-proBNP above the norm (125 pg/mL) was found in 16 (42.1%) subjects. NT-proBNP correlated with glomerular filtration rate (GFR) (r = −0.423, $p = 0.008$), and was significantly higher in CKD G5 (glomerular filtration rate grade) patients compared to CKD G2, G3, and G4 children ($p = 0.010$, $p = 0.004$, and $p = 0.018$, respectively). Moreover, NT-proBNP correlated positively with augmentation index (AP/PP: r = 0.451, $p = 0.018$, P2/P: r = 0.460, $p = 0.016$), cIMT (r = 0.504, $p = 0.020$), and E/E' in ECHO (r = 0.400, $p = 0.032$). In multivariate analysis, logNT-proBNP was the only significant predictor of cIMT Z-score (beta = 0.402, 95CI (0.082–0.721), $p = 0.014$) and P2/P1 (beta = 0.130, 95CI (0.082–0.721), $p = 0.014$). Conclusions: NT-proBNP may serve as a possible marker of thickening of the carotid artery wall in pediatric patients with CKD. The final role of NT-proBNP as a biomarker of arterial damage, left ventricular hypertrophy, or cardiac diastolic dysfunction in CKD children needs confirmation in prospective studies.

Keywords: chronic kidney disease; NT-proBNP; children; cardiovascular disease; common carotid artery intima-media thickness

Citation: Skrzypczyk, P.; Okarska-Napierała, M.; Pietrzak, R.; Pawlik, K.; Waścińska, K.; Werner, B.; Pańczyk-Tomaszewska, M. NT-proBNP as a Potential Marker of Cardiovascular Damage in Children with Chronic Kidney Disease. *J. Clin. Med.* **2021**, *10*, 4344. https://doi.org/10.3390/jcm10194344

Academic Editor: Katarzyna Taranta-Janusz

Received: 12 August 2021
Accepted: 22 September 2021
Published: 24 September 2021

Publisher's Note: MDPI stays neutral with regard to jurisdictional claims in published maps and institutional affiliations.

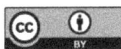

Copyright: © 2021 by the authors. Licensee MDPI, Basel, Switzerland. This article is an open access article distributed under the terms and conditions of the Creative Commons Attribution (CC BY) license (https://creativecommons.org/licenses/by/4.0/).

1. Introduction

Children with chronic kidney disease (CKD) have been recognized as the pediatric group with the highest risk of cardiovascular disease (CVD) [1]. Assessment of cardiovascular risk in children with CKD is difficult, as early stages of CVD do not cause symptoms and can progress undetected [2]. Direct evaluation of subclinical target organ damage in children with CKD requires expensive and not widely accessible devices, experienced and skilled personnel, is time-consuming and, commonly, operator-dependent. Hence, research has been conducted, aimed at finding serological markers of increased cardiovascular burden. Great expectation has been associated with the N-terminal pro-brain natriuretic peptide or the pro-B-type natriuretic peptide (NT-proBNP). As a response to increased left ventricular wall stretch due to volume overloads, and to structural damage of the myocardium, there is an increased expression of a proBNP in myocardial cells [3]. After cleavage to BNP and non-active NT-proBNP, both these particles are released to the bloodstream. Then NT-proBNP is excreted in urine without being metabolized further, while BNP can be captured by natriuretic peptide receptor types A–C, where it exerts its actions or is inactivated by neutral endopeptidase [4,5]. Physiological actions of BNP include the impact on kidneys (dilation of afferent arteriole and constriction of efferent arteriole, relaxation of mesangial cells, increased blood flow through vasa recta, decreased sodium reabsorption in the distal convoluted tubule and cortical collecting duct, inhibition of renin secretion), adrenal glands (reduction of aldosterone secretion), blood vessels (relaxation of vascular smooth muscles), myocardium (inhibition of maladaptive cardiac hypertrophy), and adipose tissue (release of free fatty acids) [4,6].

NT-proBNP is widely used to diagnose, screen, and stratify patients with heart failure and detect systolic and diastolic left ventricular dysfunction [3,7]. Its usefulness has already been investigated in adult CKD patients [8–10]. There are only scarce data on the prognostic value of BNP and NT-proBNP in pediatric patients with kidney impairment [11,12]. There are no data on the relationship between central blood pressure, arterial damage, and detailed echocardiographic evaluation and NT-proBNP in these children. Thus, this study aimed to determine the relationship between NT-proBNP and cardiovascular complications in children with CKD.

2. Materials and Methods

2.1. Study Group

This single-center cross-sectional study involved 38 pediatric CKD subjects hospitalized during two years in one tertiary center of pediatric nephrology. The inclusion criteria were: age ≥ five years and CKD stages G2-5 (glomerular filtration rate grade) according to the Kidney Disease: Improving Global Outcomes (KDIGO) guidelines [13]. The following exclusion criteria were applied: coexisting cardiovascular diseases (e.g., congenital heart defects), treatment with recombinant human growth hormone, and acute infections (temporary exclusion for two weeks).

Participants were included in the study consecutively from among the patients after considering inclusion and exclusion criteria to exclude selection bias. The flowchart of the patients included in the study group is presented in Figure 1.

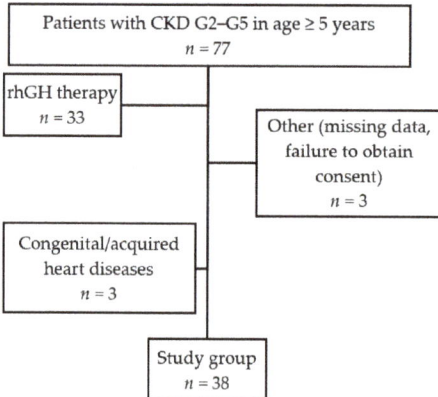

Figure 1. Flowchart of the patients' recruitment (CKD—chronic kidney disease, G—Grade, rhGH—recombinant human growth hormone).

2.2. Ethical Issues

All procedures were in accordance with the ethical standards of the institutional review board (approval no. KB/89/2013) and with the 1964 Helsinki declaration and its later amendments. Informed consent was obtained from all legal representatives and individuals ($\geq$16 years).

2.3. Clinical Parameters

The following clinical data were collected: age (years), gender, CKD etiology [14], and stage [13] based on estimated glomerular filtration rate (GFR) [15], method of renal replacement therapy, body mass (kg), height [m] and body mass index (BMI) (kg/m^2), Z-score [16], presence of arterial hypertension, and medications used.

2.4. NT-proBNP and Biochemical Parameters

Concentration of NT-proBNP (pg/mL) was determined in serum using the VITROS 5600 Integrated System (Ortho Clinical Diagnostics, Raritan, NJ, USA) with the upper limit taken from the manufacturer's normative values (125 (pg/mL)). The following biochemical parameters were evaluated: creatinine (mg/dL), urea (mg/dL), uric acid (mg/dL), hemoglobin (g/dL), albumins (g/dL), calcium (mg/dL), inorganic phosphate (mg/dL), alkaline phosphatase (IU/mL), intact parathormone (pg/mL), 25-hydroxy-vitamin D (25(OH)D) (ng/mL), total, low-density (LDL) and high-density lipoprotein (HDL) cholesterol (mg/dL), triglycerides (mg/dL), and parameters of acid base balance from arterialized capillary blood: pH, and HCO_3^- (mmol/L). All biochemical parameters were measured in the morning, on fasting, simultaneously. Normal values of hemoglobin and calcium–phosphorus metabolism parameters were taken from the Kidney Disease: Improving Global Outcome (KDIGO) guidelines [17,18], and the normal value of cholesterol and triglycerides from Stewart et al. [19]; hyperuricemia was recognized when uric acid was $\geq$5.5 (mg/dL) [20].

2.5. Blood Pressure and Parameters of Cardiovascular Damage

Peripheral office arterial blood pressure was measured with Welch Allyn VSM 300 Patient Monitor (Welch Allyn Inc., Skaneateles Falls, NY, USA) and expressed in (mmHg) and Z-score values [21]. Common carotid artery intima-media thickness (cIMT) was evaluated with a 13-MHz linear transducer (Aloka Prosound Alpha 6, Hitachi Aloka Medical, Mitaka, Japan), using methods described previously [22] and expressed in (mm) and Z-score [23]. Central blood pressure, arterial pulse waveform, and aortal pulse wave velocity (PWV) were assessed with SphygmoCor (AtCor Medical Pty Ltd., Sydney, Australia) using methods described in detail in our previous study [22]. The following parameters were analyzed: aortic (central) office systolic, diastolic, mean, and pulse pressure (AoSBP, AoDBP, AoMAP, AoPP (mm Hg)), augmentation pressure (AP = P2 − P1, where P2 is the amplitude of late, i.e., returning systolic peak pressure, and P1 is early systolic peak pressure (mm Hg)), augmentation index (AIx) expressed as AP divided by pulse pressure (AP/PP (%)), and P2/P1 ratio (%), as well as AIx (AP/PP) normalized to heart rate of 75 beats per minute (AIx75HR (%)), and aortic (carotid–femoral) pulse wave velocity. PWV was presented as (m/s) and (Z-score) based on normative pediatric data [24].

All children underwent transthoracic two-dimensional (2D), conventional Doppler, and tissue Doppler (TD) echocardiography (ECHO) with M-mode assessment of left ventricular parameters and simultaneous recording of ECG in the second limb lead with Philips iE33, transducer S5-1 (Philips, Amsterdam, The Netherlands). The following parameters were evaluated using a classical echocardiography and conventional Doppler technique. In the end-diastolic phase: the interventricular septum transverse diameter (IVSDd) (mm), left ventricular diastolic diameter (LVDd) (mm), left ventricular posterior wall diameter (LVPWd) (mm)), left atrial transverse diameter (LAD) (mm), relative wall thickness (RWT) calculated as 2 × LVPWd divided by LVDd, left ventricular mass calculated from the Deveraux equation, and left ventricular mass (LVMI) were indexed according to DeSimone [g/m$^{2.7}$] [25], as well as shortening and ejection fraction (SF, EF) (%), peak wave velocity in early and late diastole caused by atrial contraction (the E and A waves) (cm/s), and E deceleration time (Edt) [s]. The TD was used to assess the mean value of peak medial and lateral mitral annular velocity during early filling (E') (m/s), the mean value of peak medial and lateral mitral annular velocity during late filling (A') (m/s), E/E' ratio, isovolumetric relaxation time (IVRT) [s], isovolumetric contraction time (IVCT) [s], and a maximum speed of the systolic wave (C') (m/s). Left ventricular hypertrophy (LVH) was defined as LVMI $\geq$ 95c. for age and sex [26], abnormal RWT was defined as >0.42. Mildly reduced and reduced ejection fraction was defined as EF between 41% and 49% and EF $\leq$ 40%, respectively, according to the 2021 European Society of Cardiology guidelines [27].

2.6. Statistical Analysis

Statistica 13.0 PL software (TIBCO Software Inc., Palo Alto, CA, USA) was used for calculations. The normality of the distribution of the analyzed variables was assessed using the Shapiro–Wilk test. Normally distributed data were presented as mean ± standard deviation (SD) and non-normally distributed variables as median and interquartile range (Q1–Q3). Differences between data were tested using the U Mann–Whitney test. The relationship between two variables was analyzed using Pearson's linear correlation or Spearman's correlation rank, depending on the distribution. Multivariate analysis was performed using forward stepwise regression analysis. Parameters that correlated with arterial and heart damage markers with p < 0.100 in univariate analysis were included in the final model. Parameters that correlated with each other with r > 0.650 were excluded from regression models to avoid collinearity. Logarithmic transformation of non-normally distributed data was performed prior to the analysis. As NT-proBNP and cardiovascular complications of CKD are significantly correlated to GFR, the latter variable was forced into the final model. A p-value < 0.05 was considered statistically significant.

3. Results

3.1. Clinical Characteristics

Clinical characteristics of children included in the study are summarized in Table 1. Most of the subjects were in CKD grades 2 and 3, and congenital anomalies of the kidney and urinary tract (CAKUT) were the leading primary kidney pathology. Among seven patients in grade G5, six were chronically dialyzed: five were treated with peritoneal dialysis (PD), one was treated with hemodialysis (HD), and one child with eGFR of 13.45 mL/min/1.73 m^2 did not receive renal replacement therapy yet. Arterial hypertension was present in 26 patients, usually treated with one antihypertensive drug, most commonly calcium channel blockers or angiotensin-converting enzyme inhibitors.

Table 1. Clinical and biochemical data of the studied children.

Analyzed Parameter	Value (Mean ± SD or Median and Q1–Q3)
Age (years)	12.3 (8.6–16.3)
Gender (males/females)	21/17 (55%/45%)
CKD GRADE (n (%))	
G2	14 (37%)
G3	11 (29%)
G4	6 (16%)
G5	7 (18%)
Primary kidney disease (n (%))	
CAKUT	18 (47%)
Glomerulonephritis	7 (18%)
Hereditary nephropathy	3 (8%)
Toxic/ischemic kidney injury	3 (8%)
Cystic kidney disease	2 (5%)
Hemolytic uremic syndrome	1 (3%)
Other	1 (3%)
Unknown	3 (8%)
BMI Z-score	−0.1 ± 1.3

Table 1. Cont.

Analyzed Parameter	Value (Mean ± SD or Median and Q1–Q3)
Overweight (BMI Z-score 1–2)	6 (16%)
Obesity (BMI Z-score > 2)	2 (5%)
Underweight (BMI Z-score < 2)	3 (8%)
Arterial hypertension	26 (68%)
Number of antihypertensive medications	1 (1–2)
Medications [1]	
Angiotensin-converting enzyme inhibitor	16 (42%)
Angiotensin receptor antagonist	2 (5%)
Calcium channel antagonist	19 (50%)
Beta-adrenolytic	7 (18%)
Erythropoiesis-stimulating agents	11 (29%)
Vitamin D3	29 (76%)
Alfacalcidol	12 (32%)
Calcium carbonate	18 (47%)
Erythropoiesis-stimulating agents	11 (29%)

SD—standard deviation, Q1—the first quartile, Q3—the third quartile, CKD—chronic kidney disease, G—grade, CAKUT—congenital anomalies of kidney and urinary tract, BMI—body mass index. [1] number of patients.

3.2. NT-proBNP and Biochemical Parameters

The concentration of NT-pro BNP and remaining biochemical parameters are depicted in Table 2. The median value of NT-proBNP in patients with CKD was 95 (pg/mL) and varied from 15 up to 28,382 (pg/mL). NT-proBNP value above the norm (i.e., >125 pg/mL) was found in 16 (42.1%) children with CKD. NT-proBNP values did not differ significantly among children with CKD G2, G3, and G4. The highest values of NT-proBNP, significantly higher than children with CKD G2–G4, were found in children with CKD in stage G5 (Figure 2). In three of them, the NT-proBNP value exceeded 1000 (pg/mL). NT-proBNP at the concentration of 1579 (pg/mL) was detected in a 16.5-year-old boy with CKD and membranoproliferative glomerulonephritis, treated with hemodialysis. The boy had arterial hypertension treated with two drugs and left ventricular hypertrophy (LVH)—his LVMI was 40.2 g/m$^{2.7}$. NT-proBNP at 5146 (pg/mL) was noted in a 14.5-year-old girl with CKD and steroid-resistant nephrotic syndrome treated with PD, with arterial hypertension treated with three drugs and LVH—her LVMI was 50.0 g/m$^{2.7}$. The highest NT-proBNP concentration (28,382 (pg/mL)) was found in a 7.5-year-old female patient with unknown etiology of kidney disease, treated with PD, with arterial hypertension treated with two drugs, and LVH (LVMI—46.5 g/m$^{2.7}$).

Table 2. NT-pro BNP and biochemical characteristics of the study group (NT-proBNP—N-terminal pro-brain natriuretic peptide).

Analyzed Parameter	Value (Mean ± SD or Median and Q1–Q3)
NT-proBNP (pg/mL)	95.0 (52–298)
NT-proBNP G2 (pg/mL)	84.5 (32–140) [1]
NT-proBNP G3 (pg/mL)	88.0 (44–174) [2]
NT-proBNP G4 (pg/mL)	103.0 (72–171) [3]
NT-proBNP G5 (pg/mL)	391.0 (317–5146) [1,2,3]
Creatinine (mg/dL)	1.4 (0.9–2.4)
GFR (mL/min/1.73 m^2)	43.7 ± 27.3
Urea (mg/dL)	45.0 (37.0–89.0)
Hemoglobin (g/dL)	12.4 ± 1.4
Albumin (g/dL)	4.4 (4.2–4.7)
cholesterol (mg/dL)	170.0 (157.0–208.0)
LDL-cholesterol (mg/dL)	96.0 (74.2–115.0)

Table 2. Cont.

Analyzed Parameter	Value (Mean ± SD or Median and Q1–Q3)
HDL-cholesterol (mg/dL)	58.2 ± 16.9
Triglyceride (mg/dL)	101.0 (77.0–152.0)
Calcium (mg/dL)	10.0 ± 0.4
Inorganic phosphate (mg/dL)	4.7 ± 0.8
Intact parathormone (pg/mL)	53.5 (29.6–111.0)
Alkaline phosphatase (IU/L)	180.1 ± 77.6
25(OH)D (ng/mL)	21.2 (16.3–29.6)
Uric acid (mg/dL)	6.3 ± 1.3
pH	7.41 ± 0.04
HCO_3^- (mmol/L)	24.6 (22.8–25.6)
BE (mmol/L)	−0.35 ± 3.16

SD—standard deviation, Q1—the first quartile, Q3—the third quartile, NT-proBNP—N-terminal pro-brain natriuretic peptide, GFR—glomerular filtration rate according to Schwartz formula, LDL—low-density lipoprotein, HDL—high-density lipoprotein, 25(OH)D—25-hydroxy-vitamin D, pH—power of hydrogen, HCO_3^-—bicarbonate, BE—base excess. [1] $p = 0.010$, [2] $p = 0.004$, [3] $p = 0.018$.

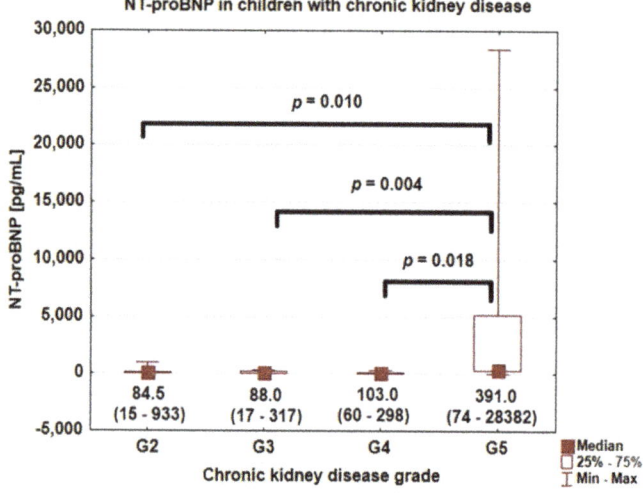

Figure 2. NT-proBNP in children with chronic kidney disease (median value and range) (G—chronic kidney disease grade).

Relevant biochemical disturbances were found in the following numbers of CKD children—anemia in 13 (34%), hypercholesterolemia in 11 (29%), hypertriglyceridemia in 14 (37%), hypercalcemia in 1 (2.6%), hyperphosphatemia in 2 (5.2%), and elevated iPTH in 8 (21.1%) patients.

3.3. Blood Pressure and Markers of Arterial and Heart Damage

Blood pressure and markers of arterial and heart damage are shown in Table 3. At the time of the study, elevated office systolic blood pressure was found in 6 (15.8%) and elevated DBP in 4 (10.5%) children. Abnormal (i.e., ≥95c.) PWV was found in 1 (2.6%), and abnormal cIMT in 12 (31.6%) CKD children. LVH was found in 4 (10.5%) and abnormal RWT in none of the subjects. None of the children had mildly reduced or reduced EF.

Table 3. Blood pressure, arterial, and heart parameters in the study group.

Parameter	Children with Primary Hypertension
Blood pressure and heart rate	
Peripheral office SBP (mmHg)	116.4 ± 12.9
Peripheral office SBP Z-score	0.99 ± 1.28
Peripheral office DBP (mmHg)	71.7 ± 12.7
Peripheral office DBP Z-score	0.82 ± 1.1
Peripheral office MAP (mmHg)	87.5 ± 12.3
Peripheral office PP (mmHg)	44.7 ± 7.7
Aortic office SBP (mmHg)	101.5 ± 13.9
Aortic office DBP (mmHg)	73.4 ± 12.8
Aortic office MAP (mmHg)	87.5 ± 12.3
Aortic office PP (mmHg)	27.4 ± 5.3
Heart rate [bpm]	82 ± 14.2
Arterial structure and function	
cIMT (mm)	0.47 ± 0.06
cIMT Z-score	1.77 ± 1.21
AP (mmHg)	1.5 (−1.3–5.3)
AP/PP (AIx) (%)	6.5 ± 16.2
P2/P1 (AIx) (%)	108.3 ± 25.4
AIx75HR (%)	12.4 ± 18.9
SEVR (%)	151.3 (139.3–173)
PWV (m/s)	4.56 ± 0.86
PWV Z-score	−0.37 ± 1.27
Heart structure and function	
IVSDd (mm)	6.0 (5–7)
LVDd (mm)	44.3 ± 7.0 (39–50)
LVPWd (mm)	6.0 (4.6–6.5)
LAD (mm)	28.2 ± 4.3
RWT	0.24 (0.22–0.28)
LVM (g)	79.8 (53.4–114.5)
LVMI (g/m$^{2.7}$)	28.7 (26.4–33.3)
SF (%)	40.1 ± 5.8
EF (%)	70.5 ± 6.69
E (cm/s)	89.38 ± 13.43
A (cm/s)	59.97 ± 11.4
E/A	1.55 ± 0.37
Edt (ms)	165 (148–192)
E' (cm/s)	13.11 ± 2.67
A' (cm/s)	6.20 (5.5–6.5)
E/E'	6.94 (5.83–7.49)
IVRT (ms)	68.4 ± 22.2
IVCT (ms)	77.2 ± 19.58
C' (m/s)	6.0 ± 1.2

SD—standard deviation, Q1—the first quartile, Q3—the third quartile, SBP—systolic blood pressure, DBP—diastolic blood pressure, MAP—mean arterial pressure, PP—pulse pressure, cIMT—common carotid artery intima media thickness, AP—augmentation pressure, P—peak pressure, Aix—augmentation index, AIx75HR—augmentation index normalized to heart rate 75 beats per minute, SEVR—subendocardial viability ratio, PWV—aortic pulse wave velocity, d—end-diastolic phase, IVS—interventricular septum transverse diameter, LVD—left ventricular diastolic diameter, LVPW—left ventricular posterior wall diameter, LAD—left atrial transverse diameter, RWT—relative wall thickness, LVM—left ventricular mass, LVMI—left ventricular mass index, SF—shortening fraction, EF—ejection fraction, E—peak wave velocity in early diastole, A—peak wave velocity in late diastole caused by atrial contraction, Edt—E deceleration time, E'—mean value of peak medial and lateral mitral annular velocity during early filling, A'—mean value of peak medial and lateral mitral annular velocity during late filling, IVRT—isovolumetric relaxation time, IVCT—isovolumetric contraction time, C'—maximum speed of systolic wave.

3.4. Correlations of NT-proBNP and Markers of Arterial and Heart Damage

Significant correlations of NT-proBNP are depicted in Table 4. In CKD children, NT-proBNP correlated positively with markers of arterial damage: AP/PP, P2/P1, cIMT Z-score, and with the marker of diastolic dysfunction—E/E'. NT-proBNP concentration correlated negatively with the alfacalcidol dose and GFR. No significant relations were found among NT-proBNP and blood pressure, PWV ((m/s) and Z-score), AIx75HR, LVMI, RWT, SF, EF, and E/A.

Table 4. Significant correlations of NT-proBNP with analyzed clinical, biochemical, and cardiovascular parameters in children with CKD (Spearman's rank correlations).

Analyzed Parameter	R	p
Alfacalcidol dose (μg/24 h)	−0.365	0.043
Creatinine (mg/dL)	0.367	0.023
GFR (mL/min/1.73 m^2)	−0.423	0.008
Urea (mg/dL)	0.407	0.008
Inorganic phosphate (mg/dL)	0.443	0.005
Intact parathormone (pg/mL)	0.435	0.006
Triglyceride (mg/dL)	0.492	0.002
AP/PP (AIx) (%)	0.451	0.018
P2/P1 (AIx) (%)	0.460	0.016
cIMT Z-score	0.504	0.020
E/E'	0.400	0.032

GFR—glomerular filtration rate, AP—augmentation pressure, PP—pulse pressure, Aix—augmentation index, P—peak pressure, cIMT—carotid intima-media thickness, E—peak wave velocity in early diastole, E'—mean value of peak medial and lateral mitral annular velocity during early filling by tissue Doppler.

PWV correlated significantly with peripheral and central DBP (r = 0.417, p = 0.034 and r = 0.406, p = 0.04, respectively), LVPWd (r = 0.506, p = 0.010), LVM (r = 0.482, p = 0.015), and A' (r = 0.467, p = 0.038); PWV Z-score correlated with heart rate (r = 0.519, p = 0.013), A (r = 0.600, p = 0.011), and E/A (r = −0.578, p = 0.015); there was also trend towards a positive correlation between PWV Z-score and triglycerides (r = 0.404, p = 0.503); AP/PP correlated positively with PTH (r = 0.383, p = 0.048), cIMT Z-score (r = 0.533, p = 0.016), and A (r = 0.495, p = 0.031); P2/P1 correlated positively with calcium (r = 0.489, p = 0.010), alkaline phosphatase (r = 0.452, p = 0.020), PTH (r = 0.423, p = 0.028), cIMT Z-score (r = 0.510, p = 0.022), A (r = 0.616, p = 0.005), and negatively with E/A (r = −0.511, p = 0.026); cIMT correlated also positively with triglycerides (r = 0.461, p = 0.016) and negatively with calcium (r = −0.392, p = 0.043); cIMT Z-score correlated positively with triglycerides (r = 0.546, p = 0.011) and with RWT (r = 0.573, p = 0.008), negatively with E' (r = −0.543, p = 0.030) and C' (r = −0.733, p = 0.001).

LVMI correlated positively with triglycerides (r = 0.377, p = 0.030) and uric acid (r = 0.370, p = 0.031); RWT with C' (r = −0.466, p = 0.011); E/A with calcium (r = −0.38, p = 0.043), alkaline phosphatase (r = −0.623, p < 0.001), and triglycerides (r = −0.450, p = 0.016); A' with number of antihypertensive medications (r = 0.508, p = 0.013); E/E' with calcium (r = 0.466, p = 0.011); and C' correlated positively with hemoglobin (r = 0.413, p = 0.026), and negatively with AP/PP (r = −0.455, p = 0.044) and P2/P1 (r = −0.489, p = 0.029).

The correlations of the analyzed parameters with age are presented in Supplementary Materials Tables S1 and S2. In the studied children, there was no significant association between age and NT-proBNP (r = −0.166, p = 0.320). Age correlated negatively with serum calcium, inorganic phosphate, alkaline phosphatase, and pH (r = −0.336, p = 0.039; r = −0.397, p = 0.014; r = −0.590, p = 0.001, and r = −0.459, p = 0.001, respectively), and positively with both peripheral and central systolic and diastolic blood pressures expressed in (mm Hg) (r = 0.388–0.493, p = 0.046–0.009); no significant associations were found between age and blood pressure Z-scores. Age correlated also positively with PWV (m/s) (r = 0.490, p = 0.011), but not with PWV Z-score (r = 0.090, p = 0.677), and negatively with augmentation indices (r = −0.396–−0.521, p = 0.040–0.005). Moreover, numerous cardiac dimensions (IVSDd, LVDd, LVPWd, LAD) correlated positively with age (r = 0.459–0.727, p = 0.012–<0.001); LV mass was positively related to age, too (r = 0.703, p < 0.001). In addition, age correlated negatively with A and positively with E/A and E' (r = −0.393, p = 0.035; r = 0.464, p = 0.011 and r = 0.438, p = 0.017, respectively).

In the multivariate analysis, logNT-proBNP was the only significant predictor of the cIMT Z-score (beta = 0.402, 95CI (0.082–0.721), p = 0.014), and P2/P1 (beta = 0.130, 95CI (0.082–0.721), p = 0.014).

4. Discussion

Chronic kidney disease and cardiovascular disease are conditions that inter-influence. In CKD patients, a gradual decline in GFR leads to overhydration and accumulation of uremic toxins. Besides fluid overload, CKD patients are exposed to numerous other traditional (hyperlipidemia, volume-independent arterial hypertension) and non-traditional, i.e., "uremia-specific" risk factors, such as malnutrition, calcium–phosphorus disturbances, anemia, and hyperhomocysteinemia. Together, they contribute to cardiovascular damage and significant shortening of estimated lifespan [1,28]. Thus, it is crucial to establish the individual CVD risk to stratify patients to particular risk groups, diagnose the disease early, improve the treatment process, and initiate cardio- and renoprotective measures. NT-proBNP is one possible biomarker of increased cardiovascular risk.

In our cohort of 38 children, we observed an abnormally elevated value of NT-proBNP in almost half of the individuals. As there is no final consensus on normal pediatric NT-proBNP values, we used the manufacturer's range. Nir and Lam proposed slightly higher normal values of the marker in the pediatric population, but they used a different kit [29,30]. NT-proBNP accumulates during CKD because of impaired renal clearance [31,32]. In our study group, NT-proBNP correlated negatively with GFR, and a gradual increase in NT-proBNP following CKD grades was found. A high concentration of NT-proBNP may contribute to cardiac strain in CKD, indicating vascular system overload. NT-proBNP provided essential prognostic and diagnostic information on fluid overload and cardiovascular damage in adults with CKD [9,33,34], despite its strong relation to kidney function. It was proven that elevated NT-proBNP concentration is correlated twofold with mortality risk [33]. NT-proBNP level indicating increased CVD risk in CKD population seems to be substantially higher in comparison to healthy people [9].

There are limited data on the usefulness of NT-proBNP as a marker of cardiovascular damage in pediatric CKD patients. A positive correlation between NT-proBNP concentration and E/A, left atrial diameter, and left ventricle hypertrophy (LVH) was reported in small pediatric CKD cohorts [11,12]. We have observed a positive correlation between NT-proBNP and the degree of diastolic dysfunction measured by tissue Doppler echocardiography. Similarly, Kim et al. outlined the correlation between NT-proBNP and E/E′ in adults, suggesting that NT-proBNP might be an early marker of diastolic dysfunction in CKD patients [34]. No correlation among LV mass, LV ejection fraction, and NT-proBNP was found in our children. We hypothesize that this might be a derivative of a relatively good kidney function (66% of the studied subjects were in CKD grade G2 or G3) and a low prevalence of LV hypertrophy in the analyzed cohort. Of note, none of the patients had even mildly reduced left ventricular ejection fraction. In turn, mild heart damage in our cohort could be explained by a low grade of renal impairment and good control of arterial hypertension. This is a significant difference compared to studies in adult patients with CKD and might explain the failure to demonstrate a statistically significant relationship between left ventricular mass, systolic function, and NT-proBNP in the studied children.

Arterial damage is the earliest indicator of cardiovascular disease in CKD children. Unique, uremia-related biochemical milieu leads to Mönckeberg's arteriosclerosis characterized by intramural calcium–phosphorus deposition, the osteoblast-like transformation of fibroblast, and a high risk of stroke or myocardial infarction [35]. We found numerous correlations among arterial damage and heart dimensions and function parameters, suggesting a strict interplay between arterial and cardiac dysfunctions in these patients.

We have found positive correlations among NT-proBNP, vascular stiffness indicators (AP/PP, P2/P1), and cIMT. NT-proBNP concentrations (expressed as decimal logarithms) were also significant predictors of cIMT and P2/P1 in multivariate analysis. While cIMT is a well-established marker of cardiovascular disease, P2/P1 and its derivative—the augmentation index shows a weaker correlation with hard-end points than the gold standard of arterial stiffness—aortic pulse wave velocity [36,37]. Little is known about pathophysiological relations between intimal and medial thickening and the heart. Sasaki found no significant associations between cIMT or the presence of atherosclerotic plaques and NT-proBNP level [38]. On the other hand, Asian authors found a positive correlation between cIMT and the concentration of this biomarker in adults with CKD [10,39,40].

NT-proBNP influences adipocyte function and was found to be negatively related to total and LDL-cholesterol concentrations [41,42]. These data suggest that NT-proBNP may have protective actions against arteriosclerosis and atherosclerotic plaque formation. It is possible that this compensatory mechanism is ineffective in CKD despite NT-proBNP accumulation. Our results suggest that NT-proBNP might serve in CKD pediatric patients as a valuable tool assessing the risk of arterial damage. Because of the cross-sectional study design, a causal relationship between cIMT thickening and NT-proBNP rise cannot be established. There is a need for prospective studies to establish its position as a biomarker of cIMT in this and other high-risk pediatric populations.

Numerous associations between NT-proBNP and calcium–phosphate metabolism parameters were observed in our study group, suggesting cardiovascular damage induced by these metabolic derangements. Similar relations were revealed in research conducted among pediatric CKD G3–G5 patients by Rinat [11]. In both adult [43] and pediatric [11,12] studies, NT-proBNP correlated positively with blood pressure. Despite evaluation of both peripheral and central blood pressure, no such relation was revealed in our cohort. We think that relatively mild kidney impairment and the common use of antihypertensive medications could mask this relationship. Furthermore, we evaluated blood pressure based on individual office measurements, which could be a source of potential bias.

Moreover, one should remember that, according to literature data, other factors may influence NT-proBNP levels, such as anemia, BMI (especially obesity), and gender [44–46]. None of these variables influenced NT-proBNP in our cohort, except for BMI. Nevertheless, this marker ought to be carefully interpreted in CKD patients considering factors that might affect it.

In our cohort of CKD patients, we revealed numerous significant correlations among biochemical parameters, heart dimensions, arterial stiffness parameters, and age. Of note, there was no significant association between age and NT-proBNP. A negative association between age and parameters of calcium–phosphorus metabolism reflects normal bone metabolism, varying with age, observed in both healthy [47] and CKD children [48]. As age and body size are crucial determinants of blood pressure and cardiac dimensions, proper indexation and comparison of the measured value with population-based norms is necessary in pediatric patients [21,26]. Noteworthy, age-normalized blood pressure and left ventricular mass index did not show any significant correlations with age.

Progressive stiffening of the arteries (measured as aortic PWV) is a well-known phenomenon, responsible, e.g., for isolated systolic hypertension in the elderly [49]. Age-dependent increase in PWV is seen already in the first two decades of life and was confirmed in large cohorts of healthy children [24,50]. On the other hand, the inverse relationship among age, body dimensions, and augmentation index was observed in the general population, similar to our cohort. In younger (and therefore shorter) patients, the pulse wave reflected from the peripheral arteries reaches back to the aorta more quickly due to its shorter pathway, resulting in an increase in the augmentation index in the youngest children, as revealed by Hidvegi et al. [51].

Some limitations of our study may be identified. We reported only a single-center study with a limited number of CKD patients, and broader research should be carried out, including a comparison of the NT-proBNP level in a control group. In addition, the vast majority of the subjects were in CKD G2 and G3 with minor biochemical and cardiovascular abnormalities, which might have influenced the number of NT-proBNP correlations. Finally, the study's cross-sectional nature precludes drawing final casual relationships between NT-proBNP and the measured parameters.

5. Conclusions

Our cross-sectional analysis revealed numerous correlations between NT-proBNP and arterial and heart damage indices in children with chronic kidney disease. As NT-proBNP was a significant determinant of cIMT and P2/P1 in the multivariate analysis, we conclude that NT-proBNP may serve as a possible marker of thickening of the carotid artery wall in pediatric patients with kidney function impairment. NT-proBNP could be used in everyday clinical practice to assess cardiovascular risk in these subjects as evaluation of its serum concentration is easy accessible, relatively cheap, and repeatable. Conversely, due to our study's limitations, the final role of NT-proBNP as a biomarker of arterial damage, left ventricular hypertrophy or diastolic cardiac dysfunction in children with CKD needs confirmation in prospective studies.

Supplementary Materials: The following are available online at https://www.mdpi.com/article/10.3390/jcm10194344/s1, Table S1: Correlations of age with NT-proBNP, clinical, and biochemical parameters in the study group. Table S2: Correlations of age with blood pressure, arterial, and heart parameters in the study group.

Author Contributions: Conceptualization, P.S., M.O.-N. and M.P.-T.; methodology, P.S., M.O.-N., R.P.; validation, P.S., B.W., M.P.-T.; formal analysis, P.S., M.O.-N.; investigation, P.S., M.O.-N., R.P.; resources, B.W., M.P.-T.; data curation, P.S., M.O.-N.; writing—original draft preparation, P.S., M.O.-N., K.P., K.W.; writing—review and editing, B.W., M.P.-T.; visualization, P.S., M.O.-N., K.P., K.W.; supervision, M.P.-T.; project administration, P.S., M.O.-N. and M.P.-T.; funding acquisition, M.P.-T. All authors have read and agreed to the published version of the manuscript.

Funding: This research was funded from the statutory funds of the Department of Pediatrics and Nephrology, Medical University of Warsaw.

Institutional Review Board Statement: The study was conducted according to the guidelines of the Declaration of Helsinki and approved by the Local Bioethics Committee of the Medical University of Warsaw (approval no. KB/89/2013).

Informed Consent Statement: Informed consent was obtained from all subjects ($\geq$16 years) and their representatives involved in the study.

Data Availability Statement: The data presented in this study are available upon request from the corresponding author.

Conflicts of Interest: The authors declare no conflict of interest.

References

1. Weaver, D.J.; Mitsnefes, M. Cardiovascular Disease in Children and Adolescents with Chronic Kidney Disease. *Semin. Nephrol.* **2018**, *38*, 559–569. [CrossRef] [PubMed]
2. Shroff, R.; Dégi, A.; Kerti, A.; Kis, E.; Cseprekál, O.; Tory, K.; Szabó, A.J.; Reusz, G.S. Cardiovascular risk assessment in children with chronic kidney disease. *Pediatr. Nephrol.* **2013**, *28*, 875–884. [CrossRef] [PubMed]
3. Maisel, A.S.; Duran, J.M.; Wettersten, N. Natriuretic Peptides in Heart Failure: Atrial and B-type Natriuretic Peptides. *Heart Fail. Clin.* **2018**, *14*, 13–25. [CrossRef] [PubMed]
4. Goetze, J.P.; Bruneau, B.G.; Ramos, H.R.; Ogawa, T.; de Bold, M.K.; de Bold, A.J. Cardiac natriuretic peptides. *Nat. Rev. Cardiol.* **2020**, *17*, 698–717. [CrossRef] [PubMed]
5. Han, X.; Zhang, S.; Chen, Z.; Adhikari, B.K.; Zhang, Y.; Zhang, J.; Sun, J.; Wang, Y. Cardiac biomarkers of heart failure in chronic kidney disease. *Clin. Chim. Acta* **2020**, *510*, 298–310. [CrossRef]
6. Forte, M.; Madonna, M.; Schiavon, S.; Valenti, V.; Versaci, F.; Zoccai, G.B.; Frati, G.; Sciarretta, S. Cardiovascular Pleiotropic Effects of Natriuretic Peptides. *Int. J. Mol. Sci.* **2019**, *20*, 3874. [CrossRef]
7. Felker, G.M.; Petersen, J.W.; Mark, D.B. Natriuretic peptides in the diagnosis and management of heart failure. *CMAJ* **2006**, *175*, 611–617. [CrossRef]
8. Colbert, G.; Jain, N.; de Lemos, J.A.; Hedayati, S.S. Utility of traditional circulating and imaging-based cardiac biomarkers in patients with predialysis CKD. *Clin. J. Am. Soc. Nephrol.* **2015**, *10*, 515–529. [CrossRef]
9. Harrison, T.G.; Shukalek, C.B.; Hemmelgarn, B.R.; Zarnke, K.B.; Ronksley, P.E.; Iragorri, N.; Graham, M.M.; James, M.T. Association of NT-proBNP and BNP with Future Clinical Outcomes in Patients with ESKD: A Systematic Review and Meta-analysis. *Am. J. Kidney Dis.* **2020**, *76*, 233–247. [CrossRef]

10. Li, X.; Yang, X.C.; Sun, Q.M.; Chen, X.D.; Li, Y.C. Brain natriuretic peptide and copeptin levels are associated with cardiovascular disease in patients with chronic kidney disease. *Chin. Med. J.* **2013**, *126*, 823–827.
11. Rinat, C.; Becker-Cohen, R.; Nir, A.; Feinstein, S.; Algur, N.; Ben-Shalom, E.; Farber, B.; Frishberg, Y. B-type natriuretic peptides are reliable markers of cardiac strain in CKD pediatric patients. *Pediatr. Nephrol.* **2012**, *27*, 617–625. [CrossRef]
12. Nalcacioglu, H.; Ozkaya, O.; Kafali, H.C.; Tekcan, D.; Avci, B.; Baysal, K. Is N-terminal pro-brain natriuretic peptide a reliable marker for body fluid status in children with chronic kidney disease? *Arch. Med. Sci.* **2020**, *16*, 802. [CrossRef]
13. Kidney Disease: Improving Global Outcomes (KDIGO) CKD Work Group. KDIGO 2012 Clinical Practice Guideline for the Evaluation and Management of Chronic Kidney Disease. *Kidney Int. Suppl.* **2013**, *3*, 1–150.
14. Harambat, J.; van Stralen, K.J.; Kim, J.J.; Tizard, E.J. Epidemiology of chronic kidney disease in children. *Pediatr. Nephrol.* **2012**, *27*, 363–373. [CrossRef]
15. Schwartz, G.J.; Muñoz, A.; Schneider, M.F.; Mak, R.H.; Kaskel, F.; Warady, B.A.; Furth, S.L. New equations to estimate GFR in children with CKD. *J. Am. Soc. Nephrol.* **2009**, *20*, 629–637. [CrossRef]
16. Kułaga, Z.; Litwin, M.; Tkaczyk, M.; Palczewska, I.; Zajączkowska, M.; Zwolińska, D.; Krynicki, T.; Wasilewska, A.; Moczulska, A.; Morawiec-Knysak, A.; et al. Polish 2010 growth references for school-aged children and adolescents. *Eur. J. Pediatr.* **2011**, *170*, 599–609. [CrossRef] [PubMed]
17. Drüeke, T.B.; Parfrey, P.S. Summary of the KDIGO guideline on anemia and comment: Reading between the (guide)line(s). *Kidney Int.* **2012**, *82*, 952–960. [CrossRef] [PubMed]
18. KDIGO 2017 Clinical Practice Guideline Update for the Diagnosis, Evaluation, Prevention, and Treatment of Chronic Kidney Disease-Mineral and Bone Disorder (CKD-MBD). *Kidney Int. Suppl.* **2017**, *7*, 1–59. [CrossRef]
19. Stewart, J.; McCallin, T.; Martinez, J.; Chacko, S.; Yusuf, S. Hyperlipidemia. *Pediatr. Rev.* **2020**, *41*, 393–402. [CrossRef]
20. Feig, D.I.; Kang, D.H.; Johnson, R.J. Uric acid and cardiovascular risk. *N. Engl. J. Med.* **2008**, *359*, 1811–1821. [CrossRef]
21. Kułaga, Z.; Litwin, M.; Grajda, A.; Kułaga, K.; Gurzkowska, B.; Góźdź, M.; Pan, H. Oscillometric blood pressure percentiles for Polish normal-weight school-aged children and adolescents. *J. Hypertens.* **2012**, *30*, 1942–1954. [CrossRef]
22. Skrzypczyk, P.; Przychodzień, J.; Mizerska-Wasiak, M.; Kuźma-Mroczkowska, E.; Okarska-Napierała, M.; Górska, E.; Stelmaszczyk-Emmel, A.; Demkow, U.; Pańczyk-Tomaszewska, M. Renalase in Children with Glomerular Kidney Diseases. *Adv. Exp. Med. Biol.* **2017**, *1021*, 81–92. [CrossRef] [PubMed]
23. Doyon, A.; Kracht, D.; Bayazit, A.K.; Deveci, M.; Duzova, A.; Krmar, R.T.; Litwin, M.; Niemirska, A.; Oguz, B.; Schmidt, B.M.; et al. Carotid artery intima-media thickness and distensibility in children and adolescents: Reference values and role of body dimensions. *Hypertension* **2013**, *62*, 550–556. [CrossRef] [PubMed]
24. Reusz, G.S.; Cseprekal, O.; Temmar, M.; Kis, E.; Cherif, A.B.; Thaleb, A.; Fekete, A.; Szabó, A.J.; Benetos, A.; Salvi, P. Reference values of pulse wave velocity in healthy children and teenagers. *Hypertension* **2010**, *56*, 217–224. [CrossRef] [PubMed]
25. De Simone, G.; Daniels, S.R.; Devereux, R.B.; Meyer, R.A.; Roman, M.J.; de Divitiis, O.; Alderman, M.H. Left ventricular mass and body size in normotensive children and adults: Assessment of allometric relations and impact of overweight. *J. Am. Coll. Cardiol.* **1992**, *20*, 1251–1260. [CrossRef]
26. Khoury, P.R.; Mitsnefes, M.; Daniels, S.R.; Kimball, T.R. Age-specific reference intervals for indexed left ventricular mass in children. *J. Am. Soc. Echocardiogr.* **2009**, *22*, 709–714. [CrossRef] [PubMed]
27. McDonagh, T.A.; Metra, M.; Adamo, M.; Gardner, R.S.; Baumbach, A.; Böhm, M.; Burri, H.; Butler, J.; Čelutkienė, J.; Chioncel, O.; et al. 2021 ESC Guidelines for the diagnosis and treatment of acute and chronic heart failure. *Eur. Heart J.* **2021**, *42*, 3599–3726. [CrossRef]
28. Querfeld, U.; Schaefer, F. Cardiovascular risk factors in children on dialysis: An update. *Pediatr. Nephrol.* **2020**, *35*, 41–57. [CrossRef]
29. Nir, A.; Lindinger, A.; Rauh, M.; Bar-Oz, B.; Laer, S.; Schwachtgen, L.; Koch, A.; Falkenberg, J.; Mir, T.S. NT-pro-B-type natriuretic peptide in infants and children: Reference values based on combined data from four studies. *Pediatr. Cardiol.* **2009**, *30*, 3–8. [CrossRef]
30. Lam, E.; Higgins, V.; Zhang, L.; Chan, M.K.; Bohn, M.K.; Trajcevski, K.; Liu, P.; Adeli, K.; Nathan, P.C. Normative Values of High-Sensitivity Cardiac Troponin T and N-Terminal pro-B-Type Natriuretic Peptide in Children and Adolescents: A Study from the CALIPER Cohort. *J. Appl. Lab. Med.* **2020**, *6*, 344–353. [CrossRef] [PubMed]
31. Niizuma, S.; Iwanaga, Y.; Yahata, T.; Tamaki, Y.; Goto, Y.; Nakahama, H.; Miyazaki, S. Impact of left ventricular end-diastolic wall stress on plasma B-type natriuretic peptide in heart failure with chronic kidney disease and end-stage renal disease. *Clin. Chem.* **2009**, *55*, 1347–1353. [CrossRef]
32. Apple, F.S.; Murakami, M.M.; Pearce, L.A.; Herzog, C.A. Multi-Biomarker Risk Stratification of N-Terminal Pro-B-Type Natriuretic Peptide, High-Sensitivity C-Reactive Protein, and Cardiac Troponin T and I in End-Stage Renal Disease for All-Cause Death. *Clin. Chem.* **2004**, *50*, 2279–2285. [CrossRef] [PubMed]
33. Shafi, T.; Zager, P.G.; Sozio, S.M.; Grams, M.E.; Jaar, B.G.; Christenson, R.H.; Boulware, L.E.; Parekh, R.S.; Powe, N.R.; Coresh, J. Troponin I and NT-proBNP and the association of systolic blood pressure with outcomes in incident hemodialysis patients: The Choices for Healthy Outcomes in Caring for ESRD (CHOICE) Study. *Am. J. Kidney Dis.* **2014**, *64*, 443–451. [CrossRef] [PubMed]
34. Kim, J.S.; Yang, J.W.; Yoo, J.S.; Choi, S.O.; Han, B.G. Association between E/e ratio and fluid overload in patients with predialysis chronic kidney disease. *PLoS ONE* **2017**, *12*, e0184764. [CrossRef] [PubMed]

35. Litwin, M.; Niemirska, A. Intima-media thickness measurements in children with cardiovascular risk factors. *Pediatr. Nephrol.* **2009**, *24*, 707–719. [CrossRef] [PubMed]
36. Scandale, G.; Dimitrov, G.; Recchia, M.; Carzaniga, G.; Perilli, E.; Carotta, M.; Catalano, M. Arterial stiffness and 5-year mortality in patients with peripheral arterial disease. *J. Hum. Hypertens.* **2020**, *34*, 505–511. [CrossRef]
37. Willeit, P.; Tschiderer, L.; Allara, E.; Reuber, K.; Seekircher, L.; Gao, L.; Liao, X.; Lonn, E.; Gerstein, H.C.; Yusuf, S.; et al. Carotid Intima-Media Thickness Progression as Surrogate Marker for Cardiovascular Risk: Meta-Analysis of 119 Clinical Trials Involving 100 667 Patients. *Circulation* **2020**, *142*, 621–642. [CrossRef]
38. Sasaki, N.; Yamamoto, H.; Ozono, R.; Maeda, R.; Kihara, Y. Association of Common Carotid Artery Measurements with N-terminal Pro B-type Natriuretic Peptide in Elderly Participants. *Intern. Med.* **2020**, *59*, 917–925. [CrossRef] [PubMed]
39. Zhou, W.; Ni, Z.; Yu, Z.; Shi, B.; Wang, Q. Brain natriuretic peptide is related to carotid plaques and predicts atherosclerosis in pre-dialysis patients with chronic kidney disease. *Eur. J. Intern. Med.* **2012**, *23*, 539–544. [CrossRef]
40. Hayashi, M.; Yasuda, Y.; Suzuki, S.; Tagaya, M.; Ito, T.; Kamada, T.; Yoshinaga, M.; Sugishita, Y.; Fujiwara, W.; Yokoi, H.; et al. Brain natriuretic peptide as a potential novel marker of salt-sensitivity in chronic kidney disease patients without cardiac dysfunction. *Heart Vessels* **2017**, *32*, 279–286. [CrossRef]
41. Sanchez, O.A.; Duprez, D.A.; Bahrami, H.; Daniels, L.B.; Folsom, A.R.; Lima, J.A.; Maisel, A.; Peralta, C.A.; Jacobs, D.R., Jr. The associations between metabolic variables and NT-proBNP are blunted at pathological ranges: The Multi-Ethnic Study of Atherosclerosis. *Metabolism* **2014**, *63*, 475–483. [CrossRef] [PubMed]
42. Schmid, A.; Albrecht, J.; Brock, J.; Koukou, M.; Arapogianni, E.; Schäffler, A.; Karrasch, T. Regulation of natriuretic peptides postprandially in vivo and of their receptors in adipocytes by fatty acids in vitro. *Mol. Cell. Endocrinol.* **2018**, *473*, 225–234. [CrossRef] [PubMed]
43. Hirata, Y.; Matsumoto, A.; Aoyagi, T.; Yamaoki, K.; Komuro, I.; Suzuki, T.; Ashida, T.; Sugiyama, T.; Hada, Y.; Kuwajima, I.; et al. Measurement of plasma brain natriuretic peptide level as a guide for cardiac overload. *Cardiovasc. Res.* **2001**, *51*, 585–591. [CrossRef]
44. Redfield, M.M.; Rodeheffer, R.J.; Jacobsen, S.J.; Mahoney, D.W.; Bailey, K.R.; Burnett, J.C., Jr. Plasma brain natriuretic peptide concentration: Impact of age and gender. *J. Am. Coll. Cardiol.* **2002**, *40*, 976–982. [CrossRef]
45. Tsuji, H.; Nishino, N.; Kimura, Y.; Yamada, K.; Nukui, M.; Yamamoto, S.; Iwasaka, T.; Takahashi, H. Haemoglobin level influences plasma brain natriuretic peptide concentration. *Acta Cardiol.* **2004**, *59*, 527–531. [CrossRef] [PubMed]
46. Wang, T.J.; Larson, M.G.; Levy, D.; Benjamin, E.J.; Leip, E.P.; Wilson, P.W.; Vasan, R.S. Impact of obesity on plasma natriuretic peptide levels. *Circulation* **2004**, *109*, 594–600. [CrossRef]
47. Marwaha, R.K.; Khadgawat, R.; Tandon, N.; Kanwar, R.; Narang, A.; Sastry, A.; Bhadra, K.; Kalaivani, M. Reference intervals of serum calcium, ionized calcium, phosphate and alkaline phosphatase in healthy Indian school children and adolescents. *Clin. Biochem.* **2010**, *43*, 1216–1219. [CrossRef]
48. Bakkaloglu, S.A.; Bacchetta, J.; Lalayiannis, A.D.; Leifheit-Nestler, M.; Stabouli, S.; Haarhaus, M.; Reusz, G.; Groothoff, J.; Schmitt, C.P.; Evenepoel, P.; et al. Bone evaluation in paediatric chronic kidney disease: Clinical practice points from the European Society for Paediatric Nephrology CKD-MBD and Dialysis working groups and CKD-MBD working group of the ERA-EDTA. *Nephrol. Dial. Transplant.* **2021**, *36*, 413–425. [CrossRef]
49. Gąsowski, J.; Piotrowicz, K.; Messerli, F.H. Arterial hypertension after age 65: From epidemiology and pathophysiology to therapy Do we know where we stand? *Kardiol. Pol.* **2018**, *76*, 723–730. [CrossRef]
50. Thurn, D.; Doyon, A.; Sözeri, B.; Bayazit, A.K.; Canpolat, N.; Duzova, A.; Querfeld, U.; Schmidt, B.M.; Schaefer, F.; Wühl, E.; et al. Aortic Pulse Wave Velocity in Healthy Children and Adolescents: Reference Values for the Vicorder Device and Modifying Factors. *Am. J. Hypertens.* **2015**, *28*, 1480–1488. [CrossRef] [PubMed]
51. Hidvégi, E.V.; Illyés, M.; Molnár, F.T.; Cziráki, A. Influence of body height on aortic systolic pressure augmentation and wave reflection in childhood. *J. Hum. Hypertens.* **2015**, *29*, 495–501. [CrossRef] [PubMed]

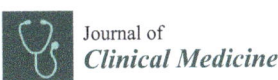

Journal of
Clinical Medicine

Article

Urinary Levels of Cathepsin B in Preterm Newborns

Monika Kamianowska [1,*], Marek Szczepański [1], Anna Krukowska [1], Aleksandra Kamianowska [2] and Anna Wasilewska [2]

1. Department of Neonatology and Neonatal Intensive Care, Medical University of Bialystok, 15-276 Białystok, Poland; szczepanski5@gazeta.pl (M.S.); anna_krukowska1@wp.pl (A.K.)
2. Department of Pediatrics and Nephrology, Medical University of Bialystok, 15-276 Białystok, Poland; olcikkam@wp.pl (A.K.); annwasil@interia.pl (A.W.)
* Correspondence: monikakamm@wp.pl; Tel.: +48-85-746-84-98; Fax: +48-85-746-86-63

Abstract: Increased investment in perinatal health in developing countries has improved the survival of preterm newborns, but their significant multiorgan immaturity is associated with short and long-term adverse consequences. Cathepsin B, as a protease with angiogenic properties, may be related to the process of nephrogenesis. A total of 88 neonates (60 premature children, 28 healthy term children) were included in this prospective study. We collected urine samples on the first or second day of life. In order to determine the concentration of cathepsin B in the urine, the commercially available enzyme immunoassay was used. The urinary concentrations of cathepsin B normalized with the urinary concentrations of creatinine (cathepsin B/Cr.) in newborns born at 30–34, 35–36, and 37–41 (the control group) weeks of pregnancy were (median, Q1–Q3) 4.00 (2.82–5.12), 3.07 (1.95–3.90), and 2.51 (2.00–3.48) ng/mg Cr, respectively. Statistically significant differences were found between the group of newborns born at 30–34 weeks of pregnancy and the control group ($p < 0.01$), and between early and late preterm babies (PTB) ($p < 0.05$). The group of children born at 35–36 weeks of pregnancy and the control group did not differ significantly. This result suggests that the elevated urinary cathepsin B/Cr. level may be the result of the kidneys' immaturity in preterm newborns.

Keywords: cathepsin B; tubular damage; premature neonates; immaturity

Citation: Kamianowska, M.; Szczepański, M.; Krukowska, A.; Kamianowska, A.; Wasilewska, A. Urinary Levels of Cathepsin B in Preterm Newborns. *J. Clin. Med.* **2021**, *10*, 4254. https://doi.org/10.3390/jcm10184254

Academic Editor: Andreas Skolarikos

Received: 23 July 2021
Accepted: 14 September 2021
Published: 19 September 2021

Publisher's Note: MDPI stays neutral with regard to jurisdictional claims in published maps and institutional affiliations.

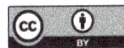

Copyright: © 2021 by the authors. Licensee MDPI, Basel, Switzerland. This article is an open access article distributed under the terms and conditions of the Creative Commons Attribution (CC BY) license (https://creativecommons.org/licenses/by/4.0/).

1. Introduction

Preterm birth (before 37 completed weeks of gestation) accounts for 11% of births worldwide [1]. Increased investment in perinatal health in developing countries and interventions such as antenatal steroids have improved survival in this group of children, but significant multiorgan immaturity is associated with short and long-term adverse consequences [2]. The first kidney glomeruli form at 9–10 weeks of gestation [3]. During the late second and third trimester, there is an exponential increase in the number of nephrons between 18 and 32 weeks [4,5]. Nephrogenesis in humans ends by approximately 34–36 weeks of gestation, with over 60% of nephrons being formed during the last trimester [6]. Hence, in premature neonates, normal nephrogenesis is interrupted, and both nephron number and kidney size are reduced [7]. While nephrogenesis may continue in premature neonates for up to 40 days following birth, these nephrons are not normal and age at an increased rate [8]. However, despite this postnatal development of the kidneys, premature children are still left with a lower number of nephrons. For example, a premature neonate born at 26 weeks of gestation, despite 40 additional days of nephrogenesis, will only have nephron development until 32 weeks as opposed to continuing nephrogenesis to 36 weeks in term gestation [9,10]. Kidney injury from hypoperfusion and drug nephrotoxicity leads to further frequently unnoticed changes in kidney structure and function. Thus, the glomerular and tubular maturation of the kidneys of preterm newborns may be confounded by the nephropathy of prematurity and acute kidney injury (AKI), whose incidence in neonates is estimated at 8–24% of children hospitalised in the Intensive Neonatal Care Units. One-third of this group are premature babies [7,11–13].

Cathepsin B is a lysosomal cysteine protease synthesized on the rough endoplasmic reticulum as a pre-proenzyme; cathepsin B in its mature, double-chain form comprises a heavy chain and a light chain [14–17]. Cathepsin B is a protein belonging to hydrolases and is involved in the processing of hormones and proteins, regulation of the cell cycle, autophagy, and cell death [18,19]. In kidneys, cathepsin B is found in proximal tubule cells. It is involved in the digestion of proteins reabsorbed from the tubular fluid following glomerular filtration. A small amount of this protease can be detected in urine under physiological conditions. Its levels increase because of tubular damage or renal dysfunction [18,20]. During pregnancy, cathepsin B is predominantly found in placental and decidual macrophages, which may be important in the mediation of villous angiogenesis and decidual apoptosis [21]. With tumours, the expression of cathepsin B correlates with angiogenesis and is thought to promote the remodeling of the extracellular matrix to permit neovascularization [22,23].

This study assessed whether cathepsin B may be involved in the maturation of the foetus' kidneys by evaluating the effect of prematurity on the concentration of cathepsin B in the urine of preterm newborns.

2. Patients and Methods

2.1. Patient Recruitment and Sample Collection

A total of 88 neonates were included in this prospective study. Sixty of them were born prematurely at 30–36 weeks of pregnancy. The neonates were hospitalized in the Department of Neonatology and Intensive Neonatal Care at the Medical University of Bialystok, Poland between December 2017 and December 2018. The study was conducted according to the guidelines of the Declaration of Helsinki, and approved by the Local Bioethics Committee of The Medical University of Bialystok (protocol code: R-I-002/360/2016, date of approval: 17 October 2016). Prior to the study written informed consent has been obtained from the parents of all the neonates. The clinical condition of the neonates was good or average; they were appropriate for gestational age (AGA), with the weight between the 10th and 90th centile of birth weight for their gestational age using normalized growth curves [24]. The group of premature babies born at 30–36 weeks of pregnancy were divided into two subgroups: 28 children born between 30 and 34 weeks of pregnancy (hospitalized in the ward for preterm babies) and 32 children born between 35 and 36 weeks of pregnancy (hospitalized in a rooming-in ward). The reference group comprised 28 healthy babies. These neonates developed through normal pregnancies, with no prenatal and perinatal complications.

The inclusion criteria for this study were normal prenatal and postnatal ultrasound examination results of the kidneys, and a good or average clinical condition. The exclusion criteria were: 1-min Apgar scores < 4; congenital abnormalities, including urinary tract defects (polycystic kidney disease, hydronephrosis, duplex kidneys/ureters, renal agenesis, or other anatomical abnormalities); inborn error of metabolism; heart disease; abnormal ultrasound examination of the kidneys and the central nervous system (hyper-echoic zones around the lateral ventricles of the brain and intraventricular hemorrhage grade I and II were accepted); abnormal laboratory tests (including elevated levels of inflammatory markers); treatment with catecholamines, antibiotics, diuretics, or mechanical ventilation. Additionally, the children of mothers with a burdened medical history were excluded from the study.

Collection of urine samples in the study group was performed using single-use sterile bags (Medres, Zabrze, Poland). Urine was collected once on the first or second day of life. The urine samples obtained after centrifugation were kept in the refrigerator (4 °C) for no longer than 2 h and then frozen at −80 °C. Repeated freeze–thaw cycles were not used. Collection of the blood samples was conducted during the first or second day of the neonate's life during routine practice in the Unit. S-Monovette 1.2 mL, Clotting Activator/Serum test tubes (Sarstedt AG & Co., Nümbrecht, Germany) for venous blood sampling were used. A blood cell morphology test and blood biochemistry tests were performed right after taking the blood samples.

2.2. Determination of Urinary Cathepsin

The levels of urinary cathepsin B were determined using a commercially available ELISA kit (Cloud–Clone Corp., Katy, TX, USA), according to manufacturer's instructions, and were expressed in nanograms per milliliter. The detection range was 0.312–20 ng/mL, according to specifications of the kit. The mean intra-assay and inter-assay coefficients of variation (CV) for cathepsin B were <10% and <12%, respectively.

In order to eliminate the potential confounding effect of urinary dilution, we normalized the urinary cathepsin B concentrations for the urinary concentration of creatinine; this was expressed in nanograms per milligram of creatinine (ng/mg Cr). The urinary concentration of creatinine was determined using Jaffé's method.

Calculation of estimated GFR was performed using the Schwartz formula (for the preterm babies, eGFR = 0.33 × L/Scr.; for term babies, eGFR = 0.45 × L/Scr., where L is the length in centimeters and Scr. is serum creatinine in milligrams per deciliter).

The determination of urinary cathepsin B was performed in the Department's Laboratory of Pediatrics and Nephrology, at the Medical University of Bialystok. The morphology and serum biochemistry tests were performed in the Department of Laboratory Diagnostics at the University Clinical Hospital in Bialystok.

2.3. Statistical Analysis

The statistical analysis was completed using Statistica 13.3 package (StatSoft, Cracow, Poland). It expressed discrete variables as counts (percentage), continuous variables as median and quartiles (Q1–Q3). In order to determine normal distribution, the Shapiro–Wilk test was used. The Mann–Whitney U test was used for intergroup comparisons of continuous variables because the data were not normally distributed. To establish the direction and power of association between urinary cathepsin B concentrations and other variables, Spearman's rank correlation coefficients were used. The results were significant at $p < 0.05$.

3. Results

Eighty-eight neonates were included in the study. Twenty-eight of them were healthy neonates, and sixty were born prematurely at 30–36 weeks of pregnancy. Both groups were sex-matched ($p > 0.05$). Birth weight, length, and head and chest circuits were significantly lower in premature neonates than in term children; however, all the children were appropriate for gestational age. Table 1 presents the characteristics of premature babies.

In both examined groups of premature babies (born at 30–34 and at 35–36 weeks of pregnancy), there were no statistically significant differences in the type of delivery (vaginal delivery or caesarean delivery). Both groups were sex-matched ($p > 0.05$). Birth weight was statistically significantly lower in neonates born at 30–34 weeks of pregnancy than in babies born at 35–36 weeks of pregnancy. All premature babies were appropriate for gestational age, and when we divided both groups of preterm neonates according to the percentile of birth weight (10–50 percentile and 51–90 percentile), they were matched according to their percentile of birth weight. Both 5-min and 10-min Apgar scores were ≥8 in all neonates, and lower 1-min and 3-min Apgar scores characterized younger children.

Table 1. Characteristics of premature babies.

Parameters	Premature			p
	(30–36 Weeks) (n = 60)	(30–34 Weeks) (n = 28)	(35–36 Weeks) (n = 32)	
	Median (Q1–Q3)			
Gestational age (weeks)	35 (33–36)	33 (32–34)	36 (35–36)	<0.01
Vaginal delivery/caesarean delivery	16/44	10/22	6/22	NS
Gender (boys/girls)	33/27	16/12	17/15	NS
Birth weight (g)	2450 (2195–2740)	2295 (1720–2450)	2620 (2415–2800)	<0.01
Birth weight (10th–50th percentile/ 51st–90th percentile)	17/43	7/21	10/22	NS
Length (cm)	50.00 (47.00–52.00)	48.00 (45.00–50.00)	52.00 (49.50–53.00)	<0.01
Chest circuit (cm)	30.00 (28.00–31.00)	28.50 (26.50–30.00)	31.00 (30.00–32.00)	<0.01
Head circuit (cm)	32.00 (31.00–33.50)	31.00 (29.00–32.00)	33.00 (32.00–34.00)	<0.01
Prenatal steroid therapy	12	12	0	<0.01
1-min Apgar score (8–10/4–7)	39/21	13/15	26/6	<0.05
3-min Apgar score (8–10/4–7)	47/13	18/10	29/3	<0.05
5-min Apgar score (8–10/4–7)	60/0	28/0	32/0	NS
10-min Apgar score (8–10/4–7)	60/0	28/0	32/0	NS
Oxygen therapy	24	19	5	<0.01
nCPAP	18	17	1	<0.01
Parenteral nutrition	29	24	5	<0.01

p—comparison of children born at 30–34 weeks and 35–36 weeks of pregnancy; NS—non statistical; nCPAP—nasal continuous positive airway pressure.

In both groups of preterm neonates, blood morphology and biochemical tests were normal. Statistically significantly higher number of leucocytes, urea, and alanine aminotransferase concentrations were found in younger children (Table 2).

Table 2. Basic laboratory results of premature neonates.

Parameters	Premature			p
	(30–36 Weeks) (n = 60)	(30–34 Weeks) (n = 28)	(35–36 Weeks) (n = 32)	
	Blood morphology			
Leukocytes ×10³/µL	14.65 (11.57–17.2)	11.57 (10.04–15.58)	16.53 (14.02–18.92)	0.01
Hemoglobin (g/dL)	17.95 (16.70–18.95)	17.75 (15.60–19.05)	18.11 (16.90–18.95)	NS
Hematocrit (%)	49.95 (46.60–52.51)	49.20 (42.55–52.75)	50.10 (47.40–52.40)	NS
Platelets ×10³/µL	258.00 (210.00–293.50)	267.00 (232.00–300.50)	247.50 (204.00–290.50)	NS
	Biochemical tests—results			
Urea (mg/dL)	25.50 (18.00–32.00)	29.50 (22.00–45.50)	22.50 (15.00–29.50)	0.01
Serum creatinine (mg/dL)	0.66 (0.61–0.75)	0.64 (0.59–0.68)	0.70 (0.63–0.76)	NS
eGFR (mL/min/1.73 m²)	24.58 (21.71–27.11)	24.38 (21.45–27.82)	24.86 (21.99–26.60)	NS
Aspartate aminotransferase (IU/L)	48.50 (38.00–59.50)	40.50 (34.50–59.00)	22.50 (15.00–29.50)	NS
Alanine aminotransferase (IU/L)	10.00 (7.00–13.00)	8.00 (6.00–11.00)	11.50 (9.00–14.50)	0.01
Bilirubin (mg/dL)	5.19 (4.05–6.20)	5.45 (3.90–6.25)	4.80 (4.10–6.13)	NS
Protein (mg/dL)	4.85 (4.40–5.20)	4.85 (4.55–5.20)	4.85 (4.30–5.20)	NS
Sodium (mmol/L)	141.50 (139.00–143.00)	141.00 (138.00–143.00)	141.00 (140.00–143.00)	NS
Potassium (mmol/L)	4.97 (4.5–5.48)	4.89 (4.5–5.47)	5.07 (4.47–5.48)	NS
Calcium (mmol/L)	2.12 (2.02–2.20)	2.14 (2.03–2.22)	2.12 (2.01–2.18)	NS
Magnesium (mmol/L)	0.86 (0.81–0.92)	0.86 (0.81–0.96)	0.84 (0.81–0.91)	NS
Phosphorus (mmol/L)	2.01 (1.64–2.28)	0.86 (0.81–0.96)	0.84 (0.81–0.91)	NS

p—comparison of children born at 30–34 weeks and 35–36 weeks; NS–non statistical.

All neonates had normal renal function parameters (serum and urinary concentration of creatinine, estimated GFR, and urine output). The serum concentration of creatinine did not show a statistically significant difference between the groups. The serum concentration of creatinine was higher in neonates born by cesarean delivery when compared to children born by vaginal delivery. The difference was close to being statistically significant ($p = 0.053$). Urinary creatinine was significantly lower in premature babies when compared to the reference group ($p < 0.01$). The lowest concentration of urinary creatinine was found in children born at 30–34 weeks. Similarly, eGFR was significantly lower in premature children compared to healthy controls ($p < 0.01$); however, we did not notice any difference in eGFR between children born at 30–34 weeks and 35–36 weeks ($p > 0.05$) (Table 3).

Table 3. Examined parameters in premature neonates and the reference group—median values and interquartile range (IQR).

Parameters	Premature Neonates (Weeks) (n)			Reference Group	p_1	p_2	p_3	p_4
	(30–36) (60)	(30–34) (28)	(35–36) (32)	(≥37) (28)				
	Median (Q1–Q3)							
Urinary creatinine (mg/dL)	23.88 (3.43–43.58)	14.95 (9.47–25.05)	35.26 (21.38–57.73)	82.32 (38.99–118.66)	<0.01	<0.01	<0.01	<0.01
Serum creatinine (mg/dL)	0.66 (0.61–0.75)	0.64 (0.59–0.68)	0.70 (0.63–0.76)	0.68 (0.55–0.80)	NS	NS	NS	NS
eGFR (mL/min/1.73 m²)	24.58 (21.71–27.11)	24.38 (21.45–27.82)	24.86 (21.99–26.60)	37.62 (33.75–47.97)	<0.01	<0.01	<0.01	NS
Cathepsin B/creatinine (ng/mg Cr.)	3.41 (2.33–4.47)	4.00 (2.82–5.12)	3.07 (1.95–3.90)	2.51 (2.00–3.48)	<0.05	<0.01	NS	<0.05

p_1—comparison of children born at 30–36 weeks and the reference group; p_2—comparison of children born at 30–34 weeks and the reference group; p_3—comparison of children born at 35–36 weeks and the reference group; p_4—comparison of children born at 30–34 weeks and 35–36 weeks. Cr.—creatinine; eGFR—estimated glomerular filtration rate; NS—non statistical.

In the entire group of premature neonates, the urinary level of cathepsin B/Cr. was higher compared to the reference group ($p < 0.05$). The highest urinary excretion of cathepsin B/Cr. was found in babies born at 30–34 weeks of pregnancy, and the difference was statistically significant when compared to the reference group ($p < 0.01$) and when compared to babies born at 35–36 weeks.($p < 0.05$). However, no statistically significant difference in the urinary level of cathepsin B/Cr. was observed between children born at 35–36 weeks of pregnancy and the reference group.

The analysis did not show any relationship between the concentration of urinary cathepsin B/Cr. and the way of delivery (vaginal delivery or caesarean delivery), Apgar score, prenatal steroid therapy, use of parenteral nutrition, use of nCPAP, or oxygen therapy. No statistically significant differences in the concentrations of urinary cathepsin B/Cr. were found between the groups of boys and girls.

4. Discussion

Kidney immaturity as a consequence of preterm delivery and perinatal problems connected to prematurity such as respiratory and circulatory failure, asphyxia, and antibiotic therapy are risk factors of renal tubular injury in premature neonates. The aim of this prospective study was to determine the values of urinary cathepsin B in premature neonates. It was hypothesized that cathepsin B may be involved in the processes of kidney maturation in the foetus.

Normally, cathepsin B is highly expressed in the proximal tubule. It is the main enzyme involved in the lysosomal digestion of proteins, which are reabsorbed via endocytosis from the glomerular ultrafiltrate. This protease has long been taken under consideration as a biomarker of tubular damage because in response to damages, its levels are lower in tubules and higher in urine [18]. It has recently been shown that the excessive reabsorption of ultrafiltered proteins by proximal tubular cells induces tubular damage and apoptosis/necrosis through the exhaustion of the lysosomal degradation pathway and the leakage of lysosomal enzymes such as cathepsin B into the cytoplasm and urine [20]. The prominent cytoplasmic release of cathepsin B in tubular epithelial cells is crucial for tubular cell injury and the activation of a cytoplasmic macromolecular complex involved in the progression of kidney diseases [25]. Studies conducted on animals showed that cathepsin B is involved in kidney diseases [26–29]. Wang et al. showed that in human proximal tubular epithelial cells undergoing apoptosis, expression levels and the activation of cathepsin B are increased, and that the serum cathepsin B level was associated with aging-related cardiovascular-renal parameters even in healthy people [30–32]. In the study conducted by Piwowar et al., cathepsin B activity increased significantly ($p < 0.001$) in the urine of diabetic patients as compared to the control group, and they concluded that it may be useful as a non-invasive surrogate marker of incipient nephropathy [33].

Knowing that many factors can contribute to tubular damage, we identified a group of sixty children with birth weights appropriate for the gestational age and clinical conditions assessed as good or medium. The children included in this study did not need drugs and mechanical ventilation. Their prenatal and postnatal ultrasound examination of kidneys was normal, and no deviations in laboratory tests and in parameters of renal function were found.

The significantly highest urinary level of cathepsin B/Cr. was observed in neonates born at 30–34 weeks of pregnancy. The lack of statistically significant differences between the urinary level of cathepsin B/Cr. in children born at 35–36 weeks of pregnancy and the reference group was caused by the fact that these neonates were born close to the term of delivery. Thus, it may be supposed that the stages of development of the kidneys in both groups were similar. The significantly highest urinary level of cathepsin B/Cr. was found in neonates born at 30–34 weeks. This may have resulted from the fact that cathepsin B may take part in the process of nephrogenesis as a protease with angiogenic properties [21–23,34].

Aisa et al. studied cathepsin B activity in the urine of neonates with intrauterine growth-restricted (IUGR) (median gestational age—36 weeks) and preterm neonates (median gestational age—35 weeks), both at 30–40 days of the corrected age. They found that cathepsin B activity in the urine was statistically significantly increased in preterm children, and even more increased in neonates with IUGR, when compared to the control group (median, (Q1–Q3)): 2.303, (1.7–2.582); 3.633, (2.146–4.848); 1.044, (0.8335–1.372) IU/min mmol, respectively. Taking into consideration significantly lower total renal volume, cortical volume, and observed proteinuria in the IUGR and preterm neonates, they suggested that cathepsin B activity may be useful in the early prediction of renal susceptibility to damage in this group of children [35].

In order to determine if other factors besides immaturity could affect the renal tubules' functions, the relationship of the concentration of urinary cathepsin B and urinary cathepsin B/Cr. with gender, way of delivery, birth weight, centile of birth weight, Apgar score, prenatal steroid therapy, respiratory disorders (use of nCPAP, oxygen therapy), and the use of parenteral nutrition was examined. However, no correlations were found between them. This result suggests that elevated urinary cathepsin B/Cr. level may be the result of the kidneys' immaturity in preterm newborns.

The main limitation for this study was the sample size of recruited children, which was quite small, as it was very difficult to get study consent from some parents.

5. Conclusions

In conclusion, the results showed that preterm neonates born at 30–34 weeks of gestation had elevated urinary cathepsin B/Cr. levels, which may be a result of the immaturity of kidneys. This preliminary observation should be confirmed in a multicenter study, which would consider not only preterm neonates with birth weights appropriate for gestational age and clinical conditions assessed as good or medium, but also those with clinical conditions assessed as bad, with or without AKI. Certainly, extending the study to the following weeks of life of the studied children, performing them both during hospitalization and after discharge from the hospital, would provide valuable information, confirming the role of cathepsin B as a biomarker of kidney maturity.

Author Contributions: M.K.—had primary responsibility for protocol development, patient screening, enrolment, outcome assessment, preliminary data analysis, and the writing of the manuscript. M.S.—took part in the protocol's development and contributed to the writing of the manuscript. A.K. (Anna Krukowska)—had primary responsibility for collecting a specimen. A.K. (Aleksandra Kamianowska)—took part in outcome assessment and the writing of the manuscript. A.W.—took part in the protocol's development and the analytical framework for the study, and contributed to the writing of the manuscript. All authors have read and agreed to the published version of the manuscript.

Funding: The grant of the Medical University of Bialystok funded this study.

Institutional Review Board Statement: The study was conducted according to the guidelines of the Declaration of Helsinki, and approved by the Local Bioethics Committee of The Medical University of Bialystok (protocol code: R-I-002/360/2016, date of approval: 17 October 2016).

Informed Consent Statement: Prior to the study written informed consent has been obtained from the parents of all the neonates to publish this paper.

Acknowledgments: We thank the employees of the Laboratory of the Department of Pediatrics and Nephrology, Medical University of Bialystok, Poland for participating in the study.

Conflicts of Interest: The authors have no conflict of interest to declare.

References

1. Vogel, J.P.; Chawanpaiboon, S.; Moller, A.-B.; Watananirun, K.; Bonet, M.; Lumbiganon, P. The global epidemiology of preterm birth. *Best Pract. Res. Clin. Obstet. Gynaecol.* **2018**, *52*, 3–12. [CrossRef] [PubMed]
2. Roberts, D.; Brown, J.; Medley, N.; Dalziel, S.R. Antenatal corticosteroids for accelerating fetal lung maturation for women at risk of preterm birth. *Cochrane Database Syst. Rev.* **2017**, *3*, CD004454. [CrossRef]
3. Kreidberg, J.A. Podocyte differentiation and glomerulogenesis. *J. Am. Soc. Nephrol.* **2003**, *14*, 806–814. [CrossRef] [PubMed]
4. Potter, E.L. *Normal and Abnormal Development of the Kidney*; Year Book Medical Publishers: Chicago, IL, USA, 1972.
5. Hinchliffe, S.A.; Sargent, P.H.; Howard, C.V.; Chan, Y.F.; van Velzen, D. Human intrauterine renal growth expressed in absolute number of glomeruli assessed by the disector method and Cavalieri principle. *Lab. Investig.* **1991**, *64*, 777–784. [PubMed]
6. Abitbol, C.L.; Rodriguez, M.M. The long-term renal and cardiovascular consequences of prematurity. *Nat. Rev. Nephrol.* **2012**, *8*, 265–274. [CrossRef]
7. Stritzke, A.; Thomas, S.; Amin, H.; Fusch, C.; Lodha, A. Renal consequences of preterm birth. *Mol. Cell. Pediatr.* **2017**, *4*, 2. [CrossRef]
8. Hughson, M.; Farris, A.B., III; Douglas-Denton, R.; Hoy, W.; Bertram, J. Glomerular number and size in autopsy kidneys: The relationship to birth weight. *Kidney Int.* **2003**, *63*, 2113–2122. [CrossRef]
9. Rodríguez, M.M.; Gómez, A.H.; Abitbol, C.L.; Chandar, J.J.; Duara, S.; Zilleruelo, G.E. Histomorphometric analysis of postnatal glomerulogenesis in extremely preterm infants. *Pediatr. Dev. Pathol.* **2004**, *7*, 17–25. [CrossRef]
10. Sutherland, M.R.; Gubhaju, L.; Moore, L.; Kent, A.L.; Dahlstrom, J.; Horne, R.; Hoy, W.; Bertram, J.; Black, M.J. Accelerated maturation and abnormal morphology in the preterm neonatal kidney. *J. Am. Soc. Nephrol.* **2011**, *22*, 1365–1374. [CrossRef]
11. Stapleton, F.B.; Jones, D.P.; Green, R.S. Acute renal failure in neonates: Incidence, etiology and outcome. *Pediatr. Nephrol.* **1987**, *1*, 314–320. [CrossRef]
12. Hentschel, R.; Lodige, B.; Bulla, M. Renal insufficiency in the neonatal period. *Clin. Nephrol.* **1996**, *46*, 54–58.
13. Agras, P.I.; Tarcan, A.; Baskin, E.; Cengiz, N.; Gurakan, B.; Saatci, U. Acute renal failure in the neonatal period. *Ren. Fail.* **2004**, *26*, 305–309. [CrossRef] [PubMed]
14. Turk, V.; Stoka, V.; Vasiljeva, O.; Renko, M.; Sun, T.; Turk, B.; Turk, D. Cysteine cathepsins: From structure, function and regulation to new frontiers. *Biochim. Biophys. Acta* **2012**, *1824*, 68–88. [CrossRef] [PubMed]
15. Kirschke, H.; Barrett, A.J.; Rawlings, N.D. Proteinases 1: Lysosomal cysteine proteinases. *Protein Profile* **1995**, *2*, 1581–1643.
16. Mort, J.S.; Buttle, D.J. Cathepsin B. *Int. J. Biochem. Cell Biol.* **1997**, *29*, 715–720. [CrossRef]
17. Cavallo-Medved, D.; Moin, K.; Sloane, B. Cathepsin B. *UCSD Nat. Mol. Pages* **2011**, *2011*, A000508.
18. Schaefer, L.; Gilge, U.; Heidland, A.; Schaefer, R.M. Urinary excretion of cathepsin B and cystatins as parameters of tubular damage. *Kidney Int. Suppl.* **1994**, *46*, 64–67.
19. Ciechanover, A. Intracellular protein degradation: From a vague idea thru the lysosome and the ubiquitin-proteasome system and onto human diseases and drug targeting. *Biochim. Biophys. Acta* **2012**, *1824*, 3–13. [CrossRef] [PubMed]
20. Liu, W.J.; Xu, B.H.; Ye, L.; Liang, D.; Wu, H.L.; Zheng, Y.Y.; Deng, J.K.; Li, B.; Liu, H.F. Urinary proteins induce lysosomal membrane permeabilization and lysosomal dysfunction in renal tubular epithelial cells. *Am. J. Physiol. Renal Physiol.* **2015**, *308*, 639–649. [CrossRef]
21. Varanou, A.; Withington, S.L.; Lakasing, L.; Williamson, C.; Burton, G.J.; Hemberger, M. The importance of cysteine cathepsin proteases for placental development. *J. Mol. Med.* **2006**, *84*, 305–317. [CrossRef]

22. Buck, M.R.; Karustis, D.G.; Day, N.A.; Honn, K.V.; Sloane, B.F. Degradation of extracellular-matrix proteins by human cathepsin B from normal and tumour tissues. *Biochem. J.* **1992**, *282*, 273–278. [CrossRef]
23. Mai, J.; Sameni, M.; Mikkelsen, T.; Sloane, B.F. Degradation of extracellular matrix protein tenascin-C by cathepsin B: An interaction involved in the progression of gliomas. *Biol. Chem.* **2002**, *383*, 1407–1413. [CrossRef] [PubMed]
24. Fenton. Available online: http://www.ucalgary.ca/fenton/2013chart (accessed on 1 December 2017).
25. Liu, D.; Wen, Y.; Tang, T.T.; Lv, L.L.; Tang, R.N.; Liu, H.; Ma, K.L.; Crowley, S.D.; Liu, B.C. Megalin/cubulin-lysosome-mediated albumin reabsorption is involved in the tubular cell activation of NLRP3 inflammasome and tubulointerstitial inflammation. *J. Biol. Chem.* **2015**, *290*, 18018–18028. [CrossRef]
26. Jiang, M.; Wei, Q.; Dong, G.; Komatsu, M.; Su, Y.; Dong, Z. Autophagy in proximal tubules protects against acute kidney injury. *Kidney Int.* **2012**, *82*, 1271–1283. [CrossRef] [PubMed]
27. Wyczalkowska-Tomasik, A.; Bartlomiejczyk, I.; Gornicka, B.; Paczek, L. Strong association between fibronectin accumulation and lowered cathepsin B activity in glomeruli of diabetic rats. *J. Physiol. Pharmacol.* **2012**, *63*, 525–530.
28. Huang, S.; Schaefer, R.M.; Reisch, S.; Paczek, L.; Schaefer, L.; Teschner, M.; Sebekova, K.; Heidland, A. Suppressed activities of cathepsins and metalloproteinases in the chronic model of puromycin aminonucleoside nephrosis. *Kidney Blood Press. Res.* **1999**, *22*, 121–127. [CrossRef]
29. Tao, Y.; Kim, J.; Faubel, S.; Wu, J.C.; Falk, S.A.; Schrier, R.W.; Edelstein, C.L. Caspase inhibition reduces tubular apoptosis and proliferation and slows disease progression in polycystic kidney disease. *Proc. Natl. Acad. Sci. USA* **2005**, *102*, 6954–6959. [CrossRef]
30. Wang, C.; Jiang, Z.; Yao, J.; Wu, X.; Sun, L.; Liu, C.; Duan, W.; Yan, M.; Sun, L.; Liu, J.; et al. Participation of cathepsin B in emodin-induced apoptosis in HK-2 Cells. *Toxicol. Lett.* **2008**, *181*, 196–204. [CrossRef]
31. Wang, J.; Chen, L.; Li, Y.; Guan, X.Y. Overexpression of cathepsin Z contributes to tumor metastasis by inducing epithelialmesenchymal transition in hepatocellular carcinoma. *PLoS ONE* **2011**, *6*, e24967.
32. Wang, N.; Bai, X.; Jin, B.; Han, W.; Sun, X.; Chen, X. The association of serum cathepsin B concentration with age-related cardiovascular-renal subclinical state in a healthy Chinese population. *Arch. Gerontol. Geriatr.* **2016**, *65*, 146–155. [CrossRef] [PubMed]
33. Piwowar, A.; Knapik-Kordecka, M.; Fus, I.; Warwas, M. Urinary activities of cathepsin B, N-acetyl-beta-D-glucosaminidase, and albuminuria in patients with type 2 diabetes mellitus. *Med. Sci. Monit.* **2006**, *12*, CR210–CR214. [PubMed]
34. Anık İlhan, G.; Yıldızhan, B. Evaluation of serum cathepsin B, D, and L concentrations in women with late-onset preeclampsia. *Turk. J. Obstet. Gynecol.* **2019**, *16*, 91–94. [CrossRef] [PubMed]
35. Aisa, M.C.; Cappuccini, B.; Barbati, A.; Orlacchio, A.; Baglioni, M.; Di Renzo, G.C. Biochemical parameters of renal impairment/injury and surrogate markers of nephron number in intrauterine growth-restricted and preterm neonates at 30–40 days of postnatal corrected age. *Pediatr. Nephrol.* **2016**, *31*, 2277–2287. [CrossRef] [PubMed]

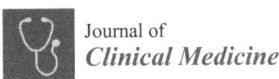

Article

Alpha-1 Acid Glycoprotein and Podocin mRNA as Novel Biomarkers for Early Glomerular Injury in Obese Children

Anna Medyńska [1,*], Joanna Chrzanowska [2], Katarzyna Kościelska-Kasprzak [3], Dorota Bartoszek [3], Marcelina Żabińska [3] and Danuta Zwolińska [1]

[1] Department of Pediatric Nephrology, Wroclaw Medical University, 50-367 Wrocław, Poland; danuta.zwolinska@umed.wroc.pl
[2] Department of Pediatric Endocrinology and Diabetology, Wroclaw Medical University, 50-367 Wrocław, Poland; joanna.chrzanowska@umed.wroc.pl
[3] Specialist Laboratory at the Department of Nephrology and Transplantation Medicine, Wroclaw Medical University, 50-367 Wrocław, Poland; katarzyna.koscielska-kasprzak@umed.wroc.pl (K.K.-K.); dorota.bartoszek@umed.wroc.pl (D.B.); marcelina.zabinska@umed.wroc.pl (M.Ż.)
* Correspondence: anna.medynska@umed.wroc.pl; Tel.: +48-71-736-4400; Fax: +48-71-736-4409

Citation: Medyńska, A.; Chrzanowska, J.; Kościelska Kasprzak, K.; Bartoszek, D.; Żabińska, M.; Zwolińska, D. Alpha-1 Acid Glycoprotein and Podocin mRNA as Novel Biomarkers for Early Glomerular Injury in Obese Children. J. Clin. Med. 2021, 10, 4129. https://doi.org/10.3390/jcm10184129

Academic Editor: Katarzyna Taranta-Janusz

Received: 13 July 2021
Accepted: 8 September 2021
Published: 13 September 2021

Publisher's Note: MDPI stays neutral with regard to jurisdictional claims in published maps and institutional affiliations.

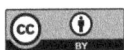

Copyright: © 2021 by the authors. Licensee MDPI, Basel, Switzerland. This article is an open access article distributed under the terms and conditions of the Creative Commons Attribution (CC BY) license (https://creativecommons.org/licenses/by/4.0/).

Abstract: Introduction: Obesity, which is a serious problem in children, has a negative impact on many organs, including kidneys, and obesity-related glomerulopathy (ORG) is an increasingly common cause of ESKD (end-stage kidney disease) in adults. Early-detected and -treated glomerular lesions are reversible, so it is important to find a useful marker of early damage. The study aimed to evaluate the albumin-to-creatinine ratio (ACR), urinary alpha-1-acid glycoprotein (α1-AGP), and mRNA of podocyte-specific proteins as indicators of glomerular injury and their relationship with the degree of obesity and metabolic disorders. Materials and Methods: A total of 125 obese children and 33 healthy peers were enrolled. Patients were divided into two groups, depending on SDS BMI values. ACR, α1-AGP, mRNA expression of nephrin, synaptopodin, podocin, and C2AP protein in urine sediment were measured. Results: ACR values did not differ between groups and were within the normal range. α1-AGP and mRNA expression were significantly higher in obese children compared with controls. mRNA expression of the remaining podocyte proteins was similar in both groups. No significant differences concerning all examined parameters were found depending on the degree of obesity. There was a positive significant correlation between α1-AGP and ACR. Conclusions: Increased α1-AGP before the onset of albuminuria suggests its usefulness as a biomarker of early glomerular damage in obese children. An increased podocin mRNA expression also indicates podocyte damage and may be linked to ORG development. The lack of increase in expression of other podocyte proteins suggests that podocin mRNA may be a more specific and sensitive biomarker. The degree of obesity has no impact on the tested parameters, but further studies are needed to confirm it.

Keywords: obesity; glomerular injury; alpha-1 acid glycoprotein; urinary mRNA expression of podocyte-associated proteins

1. Introduction

Over the past few decades, overweight and obesity have been recognized as one of the most serious public health problems worldwide, affecting not only adults but also children. It is estimated that in the United States obesity affects approximately one-fifth of the school-age population [1]. According to the World Obesity Forum, 20–35% of European children are overweight or obese [2]. Similar results were obtained by the Polish authors examining school-aged children [3]. Obesity and obesity-related metabolic diseases may lead to hypertension and diabetes, which are associated with an increased risk of chronic kidney disease (CKD).

The pathogenetic role of obesity in the development of adult CKD has been confirmed in 15–30% of patients, and a large meta-analysis showed that obesity is an independent risk factor for the development of CKD [4,5]. Moreover, it has been found that overweight and obesity are closely related to an increased risk of end-stage kidney disease (ESKD) [6]. Experimental and clinical studies have demonstrated that obesity promotes structural, hemodynamic, and metabolic alterations in the kidney, damaging different nephron segments, particularly the glomerulus. In 1974, an association was first reported between massive obesity and glomerulopathy, which is morphologically similar to focal segmental glomerulosclerosis (FSGS) [7]. Nowadays, obesity-related glomerulopathy (ORG) is an increasingly recognized cause of ESKD in the adult population.

Sodium reabsorption in the proximal tubules and in the loops of Henle plays a key pathogenic role in the development of ORG. Low sodium concentration in the macula densa dilatates afferent arterioles and leads to hyperfiltration, which increases renal plasma flow (RPF) and the glomerular filtration rate.

Abitbol et al., who studied a group of children with kidney disease and proteinuria, found that the glomerular volume was significantly greater in obese children than in the non-obese control [8]. It should be emphasized that reduced kidney function is for a long time asymptomatic and detected only incidentally.

Given that obese children often remain obese in adulthood, and obesity-related complications, including the kidney, begin in childhood, efforts should be made to detect them as soon as possible. In the era of the obesity epidemic, this should be a special health challenge for pediatric nephrologists.

It has long been known that albuminuria, not detectable in standard urinalysis, is a useful early marker of glomerular damage, as it precedes the development of overt proteinuria. Recent studies indicate that alpha-1-acid glycoprotein (α1-AGP) is a better indicator of the permeability of the glomerular filtration barrier than albuminuria [9]. Alpha-1-acid glycoprotein is an acute-phase protein synthesized primarily in the liver. It has immunomodulatory properties and participates in pro- and anti-inflammatory activities by affecting the release or inhibition of cytokines (TNF-α, IL-1, IL-6) [10]. Experimental studies in mice have shown that increased α1-AGP levels help maintain metabolic balance by suppressing inflammation [11]. In humans, α1-AGP mRNA expression correlates with mRNA expression of both pro- and anti-inflammatory cytokines released by adipose tissue (TNF-α, IL-6, adiponectin) [12]. Authors suggest that α1-AGP attenuates the inflammatory process in human adipose tissue. However, El-Beblawy et al., who studied children and adolescents with type 1 diabetes, found that α1-AGP is an independent factor for diabetic microvascular complications and that its urinary concentration increases with overt nephropathy [13].

Podocytes are terminally differentiated and highly specialized cells of the visceral epithelium, which play a major role in maintaining the structure and function of the glomerular filtration barrier. A slit diaphragm, consisting of structural and signaling proteins, is a junction connecting foot processes of neighboring podocytes. In many glomerulopathies, injured podocytes detach from the glomerular basement membrane into the urine and cause filtration barrier leakage [14–16]. This process has been used to assess the activity and progression of glomerulonephritis in adults and children [15–17]. Alternatively, urinary mRNA expression of podocyte-associated proteins (synaptopodin, nephrin, podocin, podocalyxin, and CD2AP) can be assessed.

2. Objectives

The study aimed to evaluate the urinary excretion of albumin, α1-AGP, and mRNA of podocyte-specific proteins as indicators of glomerular injury in obese children and their association with the degree of obesity SDS BMI reference ranges and metabolic disorders.

3. Materials

We examined 125 children (68 girls) aged 8–17.9 years (mean 13.7 ± 2.84) treated for obesity in the outpatient clinic at the Department of Pediatric Endocrinology and Diabetology (Wroclaw Medical University, Wrocaw, Poland). We enrolled only children with simple obesity or without concomitant chronic or acute infectious diseases. We excluded patients with secondary obesity associated with endocrine disorders, genetic syndromes, or central nervous system diseases. The control group included 33 healthy peers (18 girls) aged 7.6–17.8 years (mean 12.9 ± 3) with normal body weight. Patients were divided into two groups, depending on their SDS BMI values. Patients' characteristics are presented in Table 1.

Table 1. Patients' characteristics according to the SDS BMI values.

	Subgroup I 2 ≤ SDS BMI ≤ 4	Subgroup II SDS BMI > 4	p
Number of patients	65	60	
Age (years) (mean ± SD) range	13.7 ± 2.8 8–17.9	13.5 ± 2.9 8.2–17.8	NS
Sex (F/M) (%)	29/31 48.3/51.7	29/21 58/42	NS

NS—insignificant statistical difference, SD—standard deviation.

The study was conducted according to the guidelines of the Declaration of Helsinki, and approved by the Bioethics Committee of the Wroclaw Medical University (No. KB-376/2016). Informed consent was obtained from the parents and subjects above 16 years old.

4. Methods

Anthropometric parameters in all enrolled patients were measured: height with Harpenden Stadiometer with 0.1 cm precision and weight with an electronic weight scale (SECA, Hamburg, Germany) with an accuracy of 0.05 kg. Body mass index was calculated according to the following formula: BMI = body weight (kg)/(height (m))^2. According to the WHO recommendations, obesity was defined as 2 standard deviations (SD) above the reference median, and overweight as 1 SD above the reference median. BMI charts for Polish children population were used [3].

Serum and urine samples were tested to measure baseline serum lipid parameters (total cholesterol, HDL cholesterol, LDL cholesterol, and triglycerides), carbohydrate parameters (fasting glucose), renal function (creatinine), and hsCRP. Estimated creatinine clearance (eGFR), using the Schwartz formula [18], and insulin resistance index were calculated. In all patients, albuminuria, α1-AGP, and urinary creatinine levels and the glucose loading test were performed. Additionally, mRNA expression of podocyte-associated molecules (nephrin, synaptopodin, podocin, and C2AP protein) in urinary sediments were assessed, as markers for the presence of detachment podocyte in the urine.

Blood samples were drawn from cubital veins after an overnight fast, during routinely performed laboratory tests. Samples were clotted for 30 min, and centrifuged for 15 min at 3000 rpm. After separation, the serum was frozen at −80 °C until assayed. Serum creatinine, total cholesterol, HDL cholesterol, LDL cholesterol, glucose, insulin levels, and blood were assessed on the same day.

Urine was collected from the first morning void (50–150 mL), which was then centrifuged at 800× g for 30 min at 4 °C. The supernatant was frozen at <−80 °C until assayed. The pellet was washed in 50 mL PBS and centrifuged at 800× g for 10 min at 4 °C. Then, the pellet was analyzed for mRNA expression of structural genes, and stabilized in RNA later fluid (24 h, 4 °C). Samples were stored at <−70 °C until assayed. Creatinine and α1-AGP were measured by ELISA kits supplied by R&D Systems, Inc. (Minneapolis, MN, USA). Urinary albumin was measured by ELISA kits supplied by Wuhan (EIAab Science Co., Ltd., Wuhan, China).

All assays were performed according to the manufacturers' instructions. The concentration of parameters was expressed per milligram of creatinine in urine, except for albuminuria, which was expressed in milligrams per gram of urinary creatinine (mg/g).

5. Gene Expression

The research involved a real-time PCR analysis of urine sediment gene expression of NPHS1, NPHS2, CD2AP, and SYNPO genes, referenced to 18S rRNA or GAPDH. Total RNA was isolated from urine sediments with a QIAamp RNA Blood Mini Kit (Qiagen, Germany) according to the manufacturer protocol, including genomic DNA removal with RNase-free DNase (Qiagen, Germany). The samples were reversely transcribed with a High-Capacity RNA-to-cDNA Kit (Applied Biosystems, USA) according to the manufacturer protocol. The reaction mixes containing 0.9 µL of reverse transcription product in 10 µL of Taqman Fast Advanced Master Mix were applied to each well of custom-designed plates (Taqman), including the following assays in triplicate: Hs00190446_m1 (NPHS1), Hs00387817_m1 (NPHS2), Hs00961458_m1 (CD2AP), Hs00200768_m1 (SYNPO), Hs99999905_m1 (GAPDH), and Hs99999901_s1 (18S rRNA). Amplification reaction was performed on Taqman 7900 HT instrument with a fast protocol and analyzed with SDS 2.2.2 software. The results are presented as $\Delta CT = CT_{target} - CT_{reference}$, or as $\Delta\Delta CT = \Delta CT_{mean\ control\ sample} - \Delta CT_{test\ sample}$. Mean control sample was the mean value of ΔCTs in the healthy control group.

6. Statistical Analyses

The results are expressed as mean (x), median (M), range (min–max), lower and upper quartiles (25–75 Q), and standard deviations (SD). The equality of means in independent groups was tested with ANOVA analysis of variance and in heterogeneous groups with a Mann-Whitney non-parametric U-test; homogeneity of variance was assessed by Bartlett's test. For discrete parameters, we analyzed the frequency of trait occurrence using the c2df test with Yates' correction with an appropriate number of degrees of freedom df (df = (m − 1) * (n − 1), where m—the number of rows, n—the number of columns). For correlation analysis of selected variables, we used the Pearson or Spearman's correlation coefficient. A value of $p \leq 0.05$ was considered statistically significant. Statistical analysis was performed with EPIINFO v. 7.1.1.14 statistical software package.

7. Results

The parameters of lipid metabolism differed significantly between the study group and the control group in terms of triglycerides and HDL cholesterol values. Total cholesterol and LDL cholesterol levels in both groups were comparable. Estimated creatinine clearance values also differed between the groups and were significantly higher in the obese child population. Fasting glucose was above normal in only four children in the study group. Detailed data are presented in Table 2.

Table 2. Biochemical parameters in study and control group.

		Control Group F/M 18/15	Study Group F/M 68/57	p
Total cholesterol (mg/dL)	mean ± SD	164.1 ± 14.8	179.2 ± 134.9	0.537
	range (min–max)	133–188	111–1611	
	median	165	166	
	quartile (25–75 Q)	155–175	145–187.5	
HDL cholesterol (mg/dL)	mean ± SD	59 ± 9.6	42.2 ± 8.4	0.00000
	range (min–max)	34–78	27–65	
	median	62	42	
	quartile (25–75 Q)	50–67	36–48	

Table 2. Cont.

		Control Group F/M 18/15	Study Group F/M 68/57	p
LDL-cholesterol (mg/dL)	mean ± SD	94.1 ± 14.9	100.4 ± 24.4	0.175
	range (min–max)	65–121	49–184	
	median	97	99	
	quartile (25–75 Q)	81–105	82–118	
Triglycerides (mg/dL)	mean ± SD	90.3 ± 17.8	122.5 ± 62.1	0.00216 *
	range (min–max)	57–120	39–469	
	median	94	107	
	quartile (25–75 Q)	74–105	83.5–141	
Creatinine (mg/dL)	mean ± SD	0.736 ± 0.144	0.629 ± 0.123	0.00004
	range (min–max)	0.54–1.19	0.37–0.89	
	median	0.69	0.615	
	quartile (25–75 Q)	0.65–0.81	0.54–0.71	
eGFR (mL/min/1.73 m^2)	mean ± SD	125 ± 13.2	154 ± 25.1	0.00000
	range (min–max)	96.0–160.0	109–235	
	median	123.5	152	
	quartile (25–75 Q)	117.5–132	137–169	
Fasting glucose (mg/dL)	mean ± SD		82.5 ± 10.4	0.0118 *
	range (min–max)	75–94	56–153	
	median	88	82	
	quartile (25–75 Q)	85–91	77–82	

For a distribution deviating from the normal distribution, no mean was calculated. * analysis with the non-parametric Mann-Whitney U test.

Albumin excretion rate did not differ between the study and control groups, with values within normal range in all children (<30 mg/g creatinine). The excretion of α1-AGP was significantly higher in obese children compared with the healthy control. Detailed results are presented in Table 3.

Table 3. ACR, α-1AGP, and hsCRP in the study and control groups.

		Control Group n = 33	Study Group n = 125	p
ACR (mg/g) albumin-to-creatinine ratio	mean ± SD	14.53 ± 1.11	13.71 ± 2.75	0.168 *
	range (min–max)	12.86–16.02	12.78–18.03	
	median	15.17	14.7	
	quartile (25–75 Q)	13.42–15.51	12–15.64	
α-1 acid glycoprotein (ng/mg)	mean ± SD	447.9 ± 37.9	578.5 ± 165.2	0.00000 *
	range (min–max)	378.5–500	126.3–1783	
	median	463.3	631.4	
	quartile (25–75 Q)	407.7–479.2	470.1–672.6	
Serum hsCRP (μg/mL)	mean ± SD	1.22 ± 0.11	3.24 ± 0.44	0.00000 *
	range (min–max)	1.02–1.45	2.36–4.46	
	median	1.2	3.22	
	quartile (25–75 Q)	1.14–1.32	2.86–3.54	

* analysis with the non-parametric Mann-Whitney U test.

However, no differences were shown between the degree of obesity and albumin, and α-1-AGP levels (Table 4).

Table 4. Glomerular damage indicators between groups of children depending on the degree of obesity.

		2 ≤ SDS BMI ≤ 4	SDS BMI > 4	p
		n = 60	n = 50	
ACR (mg/g)	mean ± SD	13.6 ± 2.6	13.7 ± 3.2	0.945
	range (min–max)	1.89–6.4	1.8–18	
	median	14.6	15.1	
	quartile (25–75 Q)	12–15.7	12–15.6	
α-1 acid glycoprotein (ng/mg)	mean ± SD	590.7 ± 197.2	564 ± 137.6	0.421
	range (min–max)	131–1783	126.3–727.8	
	median	631.8	633.3	
	quartile (25–75 Q)	469.4–674.1	472.8–679.9	
Serum hsCRP (µg/mL)	mean ± SD	3.17 ± 0.41	3.31 ± 0.45	0.103
	range (min–max)	2.36–4.08	2.55–4.64	
	median	3.19	3.29	
	quartile (25–75 Q)	2.84–3.46	3.05–3.59	

Analysis with the non-parametric Mann-Whitney U test.

The mRNA expression of nephrin, synaptopodin, and CD2AP in urine sediment was not significantly different between the groups, irrespective of the degree of obesity. Podocin mRNA expression was significantly higher in the group of obese patients compared with the non-obese group. Unexpectedly, it was significantly higher in children with a lower degree of obesity than in those with a higher degree of obesity. The results are shown in Table 5.

Table 5. The level of mRNA expression of the podocin gene between groups of children depending on the degree of obesity, expressed as ΔΔCt.

Gene Examined	Gene Reference	Examined Value	2 ≤ SDS BMI ≤ 4 n = 17	SDS BMI > 4 n = 16	p
NPHS2	18S	range (min–max)	0.51–10.24	(−1.01)–5.48	0.017 *
		median	2.21	1.2	
		quartile (25–75 Q)	1.68–7.5	0.00–2.12	
NPHS2	GAPDH	range (min–max)	1.13–8.44	(−2.03)–7.13	0.001 *
		median	2.56	0.085	
		quartile (25–75 Q)	1.83–5.18	(−0.005)–1.815	

For a distribution deviating from the normal distribution, no mean was calculated. * analysis with the non-parametric Mann-Whitney U test.

We found a positive correlation only between α1-AGP and albuminuria ($r = 0.95$; $p = 0.000$), and between α1-AGP and hsCRP ($r = 0.54$; $p = 0.000$).

8. Discussion

The study showed for the first time significantly increased α1-AGP excretion in the urine of obese children as compared with non-obese peers in the absence of overt albuminuria, considered so far as an early marker of glomerular damage. Burgert et al., among others, reported microalbuminuria in more than 10% of obese American children without other comorbidities [19]. According to the authors, the appearance of albuminuria depends primarily on hyperglycaemia, which was found in our study only in four children, which may have had an impact on the ACR result.

In the study by Lurbe et al., the prevalence of microalbuminuria in obese children was only 2.4%. These authors showed no relationship between the degree of obesity and increased albumin-to-creatinine ratio (ACR), which is consistent with our observations [20]. Sawamura et al. observed albuminuria in 21% of 64 overweight and obese children and adolescents, which did not correlate with eGFR, indicating that hyperfiltration is not the only factor that damages the glomerular filtration barrier in obesity [21].

Recent studies indicate that α1-AGP is a more sensitive marker of glomerular filtration barrier injury than albuminuria. This was proved, among others, by Talks et al., who studied the urinary α1-AGP and albumin leakage in healthy volunteers in an altitude-induced hypoxia (5023 m). These authors reported a significant increase in urinary leakage of albumin and α1-AGP, but the percentage of increase was significantly higher for α1-AGP. They observed no increase for positively charged dimeric lambda free light chains (λ-FLCs) [9]. It should be emphasized that the molecule of α1-AGP is smaller than the molecule of albumin (43 kDA vs. 66 kDA) and similar in size to the podocyte slit diaphragm pore. Similar observations were reported in adult patients with type 2 diabetes. Both Christiansen et al. [22] and Narita et al. [23] have shown increased urinary α1-AGP excretion in diabetic patients with normoalbuminuria. Similarly, in a study of 60 children with type 1 diabetes, α1-AGP excretion preceded the onset of microalbuminuria and significantly increased with its onset [13]. Moreover, these authors reported a significant positive correlation between α1-AGP excretion and albuminuria, which is in line with our observations. Therefore, it seems that urinary α1-AGP may be a useful marker for assessing glomerular injury in obese children. However, in our study we did not show any significant differences in urinary α1-AGP according to the degree of obesity.

The mechanism of glomerular injury in obese patients is complex and not fully understood. Certainly, hemodynamic and metabolic as well as endocrine disturbances are interconnected. For this reason, the effect of damage to individual kidney structures may not be the same in all obese patients. Although, according to Tsuboi et al., severe forms of ORG affect mainly morbidly obese patients, the severity of kidney damage is not necessarily related to the severity of obesity [24].

Alpha-1-acid glycoprotein, a major acute-phase protein, displays a number of antioxidative and anti-inflammatory properties [25]. For this reason, its increased levels in serum and urine have been linked to vascular inflammation and subclinical atherosclerosis. This has been confirmed by El-Beblawy et al., who found a significant correlation of serum and urinary α1-AGP with hsCRP and cartoid intima-media thickness (IMT) in children with type 1 diabetes [13].

It is very likely that in obese children, α1-AGP may be a good marker not only of glomerular injury but also of very early atherosclerotic lesions. In this study, we found also a significant positive correlation between the α1-AGP and hsCRP.

Yang et al. have shown that in patients with cardiovascular disease, elevated levels of high-sensitivity CRP increase the risk of developing microalbuminuria [26]. It cannot be excluded that we would observe a similar association with longer duration of obesity. In fact, we found significantly higher hsCRP concentrations in obese children compared with non-obese children.

Many studies have demonstrated an association of podocyturia and mRNA expression of podocyte proteins in urinary sediment with an activity and progression of different glomerulopathies, including adult diabetic nephropathy [27] and lupus nephropathy [28].

However, only a few studies have demonstrated this association with ORG and the "silent" glomerular damage in obesity. For instance, Chen et al. reported a significantly lower number of podocyte density in 46 adults with clinically overt ORG compared with healthy controls [29]. Moreover, these changes were strongly associated with proteinuria and abnormalities in fasting glucose and insulin levels [29]. However, Pereira et al., who studied urinary expression of podocyte-associated mRNAs, showed higher expression levels of podocin and nephrin mRNAs in obese and overweight adults as compared with healthy controls. Moreover, it was associated with the severity of obesity and metabolic syndrome. What is, however, worth emphasizing is that they did not detect albuminuria [30].

However, higher serum insulin levels were related to podocyturia, regardless of obesity. Our study, which is, to our knowledge, the first one conducted in a population of obese children, is consistent with the previous results only with regard to podocin mRNA, because the mRNA expression of other podocyte proteins did not differ between the obese children and the healthy control. Moreover, our study did not confirm the association of podocin mRNA with weight gain or metabolic disorders, which may be due to the fact that our population was younger as compared with the obese population in other studies. The above results confirm that glomerular lesions assessed by mRNA expression of podocyte proteins occur even before the onset of albuminuria. The significantly higher mRNA expression levels of podocin, and not of other proteins, are difficult to explain. Some suggest that podocin may be a more specific and sensitive marker in podocyte damage than nephrin, podocalyxin, or synaptopodin. This was confirmed, among others, by Garovic et al., who conducted investigations in pregnant women with preeclampsia [31]. This is also suggested by the results of experimental studies on rats with diphtheria-induced kidney damage with a subsequent increase in urine podocin and nephrin mRNA expression [32]. After 8 days of observation, the presence of podocin mRNA was still detected, and no expression of nephrin mRNA was found. Given the fact that obese patients may develop ORG, podocyturia measured with urinary mRNA expression levels of podocyte-assosiated proteins may be one of the first indicators of ORG development.

9. Conclusions

Increased α1-AGP before the onset of albuminuria suggests its usefulness as a biomarker of early glomerular damage in obese children. An increased podocin mRNA expression also indicates podocyte damage and may be linked to ORG development. The lack of increase in expression of other podocyte proteins suggests that podocin mRNA may be a more specific and sensitive biomarker. The degree of obesity has no impact on the tested parameters, but further studies are needed to confirm it.

Author Contributions: Conceptualization, A.M. and D.Z.; Data curation, A.M., J.C., K.K.-K., D.B. and M.Ż.; Investigation, A.M., J.C.; Methodology, A.M., K.K.-K., D.B. and M.Ż.; Writing—original draft, A.M., K.K.-K. and D.Z.; Writing—review and editing, A.M. and D.Z. All authors have read and agreed to the published version of the manuscript.

Funding: This work was financed by a grant from Wroclaw Medical University, Poland (grant number ST-C210.16.082).

Institutional Review Board Statement: The study was conducted according to the guidelines of the Declaration of Helsinki, and approved by the Bioethics Committee of the Wroclaw Medical University (No. KB-376/2016).

Informed Consent Statement: Informed consent was obtained from all subjects ($\geq$16 years) and their representatives involved in the study.

Data Availability Statement: Data associated with the paper are not publicly available but are available from the corresponding author at reasonable request.

Conflicts of Interest: The authors declare no conflict of interest.

References

1. Wang, Y.; Beydoun, M.A.; Min, J.; Xue, H.; Kaminsky, L.; Cheskin, L.J. Has the prevalence of overweight, obesity and central obesity levelled off in the United States? Trends, patterns, disparities, and future projections for the obesity epidemic. *Int. J. Epidemiol.* **2020**, *49*, 810–823. [CrossRef] [PubMed]
2. World Health Organization. *Obesity: Preventing and Managing the Global Epidemic. WHO Expert Consultation*; Technical Report Series No. 894; WHO: Geneva, Switzerland, 2000. Available online: http://whqlibdoc.who.int/trs/WHO_TRS_894.pdf?ua=1 (accessed on 7 November 2016).
3. Kułaga, Z.; Grajda, A.; Gurzkowska, B.; Wojtyło, M.; Gozdz, M.; Litwin, M. The prevalence of overweight and obesity among Polish school-aged children and adolescents. *Prz. Epidemiol.* **2017**, *70*, 641–651.
4. Rhee, C.; Ahmadi, S.F.; Kalantar-Zadeh, K. The dual roles of obesity in chronic kidney disease: A review of the current literature. *Curr. Opin. Nephrol. Hypertens.* **2016**, *25*, 208–216. [CrossRef] [PubMed]
5. Sandino, J.; Luzardo, L.; Morales, E.; Praga, M. Which Patients with Obesity Are at Risk for Renal Disease? *Nephron* **2021**, *5*, 1–9. [CrossRef] [PubMed]
6. Assadi, F. The Growing Epidemic of Chronic Kidney Disease: Preventive Strategies to Delay the Risk for Progression to ESRD. *Adv. Exp. Med. Biol.* **2019**, *1121*, 57–59.

7. Weisinger, J.R.; Kempson, R.L.; Eldridge, F.L.; Swenson, R.S. The nephrotic syndrome: A complication of massive obesity. *Ann. Intern. Med.* **1974**, *81*, 440–447. [CrossRef] [PubMed]
8. Abitbol, C.L.; Chandar, J.; Rodríguez, M.M.; Berho, M.; Seeherunvong, W.; Freundlich, M.; Zilleruelo, G. Obesity and preterm birth: Additive risks in the progression of kidney disease in children. *Pediatr. Nephrol.* **2009**, *24*, 1363–1370. [CrossRef]
9. Talks, B.J.; Bradwell, S.B.; Delamere, J.; Rayner, W.; Clarke, A.; Lewis, C.T.; Thomas, O.D.; Bradwell, A.R. Urinary Alpha-1-Acid Glycoprotein Is a Sensitive Marker of Glomerular Protein Leakage at Altitude. *High Alt. Med. Biol.* **2018**, *19*, 295–298. [CrossRef]
10. Hochepied, T.; Berger, F.G.; Baumann, H.; Libert, C. Alpha(1)-acid glycoprotein: An acute phase protein with inflammatory and immunomodulating properties. *Cytokine Growth Factor Rev.* **2003**, *14*, 25–34. [CrossRef]
11. Lee, Y.S.; Choi, J.W.; Hwang, I.; Lee, J.W.; Lee, J.H.; Kim, A.Y.; Huh, J.Y.; Koh, Y.J.; Koh, G.Y.; Son, H.J.; et al. Adipocytokine orosomucoid integrates inflammatory and metabolic signals to preserve energy homeostasis by resolving immoderate inflammation. *J. Biol. Chem.* **2010**, *285*, 22174–22185. [CrossRef]
12. Alfadda, A.A.; Fatma, S.; Chishti, M.A.; Al-Naami, M.Y.; Elawad, R.; Mendoza, C.D.; Jo, H.; Lee, Y.S. Orosomucoid serum concentrations and fat depot-specific mRNA and protein expression in humans. *Mol. Cells* **2012**, *33*, 35–41. [CrossRef]
13. El-Beblawy, N.M.; Andrawes, N.G.; Ismail, E.A.; Enany, B.E.; El-Seoud, H.S.; Erfan, M.A. Serum and Urinary Orosomucoid in Young Patients With Type 1 Diabetes: A Link Between Inflammation, Microvascular Complications, and Subclinical Atherosclerosis. *Clin. Appl. Thromb. Hemost.* **2016**, *22*, 718–726. [CrossRef]
14. Hara, M.; Yanagihara, T.; Takada, T.; Itoh, M.; Matsuno, M.; Yamamoto, T.; Kihara, I. Urinary excretion of podocytes reflects disease activity in children with glomerulonephritis. *Am. J. Nephrol.* **1998**, *18*, 35–41. [CrossRef] [PubMed]
15. Hara, M.; Yanagihara, T.; Kihara, I. Urinary podocytes in primary focal segmental glomerulosclerosis. *Nephron* **2001**, *89*, 342–347. [CrossRef]
16. Nakamura, T.; Ushiyama, C.; Suzuki, S.; Hara, M.; Shimada, N.; Sekizuka, K.; Ebihara, I.; Koide, H. Urinary podocytes for the assessment of disease activity in lupus nephritis. *Am. J. Med. Sci.* **2000**, *320*, 112–116. [CrossRef] [PubMed]
17. Nakamura, T.; Ushiyama, C.; Suzuki, S.; Hara, M.; Shimada, N.; Ebihara, I.; Koide, H. Urinary excretion of podocytes in patients with diabetic nephropathy. *Nephrol. Dial. Transplant.* **2000**, *15*, 1379–1383. [CrossRef] [PubMed]
18. Schwartz, G.J.; Haycock, G.B.; Edelmann, C.M., Jr.; Spiter, A. A simple estimate of glomerular filtration rate in children derived from body length and plasma create—Nine. *Pediatrics* **1976**, *58*, 259–263. [PubMed]
19. Burgert, T.S.; Dziura, J.; Yeckel, C.; Taksali, S.E.; Weiss, R.; Tamborlane, W.; Caprio, S. Microalbuminuria in pediatric obesity: Prevalence and relation to other cardiovascular risk factors. *Int. J. Obes.* **2006**, *30*, 273–280. [CrossRef]
20. Lurbe, E.; Torro, M.I.; Alvarez, J.; Aguilar, F.; Fernandez-Formoso, J.A.; Redon, J. Prevalence and factors related to urinary albumin excretion in obese youths. *J. Hypertens.* **2013**, *31*, 2230–2236. [CrossRef]
21. Sawamura, L.S.; Gomes de Souza, G.; Dos Santos, J.D.G.; Suano-Souza, F.I.; Del Vecchio Gessullo, A.; Saccardo Sarni, R.O. Albuminuria and glomerular filtration rate in obese children and adolescents. *J. Bras. Nefrol.* **2019**, *41*, 193–199. [CrossRef] [PubMed]
22. Christiansen, M.S.; Iversen, K.; Larsen, C.T.; Goetze, J.P.; Hommel, E.; Mølvig, J.; Pedersen, B.K.; Magid, E.; Feldt-Rasmussen, B. Increased urinary orosomucoid excretion: A proposed marker for inflammation and endothelial dysfunction in patients with type 2 diabetes. *Scand. J. Clin. Lab. Investig.* **2009**, *69*, 272–281. [CrossRef]
23. Narita, T.; Sasaki, H.; Hosoba, M.; Miura, T.; Yoshioka, N.; Morii, T.; Shimotomai, T.; Koshimura, J.; Fujita, H.; Kakei, M.; et al. Parallel increase in urinary excretion rates of immunoglobulin G, ceruloplasmin, transferrin, and orosomucoid in normoalbuminuric type 2 diabetic patients. *Diabetes Care* **2004**, *27*, 1176–1181. [CrossRef]
24. Tsuboi, N.; Okabayashi, Y.; Shimizu, A.; Yokoo, T. The renal pathology of obesity. *Kidney Int. Rep.* **2017**, *2*, 251–260. [CrossRef]
25. Luo, Z.; Lei, H.; Sun, Y.; Liu, X.; Su, D.F. Orosomucoid, an acute response protein with multiple modulating activities. *J. Physiol. Biochem.* **2015**, *71*, 329–340. [CrossRef]
26. Yang, S.K.; Li, J.; Yi, B.; Mao, J.; Zhang, X.M.; Liu, Y.; Lei, D.D.; Gui, M.; Zhang, H. Elevated High Sensitivity C-Reactive Protein Increases the Risk of Microalbuminuria in Subjects With Cardiovascular Disease Risk Factors. *Ther. Apher. Dial.* **2017**, *21*, 387–394. [CrossRef]
27. Fayed, A.; Tohamy, I.A.R.; Kahla, H.; Elsayed, N.M.; El Ansary, M.; Saadi, G. Urinary podocyte-associated mRNA profile in Egyptian patients with diabetic nephropathy. *Diabetes Metab. Syndr.* **2019**, *13*, 2849–2854. [CrossRef] [PubMed]
28. Wang, G.; Lai, F.M.; Tam, L.S.; Li, K.M.; Lai, K.B.; Chow, K.M.; Li, K.T.; Szeto, C.C. Messenger RNA expression of podocyte-associated molecules in urinary sediment of patients with lupus nephritis. *J. Rheumatol.* **2007**, *34*, 2358–2364.
29. Chen, H.M.; Liu, Z.H.; Zeng, C.H.; Li, S.J.; Wang, Q.W.; Li, L.S. Podocyte lesions in patients with obesity-related glomerulopathy. *Am. J. Kidney Dis.* **2006**, *48*, 772–779. [CrossRef] [PubMed]
30. Pereira, S.V.; Dos Santos, M.; Rodrigues, P.G.; do Nascimento, J.F.; Timm, J.R.; Zancan, R.; Friedman, R.; Veronese, F.V. Increased urine podocyte-associated messenger RNAs in severe obesity are evidence of podocyte injury. *Obesity* **2015**, *23*, 1643–1649. [CrossRef]

31. Garovic, V.D.; Wagner, S.J.; Turner, S.T.; Rosenthal, D.W.; Watson, W.J.; Brost, B.C.; Rose, C.H.; Gavrilova, L.; Craigo, P.; Bailey, K.R.; et al. Urinary podocyte excretion as a marker for preeclampsia. *Am. J. Obstet. Gynecol.* **2007**, *196*, 320.e1–320.e7. [CrossRef] [PubMed]
32. Sato, Y.; Wharram, B.L.; Lee, S.K.; Wickman, L.; Goyal, M.; Venkatareddy, M.; Chang, J.W.; Wiggins, J.E.; Lienczewski, C.; Kretzler, M.; et al. Urine podocyte mRNAs mark progression of renal disease. *J. Am. Soc. Nephrol.* **2009**, *20*, 1041–1052. [CrossRef] [PubMed]

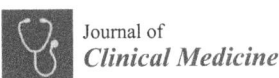

Article

Differences between Obese and Non-Obese Children and Adolescents Regarding Their Oral Status and Blood Markers of Kidney Diseases

Katarzyna Maćkowiak-Lewandowicz [1,*], Danuta Ostalska-Nowicka [1], Jacek Zachwieja [1,†] and Elżbieta Paszyńska [2,†]

[1] Department of Pediatric Nephrology and Hypertension, Poznan University of Medical Sciences, 60-572 Poznan, Poland; dostalska@ump.edu.pl (D.O.-N.); jacekzachwieja@ump.edu.pl (J.Z.)
[2] Department of Integrated Dentistry, Poznan University of Medical Sciences, 60-812 Poznan, Poland; paszynska@ump.edu.pl
* Correspondence: kasiamackowiak@poczta.onet.pl
† These authors contributed equally to this work as the last authors.

Abstract: (1) Background: A rarely discussed effect of obesity-related glomerulopathy (ORG) may slowly lead to irreversible glomerular damage and the development of chronic kidney disease. These patients need to undertake medical care, but whether they should be included in intensive oral care is still not mandatory. The study aimed to assess a relationship between renal, metabolic, and oral health indicators among pediatric patients affected by simple obesity. (2) Methods: 45 children and adolescents with simple obesity hospitalized (BMI 34.1 ± 4.8 kg/m^2, age 15.4 ± 2.3) and compared with 41 aged-matched healthy controls (BMI 16.4 ± 2.4 kg/m^2, age 15.4 ± 2.7). Echocardiography, 24-h ambulatory blood pressure monitoring, ultrasound exam with Doppler, and laboratory tests including kidney and metabolic markers were performed. Oral status was examined regarding the occurrence of carious lesions using decay missing filling teeth (DMFT), gingivitis as bleeding on probing (BOP), and bacterial colonization as plaque control record (PCR). (3) Results: The strongest correlation was revealed between BMI and concentration of uric acid, cystatin C, GFR estimated by the Filler formula (r = 0.74; r = 0.48; r = −0.52), and between oral variables such as PCR and BOP (r = 0.54; r = 0.58). Children and adolescents with obesity demonstrated untreated dental caries, less efficient in plaque control and gingivitis. (4) Conclusions: No specific relation to markers of kidney disease were found; however, more frequent gingivitis/bacterial colonization and significant differences in oral status between obese and non-obese patients were revealed. Susceptibility to inflammation may be conducive to developing metabolic syndrome and kidney damage in the form of obesity-related glomerulopathy and contribute to future dental caries. Uric acid seems to indicate metabolic syndrome and cardiovascular complications (LVMI > 95 percentiles). Cystatin C and uric acid might aspire to be early markers of kidney damage leading to obesity-related glomerulopathy.

Keywords: obesity; childhood; dental caries; gingivitis; kidney injury; glomerulopathy; uric acid; cystatin C

1. Introduction

The COVID-19 outbreak, which contributed to a decrease in physical activity and strengthening of harmful eating habits resulting from remote learning and lockdown, has significantly accelerated an increase in the number of obese patients in Poland. It seems to be a necessary task of the medical environment to address a high risk of obesity complications among pediatric patients with obesity. Typical complications of obesity in children and adolescents, for example, arterial hypertension and dyslipidemia, are well known. A rarely discussed effect is obesity-related glomerulopathy (ORG). Despite its initial asymptomatic course, it slowly leads to irreversible glomerular damage and development of chronic kidney disease, with end-stage renal failure in 1 per 3 patients. In the first period of ORG, obesity leads to hyperfiltration. An increased tubular flow decreases the contact time between proteins and tubular epithelium and produces an increased radial gradient of albumin concentration, resulting in reduced protein reabsorption that may occur without evidence for glomerular dysfunction. The excessive reabsorption of proteins generates apoptosis, renal oxidative stress, inflammation, hypoxia, and lipid accumulation, leading to fibrosis [1,2]. Clinically, ORG is manifested with proteinuria of various severity, depending on the extension of glomerular structural changes: from permanent, mild proteinuria to nephrotic proteinuria [3]. A final diagnosis of obesity-related glomerulopathy is based on biopsy, which carries a higher risk of complications than standard diagnosis due to the patient's obesity and more difficult access to the material collected during a biopsy [4]. It is not a routine procedure and selecting a group of ORG patients without this type of invasive diagnostic procedure is a big challenge for physicians [5]. ORG is suspected in obese patients with proteinuria and concomitant arterial hypertension and lipid metabolism disorders [6,7]. Significant underestimation of ORG patients stems from the fact that markers of this disease revealed by thin-needle biopsy are also found in patients without proteinuria [8]; therefore, new, early markers of kidney damage that would find use in diagnosing ORG are searched for, such as urine megalin and expression of connexin 43 [9,10]. Pediatric patients affected by obesity should be encouraged to undertake medical care, but whether they should be included in oral care because of dental or gingival diseases remains still an uncertain requirement; however, more and more information concerning overlapping relationships with oral cavity homeostasis is available in the literature. Proinflammatory cytokines, produced by adipose cells, lead to low-grade chronic inflammation in the salivary glands [11]. The cause of the imbalance of salivary substances is a significant increase in susceptibility to caries, even in very young patients [12]. A diet rich in carbohydrates favors bacterial colonization, creating favorable conditions for caries promotion. Another oral manifestation of obesity may take the form of gingival inflammation due to poor oral hygiene. Then gingivitis may generate periodontal tissues response and intensify metabolic disorders or even promote weight gain. Combining the above-mentioned dental complications of obesity, such as dental caries, microbial imbalance, and defective salivary composition stimulates potential risk for systemic diseases [11]. It will most likely be connected with an inflammatory response to bacterial pathogens and the generation of reactive oxygen species. Oxidative imbalance contributes to generating lipid peroxide, which can diffuse into the bloodstream [12]. The components of the oxidative stress cascade interact with glomeruli and contribute to obesity-related glomerulopathy [12].

The aim of the study was to assess a correlation between renal, metabolic, and oral health indicators among pediatric patients affected by simple obesity.

2. Materials and Methods

2.1. Study and Control Groups

The study group finally consisted of 45 children and adolescents with simple obesity, admitted to the Department of Pediatric Nephrology and Hypertension in Poznań between 1 January 2019 and 31 December 2020. A reason for hospitalization was the verification of primary hypertension. The control group consisted of 41 age-matched healthy children and adolescents. The flow chart of the study is presented as Supplemental Material in Figure S1.

Echocardiography was performed on all patients with the assessment of left ventricular hypertrophy marker (left ventricular mass index—LVMI > 95 centile), as were abdominal ultrasound exam with Doppler test to evaluate the blood flow through kidneys' arteries and blood laboratory analysis to exclude comorbidities [13]:

1. Peripheral blood morphology, blood gases, C-reactive protein.
2. Concentrations of creatinine, cystatin C, uric acid (UA), urea, Na, K, Ca, Mg.

3. Total cholesterol, LDL-cholesterol, HDL-cholesterol, triglycerides, glucose, glycated hemoglobin, insulin profile.
4. Thyroid-stimulating hormone, triiodothyronine.
5. Liver enzymes, brain natriuretic peptide, troponin.
6. Urine analysis, 24-h urine concentrations of protein and albumin, Na.

All patients were fasting for twelve hours for an ultrasound exam and laboratory tests. During next twenty four hours, urine collection was carried out by collecting every urine sample in a container, starting with the second urinating on the first day of hospitalization, ending the next day with the first portion of urine. Laboratory tests were performed using a standardized method, according to the manufacturer's instructions. Glomerular filtration rate was estimated by Schwartz and Filler formula [14]. Based on the Filler formula, hyperfiltration was defined as GFR > 130 mL/min/1.73 m^2 and hypofiltration when GFR was less than 90 mL/min/1.73 m^2. Arterial blood pressure was assessed by 24-h ambulatory blood pressure monitoring [15]. Atrial hypertension was diagnosed when average systolic or diastolic blood pressure or both, obtained in the course of over three different medical visits was at/above the 95th percentile for age, sex, and height [16]. Simple obesity (BMI > 95 percentiles, BMI Z-score > 1.4) was diagnosed when secondary obesity was excluded. BMI values were transformed into BMI Z-scores using WHO reference values for pediatric BMI [17].

Inclusion and exclusion criteria for study and control groups are described in Table 1 [18]. The protocol allowed 45 children and adolescents with simple obesity; 25 patients additionally with primary hypertension within this group; therefore, the obesity group was divided into two subgroups: suspicion of obesity-related glomerulopathy (sORG) and without ORG group (without ORG). The selection of obesity patients with sORG was based on scientific reports [4,7]: the presence of significant clinical microalbuminuria (>30 mg/day), primary hypertension (revealed during hospitalization), and lipid disorders (decreased concentration of HDL and increased concentration of triglycerides). Seven adolescents met the whole inclusion criteria for suspicion of obesity-related glomerulopathy group. Forty-one healthy children and adolescents enrolled in the control group had to fulfill the inclusion criteria presented in Table 1.

2.2. Dental Examination

A dental assessment was carried out at the dental office by one qualified dentist (E.P.) during hospitalization in the Department of Pediatric Nephrology and Hypertension, in a blind fashion for each child, before the final diagnosis. Before this study, the dental examiner was calibrated after a training course evaluation described in a previous project [19]. Dental evaluation of the occlusal, buccal, and lingual teeth surfaces was performed after the cleaning and drying (excluding the third molars) under visual and tactile examination in artificial light, without magnification, using a dental mirror and blunt probe [20]. The dental assessment included the number of milk/permanent (using lower case letter for primary teeth/capital letters for permanent teeth) decayed teeth (d/D), the number of missed teeth (m/M), the number of filled teeth (f/F), as a dmft/DMFT score [20]. Active dental caries was scored when the lesion manifested a visible cavity, undermined enamel, or softened area. A tooth rebuilt due to dental caries was recorded when a tooth had at least one final restoration applied to cure decay. The missing constituent of the DMFT index was estimated when a tooth had been removed due to dental caries failures. A manual graded periodontal explorer assessed dental plaque and gingival inflammation (LM-instruments, LM8 5050 probe, Osakeyhtiö, Parainen, Finland). Plaque deposit was estimated by the plaque control record index (PCR) [21]. Gingival inflammation was determined using the bleeding on probing index (BOP) [22], measured in six points of the gingival sulcus of all teeth (excluding the third molars). The proportion of surfaces (%) with dental plaque or bleeding-on-probing gums, respectively, were calculated for each subject as % of sites [23]. STROBE protocol was included and attached in the Supplemental Material.

Table 1. Inclusion and exclusion criteria for study and control groups.

Criteria for Inclusion into the Obesity Group	Criteria for Inclusion into the Control Group	Criteria for Exclusion from Study and Control Groups
aged 9–18	aged 9–18	interview: prematurity, congenital abnormalities of urinary tract such as unilateral or bilateral kidney hypoplasia, unilateral kidney aplasia; incorrect kidney location in abdomen; unilateral, bilateral vesicoureteral refluxmedical history: recurrent urinary tract infections
simple obesity	normal weight	genetic obesity, diabetes mellitus, familial hyperlipidemia
normal blood pressure/primary hypertension	normal blood pressure	secondary hypertension (based on kidney diseases, coarctation of the aorta, endocrine disorders, iatrogenic–medications such as steroids)
BMI > 95 percentiles, BMI Z-score ≥ 1.4	BMI < 85 percentiles BMI Z-score < 1.3	BMI < 25 percentiles
		clinical or laboratory markers of previously acute or chronic diseases
		no aberrations in ECHO, USG
a patient, parent, or legal guardian approval	a patient, parent, or legal guardian approval	lack of acceptance from patients, parents, or legal guardians

Abbreviations: BMI—Body Mass Index, BMI Z-score—were transformed from BMI values using WHO reference values for pediatric BMI, ECHO—echocardiogram.

2.3. Statistical Analysis

The Shapiro–Wilk test was used to assess the normality of the data. The homogeneity of variance of each variable was calculated with Levene's test. Non-parametric Mann–Whitney U-test was applied in the analyses of data with non-normal distribution. Student t-test was employed in the analyses of variables with normal distribution. Spearman's correlation rank test was performed to analyze the correlation of parameters with non-normal distribution. Pearson test was employed to test the correlation of normal distribution variables. The statistical significance level was set at $p < 0.05$. Statistical analyses were conducted using Statistica 13.3 (TIBCO Software Inc., Palo Alto, CA, USA).

3. Results

This section may be divided into subheadings. It should provide a concise and precise description of the experimental results, their interpretation, and the empirical conclusions that can be drawn.

3.1. Anthropometric, Clinical, and Biochemical Evaluation

The final group consisted of 86 participants (45 with obesity and 41 control subjects). The mean age of the obese patients was 15.4 ± 2.33 years, the mean age of the controls was 15.4 ± 2.74 years, with no statistically significant difference. BMI and BMI Z-score were statistically different between patients and controls ($p = 0.001$; $p = 0.001$). The clinical and biochemical characteristics of all patients are presented in Table 2.

Table 2. Anthropometric, biochemical, and oral data for obesity group and control individuals.

Variables	Obesity Group (n = 45) Mean ± SD Median (Min-Max)	Control Group (n = 41) Mean ± SD Median (Min-Max)	p-Value
age [years]	15.40 ± 2.33 16 (8–19)	15.36 ± 2.74 16 (9–18)	ns
BMI [kg/m^2]	34.05 ± 4.75 33.80 (26–47)	16.43 ± 2.43 20.00 (15–24)	0.001
BMI Z-score	2.30 ± 0.38 2.32 (1.4–3.0)	−0.10 ± 0.65 0.07 (−1.7–0.74)	0.001
creatinine [mg/dL]	0.63 ± 0.12 0.63 (0.33–0.91)	0.59 ± 0.19 0.57 (0.30–1.06)	ns
BUN [mg/dL]	24.17 ± 5.45 24 (16–36)	25.27 ± 6.42 24 (17–41)	ns
UA [mg/dL]	6.38 ± 1.33 6.70 (3.7–9.1)	4.40 ± 1.07 3.90 (2.9–6.2)	0.001
cystatin C [mg/L]	0.88 ± 0.16 0.91 (0.4–1.2)	0.76 ± 0.11 0.75 (0.6–0.9)	0.028
GFR F [ml/min/1.73 m^2]	111.26 ± 31.15 102 (75–249)	127.18 ± 22.54 127 (101–163)	0.019
GFR S [ml/min/1.73 m^2]	115.57 ± 20.54 113 (80–175)	118.02 ± 36.02 111 (53–199)	ns
microalbuminuria [mg/day]	20.56 ± 17.90 14.17 (5–87)	11.70 ± 7.03 10.92 (6–29)	ns
total cholesterol [mg/dL]	184.83 ± 33.67 187 (112–260)	173.08 ± 32.44 177 (122–243)	ns
HDL [mg/dL]	42.88 ± 7.90 42 (31–60)	55.47 ± 10.02 56 (34–75)	0.001
LDL [mg/dL]	112.79 ± 28.31 113 (34–169)	105.73 ± 27.55 103 (70–162)	ns

Table 2. Cont.

Variables	Obesity Group (n = 45) Mean ± SD Median (Min-Max)	Control Group (n = 41) Mean ± SD Median (Min-Max)	p-Value
triglycerides [mg/dL]	161.28 ± 131.40 132 (44–785)	76.41 ± 25.39 80 (27–130)	0.001
glucose [mg/dL]	92.57 ± 6.14 91 (79–108)	88.79 ± 5.45 89 (80–99)	0.029
LVMI [g/m$^{2.7}$]	37.30 ± 9.12 34.01 (29–54)	25.04 ± 3.28 24.16 (20–29)	0.001
D	1.91 ± 2.93 1 (0–11)	0.12 ± 0.33 0 (0–1)	0.001
M	0.08 ± 0.28 0 (0–1)	0 ± 0 0 (0)	0.054
F	2.03 ± 3.39 1 (0–15)	1.71 ± 1.94 1 (0–6)	ns
DMFT	4.03 ± 4.18 2 (0–16)	1.83 ± 1.99 1.5 (0–7)	0.016
d	0.40 ± 1.65 0 (0–9)	0.02 ± 0.15 0 (0–1)	ns
mt	0 ± 0 0 (0)	0.02 ± 0.15 0 (0–1)	ns
f	0 ± 0 0 (0)	0.26 ± 0.77 0 (0–3)	0.037
dmft	0.40 ± 1.65 0 (0–9)	0.31 ± 0.87 0 (0–3)	ns
DMFT + dmft	4.31 ± 4.39 3 (0–17)	2.14 ± 2.04 2 (0–7)	ns
PCR [%]	56.40 ± 34.16 50 (5–100)	15.87 ± 19.27 9.5 (0–80)	0.001
BOP [%]	46.46 ± 33.68 50 (0–100)	7.19 ± 10.64 0 (0–40)	0.001

Results are expressed as mean ± standard deviation, median (min-max ranges). Statistical significance is given according to p-value ($p \leq 0.05$) vs. non-significance (ns). Statistical tests used were Mann–Whitney U test, t-test, and Welch test. Abbreviations: BMI—body max index; BUN—blood urea nitrogen; UA—uric acid; GFR F—glomerular filtration rate estimated by the Filler formula; GFR S—glomerular filtration rate calculated by the Schwartz formula; LVMI—left ventricular mass index, D—number of decayed secondary teeth; M—number of missing secondary teeth; F—number of filled secondary teeth; DMFT—decayed, missing, filled teeth score, evaluating dental caries in permanent teeth; d—number of decayed primary teeth; m—number of missing primary teeth; f—number of filled primary teeth; dmft score—total score evaluating the number of decayed, missing, filled primary teeth; PCR [%]—plaque control record index; BOP [%]—bleeding on probe index.

The study and control group did not differ in serum concentrations of creatinine and urea. Significantly higher concentrations of uric acid and cystatin C were observed in obesity group ($p = 0.001$; $p = 0.028$). According to the Schwartz formula, GFR values did not differ significantly between the study and control group (115.57 ± 20.54 mL/min/1.73 m^2 and 118.02 ± 36.02 mL/min/1.73 m^2, respectively). Mean GFR estimated by Filler formula in the obesity group was 111.26 ± 31.15 mL/min/1.73 m^2 and 127.18 ± 22.54 mL/min/1.73 m^2 in the control group ($p = 0.019$). The study and control group presented no proteinuria in urine analysis. Clinically significant microalbuminuria (>30 mg/d) was observed in 7 patients with obesity, while in the control group, microalbuminuria >30 mg/d was not detected ($p = 0.183$).

In the study group, 25 patients presented primary hypertension, while AH was not observed in the control group. Obesity and control groups did not differ in serum concentrations of total cholesterol and LDL. Significantly higher concentrations of HDL, triglycerides and glucose were observed in study group ($p = 0.001$; $p = 0.001$; $p = 0.029$). Median LVMI was significantly different between obesity and control groups ($p = 0.001$).

3.2. Oral Data

Analysis of the oral cavity revealed that obesity group presented a significantly higher number of D ($p = 0.001$) and DMFT score ($p = 0.016$), amount of dental plaque (PCR), ($p = 0.001$), and gingival inflammation (BOP), ($p = 0.001$). No differences in the results of the dental examination of the primary dentition were detected between the study and the control group (Table 2).

3.3. Correlations between the Variables

In the obesity group, Spearman analysis evidenced a significant correlation between BMI and concentrations of creatinine, urea, cystatin C, GFR estimated by the Filler formula, microalbuminuria, and the number of decayed teeth D. The strongest correlation was revealed between BMI and concentration of uric acid ($r = 0.737$), and oral variables such as PCR and BOP ($r = 0.539$; $r = 0.583$). Additionally, the most significant correlation was found between BMI Z-score and oral status estimated by BOP and DMFT scores ($r = 0.499$; $r = 0.499$). In the study group, statistical analysis evidenced a significant correlation between uric acid and HDL, triglycerides, and BOP. The strongest correlation was revealed between UA and LVMI ($r = 0.616$). There was a significant correlation between cystatin C and BOP, LVMI, and between BOP and triglycerides, glucose, HDL, and GFR estimated by the Filler formula (Table 3).

Table 3. Significant results of the Spearman's and Pearson's correlation rank tests regarding clinical and biochemical parameters ($p < 0.05$) for the obesity group.

Obesity Group $n = 45$	p-Value	Spearman R/Pearson r
BMI and D	0.001	R 0.433
BMI and PCR	0.001	R 0.539
BMI and BOP	0.001	R 0.583
BMI and creatinine	0.033	r 0.286
BMI and urea	0.007	R 0.256
BMI and UA	0.001	R 0.737
BMI and cystatin C	0.001	R 0.480
BMI and GFR F	0.001	R −0.524
BMI and microalbuminuria	0.004	R 0.419
BMI Z-score and D	0.025	R 0.316
BMI Z-score and BOP	0.001	R 0.499
BMI Z-score and DMFT	0.001	R 0.499
BMI Z-score and UA	0.000	r 0.606
BMI Z-score and cystatin C	0.000	R 0.477
BMI Z-score and GFR F	0.000	R −0.478
BMI Z-score and microalbuminuria	0.020	R 0.348
UA and BOP [%]	0.001	R 0.481
UA and HDL	0.001	r −0.582
UA and triglycerides	0.001	r 0.479
UA and LVMI	0.004	R 0.616
cystatin C and BOP [%]	0.005	R 0.407
cystatin C and LVMI	0.039	r 0.475
microalbuminuria and HDL	0.001	R −0.054
microalbuminuria and triglycerides	0.009	R 0.398
creatinine and HDL	0.014	R 0.337

Table 3. Cont.

Obesity Group n = 45	p-Value	Spearman R/Pearson r
BOP and GFR F	0.005	R −0.413
BOP and HDL	0.001	R −0.439
BOP and triglycerides	0.004	R −0.394
BOP and glucose	0.004	R 0.388
DMFT and total cholesterol	0.034	R 0.307
DMFT and triglycerides	0047	R 0.277
DMFT and glucose	0.041	R 0.279

Abbreviations: BMI—body max index; UA—uric acid; GFR F—glomerular filtration rate estimated by the Filler formula; LVMI—left ventricular mass index. D—number of decayed secondary teeth; DMFT—decayed, missing, filled teeth score, evaluating dental caries in permanent teeth; PCR [%]—plaque control record index; BOP [%]—bleeding on probe index.

3.4. Clinical and Biochemical Characteristics: Suspicion of Obesity-Related Glomerulopathy Group and without ORG Group

Individuals composing the suspicion of ORG and without ORG group did not differ in serum concentrations of creatinine, urea, cystatin C and GFR estimated by the Filler formula. Significantly higher concentrations of uric acid were observed in the suspicion ORG group ($p = 0.002$). Mean GFR calculated by the Filler formula in the suspicion of ORG group was 130.14 ± 54.88 mL/min/1.73 m^2 and 106.37 ± 20.38 mL/min/1.73 m^2 in the without ORG group. Median microalbuminuria was significantly different between the probable ORG group and without ORG group ($p = 0.001$) (Table 4).

Table 4. Anthropometric, biochemical, and oral data under suspicion of ORG (sORG) and without ORG among individuals.

Variables	sORG (n = 7) Mean ± SD Median (Min-Max)	Without ORG (n = 38) Mean ± SD Median (Min-Max)	p-Value
age	16.14 ± 1.77 16 (14–19)	15.16 ± 1.77 16 (8–18)	ns
BMI	35.78 ± 3.65 36.6 (29.5–40)	33.62 ± 4.94 32.61 (26–47)	ns
BMI Z-score	2.42 ± 0.25 2.32 (2.06–2.7)	2.28 ± 0.41 2.33 (1.36–3.03)	ns
creatinine	0.66 ± 0.09 0.7 (0.53–0.77)	0.62 ± 0.13 0.61 (0.33–0.91)	ns
BUN	23 ± 4.43 22 (19–32)	24.5 ± 5.71 24 (16–36)	ns
UA	7.31 ± 0.59 7.3 (6.3–8.2)	6.14 ± 1.36 6 (3.7–9.1)	0.002
cystatin C	0.79 ± 0.21 0.78 (0.41–1)	0.9 ± 0.15 0.92 (067–1.2)	ns
GFR F	130.14 ± 54.88 121 (92–249)	106.37 ± 20.38 101 (75–144)	ns
GFR S	112.83 ± 19.19 103 (92–144)	116.26 ± 21.14 113.5 (80–175)	ns
microalbuminuria	51.41 ± 22.65 41.5 (30–87)	13.95 ± 6.32 13.45 (5–28)	0.001
total cholesterol	195 ± 49.1 218 (112–240)	182.28 ± 29.3 185 (128–260)	ns

Table 4. Cont.

Variables	sORG (n = 7) Mean ± SD Median (Min-Max)	Without ORG (n = 38) Mean ± SD Median (Min-Max)	p-Value
HDL	39.28 ± 6.68 39 (33–51)	43.78 ± 8.03 43 (31–60)	ns
LDL	122.28 ± 48.65 141 (34–169)	110.23 ± 20.64 111 (60–153)	ns
triglycerides	167 ± 56.07 155 (108–259)	159.85 ± 145.03 129 (44–785)	ns
glucose	91.43 ± 6.37 95 (79–97)	92.86 ± 6.17 91 (82–108)	ns
LVMI	53.4 ± 40 53.4 (50–63)	35.96 ± 8.08 33.06 (29–54)	ns
D	2.14 ± 3.34 0 (0–9)	1.86 ± 2.89 1 (0–11)	ns
DMFT	3 ± 4.16 1 (0–11)	4.28 ± 4.21 2 (0–16)	ns
PCR [%]	67.42 ± 33.16 80 (20–100)	53.64 ± 34.44 50 (50–100)	ns
BOP [%]	50 ± 36.51 50 (0–100)	45.57 ± 33.59 45 (0–100)	ns

Results are expressed as mean ± standard deviation, median (min-max ranges). Statistical significance is given according to p-value ($p \leq 0.05$) vs. non-significance (ns). Abbreviations: sORG—suspicion of obesity-related glomerulopathy. BMI—body max index; BUN—blood urea nitrogen; UA—uric acid; GFR F—glomerular filtration rate estimated by the Filler formula; GFR S—glomerular filtration rate calculated by the Schwartz formula; LVMI—left ventricular mass index. D—number of decayed secondary teeth; DMFT—decayed, missing, filled teeth score, evaluating dental caries in permanent teeth; PCR [%]—plaque control record index; BOP [%]—bleeding on probe index.

4. Discussion

4.1. Dental Caries

In this study, no specific relations between oral status and markers of kidney disease were found; however, more frequent gingivitis/bacterial colonization and significant differences in oral status between obese and non-obese children were revealed. Obese patients demonstrated a higher incidence of oral-related complications according to dental status and less efficient oral biofilm control and gingival inflammation than non-obese subjects.

Based on the literature review on childhood obesity, cause-and-effect relationships to oral diseases show strong associations with periodontal diseases and different relationships to caries progression, such as confirming [24–26] or denying [27–30]. It seems to depend on multiple factors contributing to the disease progress and the risk of dental caries in primary and permanent dentition among pediatric patients affected by simple obesity. This is, to the best of our knowledge, the third study related to obese children in our country [31,32]. In comparison to the first study carried out on obese children in the similar age group of 7 and 12 years old, in the group of younger children, no difference was found between healthy and obese children (82.2% versus 95.0%; ns), while in the group of children aged 12, the incidence of caries was significantly higher in the group of obese children (53.2% versus 84.2%; $p = 0.004$) [31]. In addition, obese adolescents revealed a correlation with the number of surfaces affected by caries, dental plaque, and gingivitis ($p = 0.001$). The second survey confirmed high caries incidence of obese children aged 6–12 years old, but the relationship between BMI and insufficient oral hygiene has not been demonstrated [32]. A similar study of 91 participants divided on normal and overweight children between 6–12 years old revealed a low caries experience and risk classification CAMBRA [30]. The lack of differences in the group consisted of younger children may be explained by the very high caries prevalence among Polish children under 7 years old, estimated at 85.0% [33].

In contrast, older children aged 12–18 have easier access to dental operatory offices and school oral health education/promotion facilities. Other co-factors such as preferred diet, socioeconomic class, industrialized origin life conditions may be found as moderators [29,34,35]. Assuming the present trial's statistical differences between DMFT values at age 15, obese children revealed that increasing body weight boosts caries prevalence.

At this point, it is worth emphasizing the role of dentistry in the monitoring of childhood obesity [36,37]. Frequent contact with children and young adults in the dental setting makes it possible for them to prevent obesity. The overweight parent and child–dentist relationship in an extended period may allow that dietary advice may be given to reduce sugar consumption and meal frequency. This could be valid from the oral diseases and BMI reduction points of view. Moreover, becoming aware of the oral indicators of obesity may strengthen motivation to alter any unhealthy behaviors [36,37].

4.2. Dental Plaque and Gingival Bleeding

It is noteworthy that the relationship between obesity and periodontal inflammation is reported wider than dental caries and gingivitis experience, probably because of exposure to a number of factors [38–40]. Based on the literature mentioned above, a failure in periodontal health maintenance is due to an influence of blood proinflammatory cytokines, such as IL-1, IL-6, TNF-α, CRP, and oxidative stress activity [12]. Proinflammatory mediators secreted by adipose cells, interfering with the immune system, may modify the host's response to plaque antigens and contribute to blocking periodontal protection [41]; therefore, focusing on gingivitis observed in obese children results from metabolic disturbances, inflammatory factors, and poor oral hygiene habits. Additionally, predisposition to gingivitis may be related to circulating sex hormones as higher estrogen levels owing to androgen disturbances in adipose tissue [42,43]. Even if a clinical survey did not show significant deviations in periodontal tissues, such as the number and depth of gingival pockets or periodontal attachment loss, poor cleaning habits with gingival inflammation may be observed among obese children [44].

At such a young age, periodontal health elements such as depth and attachment level are usually not examined because of their developmental status; however, it is known that high inflammatory scores and poor oral hygiene are more likely to generate permanent periodontal inflammation in the future. Moreover, the effectiveness of periodontal surgical treatment coexisting with obesity may have an uncertain recovery prognosis [45–47]. In this study, we demonstrated the adolescent patients affected by gingivitis, defined by the BOP index. This local manifestation of systemic inflammation accompanying obesity may suggest the development of metabolic syndrome and kidney damage in the form of obesity-related glomerulopathy.

Notably, obesity in pediatric patients may promote oral colonization with pathogens, which the PCR index may assess. This is in line with current literature concerning weight gain in childhood, where it is reported how excessive bacterial plaque increases unfavorable microbiota composition in the oral cavity [48,49]. In this context, Craig et al. revealed how oral microbiota trajectories varied in childhood according to weight gain [50]. Zeigler et al. documented an increase in both *Firmicutes* and *Bacteroidetes* sp. in obese patients compared to normal-weight individuals [43]. Nagawa et al. demonstrated that some species might support progesterone and estrogen access to vitamin K production needed for bacterial growth factors [51]. It seems that the role of oral bacteria in the formation and maintenance of inflammation in obesity may help to understand not only quantity but quality effects on microbial colonization or abundance in the oral cavity [50]. Changes leading to oral microbial dysbiosis need further microbiota investigations.

4.3. BMI and Obesity-Related Glomerulopathy

The study revealed significantly higher concentrations of uric acid, cystatin C, and mean GFR estimated by Filler formula in the obesity group than in the control group. These laboratory results showed the early, asymptomatic kidney injury without clinically important microalbuminuria in obese patients. The initial hypothesis could be that serum cystatin C and uric acid might aspire to be early markers of kidney damage in obesity, getting ahead of an increase in the concentration of creatinine, urea, and hypofiltration. Moreover, GFR calculated with the Filler formula based on serum concentration of cystatin C represents a more precise index of hyperfiltration, which is characteristic of ORG [52].

Additionally, our study presented the markers of metabolic syndrome in the study group and no hypertension, hypertriglyceridemia, low concentrations of HDL in the control group, which confirms the representative group of patients with obesity. In addition, uric acid is considered a marker connecting obesity with metabolic syndrome and is also indicative of the development of cardiovascular diseases, including arterial hypertension, atherosclerosis, and renal impairment [53]. The above reports are confirmed in the present study by a positive correlation between the uric acid level and markers of the metabolic syndrome: concentration of triglycerides, HDL, and LVMI indicating left ventricular hypertrophy and as a risk factor of cardiovascular diseases, including arterial hypertension.

In the present study, the BMI, describing simple obesity in children and adolescents, correlated the most with two oral status markers: PCR and BOP. Additionally, the project revealed a high correlation between BMI Z-score and gingivitis, estimated by the BOP index. The presented results may initiate the discussion and our future studies of the role of gingivitis in the progression of obesity. Moreover, the study evidenced a significant correlation between BOP index and concentration of kidney markers: uric acid, cystatin C, and indicators of metabolic syndrome: concentration of triglycerides, HDL, and glucose. Based on the above information and other reports [54], we suggest that gingivitis may represent an early marker of metabolic syndrome and kidney injury such as obesity-related glomerulopathy. In particular, the strongest correlation was found between the BOP index and uric acid. It seems to be the link between local inflammation in the oral cavity and systemic inflammatory response, which occurs in patients with obesity and morphological or functional changes in kidneys, described as obesity-related glomerulopathy.

Showing the usefulness of dental and biochemical markers, which are routinely assessed during diagnostics of obesity complications, may contribute to improved identification of the group of children with a risk of ORG and, therefore, chronic kidney disease in adulthood. In this way, invasive diagnostics of kidney damage, i.e., kidney biopsy, could be avoided. Early introduction of nephroprotective treatment and intensification of body weight reduction in this group of patients may significantly contribute to a decrease in the number of patients with obesity who may develop end-stage renal failure later in adulthood.

4.4. Limitations of the Study

The study has other limitations that have to be underlined in our interpretation of the results. No renal biopsies were performed in the group of patients with obesity-related glomerulopathy and healthy children and adolescents to confirm the clinical results received from the study. ORG is defined by glomerular hypertrophy (glomerulomegaly), adaptive focal segmental glomerulosclerosis, and tubulointerstitial fibrosis with tubular atrophy [55,56]. Renal biopsy is too invasive a procedure in children and adolescents (in Poland, it is usually used in case of acute renal failure without the onset point). At the time of the survey, the hormonal profiles of the subjects were not investigated, and oral status was examined without any pre-diagnostic dental history (baseline). Further, family members were not studied at all, and even they presented with overweight body mass. Finally, fewer than 100 participants may not be a representative study group for distinct conclusions. On the other hand, a homogenous group of children affected by obesity was collected, which was examined in one hospital and tested by the same diagnostic laboratory.

Further, the assessment of salivary levels of such markers as cystatin C and uric acid should be considered in search of an alternative, still non-invasive method of ORG diagnosis in children [57]. The circumstances mentioned above would add valuable data to general analysis. Oral health indicators may motivate to begin obesity treatment and support diminishing the risk of developing or progressing obesity-related glomerulopathy and metabolic syndrome in pediatric patients. Obtained results highlight the differences in oral status between obese and non-obese young patients, as well as the need for prophylactic programs, especially in times of pandemic, with unpredictable access to public spaces and enforced lockdowns [58].

5. Conclusions

No specific relation to markers of kidney disease was found; however, more frequent gingivitis/bacterial colonization and significant differences in oral status between obese and non-obese patients were revealed. Susceptibility to inflammation may be conducive to developing metabolic syndrome and kidney damage in the form of obesity-related glomerulopathy and contribution to dental caries progression in the future.

Increased serum cystatin C and uric acid might aspire to be early markers of kidney damage leading to obesity-related glomerulopathy. GFR based on serum concentration of cystatin C represents a more precise index of hyperfiltration, which is characteristic of ORG. Uric acid seems to indicate metabolic syndrome and cardiovascular complications (LVMI > 95 percentiles).

Since the group with suspicion of ORG is small and comparisons with non-ORG patients are inconclusive, an analysis of the relationship between renal, metabolic, and oral health indicators among pediatric patients affected by simple obesity needs to be continued in future clinical trials.

Supplementary Materials: The following are available online at https://www.mdpi.com/article/10.3390/jcm10163723/s1, Figure S1: Flow chart of the study. Figure S2: STROBE Protocol Checklist.

Author Contributions: K.M.-L.: data curation, investigation, and software; D.O.-N.: conceptualization, funding acquisition, supervision, and revising the manuscript; J.Z.: supervision; E.P.: conceptualization, investigation, writing review, and editing the manuscript. All authors have read and agreed to the published version of the manuscript.

Funding: This research and the APC were funded only by the Poznan University of Medical Sciences.

Institutional Review Board Statement: Before the experiment was started, approval was obtained from the Bioethics Committee at the Poznan University of Medical Sciences (protocol code No. 679/17 and date of approval 22 June 2017). The study followed the rules of the Declaration of Helsinki and complied with Good Clinical Practice guidelines. Before the subject evaluation, the whole course of the study was explained to all patients, and they were asked to express their opinion.

Informed Consent Statement: Written informed consent was obtained from all patients and their parents or legal guardians, or both for study participation and publication of this paper. Additionally, a parent or legal guardian approval was needed for inclusion in the study. A lack of acceptance from patients and their parents/legal guardians resulted in exclusion from the study.

Data Availability Statement: Data associated with the paper are not publicly available but are available from the corresponding author at reasonable request.

Acknowledgments: We appreciate any technical support in editing performed by Tomasz Maksymiuk.

Conflicts of Interest: The authors declare no conflict of interest. The funders had no role in the design of the study, in the collection, analyses, or interpretation of data, in the writing of the manuscript, or in the decision to publish the results.

References

1. Zoja, C.; Abbate, M.; Remuzzi, G. Progression of renal injury toward interstitial inflammation and glomerular sclerosis is dependent on abnormal protein filtration. *Nephrol. Dial. Transplant.* **2015**, *30*, 706–712. [CrossRef] [PubMed]
2. Chagnac, A.; Zingerman, B.; Rozen-Zvi, B.; Herman-Edelstein, M. Consequences of glomerular hyperfiltration: The role of physical forces in the pathogenesis of chronic kidney disease in diabetes and obesity. *Nephron* **2019**, *143*, 38–42. [CrossRef]
3. Kambham, N.; Markowitz, G.S.; Valeri, A.M.; Lin, J.; D'Agati, V.D. Obesity-related glomerulopathy: An emerging epidemic. *Kidney Int.* **2011**, *59*, 1498–1509. [CrossRef]
4. Praga, M.; Morales, E. The Fatty Kidney: Obesity and renal disease. *Nephron* **2017**, *136*, 273–276. [CrossRef]
5. Serra, A.; Romero, R.; Lopez, D.; Navarro, M.; Esteve, A.; Perez, N.; Alastrue, A.; Ariza, A. Renal injury in the extremely obese patients with normal renal function. *Kidney Int.* **2008**, *73*, 947–955. [CrossRef]
6. Ostalska-Nowicka, D.; Mackowiak-Lewandowicz, K.; Perek, B.; Zaorska, K.; Zachwieja, J.; Nowicki, M. Megalin—A facultative marker of obesity-related glomerulopathy in children. *J. Biol. Regul. Homeost. Agents* **2019**, *33*, 415–420.
7. Zhao, Y.; Li, G.; Wang, Y.; Liu, Z. Alteration of Connexin43 expression in a rat model of obesity-related glomerulopathy. *Exp. Mol. Pathol.* **2018**, *104*, 12–18. [CrossRef] [PubMed]
8. Modéer, T.; Blomberg, C.; Wondimu, B.; Lindberg, T.Y.; Marcus, C. Association between obesity and periodontal risk indicators in adolescents. *Int. J. Pediatr. Obes.* **2011**, *6*, 264–270. [CrossRef]
9. Guaré, R.O.; Ciamponi, A.L.; Santos, M.T.B.R.; Gorjão, R.; Diniz, M.B. Caries experience and salivary parameters among overweight children and adolescents. *Dent. J.* **2013**, *1*, 31–40. [CrossRef]
10. Prpic, J.; Kuis, D.; Pezelj-Ribaric, S. Obesity and oral health—Is there an association? *Coll. Antropol.* **2012**, *36*, 755–759.
11. Goodson, J.M. Disease reciprocity between gingivitis and obesity. *J. Periodontol.* **2020**, *91*, 26–34. [CrossRef] [PubMed]
12. Tomofuji, T.; Ekuni, D.; Irie, K.; Azuma, T.; Tamaki, N.; Maruyama, T.; Yamamoto, T.; Watanabe, T.; Morita, M. Relationships between periodontal inflammation, lipid peroxide and oxidative damage of multiple organs in rats. *Biomed Res.* **2011**, *32*, 343–349. [CrossRef] [PubMed]
13. Weaver, D.J. Hypertension in children and adolescents. *Pediatr. Rev.* **2017**, *38*, 369–382. [CrossRef] [PubMed]
14. Bacchetta, J.; Cochat, P.; Rognant, N.; Ranchin, B.; Hadj-Aissa, A.; Dubourg, L. Which creatinine and cystatin C equations can be reliably used in children? *Clin. J. Am. Soc. Nephrol.* **2011**, *6*, 552–560. [CrossRef] [PubMed]
15. Tykarski, A.; Filipiak, K.J.; Januszewicz, A.; Litwin, M.; Narkiewicz, K.; Prejbisz, A.; Ostalska-Nowicka, D.; Widecka, K.; Kostka-Jeziorny, K. Guidelines for the Management of Hypertension. *Arter. Hypertens.* **2019**, *23*, 41–87. [CrossRef]
16. Lurbe, I.; Ferrer, E. 2016 European society of hypertension guidelines for the management of high blood pressure in children and adolescents. *An. Pediatr.* **2016**, *85*, 167–169. (In Spanish)
17. Kêkê, L.M.; Samouda, H.; Jacobs, J.; di Pompeo, C.; Lemdani, M.; Hubert, H.; Zitouni, D.; Guinhouya, B. Body mass index and childhood obesity classification systems: A comparison of the French, International Obesity Task Force (IOTF) and World Health Organization (WHO) references. *Rev. Epidemiol. Sante Publique* **2015**, *63*, 173–182. [CrossRef] [PubMed]
18. Abitbol, C.L.; Ingelfinger, J.R. Nephron mass and cardiovascular and renal disease risks. *Semin. Nephrol.* **2009**, *29*, 445–454. [CrossRef]
19. Paszynska, E.; Pawinska, M.; Gawriolek, M.; Kaminska, I.; Otulakowska-Skrzynska, J.; Marczuk-Kolada, G.; Rzatowski, S.; Sokolowska, K.; Olszewska, A.; Schlagenhauf, U.; et al. Impact of a toothpaste with microcrystalline hydroxyapatite on the occurrence of early childhood caries: A 1-year randomized clinical trial. *Sci. Rep.* **2021**, *11*, 2650. [CrossRef] [PubMed]
20. Bischoff, J.I.; van der Merwe, E.H.; Retief, D.H.; Barbakow, F.H.; Cleaton-Jones, P.E. Relationship between fluoride concentration in enamel, DMFT index, and degree of fluorosis in a community residing in an area with a high level of fluoride. *J. Dent. Res.* **1976**, *55*, 37–42. [CrossRef]
21. O'Leary, T.J.; Drake, R.B.; Naylor, J.E. The plaque control record. *J. Periodontol.* **1972**, *43*, 38. [CrossRef] [PubMed]
22. Ainamo, J.; Bay, I. Periodontal indexes for and in practice. *Tandlaegebladet* **1976**, *80*, 149–152.
23. Ainamo, J.; Bay, I. Problems and proposals for recording gingivitis and plaque. *Int. Dent. J.* **1975**, *25*, 229–235.
24. Paszynska, E.; Dmitrzak-Weglarz, M.; Ostalska-Nowicka, D.; Nowicki, M.; Gawriolek, M.; Zachwieja, J. Association of oral status and early primary hypertension biomarkers among children and adolescents. *Int. J. Environ. Res. Public Health* **2020**, *17*, 7981. [CrossRef]
25. Paszynska, E.; Dmitrzak-Węglarz, M.; Perczak, A.; Gawriolek, M.; Hanć, T.; Bryl, E.; Mamrot, P.; Dutkiewicz, A.; Roszak, M.; Tyszkiewicz-Nwafor, M.; et al. Excessive weight gain and dental caries experience among children affected by ADHD. *Int. J. Environ. Res. Public Health* **2020**, *17*, 5870. [CrossRef]
26. Manohar, N.; Hayen, A.; Fahey, P.; Arora, A. Obesity and dental caries in early childhood: A systematic review and meta-analyses. *Obes. Rev.* **2020**, *21*, e12960. [CrossRef]
27. Alves, L.S.; Susin, C.; Damé-Teixeira, N.; Maltz, M. Overweight and obesity are not associated with dental caries among 12-year-old South Brazilian schoolchildren. *Commun. Dent. Oral Epidemiol.* **2013**, *41*, 224–231. [CrossRef]
28. Alshihri, A.A.; Rogers, H.J.; Alqahtani, M.A.; Aldossary, M.S. Association between dental caries and obesity in children and young people: A narrative review. *Int. J. Dent.* **2019**, *2019*, 9105759. [CrossRef]
29. Hayden, C.; Bowler, J.O.; Chambers, S.; Freeman, R.; Humphris, G.; Richards, D.; Cecil, J.E. Obesity and dental caries in children: A systematic review and meta-analysis. *Commun. Dent. Oral. Epidemiol.* **2013**, *41*, 289–308. [CrossRef]

30. Guaré, R.O.; Perez, M.M.; Novaes, T.F.; Ciamponi, A.L.; Gorjão, R.; Diniz, M.B. Overweight/obese children are associated with lower caries experience than normal-weight children/adolescents. *Int. J. Paediatr. Dent.* **2019**, *29*, 756–764. [CrossRef] [PubMed]
31. Chłapowska, J.; Rataj-Kulmacz, A.; Krzyżaniak, A.; Borysewicz-Lewicka, M. Zaleznosc wystepowania prochnicy od stanu odzywienia u dzieci 7-i 12-letnich. [Association between dental caries and nutritional status of 7-and 12-years-old children]. *Dev. Period. Med.* **2014**, *18*, 349–355. (In Polish)
32. Kaczmarek, U.; Szymonajtis, A.; Kłaniecka, B. Prochnica zebow i higiena jamy ustnej u dzieci szkolnych z prawidłowa i nadmierna masa ciała. [Dental caries and oral hygiene in normal and overweight schoolchildren]. *Nowa Stomatol.* **2014**, *1*, 15–19. (In Polish)
33. Olczak-Kowalczyk, D.; Gozdowski, D.; Kaczmarek, U. Próchnica zębów stałych u dzieci w wieku 5 i 7 lat w Polsce i jej związek z próchnicą zębów mlecznych. [Dental caries in permanent dentition in children aged 5 and 7 in Poland and its association with dental caries in primary dentition]. *Nowa Stomatol.* **2017**, *3*, 129–141. (In Polish)
34. Costa, L.R.; Daher, A.; Queiroz, M.G. Early childhood caries and body mass index in young children from low income families. *Int. J. Environ. Res. Public Health* **2013**, *10*, 867–878. [CrossRef]
35. Modéer, T.; Blomberg, C.C.; Wondimu, B.; Julihn, A.; Marcus, C. Association between obesity, flow rate of whole saliva and dental caries in adolescents. *Obesity* **2010**, *18*, 2367–2373. [CrossRef]
36. Greenberg, B.L.; Glick, M.; Tavares, M. Addressing obesity in the dental setting: What can be learned from oral health care professionals' efforts to screen for medical conditions. *J. Public Health Dent.* **2017**, *77* (Suppl. 1), S67–S78. [CrossRef]
37. Nainar, S.M. Five-minute nutrition workup for children in dental practice. *Gen. Dent.* **2013**, *61*, e2–e3.
38. Genco, R.J.; Borgnakke, W.S. Risk factors for periodontal disease. *Periodontol. 2000* **2013**, *62*, 59–94. [CrossRef]
39. Suvan, J.; Petrie, A.; Moles, D.R.; Nibali, L.; Patel, K.; Darbar, U.; Donos, N.; Tonetti, M.; D'Aiuto, F. Body mass index as a predictive factor of periodontal therapy outcomes. *J. Dent. Res.* **2014**, *93*, 49–54. [CrossRef]
40. Gorman, A.; Kaye, E.K.; Apovian, C.; Fung, T.T.; Nunn, M.; Garcia, R.I. Overweight and obesity predict time to periodontal disease progression in men. *J. Clin. Periodontol.* **2012**, *39*, 107–114. [CrossRef] [PubMed]
41. Jimenez, M.; Hu, F.B.; Marino, M.; Li, Y.; Joshipura, K.J. Prospective associations between measures of adiposity and periodontal disease. *Obesity* **2012**, *20*, 1718–1725. [CrossRef]
42. von Bremen, J.; Lorenz, N.; Ruf, S. Impact of body mas index on oral health during orthodontic treatment: An explorative pilot study. *Eur. J. Orthod.* **2016**, *38*, 386–392. [CrossRef] [PubMed]
43. Zeigler, C.C.; Persson, G.R.; Wondimu, B.; Marcus, C.; Sobko, T.; Modéer, T. Microbiota in the oral subgingival biofilm is associated with obesity in adolescence. *Obesity* **2012**, *20*, 157–164. [CrossRef]
44. Pussinen, P.J.; Paju, S.; Viikari, J.; Salminen, A.; Taittonen, L.; Laitinen, T.; Burgner, D.; Kähönen, M.; Lehtimäki, T.; Hutri-Kähönen, N.; et al. Childhood oral infections associate with adulthood metabolic syndrome: A longitudinal cohort study. *J. Dent. Res.* **2020**, *99*, 1165–1173. [CrossRef] [PubMed]
45. Altay, U.; Gurgan, C.A.; Ağbaht, K. Changes in inflammatory and metabolic parameters after periodontal treatment in patients with and without obesity. *J. Periodontol.* **2013**, *84*, 13–23. [CrossRef]
46. Lakkis, D.; Bissada, N.F.; Saber, A.; Khaitan, L.; Palomo, L.; Narendran, S.; Al-Zahrani, M.S. Response to periodontal therapy in patients who had weight loss after bariatric surgery and obese counterparts: A pilot study. *J. Periodontol.* **2012**, *83*, 684–689. [CrossRef] [PubMed]
47. Goncalves, T.E.; Zimmermann, G.S.; Figueiredo, L.C.; Souza, M.D.C.; da Cruz, D.F.; Bastos, M.F.; da Silva, H.D.; Duarte, P.M. Local and serum levels of adipokines in patients with obesity after periodontal therapy: One-year follow-up. *J. Clin. Periodontol.* **2015**, *42*, 431–439. [CrossRef]
48. Goodson, J.M.; Groppo, D.; Halem, S.; Carpino, E. Is obesity an oral bacterial disease? *J. Dent. Res.* **2009**, *88*, 519–523. [CrossRef]
49. Haffajee, A.D.; Socransky, S.S. Relation of body mass index, periodontitis and Tannerella forsythia. *J. Clin. Periodontol.* **2009**, *36*, 89–99. [CrossRef] [PubMed]
50. Craig, S.J.C.; Blankenberg, D.; Parodi, A.C.L.; Paul, I.M.; Birch, L.L.; Savage, J.S.; Marini, M.E.; Stokes, J.L.; Nekrutenko, A.; Reimherr, M.; et al. Child weight gain trajectories linked to oral microbiota composition. *Sci. Rep.* **2018**, *8*, 14030. [CrossRef] [PubMed]
51. Nakagawa, S.; Fujii, H.; Machida, Y.; Okuda, K. A longitudinal study from prepuberty to puberty of gingivitis. Correlation between the occurrence of Prevotella intermedia and sex hormones. *J. Clin. Periodontol.* **1994**, *21*, 658–665. [CrossRef]
52. Porrini, E.; Ruggenenti, P.; Luis-Lima, S.; Carrara, F.; Jiménez, A.; de Vries, A.P.J.; Torres, A.; Gaspari, F.; Remuzzi, G. Estimated GFR: Time for a critical appraisal. *Nat. Rev. Nephrol.* **2019**, *15*, 177–190. [CrossRef] [PubMed]
53. Feig, D.; Mazzali, M.; Kang, D.H.; Nakagawa, T.; Price, K.; Kannelis, J.; Johnson, R.J. Serum uric acid: A risk factor and a target for treatment? *J. Am. Soc. Nephrol.* **2006**, *17*, 69–73. [CrossRef] [PubMed]
54. Lamster, I.; Pagan, M. Periodontal disease and the metabolic syndrome. *Int. Dent. J.* **2017**, *67*, 67–77. [CrossRef]
55. Xu, T.; Sheng, Z.; Li Yao, L. Obesity-related glomerulopathy: Pathogenesis, pathologic, clinical characteristics and treatment. *Front. Med.* **2017**, *11*, 340–348. [CrossRef] [PubMed]
56. D'Agati, V.D.; Chagnac, A.; de Vries, A.P.; Levi, M.; Porrini, E.; Herman-Edelstein, M.; Praga, M. Obesity-related glomerulopathy: Clinical and pathologic characteristics and pathogenesis. *Nat. Rev. Nephrol.* **2016**, *12*, 453–471. [CrossRef]
57. Bigler, L.R.; Streckfus, C.F.; Copeland, L.; Burns, R.; Dai, X.; Kuhn, M.; Martin, P.; Bigler, S.A. The potential use of saliva to detect recurrence of disease in women with breast carcinoma. *J. Oral Pathol. Med.* **2002**, *31*, 421–431. [CrossRef] [PubMed]
58. Olszewska, A.; Paszynska, E.; Roszak, M.; Czajka-Jakubowska, A. Management of the oral health of children during the COVID-19 pandemic in Poland. *Front. Public Health* **2021**. [CrossRef] [PubMed]

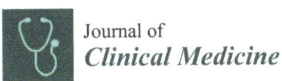

Article

Serum Sclerostin Is Associated with Peripheral and Central Systolic Blood Pressure in Pediatric Patients with Primary Hypertension

Piotr Skrzypczyk [1,*], Anna Ofiara [1], Michał Szyszka [2], Anna Stelmaszczyk-Emmel [3], Elżbieta Górska [3] and Małgorzata Pańczyk-Tomaszewska [1]

1. Department of Pediatrics and Nephrology, Medical University of Warsaw, 02-091 Warsaw, Poland; aniaofi@gmail.com (A.O.); mpanczyk1@wum.edu.pl (M.P.-T.)
2. Department of Pediatrics and Nephrology, Doctoral School, Medical University of Warsaw, 02-091 Warsaw, Poland; michalszyszkaa@gmail.com
3. Department of Laboratory Diagnostics and Clinical Immunology of Developmental Age, Medical University of Warsaw, 02-091 Warsaw, Poland; anna.stelmaszczyk-emmel@wum.edu.pl (A.S.-E.); elzbieta.gorska@uckwum.pl (E.G.)
* Correspondence: pskrzypczyk@wum.edu.pl; Tel.: +48-22-317-96-53; Fax: +48-22-317-99-54

Abstract: Recent studies showed the significance of the canonical Wnt/beta-catenin pathway and its inhibitor—sclerostin, in the formation of arterial damage, cardiovascular morbidity, and mortality. The study aimed to assess serum sclerostin concentration and its relationship with blood pressure, arterial damage, and calcium-phosphate metabolism in children and adolescents with primary hypertension (PH). Serum sclerostin concentration (pmol/L) was evaluated in 60 pediatric patients with PH and 20 healthy children. In the study group, we also assessed calcium-phosphate metabolism, office peripheral and central blood pressure, 24 h ambulatory blood pressure, and parameters of arterial damage. Serum sclerostin did not differ significantly between patients with PH and the control group (36.6 ± 10.6 vs. 41.0 ± 11.9 (pmol/L), $p = 0.119$). In the whole study group, sclerostin concentration correlated positively with height Z-score, phosphate, and alkaline phosphatase, and negatively with age, peripheral systolic and mean blood pressure, and central systolic and mean blood pressure. In multivariate analysis, systolic blood pressure (SBP) and height expressed as Z-scores were the significant determinants of serum sclerostin in the studied children: height Z-score ($\beta = 0.224$, (95%CI, 0.017–0.430)), SBP Z-score ($\beta = -0.216$, (95%CI, −0.417 to −0.016)). In conclusion, our results suggest a significant association between sclerostin and blood pressure in the pediatric population.

Keywords: sclerostin; primary hypertension; children; adolescents; arterial damage; blood pressure

1. Introduction

It is estimated that arterial hypertension (AH) affects 3–5% of the pediatric population, and its frequency increases with the age of the children studied [1]. Today, in Western countries, with adverse lifestyle changes, the incidence of primary hypertension (PH) is increasing and is slowly becoming the dominant form of AH also in the developmental age [2]. PH is now believed to be not only cardiovascular disease but a multifaceted syndrome involving abnormal body fat distribution, overactive renin-angiotensin-aldosterone, sympathetic and immune systems, and premature aging (including early vascular aging) [3].

The importance of calcium-phosphate disorders, including vitamin D, in the development of AH and target-organ damage has become the subject of intensive research in recent years [4]. Although the recently published VITAL study (The Vitamin D and OmegA-3 Trial) did not demonstrate an impact of vitamin D supplementation on cardiovascular morbidity in adults [5], research is ongoing on the potential interplay between cardiovascular and bone health.

Citation: Skrzypczyk, P.; Ofiara, A.; Szyszka, M.; Stelmaszczyk-Emmel, A.; Górska, E.; Pańczyk-Tomaszewska, M. Serum Sclerostin Is Associated with Peripheral and Central Systolic Blood Pressure in Pediatric Patients with Primary Hypertension. *J. Clin. Med.* **2021**, *10*, 3574. https://doi.org/10.3390/jcm10163574

Academic Editors: Katarzyna Taranta-Janusz, Kinga Musiał and Giuseppe Regolisti

Received: 15 June 2021
Accepted: 12 August 2021
Published: 13 August 2021

Publisher's Note: MDPI stays neutral with regard to jurisdictional claims in published maps and institutional affiliations.

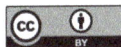

Copyright: © 2021 by the authors. Licensee MDPI, Basel, Switzerland. This article is an open access article distributed under the terms and conditions of the Creative Commons Attribution (CC BY) license (https://creativecommons.org/licenses/by/4.0/).

Sclerostin is a protein made up of 190 amino acids encoded by the *SOST* gene located on 17q12-21 chromosome, produced mainly by osteocytes, but also by chondrocytes, cementocytes, kidneys, liver, and vascular smooth muscle cells. Initially, it was thought that sclerostin belongs to the bone morphogenic protein (BMP) family [6]. However, it is now known that sclerostin, alongside the Dickkopf-1 protein (Dkk-1) is the most important inhibitor of the Wnt/beta-catenin pathway. Wnt ligands connect to the frizzled receptor and LRP5/6 (low-density lipoprotein receptor-related protein) coreceptor, stabilizing the beta-catenin structure, inducing its transfer to the nucleus, and affecting the transcription of genes encoding the proteins responsible for bone formation. Sclerostin combines with LRP5/6 coreceptors and inhibits the Wnt/beta-catenin pathway, which, in effect, reduces bone formation by inhibiting the formation of new osteoblasts and has a negative impact on the survival of already existing osteoblasts. Recent data indicate that sclerostin also stimulates osteoclast differentiation and increases bone resorption [7–9]. In 2019, the U.S. Food and Drug Administration (FDA) and European Medicines Agency (EMA) issued a positive opinion on the authorization of a monoclonal antibody against sclerostin (romosozumab) in postmenopausal women with osteoporosis and a high risk of fractures.

The Wnt/beta-catenin system might be the link between the bone and vascular system. Increased Wnt/beta-catenin activity was found in the experimental model of vascular calcification [10] and sclerostin expression was demonstrated in atherosclerotic plaques and calcifications within the human aorta [11]. The role of the Wnt/beta-catenin system and its endogenous inhibitors in circulatory system is unclear. Studies have shown both a positive [12,13] and negative [14,15] association, as well as no significant relationship [16,17] between sclerostin levels and arterial damage and cardiovascular risk in adults.

Considering the short duration of the disease and a small number of comorbidities, the population of children and adolescents with primary hypertension seems to be an ideal group to study the relationship between sclerostin, blood pressure, and subclinical arterial damage. Our study aims to assess serum sclerostin concentration in pediatric patients with PH and analyze its relationship with peripheral and central blood pressure, parameters of arterial damage, and parameters of calcium-phosphate metabolism.

2. Materials and Methods

2.1. Study Group

This single-center cross-sectional study included patients with PH treated in 2018–2020 in one tertiary center of pediatric nephrology. The criterion for inclusion in the study was confirmed AH following ESH recommendations [1]. In all patients referred to the center, we confirmed hypertension using ambulatory blood pressure monitoring. Only patients with elevated both office and 24 h ambulatory blood pressure were included in the final analysis. The exclusion criteria were: secondary forms of hypertension, the coexistence of known bone pathology, abnormalities in biochemical parameters of calcium-phosphate metabolism, diabetes mellitus, chronic inflammatory disease, or acute infectious disease. Based on available literature on sclerostin, assuming a delta of 4.5 (effect size: 0.50), a 0.05 alpha level, and 80% power, we estimated the sample size at 60 patients [13,14,16,18–20]; 20 age- and sex-matched healthy subjects were included in the control group. In the statistical analysis, the control group was smaller than the study group due to the comparable variance of key parameters in both groups.

Participants were included in the study consecutively from among the patients after considering inclusion and exclusion criteria to exclude selection bias. In the analyzed period (2018–2020), there were also 31 patients with white coat hypertension and seven patients with masked hypertension who were excluded from further analysis.

2.2. Ethical Issues

The authors obtained approval of the local Bioethical Committee before initiating the research (approval no. KB/58/2016, 15 March 2016). All procedures involving human participants were in accordance with the highest ethical standards of the institutional research committee and were performed according to the Declaration of Helsinki on the treatment of human subjects and its later amendments. Informed consent was obtained from all participants' representatives and participants (≥ 16 years) before enrolling in the study.

2.3. Clinical Parameters

In all participants, the following clinical parameters were assessed: sex, age (years), body height (cm), body weight (kg), body mass index (kg/m^2), antihypertensive medications taken, and duration of hypertension (months). Anthropometric parameters were compared with the standards for the local population and presented in the form of Z-score [21]. Overweight and obesity were defined according to WHO recommendations as a BMI Z-score above 1 and 2, respectively.

2.4. Serum Sclerostin

Serum sclerostin (ELISA enzyme-linked immunosorbent assay) was evaluated in all children studied using a kit from Biomedica Medizinprodukte GmbH, Vienna, Austria (BI-20492 Sclerostin ELISA). Blood samples were drawn on fasting from all the participants and thawed immediately after centrifugation at $-84\,^\circ$C.

2.5. Biochemical Parameters

All the participants had their calcium-phosphate metabolism evaluated on the basis of: serum concentrations of calcium (mg/dL), phosphate (mg/dL), 25-hydroxyvitamin D–25OHD (ng/mL), parathyroid hormone (pg/mL), and alkaline phosphatase activity (IU/L). In addition, the following biochemical parameters were evaluated: serum concentrations of creatinine (mg/dL), uric acid (mg/dL), total HDL- and LDL-cholesterol (mg/dL), and triglyceride (mg/dL). The estimated glomerular filtration rate (eGFR) was calculated in all patients (mL/min/1.73 m^2) according to the revised 2009 Schwartz formula [22]. In line with local recommendations, 25OHD concentration was classified as severe deficiency (0–10 ng/mL), deficiency (>10–20 ng/mL), suboptimal (>20–30), optimal (>30–50 ng/mL), high (>50–100 ng/mL), and toxic (>100 ng/mL) levels [23]. Normal calcium (8.8–10.7 mg/dL), phosphate (2.8–5.6 mg/dL), parathyroid hormone (12–95 pg/mL), and alkaline phosphatase activity (45–515 IU/L) were derived from the manufacturer's reference values.

2.6. Blood Pressure and Parameters of Arterial Damage

Each participant had their blood pressure measured three times, and the mean of the second and third measurements was taken for further analysis. Blood pressure measurements were performed oscillometrically (Welch Allyn Patient Monitor, Welch Allyn, Skaneateles Falls, NY, USA) according to ESH recommendations and were analyzed using pediatric normative values [24]. All the patients studied also had 24 h ambulatory blood pressure measurement performed (Oscar 2 Suntech, SunTech Medical Inc., Morrisville, NC, USA) according to the American Heart Association guidelines [25]. The device was programmed to perform measurement every 15 min between 7 a.m. and 10 p.m. and every 30 min between 10 p.m. and 7 a.m., giving 78 measurements per 24 h. We analyzed only reports with at least 50 readings per 24 h. The mean number of successful measures was 69.3 ± 4.5 readings (from 54 to 78 readings). Activity and resting periods were assessed according to the patient's individual diaries. Systolic, diastolic, and mean pressures (SBP, DBP, MAP, respectively), blood pressure loads, and nighttime blood pressure dipping (DIP) were analyzed. DIP below 10% was considered as disturbed circadian rhythm [25]. For both office and ambulatory monitoring, the blood pressure cuff was chosen following ESH recommendations and the devices' instructions. In all individuals, the middle upper-arm circumference was measured, and an appropriate cuff was selected from the cuffs available (Welch Allyn VSM: 20–26 cm, 25–34 cm, 32–43 cm, Oscar 2 Suntech: 17–25 cm, 23–33 cm, and 31–40 cm).

Arterial structure and function tests were performed using following methods: ultrasonographic examination of the common carotid artery (ALOKA Prosound Alpha 6, Hitachi Ltd., Tokyo, Japan)—common carotid artery intima media thickness (cIMT) (mm), Z-score [26], and common carotid artery local stiffness (E-tracking); applanation tonometry (Sphygmocor, ATCOR, Sydney, Australia)—central blood pressure, pulse wave analysis, and aortic (carotid-femoral) pulse wave velocity (aPWV) (m/s) Z-score [27]. The detailed description of the methods used was presented in the previous manuscripts of the research group [4,28]. In brief, arterial structure and function measurements were performed in a quiet room with ambient temperature (20 ± 5 °C) after 5 min of resting. Peripheral pressure waveforms were recorded from the radial artery at the right wrist (patient in sitting position, with back supported). Once 20 sequential waveforms had been acquired, the transfer function was used to generate the central aortic pressure waveform. aPWV was measured in a supine position and calculated as a difference in the carotid-to-femoral path length divided by the difference in R wave to the foot of the pressure wave taken from the superimposed ECG and pressure tracings. The distance was measured as the distance from the right carotid sampling site to the jugular notch, subtracted from the distance from the jugular notch to the right femoral sampling site in accordance with pediatric normative values by Reusz et al. [27]. Measurements of peripheral pressure waveform and aPWV were obtained three times in each subject, and the mean value of these measurements were taken for further analysis. cIMT was measured in a patient in a supine position using a manual method approximately 1 cm proximal to the carotid bulb on the distal carotid wall. Six determinations of cIMT—three on the left and three on the right side—were obtained and averaged. All arterial measurements were performed by a single experienced investigator (P.S.).

2.7. Statistical Analysis

The results were statistically analyzed using TIBCO Statistica 13.3 software (TIBCO Software Inc., Palo Alto, CA, USA). The numerical data obtained were presented as mean, standard deviation (SD), and interquartile range (IQR, Q1, Q3). The normality of variables was studied using the Shapiro–Wilk test. Normally distributed data were compared with Student *t*-test for independent groups and non-normally distributed data using the Mann–Whitney U test. The relationship between the two groups of variables was analyzed using Pearson correlation or Spearman rank correlation (depending on the distribution). Percentages in both groups were compared using the chi-square test and Fisher's exact test. Multivariate analysis was performed using a general linear model. Parameters correlating with each other with r > 0.600 were excluded from the final model to avoid collinearity. The results of the multivariate analysis were presented with beta coefficients, confidence intervals (CI), and *p*-value. A *p*-value < 0.05 was considered statistically significant.

3. Results

3.1. Clinical, Laboratory Parameters, Blood Pressure, and Arterial Damage

Clinical and biochemical parameters in the PH and control groups are presented in Table 1, and data supporting the results can be found in Table S1. Patients with PH had significantly higher body weight, BMI, higher serum concentrations of uric acid and triglycerides, and lower concentration of HDL-cholesterol. In the PH group, 14 (23.3%) children were overweight, and 18 (30.0%) were obese. The duration of hypertension was 19.0 ± 25.4 (3–24) months. Twenty-five subjects were treated with antihypertensive medications and amlodipine was the most commonly used drug. The blood pressure and arterial parameters analysis revealed significantly higher office central and peripheral blood pressure and 24 h ambulatory blood pressure in the PH group (Table 2). Patients with PH were characterized by significantly higher cIMT, aPWV, larger diameter of common carotid artery, and slower time to maximal artery diameter.

Table 1. Clinical and biochemical data of the studied children.

Parameter	Children with Primary Hypertension	Healthy Children	p
Number of patients (n)	60	20	-
Age (years)	15.0 ± 2.9 (13.9–17.1)	14.4 ± 2.5 (12.6–16.8)	0.405
Gender (boys/girls)	37/23 (61.7%/38.3%)	9/11 (45%/55%)	0.205
Height (cm)	168.0 ± 16.2 (162–178)	164.9 ± 12.0 (158–174)	0.162
Height Z-score	0.50 ± 1.09 (−0.10–1.22)	0.54 ± 1.51 (−0.13–1.35)	0.689
Weight (kg)	71.4 ± 21.8 (60.5–82.7)	57.5 ± 15.4 (47.2–66.5)	0.010
Weight Z-score	1.20 ± 1.06 (0.39–1.95)	0.49 ± 1.14 (−0.27–1.53)	0.012
BMI (kg/m^2)	24.7 ± 5.2 (20.92–28.36)	20.8 ± 3.8 (18.1–23.3)	0.003
BMI Z-score	1.15 ± 1.11 (0.39–2.13)	0.32 ± 0.91 (−0.49–1.13)	0.002
Antihypertensive medications (n)	25 (41.7%)	-	-
Calcium channel antagonists	19		
Angiotensin convertase inhibitors	8		
Beta-adrenolytics	3		
Diuretics	2		
Alfa-adrenolytics	2		
eGFR ac. to Schwartz (mL/min/1.73 m^2)	101.9 ± 21.4 (88.8–113.1)	108.4 ± 20.8 (94.2–124.4)	0.192
Uric acid (mg/dL)	5.5 ± 1.4 (4.8–6.1)	4.5 ± 1.1 (3.8–5.5)	0.003
Total cholesterol (mg/dL)	159.9 ± 36.9 (136–171)	152.8 ± 29.5 (133–176)	0.509
HDL-cholesterol (mg/dL)	51.7 ± 14.4 (43–58)	57.7 ± 12.3 (49–64)	0.041
LDL-cholesterol (mg/dL)	88.6 ± 33.9 (66–98)	81.3 ± 25 (64–104)	0.505
Triglyceride (mg/dL)	98.4 ± 48.8 (63–121)	69.2 ± 26.3 (50–82)	0.010

BMI: body mass index; eGFR: estimated glomerular filtration rate; HDL: high-density lipoprotein; LDL: low-density lipoprotein.

Table 2. Blood pressure of the studied children.

Parameter	Children with Primary Hypertension	Healthy Children	p
Office oscillometric blood pressure			
SBP (mm Hg)	130.5 ± 11.6 (121–138)	119.0 ± 9.8 (109–126)	<0.001
SBP Z-score	1.43 ± 0.95 (0.93–2.12)	0.52 ± 0.79 (−0.17–1.13)	<0.001
DBP (mm Hg)	77.3 ± 10.8 (71–82)	67.7 ± 7.3 (65–74)	<0.001
DBP Z-score	1.65 ± 1.49 (0.88–2.28)	0.30 ± 0.91 (−0.14–1.06)	<0.001
Central blood pressure			
AoSBP (mm Hg)	109.6 ± 9.6 (102–117)	98.1 ± 8.1 (91–105)	<0.001
AoDBP (mm Hg)	79.2 ± 10.9 (72–84)	69.0 ± 7.2 (66–74)	<0.001
24 h ambulatory blood pressure			
SBP 24 h (mm Hg)	129.3 ± 9.6 (121–136)	114.8 ± 4.9 (112–117)	<0.001
DBP 24 h (mm Hg)	70.8 ± 7.7 (66–76)	64.4 ± 5.2 (62–68)	<0.001
MAP 24 h (mm Hg)	90.3 ± 7.7 (85–96)	81.1 ± 4.7 (78–85)	<0.001
SBPL 24 h (%)	44.0 ± 26.7 (27–63)	10.2 ± 6.8 (6–14)	<0.001
DBPL 24 h (%)	23.9 ± 21.0 (8–36)	7.3 ± 5.8 (2–11)	<0.001
SBP DIP (%)	10.3 ± 5.2 (8–13)	11.4 ± 3.4 (10–13)	0.383
DBP DIP (%)	15.3 ± 7.6 (11–20)	16.1 ± 3.7 (14–18)	0.642

Table 2. Cont.

Parameter	Children with Primary Hypertension	Healthy Children	p
Parameters of arterial damage			
cIMT (mm)	0.46 ± 0.07 (0.41–0.51)	0.41 ± 0.06 (0.31–0.42)	0.003
cIMT Z-score	1.47 ± 1.47 (0.45–2.41)	0.45 ± 1.08 (−0.29–0.68)	0.003
aPWV (m/s)	5.3 ± 1.0 (4.7–5.9)	4.6 ± 0.6 (4.2–5.0)	0.004
aPWV Z-score	−0.05 ± 1.17 (−0.95–0.71)	−0.88 ± 0.79 (−1.53–−0.33)	0.004
AIx75HR (%)	−2.1 ± 13.0 (−10.0–4.8)	−3.4 ± 13.0 (−9.2–3.3)	0.756
SEVR (%)	163.2 ± 41.2 (133–195)	155.6 ± 27.3 (137–169)	0.440
E-tracking beta	3.9 ± 3.3 (2.5–4.2)	3.7 ± 1.0 (3.1–4.5)	0.315
E-tracking Ep (kPa)	52.1 ± 42.3 (33–57)	44.9 ± 13.0 (34–55)	0.991
E-tracking AC (mm^2/kPa)	1.3 ± 0.5 (0.9–1.6)	1.0 ± 0.2 (0.8–1.1)	0.016
E-tracking AIx (%)	−5.5 ± 17.2 (−11.9–−0.7)	−2.7 ± 6.1 (−4.5–0.4)	0.168
E-tracking PWVbeta (m/s)	4.1 ± 1.3 (3.4–4.4)	3.9 ± 0.6 (3.5–4.5)	0.934
E-tracking D_max (mm)	6.4 ± 0.7 (6.0–6.8)	5.7 ± 0.7 (5.1–6.3)	<0.001
E-tracking D_min (mm)	5.5 ± 0.7 (4.9–5.9)	4.9 ± 0.7 (4.3–5.4)	0.003
E-tracking DAT_max (ms)	128.5 ± 39.9 (105–140)	146.0 ± 41.8 (125–152)	0.026

SBP: systolic blood pressure; DBP: diastolic blood pressure; AoSBP: aortic (central) systolic blood pressure; AoDBP: aortic (central) diastolic blood pressure; SBPL: systolic blood pressure load; DBPL: diastolic blood pressure load; DIP: dipping; cIMT: common carotid artery intima-media thickness; aPWV: aortic pulse wave velocity; AIx75HR: augmentation index normalized to heart rate of 75 beats per minute; SEVR: subendocardial viability ratio; beta: stiffness index; Ep: pressure strain elasticity modulus; AC: arterial compliance; AIx: augmentation index; D_max: maximal diameter of the right common carotid artery; D_min: minimal diameter of the right common carotid artery; DAT_max: acceleration time to the right common carotid artery maximal diameter.

3.2. Sclerostin and Parameters of Calcium-Phosphate Metabolism

The concentration of sclerostin and parameters of calcium-phosphate metabolism are shown in Table 3. The groups did not differ significantly in sclerostin concentration (Figure 1). All the patients studied had normal calcium, phosphate, parathyroid hormone, and alkaline phosphatase levels, but the serum calcium level was significantly higher in the PH group without any other differences between the groups. Severe deficiency and deficiency of vitamin D were found in more than half (56.3%) of the children studied. In children with PH, we showed no difference in serum sclerostin concentration between boys and girls (38.2 ± 10.0 vs. 34.1 ± 11.2 (pmol/L), p = 0.142) and between patients treated and untreated with antihypertensive agents (34.3 ± 10.6 vs. 38.3 ± 10.4 (pmol/L), p = 0.151).

Table 3. Sclerostin and parameters of calcium-phosphate metabolism in studied children.

Parameter	Primary Hypertension	Healthy Children	p
Sclerostin (pmol/L)	36.6 ± 10.6 (27.3–42.7)	41.0 ± 11.9 (31.9–50.3)	0.119
Calcium (mg/dL)	10.0 ± 0.3 (9.8–10.2)	9.8 ± 0.3 (9.6–9.9)	0.005
Phosphate (mg/dL)	4.4 ± 0.7 (3.9–4.9)	4.4 ± 0.5 (4.0–4.7)	0.922
25OHD (ng/mL)	20.5 ± 7.8 (15.8–23.4)	20.3 ± 7.8 (15.8–22.3)	0.859
Severe vitamin D deficiency	3 (5.0%)	0 (0.0%)	0.580
Vitamin D deficiency	30 (50.0%)	12 (60.0%)	
Suboptimal vitamin D level	20 (33.3%)	7 (35.0%)	
Optimal vitamin D level	7 (11.7%)	1 (5.0%)	
Parathyroid hormone (pg/mL)	27.5 ± 12.7 (17–35)	22.9 ± 11.4 (13–31)	0.153
Alkaline phosphate (IU/L)	125.2 ± 67.8 (74–153)	154.3 ± 80.6 (91–213)	0.153

25OHD—25-hydroxyvitamin D.

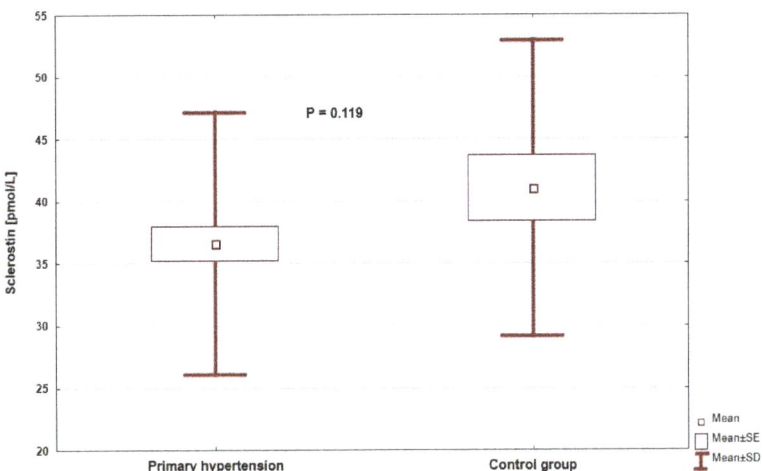

Figure 1. Serum sclerostin in children and adolescents with primary hypertension and in the control group (SE—standard error, SD—standard deviation).

3.3. Correlations of Sclerostin with Clinical and Biochemical Parameters, Blood Pressure, and Parameters of Arterial Damage

As there was no significant difference in serum sclerostin between PH and healthy children, both groups were analyzed together. Correlations of serum sclerostin concentration with analyzed clinical and biochemical parameters in 80 studied children are presented in Table 4. The serum sclerostin correlated positively with the height Z-score, serum phosphate, and alkaline phosphatase activity, and negatively with systolic and mean blood pressure. Negative correlations of serum sclerostin with peripheral and central systolic blood pressure are presented in Figure 2, Figure 3, respectively. There were no significant correlations of sclerostin and markers of arterial damage (aPWV (m/s): r = −0.065, p = 0.567, aPWV Z-score: r = −0.062, p = 0.584, AIx75HR (%): r = −0.053, p = 0.638, cIMT (mm): r = −0.084, p = 0.459, and cIMT Z-score: r = −0.092, p = 0.417).

Table 4. Significant correlations of sclerostin with clinical and biochemical parameters in the study group.

Analyzed Parameter	r	p
age (years)	−0.329	0.003
height Z-score	0.320	0.004
SBP (mm Hg)	−0.251	0.025
SBP Z-score	−0.240	0.032
MAP (mm Hg)	−0.226	0.044
AoSBP (mm Hg)	−0.296	0.008
AoMAP (mm Hg)	−0.253	0.024
phosphate (mg/dL)	0.323	0.003
alkaline phosphatase (IU/L)	0.462	<0.001

SBP: systolic blood pressure; MAP: mean arterial pressure; AoSBP: aortic (central) systolic blood pressure; AoMAP: aortic (central) mean blood pressure.

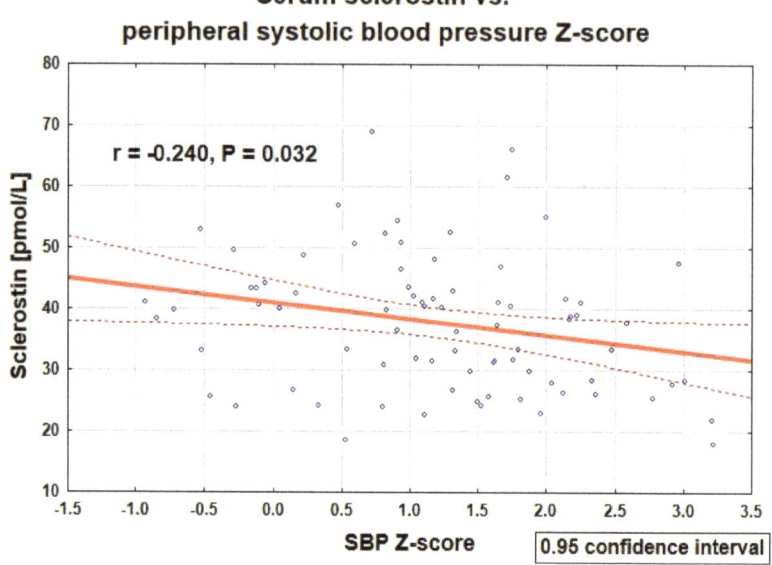

Figure 2. Correlation of serum sclerostin with peripheral systolic blood pressure Z-score in the studied children (SBP—peripheral systolic blood pressure).

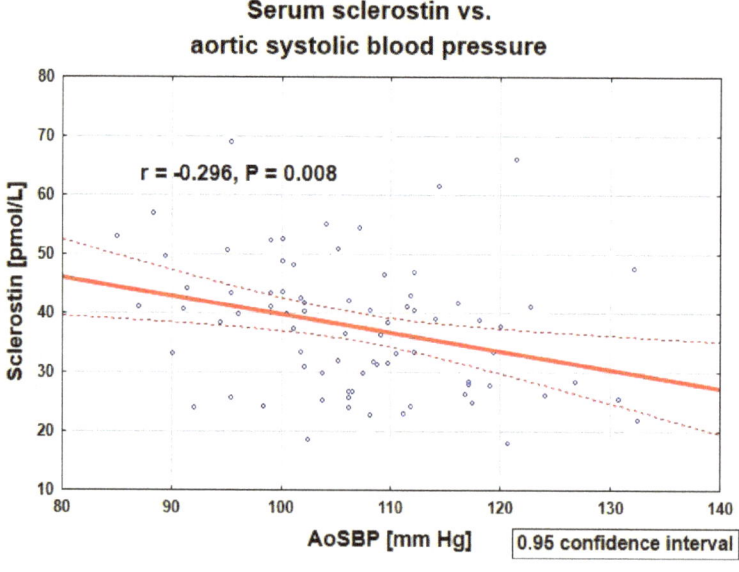

Figure 3. Correlation of serum sclerostin with central (aortic) systolic blood pressure in the studied children (AoSBP—aortic systolic blood pressure).

The results of multivariate analysis (general linear model) are shown in Table 5. Systolic blood pressure and height expressed as Z-scores were the significant independent determinants of serum sclerostin in the studied children.

Table 5. Multivariate analysis of sclerostin determinants in the studied children.

Parameter	Beta	95% Confidence Interval	p
Height Z-score	0.224	(0.017–0.430)	0.034
SBP Z-score	−0.216	(−0.417–−0.016)	0.035
Phosphate (mg/dL)	0.219	(−0.002–0.441)	0.053
Age (years)	−0.170	(−0.396–0.055)	0.137

SBP: systolic blood pressure.

In a subanalysis of 35 untreated patients with primary hypertension, we found trends towards a negative correlation between serum sclerostin and peripheral systolic blood pressure (SBP) (mm Hg) (r = −0.323, p = 0.058), SBP Z-score (r = −0.299, p = 0.081), central systolic blood pressure (AoSBP) (mm Hg)) (r = −0.311, p = 0.069), central pulse pressure (AoPP (mm Hg)) (r = −0.292, p = 0.088), E-tracking pressure strain elasticity modulus (ET Ep) (r = −0.313, p = 0.067), and alkaline phosphatase (IU/L) (r = 318, p = 0.063).

4. Discussion

In our cross-sectional single-center study, we analyzed serum sclerostin in the group of pediatric patients with primary hypertension. Serum sclerostin did not differ significantly between hypertensive and normotensive children. Additionally, antihypertensive pharmacological treatment did not influence sclerostin concentration significantly. In the whole group of studied children, sclerostin correlated negatively with peripheral and central systolic and mean blood pressure; we also found significant positive association of sclerostin and calcium and phosphate metabolism parameters. In the multivariate analysis, systolic blood pressure and height, expressed as Z-scores, were the only significant determinants of serum sclerostin concentration. There was no significant correlation between parameters of arterial damage and serum sclerostin concentration.

Research studies from recent years suggested that Wnt/beta-catenin signaling system may be a crucial player in initiating and subsequently intensifying negative changes in the arteries. Its activation leads to the proliferation and apoptosis of vascular smooth muscle cells [29] and their transformation into osteoblast-like cells [30]. In addition, Wnt/beta-catenin pathway was shown to play a vital role in developing inflammation within the arterial wall by exacerbating the adhesion of monocytes to endothelium and promoting their passage through the vascular wall [31]. Therefore, it may be justified to hypothesize that inhibition of this signaling pathway by its inhibitors (sclerostin and DKK-1) in the arteries is a compensatory and protective mechanism [11,32].

Numerous studies in adults at high cardiovascular risk seem to support this hypothesis. Thambiah et al. demonstrated a negative relationship between DKK-1 and arterial stiffness (analyzed using the photoplethysmography method). However, the authors did not find such a correlation for sclerostin [16]. Gaudio et al. showed a negative correlation between cIMT and sclerostin concentrations in postmenopausal women with type 2 diabetes mellitus [14]. The same authors revealed a negative relationship between augmentation index and sclerostin concentration in 67 healthy adults [15]. However, one should not forget that some authors have shown a positive relationship between the concentration of circulating sclerostin and cIMT and arterial stiffness in adults [12,20,33]. The latter may indicate the complexity of the interaction between the Wnt/beta-catenin system and arterial wall.

In our cohort of pediatric patients with primary hypertension, we found no significant correlations between serum sclerostin and well-established indices of arterial wall damage (cIMT, aPWV, AIx75HR). Of note, to increase the precision of our analysis, we analyzed both aortic and local carotid damage. This negative finding can be partially explained by the relatively low severity of arterial lesions in children compared with adult patients. Large multicenter analyses revealed that subclinical arterial damage observed in children and adolescents are mainly adaptations of arterial wall to increased pressure (arteriosclerosis) and do not necessarily indicate the onset of atherosclerosis and calcification of the vascular wall [26,27,34]. On the other hand, in one of our previous studies, we have revealed a significant negative correlation between cIMT and serum fetuin level in pediatric PH patients [4]. Perhaps, other determinants of calcium-phosphate metabolism (e.g., calcification inhibitors), not Wnt/beta-catenin pathway, are involved in the earliest stages of hypertension-associated arterial damage.

Conversely, our results may indicate a protective effect of Wnt/beta-catenin inhibitors on the level of blood pressure in children. We showed numerous negative correlations between sclerostin and both central and peripheral blood pressure. We confirmed these univariate relationships in multivariate analysis. Additionally, a subanalysis of a small cohort of untreated PH subjects revealed a similar trend.

Of note, the relatively low duration of hypertension in our patients excluded advanced arterial lesions. In fact, notwithstanding significantly higher values of indexes of arterial stiffness (e.g., aPWV, AIx75HR, elastic modulus) in hypertensive than in normotensive patients, this difference might reflect the effect of higher blood pressure values. The absence of a significant relationship between serum sclerostin levels and indexes of arterial stiffness in the whole study population, as opposed to a significant negative correlation between sclerostin levels and systolic blood pressure Z-score at multivariate analysis, supports this interpretation. Thus, the results of this study should certainly be considered preliminary.

Contrary to our results, a positive correlation between serum sclerostin and systolic blood pressure ($r = 0.262$, $p = 0.031$) was demonstrated in kidney transplant adult patients [33]. In contrast, no significant association was seen in adults on hemodialysis [35] or with rheumatoid arthritis [18]. Whether sclerostin could be a good marker of cardiovascular morbidity and mortality remains an open question [36].

The protective role of sclerostin on circulatory system was suggested in a recent meta-analysis focused on cardiovascular events in patients treated with romosozumab. The findings of the meta-analysis indicate that the inhibition of sclerostin might elevate cardiovascular risk. Furthermore, the same author revealed that some variants of *SOST* gene were associated with significantly higher systolic blood pressure [37]. Interestingly, similarly to our results, systolic blood pressure, not diastolic blood pressure, seems to be associated with sclerostin action. Additionally, a pharmacovigilance analysis of the Food and Drug Administration Adverse Event Reporting System (FAERS) identified a potential signal for elevated risk of myocardial infarction, stroke, or cardiovascular death in patients treated with romosozumab [38]. Further research is needed to answer the nature of the interaction between the Wnt/beta-catenin system and the circulatory system. Nevertheless, these results warrant a rigorous evaluation of the cardiovascular safety of sclerostin inhibitors.

Some experimental and clinical data suggest the interaction of sclerostin and renin-angiotensin-system (RAS) in the formation of arterial damage. Sclerostin was found to inhibit angiotensin II-induced aortic aneurysm and atherosclerotic plaque formation in mice [39]. In addition, Mayer Jr et al. found a synergistic effect of sclerostin and angiotensin II receptor 1 polymorphism on arterial stiffening in the general adult population [40]. In our cohort, we have not analyzed concentrations of RAS components. Moreover, almost half of the subjects had already been treated with antihypertensive medications, which could have influenced possible RAS and sclerostin interaction.

In the analyzed group of patients, we did not find differences between sclerostin concentrations in boys and girls. Other authors found higher serum sclerostin in males in both children [19] and adults [6,16]. Higher concentrations of sclerostin in the male sex may be explained by higher bone mass. In the adult population, there was a positive relationship between sclerostin concentrations and age [6,16]. Increasing sclerostin levels with age may be due to an imbalance between bone formation and bone resorption processes [16]. Kirmani et al. analyzed in detail the relationship between sclerostin, age, bone age, densitometric parameters, and serological markers of bone turnover in children. The authors showed that sclerostin levels increase in boys up to 10 years of age, in girls up to 14 years of age, and then steadily decrease to start rising again around 20 years of age [19].

Since the vast majority of the children studied were in the second decade of life, our results (negative relationship between sclerostin and age) can be considered consistent with the results of Kirmani et al.

The same researchers found a positive relationship between sclerostin concentrations and markers of bone turnover: a marker of bone formation—N-terminal collagen propeptide type I (PINP) and a marker of bone resorption—C-terminal collagen telopeptide type I (CTX); however, there was no correlation between sclerostin and parathyroid and 25OHD levels [19]. Our group of children showed a positive relationship between height Z-score, serum phosphate, alkaline phosphatase activity and serum sclerostin concentration, which is most likely a reflection of larger bone mass and higher bone turnover in taller children.

Some limitations to our research need to be listed. This was a cross-sectional analysis; thus, final conclusions on the nature of the relationship between blood pressure and sclerostin cannot be drawn. Secondly, we did not analyze bone mass, which was found to have a substantial impact on serum sclerostin concentration. Our research did not examine the concentration of Dickkopf-1—another important inhibitor of Wnt/beta-catenin pathway. Additionally, despite the large study sample, analysis in subgroups (healthy children, treated/untreated patients) may have been subject to error due to small numbers. As many as 25 out of 60 analyzed hypertensive subjects had already been treated with antihypertensive medications, which could have influenced the final results. Antihypertensives might have masked some of the relationships, for example, between sclerostin and target-organ damage. Moreover, the short duration of arterial hypertension in our patients excluded advanced arterial lesions and masked a possible relationship with sclerostin observed in adult studies. Of note, despite many years of our clinical and research experience with the blood pressure monitors used, it should be emphasized that both these devices had been validated only in the adult population so far. The latter may have influenced the results, although it is essential that we tested both control and study groups with the same instruments using the same protocol.

5. Conclusions

Sclerostin, an endogenous inhibitor of Wnt/beta-catenin pathway, was found to be associated with cardiovascular damage in adults. In our research, serum sclerostin was not correlated to non-invasive indices of arterial damage but was inversely associated with systolic blood pressure. These results may suggest a significant association between sclerostin and blood pressure in the pediatric population and are consistent with studies on the cardiovascular safety of sclerostin inhibitors. There is a need for further studies at both experimental and clinical levels on the relationship between cardiovascular and Wnt/beta-catenin systems.

Supplementary Materials: The following are available online at https://www.mdpi.com/article/10.3390/jcm10163574/s1, Table S1: Patient data (patient_data.xlsx).

Author Contributions: Conceptualization, P.S. and M.P.-T.; methodology, P.S., A.S.-E., and E.G.; validation, P.S. and M.P.-T.; formal analysis, P.S.; investigation, P.S., A.O., M.S., A.S.-E., and E.G.; resources, M.P.-T.; data curation, P.S. and A.O.; writing—original draft preparation, P.S., A.O., and M.S.; writing—review and editing, M.P.-T.; visualization, P.S.; supervision, M.P.-T.; project administration, P.S. and M.P.-T.; funding acquisition, M.P.-T. All authors have read and agreed to the published version of the manuscript.

Funding: This research was funded from the statutory funds of the Department of Pediatrics and Nephrology, Medical University of Warsaw.

Institutional Review Board Statement: The study was conducted according to the guidelines of the Declaration of Helsinki, and approved by the Local Bioethics Committee of the Medical University of Warsaw (approval no. KB/58/2016, 15 March 2016).

Informed Consent Statement: Informed consent was obtained from all subjects ($\geq$16 years) and their representatives involved in the study.

Data Availability Statement: Data used to support the findings of this study are included within the supplementary information files, Supplementary Table S1 (patient_data.xlsx).

Conflicts of Interest: The authors declare no conflict of interest.

References

1. Lurbe, E.; Agabiti-Rosei, E.; Cruickshank, J.K.; Dominiczak, A.; Erdine, S.; Hirth, A.; Invitti, C.; Litwin, M.; Mancia, G.; Pall, D.; et al. 2016 European Society of Hypertension guidelines for the management of high blood pressure in children and adolescents. *J. Hypertens* **2016**, *34*, 1887–1920. [CrossRef]
2. Gupta-Malhotra, M.; Banker, A.; Shete, S.; Hashmi, S.S.; Tyson, J.E.; Barratt, M.S.; Hecht, J.T.; Milewicz, D.M.; Boerwinkle, E. Essential hypertension vs. secondary hypertension among children. *Am. J. Hypertens* **2015**, *28*, 73–80. [CrossRef]
3. Litwin, M.; Feber, J.; Niemirska, A.; Michałkiewicz, J. Primary hypertension is a disease of premature vascular aging associated with neuro-immuno-metabolic abnormalities. *Pediatr. Nephrol.* **2016**, *31*, 185–194. [CrossRef]
4. Skrzypczyk, P.; Stelmaszczyk-Emmel, A.; Szyszka, M.; Ofiara, A.; Pańczyk-Tomaszewska, M. Circulating calcification inhibitors are associated with arterial damage in pediatric patients with primary hypertension. *Pediatr. Nephrol.* **2021**. [CrossRef]
5. Manson, J.E.; Cook, N.R.; Lee, I.M.; Christen, W.; Bassuk, S.S.; Mora, S.; Gibson, H.; Gordon, D.; Copeland, T.; D'Agostino, D.; et al. Vitamin D Supplements and Prevention of Cancer and Cardiovascular Disease. *N. Engl. J. Med.* **2019**, *380*, 33–44. [CrossRef]
6. Winkler, D.G.; Sutherland, M.K.; Geoghegan, J.C.; Yu, C.; Hayes, T.; Skonier, J.E.; Shpektor, D.; Jonas, M.; Kovacevich, B.R.; Staehling-Hampton, K.; et al. Osteocyte control of bone formation via sclerostin, a novel BMP antagonist. *EMBO J.* **2003**, *22*, 6267–6276. [CrossRef]
7. Rao, T.P.; Kühl, M. An updated overview on Wnt signaling pathways: A prelude for more. *Circ. Res.* **2010**, *106*, 1798–1806. [CrossRef]
8. Delgado-Calle, J.; Sato, A.Y.; Bellido, T. Role and mechanism of action of sclerostin in bone. *Bone* **2017**, *96*, 29–37. [CrossRef]
9. Tanaka, S.; Matsumoto, T. Sclerostin: From bench to bedside. *J. Bone Min. Metab.* **2021**, *39*, 332–340. [CrossRef] [PubMed]
10. Liao, R.; Wang, L.; Li, J.; Sun, S.; Xiong, Y.; Li, Y.; Han, M.; Jiang, H.; Anil, M.; Su, B. Vascular calcification is associated with Wnt-signaling pathway and blood pressure variability in chronic kidney disease rats. *Nephrology (Carlton)* **2020**, *25*, 264–272. [CrossRef]
11. Didangelos, A.; Yin, X.; Mandal, K.; Baumert, M.; Jahangiri, M.; Mayr, M. Proteomics characterization of extracellular space components in the human aorta. *Mol. Cell Proteom.* **2010**, *9*, 2048–2062. [CrossRef]
12. Morales-Santana, S.; García-Fontana, B.; García-Martín, A.; Rozas-Moreno, P.; García-Salcedo, J.A.; Reyes-García, R.; Muñoz-Torres, M. Atherosclerotic disease in type 2 diabetes is associated with an increase in sclerostin levels. *Diabetes Care* **2013**, *36*, 1667–1674. [CrossRef] [PubMed]
13. Hampson, G.; Edwards, S.; Conroy, S.; Blake, G.M.; Fogelman, I.; Frost, M.L. The relationship between inhibitors of the Wnt signalling pathway (Dickkopf-1(DKK1) and sclerostin), bone mineral density, vascular calcification and arterial stiffness in post-menopausal women. *Bone* **2013**, *56*, 42–47. [CrossRef] [PubMed]
14. Gaudio, A.; Privitera, F.; Pulvirenti, I.; Canzonieri, E.; Rapisarda, R.; Fiore, C.E. The relationship between inhibitors of the Wnt signalling pathway (sclerostin and Dickkopf-1) and carotid intima-media thickness in postmenopausal women with type 2 diabetes mellitus. *Diabetes Vasc. Dis. Res.* **2014**, *11*, 48–52. [CrossRef] [PubMed]
15. Gaudio, A.; Fiore, V.; Rapisarda, R.; Sidoti, M.H.; Xourafa, A.; Catalano, A.; Tringali, G.; Zanoli, L.; Signorelli, S.S.; Fiore, C.E. Sclerostin is a possible candidate marker of arterial stiffness: Results from a cohort study in Catania. *Mol. Med. Rep.* **2017**, *15*, 3420–3424. [CrossRef] [PubMed]
16. Thambiah, S.; Roplekar, R.; Manghat, P.; Fogelman, I.; Fraser, W.D.; Goldsmith, D.; Hampson, G. Circulating sclerostin and Dickkopf-1 (DKK1) in predialysis chronic kidney disease (CKD): Relationship with bone density and arterial stiffness. *Calcif. Tissue Int.* **2012**, *90*, 473–480. [CrossRef]
17. Gravani, F.; Papadaki, I.; Antypa, E.; Nezos, A.; Masselou, K.; Ioakeimidis, D.; Koutsilieris, M.; Moutsopoulos, H.M.; Mavragani, C.P. Subclinical atherosclerosis and impaired bone health in patients with primary Sjogren's syndrome: Prevalence, clinical and laboratory associations. *Arthritis Res. Ther.* **2015**, *17*, 99. [CrossRef]
18. Paccou, J.; Mentaverri, R.; Renard, C.; Liabeuf, S.; Fardellone, P.; Massy, Z.A.; Brazier, M.; Kamel, S. The relationships between serum sclerostin, bone mineral density, and vascular calcification in rheumatoid arthritis. *J. Clin. Endocrinol. Metab.* **2014**, *99*, 4740–4748. [CrossRef]
19. Kirmani, S.; Amin, S.; McCready, L.K.; Atkinson, E.J.; Melton, L.J., 3rd; Müller, R.; Khosla, S. Sclerostin levels during growth in children. *Osteoporos Int.* **2012**, *23*, 1123–1130. [CrossRef]
20. Chang, Y.C.; Hsu, B.G.; Liou, H.H.; Lee, C.J.; Wang, J.H. Serum levels of sclerostin as a potential biomarker in central arterial stiffness among hypertensive patients. *BMC Cardiovasc. Disord.* **2018**, *18*, 214. [CrossRef]
21. Kułaga, Z.; Litwin, M.; Tkaczyk, M.; Palczewska, I.; Zajączkowska, M.; Zwolińska, D.; Krynicki, T.; Wasilewska, A.; Moczulska, A.; Morawiec-Knysak, A.; et al. Polish 2010 growth references for school-aged children and adolescents. *Eur. J. Pediatr.* **2011**, *170*, 599–609. [CrossRef]
22. Schwartz, G.J.; Muñoz, A.; Schneider, M.F.; Mak, R.H.; Kaskel, F.; Warady, B.A.; Furth, S.L. New equations to estimate GFR in children with CKD. *J. Am. Soc. Nephrol.* **2009**, *20*, 629–637. [CrossRef]

23. Rusińska, A.; Płudowski, P.; Walczak, M.; Borszewska-Kornacka, M.K.; Bossowski, A.; Chlebna-Sokół, D.; Czech-Kowalska, J.; Dobrzańska, A.; Franek, E.; Helwich, E.; et al. Vitamin D Supplementation Guidelines for General Population and Groups at Risk of Vitamin D Deficiency in Poland-Recommendations of the Polish Society of Pediatric Endocrinology and Diabetes and the Expert Panel With Participation of National Specialist Consultants and Representatives of Scientific Societies-2018 Update. *Front. Endocrinol. (Lausanne)* **2018**, *9*, 246. [CrossRef]
24. Kułaga, Z.; Litwin, M.; Grajda, A.; Kułaga, K.; Gurzkowska, B.; Góźdź, M.; Pan, H. Oscillometric blood pressure percentiles for Polish normal-weight school-aged children and adolescents. *J. Hypertens* **2012**, *30*, 1942–1954. [CrossRef]
25. Flynn, J.T.; Daniels, S.R.; Hayman, L.L.; Maahs, D.M.; McCrindle, B.W.; Mitsnefes, M.; Zachariah, J.P.; Urbina, E.M. Update: Ambulatory blood pressure monitoring in children and adolescents: A scientific statement from the American Heart Association. *Hypertension* **2014**, *63*, 1116–1135. [CrossRef]
26. Doyon, A.; Kracht, D.; Bayazit, A.K.; Deveci, M.; Duzova, A.; Krmar, R.T.; Litwin, M.; Niemirska, A.; Oguz, B.; Schmidt, B.M.; et al. Carotid artery intima-media thickness and distensibility in children and adolescents: Reference values and role of body dimensions. *Hypertension* **2013**, *62*, 550–556. [CrossRef]
27. Reusz, G.S.; Cseprekal, O.; Temmar, M.; Kis, E.; Cherif, A.B.; Thaleb, A.; Fekete, A.; Szabó, A.J.; Benetos, A.; Salvi, P. Reference values of pulse wave velocity in healthy children and teenagers. *Hypertension* **2010**, *56*, 217–224. [CrossRef]
28. Skrzypczyk, P.; Przychodzień, J.; Mizerska-Wasiak, M.; Kuźma-Mroczkowska, E.; Okarska-Napierała, M.; Górska, E.; Stelmaszczyk-Emmel, A.; Demkow, U.; Pańczyk-Tomaszewska, M. Renalase in Children with Glomerular Kidney Diseases. *Adv. Exp. Med. Biol.* **2017**, *1021*, 81–92. [CrossRef]
29. Couffinhal, T.; Dufourcq, P.; Duplàa, C. Beta-catenin nuclear activation: Common pathway between Wnt and growth factor signaling in vascular smooth muscle cell proliferation? *Circ. Res.* **2006**, *99*, 1287–1289. [CrossRef]
30. Quasnichka, H.; Slater, S.C.; Beeching, C.A.; Boehm, M.; Sala-Newby, G.B.; George, S.J. Regulation of smooth muscle cell proliferation by beta-catenin/T-cell factor signaling involves modulation of cyclin D1 and p21 expression. *Circ. Res.* **2006**, *99*, 1329–1337. [CrossRef]
31. Arderiu, G.; Espinosa, S.; Peña, E.; Aledo, R.; Badimon, L. Monocyte-secreted Wnt5a interacts with FZD5 in microvascular endothelial cells and induces angiogenesis through tissue factor signaling. *J. Mol. Cell Biol.* **2014**, *6*, 380–393. [CrossRef]
32. Ueland, T.; Otterdal, K.; Lekva, T.; Halvorsen, B.; Gabrielsen, A.; Sandberg, W.J.; Paulsson-Berne, G.; Pedersen, T.M.; Folkersen, L.; Gullestad, L.; et al. Dickkopf-1 enhances inflammatory interaction between platelets and endothelial cells and shows increased expression in atherosclerosis. *Arter. Thromb. Vasc. Biol.* **2009**, *29*, 1228–1234. [CrossRef] [PubMed]
33. Hsu, B.G.; Liou, H.H.; Lee, C.J.; Chen, Y.C.; Ho, G.J.; Lee, M.C. Serum Sclerostin as an Independent Marker of Peripheral Arterial Stiffness in Renal Transplantation Recipients: A Cross-Sectional Study. *Medicine (Baltim.)* **2016**, *95*, e3300. [CrossRef] [PubMed]
34. Litwin, M.; Niemirska, A. Intima-media thickness measurements in children with cardiovascular risk factors. *Pediatr. Nephrol.* **2009**, *24*, 707–719. [CrossRef] [PubMed]
35. Stavrinou, E.; Sarafidis, P.A.; Koumaras, C.; Loutradis, C.; Giamalis, P.; Tziomalos, K.; Karagiannis, A.; Papagianni, A. Increased Sclerostin, but Not Dickkopf-1 Protein, Is Associated with Elevated Pulse Wave Velocity in Hemodialysis Subjects. *Kidney Blood Press Res.* **2019**, *44*, 679–689. [CrossRef] [PubMed]
36. Kanbay, M.; Solak, Y.; Siriopol, D.; Aslan, G.; Afsar, B.; Yazici, D.; Covic, A. Sclerostin, cardiovascular disease and mortality: A systematic review and meta-analysis. *Int. Urol. Nephrol.* **2016**, *48*, 2029–2042. [CrossRef] [PubMed]
37. Bovijn, J.; Krebs, K.; Chen, C.Y.; Boxall, R.; Censin, J.C.; Ferreira, T.; Pulit, S.L.; Glastonbury, C.A.; Laber, S.; Millwood, I.Y.; et al. Evaluating the cardiovascular safety of sclerostin inhibition using evidence from meta-analysis of clinical trials and human genetics. *Sci. Transl. Med.* **2020**, *12*. [CrossRef]
38. Vestergaard Kvist, A.; Faruque, J.; Vallejo-Yagüe, E.; Weiler, S.; Winter, E.M.; Burden, A.M. Cardiovascular Safety Profile of Romosozumab: A Pharmacovigilance Analysis of the US Food and Drug Administration Adverse Event Reporting System (FAERS). *J. Clin. Med.* **2021**, *10*, 1660. [CrossRef]
39. Krishna, S.M.; Seto, S.W.; Jose, R.J.; Li, J.; Morton, S.K.; Biros, E.; Wang, Y.; Nsengiyumva, V.; Lindeman, J.H.; Loots, G.G.; et al. Wnt Signaling Pathway Inhibitor Sclerostin Inhibits Angiotensin II-Induced Aortic Aneurysm and Atherosclerosis. *Arter. Thromb. Vasc. Biol.* **2017**, *37*, 553–566. [CrossRef]
40. Mayer, O., Jr.; Seidlerová, J.; Kučera, R.; Kučerová, A.; Černá, V.; Gelžinský, J.; Mateřánková, M.; Mareš, Š.; Kordíková, V.; Pešta, M.; et al. Synergistic effect of sclerostin and angiotensin II receptor 1 polymorphism on arterial stiffening. *Biomark Med.* **2020**, *14*, 173–184. [CrossRef]

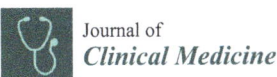

Article

Hyperuricemia Is an Early and Relatively Common Feature in Children with *HNF1B* Nephropathy but Its Utility as a Predictor of the Disease Is Limited

Marcin Kołbuc [1,*], Beata Bieniaś [2], Sandra Habbig [3], Mateusz F. Kołek [4], Maria Szczepańska [5], Katarzyna Kiliś-Pstrusińska [6], Anna Wasilewska [7], Piotr Adamczyk [8], Rafał Motyka [1], Marcin Tkaczyk [9], Przemysław Sikora [2], Bodo B. Beck [10] and Marcin Zaniew [1,*]

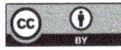

1. Department of Pediatrics, University of Zielona Góra, 65-417 Zielona Góra, Poland; rmotyka97@gmail.com
2. Department of Pediatric Nephrology, Medical University of Lublin, 20-059 Lublin, Poland; beatabienias@umlub.pl (B.B.); przemyslawsikora@umlub.pl (P.S.)
3. Department of Pediatrics, University Hospital of Cologne, 50937 Cologne, Germany; sandra.habbig@uk-koeln.de
4. Department of Animal Physiology, Faculty of Biology, University of Warsaw, 00-927 Warsaw, Poland; m.kolek@biol.uw.edu.pl
5. Department of Pediatrics, Faculty of Medical Sciences in Zabrze, Medical University of Silesia in Katowice, 41-808 Zabrze, Poland; szczep57@poczta.onet.pl
6. Department of Paediatric Nephrology, Wrocław Medical University, 50-367 Wrocław, Poland; kilis@wp.pl
7. Department of Pediatric Nephrology, University Hospital, 15-089 Białystok, Poland; annwasil@interia.pl
8. Department of Pediatrics, Faculty of Medical Sciences in Katowice, Medical University of Silesia in Katowice, 40-752 Katowice, Poland; padamczyk@gczd.katowice.pl
9. Department of Pediatrics, Immunology and Nephrology, Polish Mother's Memorial Hospital Research Institute, 93-338 Łódź, Poland; marcin.tkaczyk45@gmail.com
10. Institute of Human Genetics and Center for Molecular Medicine Cologne, University of Cologne, Faculty of Medicine and University Hospital Cologne, 50937 Cologne, Germany; bodo.beck@uk-koeln.de
* Correspondence: m.kolbuc@cm.uz.zgora.pl (M.K.); m.zaniew@cm.uz.zgora.pl (M.Z.)

Abstract: Background: Hyperuricemia is recognized as an important feature of nephropathy, associated with a mutation in the hepatocyte nuclear factor-1B (*HNF1B*) gene, and could serve as a useful marker of the disease. However, neither a causal relationship nor its predictive value have been proven. The purpose of this study was to assess this in children with renal malformations, both with (mut+) and without *HNF1B* mutations (mut-). Methods: We performed a retrospective analysis of clinical characteristics of pediatric patients tested for *HNF1B* mutations, collected in a national registry. Results: 108 children were included in the study, comprising 43 mut+ patients and 65 mut- subjects. Mean sUA was higher and hyperuricemia more prevalent (42.5% vs. 15.4%) in *HNF1B* carriers. The two groups were similar with respect to respect to age, sex, anthropometric parameters, hypertension, and renal function. Renal function, fractional excretion of uric acid and parathyroid hormone level were independent predictors of sUA. The potential of hyperuricemia to predict mutation was low, and addition of hyperuricemia to a multivariate logistic regression model did not increase its accuracy. Conclusions: Hyperuricemia is an early and common feature of *HNF1B* nephropathy. A strong association of sUA with renal function and parathyroid hormone limits its utility as a reliable marker to predict *HNF1B* mutation among patients with kidney anomalies.

Keywords: *HNF1B*; hyperuricemia; PTH; renal function; uric acid; FEUA

1. Introduction

Hepatocyte nuclear factor 1β (*HNF1B*) is a critical transcription factor (encoded by the *HNF1B* gene) that regulates the development of the kidneys, pancreas, liver, and genital tract [1–3]. Its multi-organ expression results in a wide spectrum of renal and extra-renal manifestations in patients with *HNF1B*-associated disease, which includes renal cysts, multicystic dysplastic kidney, solitary kidney, agenesis of pancreas body and tail, maturity-onset diabetes in the young type 5, genital malformations, elevated liver enzymes, electrolyte abnormalities, primary hyperparathyroidism, gout, and epilepsy [4,5]. Hyperuricemia is a key hallmark of the disease that has been repeatedly reported in patients with *HNF1B* mutation [6–15]. Although this association is described in many studies, when compared to patients without *HNF1B* mutation, the frequency of hyperuricemia in patients with *HNF1B* mutation was not significantly different [10,11]. Thus, a causal relationship between *HNF1B* mutation and elevated serum uric acid (sUA) has not been proven to date.

Abnormalities in uric acid handling were first reported in 2003 in a kindred diagnosed with familial juvenile hyperuricemic nephropathy with an underlying mutation in the *HNF1B* gene [15]. Subsequently, analysis of sUA levels in patients with *HNF1B* mutations and healthy type 2 diabetic subjects without *HNF1B* mutation demonstrated significantly higher levels in *HNF1B* mutation carriers. However, the study found no significant difference between carriers and gender-matched controls with renal impairments of other causes. Despite this, the authors concluded that gout and hyperuricemia are general features of *HNF1B* mutations. Since this publication, the finding of elevated sUA levels in *HNF1B* mutation carriers has not been adequately analyzed in other cohorts [4]. It remains unclear whether raised sUA is a feature of *HNF1B*-related disease and is directly related to mutation, or if this symptom is a byproduct of chronic kidney disease (CKD), which could be present during the course of the disease.

A search of the literature revealed that the frequency of hyperuricemia varies significantly, depending mostly on the severity of CKD and age of the cohorts [6–14]. Importantly, in studies for which a combined cohort (i.e., children and adults) has been studied, the authors used higher upper limits for sUA, usually those applicable for adult patients. This could ultimately result in a low prevalence of hyperuricemia in children [10,14]. Others utilized reference data published in 1990, which are not reliable as these were generated from a small sample, and could be regarded as outdated [16]. Thus, we hypothesized that hyperuricemia might be misdiagnosed and under-recognized, especially in children, and this could limit investigations aimed at assessing its usefulness as a predictor of *HNF1B* disease. In fact, its diagnostic value has never been formally assessed.

We aimed to assess a causal relationship between elevated sUA level and *HNF1B* defects by comparing patients with and without mutations, and to investigate the predictive value of hyperuricemia for distinguishing *HNF1B* mutation carriers among patients with a range of renal anomalies.

2. Materials and Methods
2.1. Study Population

This is a multi-center, retrospective study of patients tested for *HNF1B* mutations, whose data were collected in the Polish Registry of Inherited Tubulopathies (POLtube) between July 2012 and July 2020. A suspicion of *HNF1B* nephropathy, based on a renal phenotype with additional extra-renal features, led to the initiation of *HNF1B* mutational analysis. The referral remained at clinicians' discretion.

In total, 117 subjects suspected to have *HNF1B* nephropathy were recruited to the registry. Adults ($n = 8$) were excluded from the study to eliminate the effects of potential co-morbidities on the analyzed parameters, and to permit uniform analysis of hyperuricemia by applying the most recent pediatric norms [17]. One pediatric patient was excluded due to end-stage renal disease. Finally, the study group comprised 108 patients, of whom 43 patients were positive for *HNF1B* mutations (mut+), i.e., were carriers of a heterozygous point mutation or whole *HNF1B* gene deletion. The remaining patients ($n = 65$) were negative for *HNF1B* (mut-) and served as controls. The clinical and genetic characteristics of 14 of the mut+ patients have been reported previously [12,18,19].

2.2. Clinical Assessment and Definitions of Analyzed Parameters

Each subject's anthropometrical and biochemical parameters and urinary indices, as well as details regarding family history of diabetes and/or renal anomalies, or renal and extra-renal phenotype and genotypes, were retrieved from the registry database and anonymized. Data were analyzed cross-sectionally at the time of molecular diagnosis for all patients, and at the time of the last visit in the mut+ group. In mut- patients, data were available only from the time of genetic testing. Renal phenotypes were characterized sonographically, similarly to Faguer et al. [20]. Extra-renal features had not been studied systematically in the cohort, but had been reported to the registry by the referring physician. Plasma and urine biochemistries were established using routine laboratory procedures, according to local policies. Both spot urine samples and 24 h urine collection were used to calculate urinary indices (fractional excretion of K^+, Ca^{2+}, Mg^{2+}, and uric acid).

Serum Mg^{2+} (sMg) and sUA reference values for age and gender intervals proposed by Ridefelt et al. were applied with respect to hypomagnesemia and hyperuricemia definition [17]. Patients receiving supplementary oral Mg^{2+} ($n = 12$) and allopurinol ($n = 8$) were also considered as having low sMg or high sUA, respectively. Raw sMg/sUA values of these patients were not included in the analysis. Other parameters were defined as follows: hypokalemia as K^+ level < 3.5 mmol/L, and hyperparathyroidism if the parathyroid hormone (PTH) level exceeded the local laboratory upper reference limit. Estimated glomerular filtration rate (eGFR) was calculated using the original or modified Schwartz equation when applicable [21,22]. Staging of CKD was based on eGFR and adopted from KDIGO (Kidney Disease: Improving Global Outcomes) guidelines [23], and was as follows: CKD stage I (eGFR > 90 mL/min/1.73 m^2), stage II (eGFR between 60 and 89 mL/1.73 m^2/min), stage III (eGFR between 30 and 59 mL/min/1.73 m^2), CKD IV (eGFR between 15 and 29 mL/min/1.73 m^2), and CKD V (eGFR < 15 mL/min/1.73 m^2). Glucose metabolism disorders, i.e., impaired fasting glucose and diabetes mellitus, were defined according to the International Society of Pediatric and Adolescent Diabetes Guidelines [24]. Hypertension was defined as a systolic and/or diastolic blood pressure > 95th percentile appropriate for age, gender, and height. For children > 3 years of age, normative blood pressure values for Polish population were used [25,26], while children < 3 years reference values from the fourth report on blood pressure in children and adolescents [27]. Patients receiving antihypertensive drug was also defined as hypertensive. Standard deviation scores (SDS) for height and body mass index (BMI) were calculated from the World Health Organization growth charts (http://www.who.int/growthref/en, accessed on 26 August 2020). Growth impairment was defined as height-SDS < −2, and overweight as BMI-SDS > 1.

2.3. Molecular Analysis of HNF1B Gene

Genetic testing was performed as described elsewhere [12]. In brief, MLPA analysis was first performed to detect copy number variations (SALSA MLPA P241; MRC-Holland). If this result was negative, targeted Sanger sequencing of exons 1–9 of HNF1B was carried out. Written informed consent for the testing was obtained from parents and assent from children, where appropriate.

2.4. Statistical Analyses

Data were presented as means (95% confidence interval) for continuous variables and as counts (percentages) for categorical variables. Before proceeding to the analysis of differences, Shapiro–Wilk normality tests were performed on subgroups, and skewness was calculated. Equipotency of subgroups and variance homogeneity were determined if the normality assumption was met. To determine differences between patients with mutation at diagnosis and at follow-up, Student's t-tests for dependent samples, Wilcoxon signed rank tests for numerical variables, and McNemar's tests were performed. In order to compare this data with the control group, Student's t-tests for independent samples, Mann–Whitney U tests and Chi-squared tests were used. Yates' continuity correction and Welch's correction for non-homogenous variances were applied if necessary. Separate regression analyses were used to determine the relationships between sUA and other continuous variables in the mut+ and mut- cohorts.

To predict concentrations of sUA, linear regression models were built. Firstly, univariate models were built to determine the most statistically significant predictors. Next, a multivariate model was built and simplified using a stepwise linear regression method. Only variables whose p value was less than 0.05 in the univariate analysis were included. The quality of the models was determined with the R^2 coefficient. In order to predict mutation, an additional logistic regression model was implemented. Its quality was determined with the use of accuracy, sensitivity, and specificity coefficients. The variables included in the final model were determined using the information gain coefficient, based on conditional entropy. Data were split into training and test datasets. The level of significance was $\alpha = 0.05$. Analysis was performed using R programming language, RStudio, and IBM SPSS Statistics 25.

3. Results

3.1. Characteristics of the Study Patients

The clinical characteristics of the cohorts are presented in Table 1. Among mut+ patients, *HNF1B* whole gene deletion was detected in 22/43 patients (51.2%). At the time of molecular testing, both cohorts were comparable with respect to age, sex distribution, anthropometric parameters, prevalence of hypertension, and eGFR. In both groups, renal function was well preserved; The majority of patients had CKD stage 1 or stage 2 (91.2% and 94.1% of mut+ and mut- cohorts, respectively). As expected, well-known features of *HNF1B*-related disease, i.e., hypomagnesemia (65%) and hyperparathyroidism (38.5%) were more frequently found than in mut- subjects. The two cohorts were also different with respect to impairments in glucose metabolism (30% vs. 7.7% for mut+ and mut-, respectively), pancreatic anomalies (20.9%; exclusively found in mut+ patients), and liver involvement (14.3% vs. 1.5%).

All patients presented with renal anomalies on ultrasound. A phenotypic comparison of the two cohorts is presented in Table 2. Cystic kidney disease was the most common renal phenotype in both groups. In those with *HNF1B* mutations, increased renal echogenicity and multicystic dysplastic kidney disease were more prevalent.

For a great number of mut+ patients, follow-up data were also available. The mean record duration was 40.2 months (95% CI; 30.9–49.6). On follow-up, no significant changes were observed in these patients compared with the baseline data.

3.2. Serum Uric Acid Concentration

At the time of molecular testing, the mean sUA was higher in mut+ than in mut- subjects (5.74 mg/dL (95% CI; 5.22–6.27) vs. 4.87 mg/dL (95% CI; 4.47–5.28), $p = 0.006$). Hyperuricemia was more frequent in mut+ patients than in mut- cases (42.5% vs. 15.4%, $p = 0.002$). During the follow-up period, another four patients developed hyperuricemia. All sUA measurements for boys and girls are plotted in Figure 1. No clinical symptoms of gout were present in either cohort. Among mut+ patients, an elevated level of sUA was more frequent in those harboring point mutations than deletions of the *HNF1B* gene (57.1% vs. 29.7%, $p < 0.019$). No influence of any renal feature/phenotype on hyperuricemia prevalence was found.

A sensitivity analysis was performed after exclusion of patients with impairments in glucose metabolism. Raised sUA was present in 35.7% (in 10/28 patients) vs. 13.3% (in 8/60 patients; $p = 0.015$) of the mut+ and mut- groups, respectively. There was also a tendency for a higher mean sUA (5.33 mg/dL (95% CI; 4.89–5.76) vs. 4.75 mg/dL (95% CI; 4.34–5.15), $p = 0.052$), between mut+ and mut- subjects, respectively.

Table 1. Characteristics of the study cohorts.

Variable	mut+ at Diagnosis	mut-	p Value
Age (years)	7.84 (6.10–9.58)	8.74 (7.34–10.14)	0.436
Gender (M/F)	24/16 (60.5–39.5)	38/27 (58.5–41.5)	0.876
Height-SDS	0.04 (−0.53–0.61)	0.10 (−0.24–0.45)	0.857
Short stature	4 (11.1)	2 (3.8)	0.355 [a]
BMI-SDS	0.49 (−0.03–1.00)	0.34 (0.03–0.66)	0.324
Overweight	13 (36.1)	13 (24.5)	0.238
eGFR (mL/min/1.73 m^2)	104.09 (90.40–117.78)	115 (104.32–126.03)	0.210
CKD			—
1	21 (63.6)	36 (70.6)	0.505
2	9 (27.3)	12 (23.5)	0.699
3	3 (9.1)	3 (5.9)	0.577
4	—	—	—
5	—	—	—
sMg (mmol/L)	0.72 (0.69–0.76)	0.86 (0.84–0.88)	<0.001
Hypomagnesemia	26 (65.0)	3 (4.8)	<0.001
sUA (mg/dL)	5.74 (5.22–6.27)	4.87 (4.47–5.28)	0.006
Hyperuricemia	17 (42.5)	10 (15.40)	0.002
sK (mmol/L)	4.43 (4.26–4.60)	4.64 (4.51–4.78)	0.041
Hypokalemia	0 (0.0)	0 (0.0)	—
PTH (pg/mL)	67.78 (45.50–90.06)	33.46 (27.09–39.82)	0.001
Hyperparathyroidism	10 (38.5)	1 (3.0)	0.001
FEMg (%)	6.89 (5.54–8.24)	3.97 (3.35–4.60)	<0.001
FEUA (%)	6.88 (5.27–8.50)	6.16 (5.59–6.74)	0.888
FECa (%)	0.65 (0.29–1.01)	0.51 (0.35–0.66)	0.754
FEK (%)	7.48 (4.61–10.36)	5.68 (4.72–6.65)	0.149
Positive family history [b]	21 (51.2)	27 (58.7)	0.484
IFG/DM	10/2 (30.0)	4/1 (7.70)	0.003
Pancreatic anomalies	9 (20.9)	0 (0)	<0.001 [a]
Liver involvement	6 (14.3)	1 (1.5)	0.028 [a]
Genital tract anomaly	2 (4.7)	4 (6.2)	0.305 [a]
Developmental/speech delay	3 (7.0)	1 (1.5)	0.143
Hypertension	11 (27.5) [c]	10 (15.4) [d]	0.529

Data are presented as numbers (percentages) or as means (95% confidence interval). BMI-SDS, body mass index standard deviation score; CKD, chronic kidney disease; DM, diabetes mellitus; eGFR, estimated glomerular filtration rate; F, female; FECa, fractional excretion of Ca^{2+}; FEK, fractional excretion of K^+; FEMg, fractional excretion of Mg^{2+}; FEUA, fractional excretion of uric acid; Height-SDS, height standard deviation score; IFG, impaired fasting glucose; M, male; mut+, HNF1B positive patients; mut-, HNF1B negative patients; PTH, parathyroid hormone; sK, serum K^+; sMg, serum Mg^{2+}; and sUA, serum uric acid. [a] Yates continuity correction to Chi-squared test was performed; [b] family member with either diabetes mellitus and/or structural kidney disease; [c] medications (n): angiotensin-converting enzyme inhibitors (7), Ca^{2+} channel blockers (5), β-blocker (1); [d] medications (n): angiotensin-converting enzyme inhibitors (8); angiotensin receptor blocker (1), and Ca^{2+} channel blocker (1).

Table 2. Renal phenotype with respect to HNF1B mutation status.

	HNF1B+	HNF1B-	p Value
Renal hyperechogenicity	27 (73.0)	10 (27.0)	<0.001
Renal cysts	26 (43.4)	34 (56.7)	0.359
Multicystic dysplastic kidney	17 (60.7)	11 (39.3)	0.008
Renal hypoplasia/hypodysplasia	8 (57.1)	6 (42.9)	0.147
Urinary tract malformations	11 (91.7) [a]	1 (8.3) [b]	<0.001
Solitary kidney	5 (27.8)	13 (72.2)	0.267

Data were presented as numbers of patients (percentages). [a] pelviectasis (n = 7), posterior urethral valve-like partial bladder outlet obstruction (n = 1), kidney ectopy (n = 1), kidney malrotation (n = 1), and vesicoureteral reflux (n = 1). [b] ureteral dilatation.

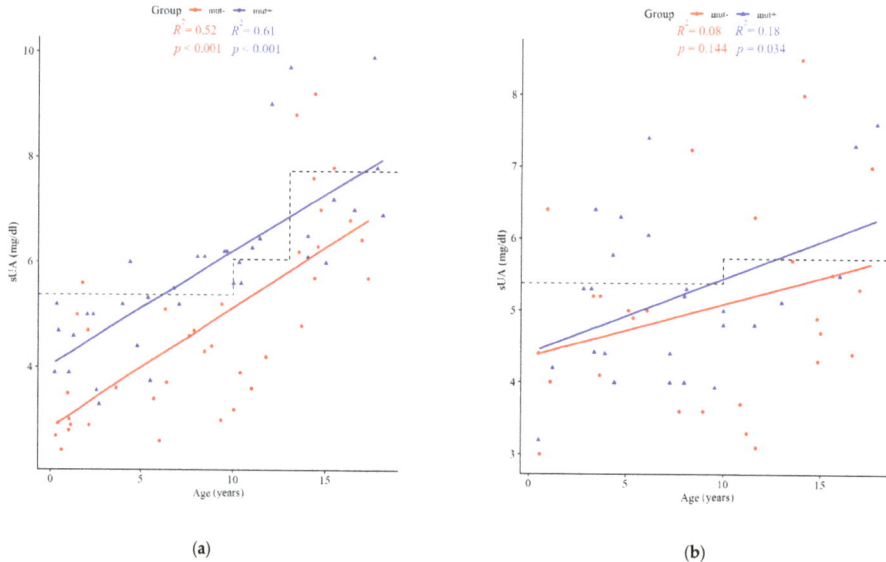

Figure 1. Scatter plots of serum uric acid (sUA) concentrations showing trends with age in children harboring *HNF1B* mutations (mut+, blue triangles) versus those without mutations (red dots). Boys (**a**) and girls (**b**) are presented separately with age-adjusted upper limits of reference values applied as dashed lines.

Due to the age dependence of sUA, the mut+ and mut- cohorts were arbitrarily divided into two age groups (0–9 and 10–18 years) and compared, with respect to sUA, eGFR, BMI-SDS, fractional excretion of uric acid (FEUA), and the frequency of hyperuricemia. Higher mean values of sUA were observed in patients harboring *HNF1B* mutations compared with mut- subjects within both age intervals ($p = 0.003$ and 0.052 for 0–9 and 10–18 years, respectively). Elevated sUA was already present at an early age, i.e., in 37.5% of *HNF1B* patients in the first decade versus 50% in the second decade of life (Table 3). In this regard, the difference between mut+ and mut- cohorts was more pronounced in younger children. Notably, there were no differences between the remaining analyzed parameters that could explain the difference in sUA. Figure 2 shows the relationships between sUA and eGFR (panel a), and between sUA and FEUA (panel b) for the mut+ and mut- groups separately.

Table 3. Differences in serum uric acid levels, frequency of hyperuricemia and fractional excretion of uric acid between *HNF1B* positive and negative patients presented for age-specific intervals.

Parameter	Age Group	HNF1B+	HNF1B-	*p* Value
BMI-SDS	0–9	0.31 (−0.19–0.81; n = 37)	0.32 (−0.26–0.90; n = 21)	0.992
	10–18	0.41 (−0.03–0.86; n = 31)	0.36 (−0.03–0.74; n = 32)	0.846
eGFR (mL/min/1.73 m^2)	1–9	112.28 (103.80–120.76; n = 33)	128.89 (109.05–148.72; n = 17)	0.119
	10–18	95.01 (80.59–109.43; n = 32)	107.89 (94.96–120.81; n = 32)	0.180
sUA (mg/dL)	0–9	4.93 (4.59–5.26; n = 35)	4.14 (3.73–4.54; n = 33)	0.003
	10–18	6.50 (5.89–7.11; n = 25)	5.63 (5.00–6.26; n = 32)	0.052
Hyperuricemia (%)	0–9	37.5% (n = 24)	8.6% (n = 35)	0.017
	10–18	50% (n = 16)	23.3% (n = 30)	0.066
FEUA (%)	0–9	7.33 (6.01–8.65; n = 25)	6.82 (5.92–7.72; n = 25)	0.511
	10–18	6.16 (4.77–7.55; n = 21)	5.60 (4.87–6.32; n = 29)	0.425

Data are presented as means (95% confidence interval) or percentages. BMI-SDS, body mass index standard deviation score; eGFR, estimated glomerular filtration rate; FEUA, fractional excretion of uric acid; and sUA, serum uric acid.

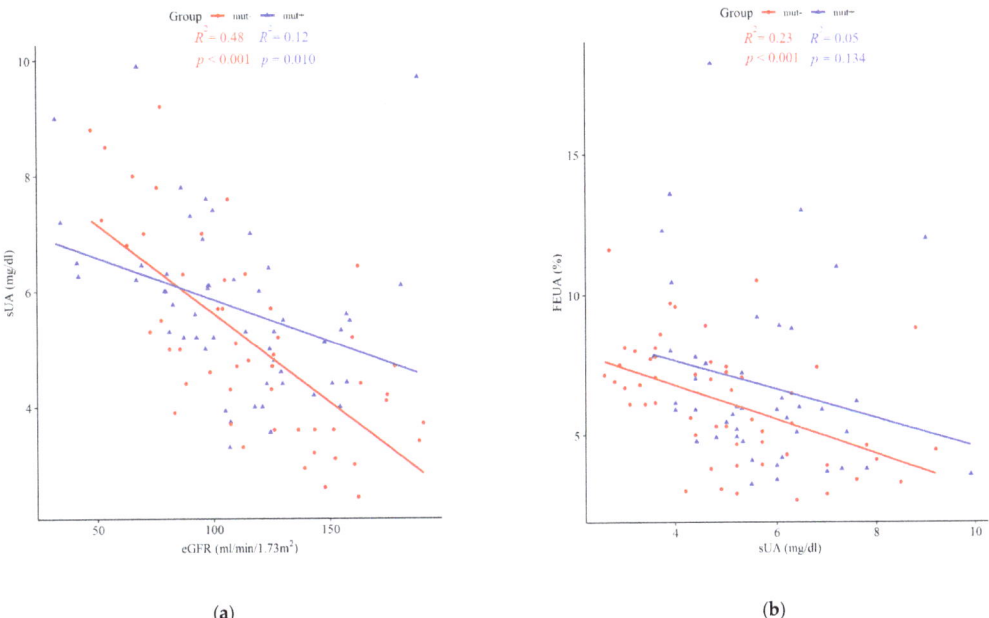

Figure 2. Correlations between serum uric acid (sUA) concentrations and estimated glomerular filtration rate (eGFR) (**a**) and fractional excretion of uric acid (FEUA) (**b**) in individuals with *HNF1B* mutations (mut+, blue triangles) and those who were negative for mutations (mut-, red dots).

3.3. Fractional Excretion of Uric Acid

FEUA was comparable between the mut+ and mut- groups (6.88% (95% CI; 5.27–8.5) vs. 6.16% (95% CI; 5.59–6.74), $p = 0.888$), respectively) when analyzing the entire cohort, as well as within age sub-groups (Table 3). Among mut+ patients, there was no difference in FEUA depending on the mutation type. Figure 3 shows the relationships between FEUA and age (panel a), and between FEUA and eGFR (panel b).

3.4. Determinants of Serum Uric Acid

In the univariate linear regression models, age, eGFR, CKD, sMg, hypomagnesemia, fractional excretion of Mg^{2+}, PTH, hyperparathyroidism, glucose metabolism disorders, hypertension, *HNF1B* mutation, and FEUA were all significantly associated with sUA (Supplementary Material–Table S1). However, in a multivariate linear stepwise regression model, only eGFR, FEUA, and PTH were independent predictive variables of sUA ($R^2 = 0.85$, F = 41.47, $p < 0.001$) (Table 4). sUA correlated positively with PTH ($R^2 = 0.18$, $p < 0.001$).

Table 4. Independent predictors of serum uric acid.

Parameter	B	SE	Beta	t	F	R^2
(Constant)	9.95	0.85	—	11.72 ***		
eGFR	−0.03	0.01	−0.60	−6.31 ***	41.47 ***	0.85
PTH	0.02	0.00	0.44	4.75 ***		
FEUA	−0.31	0.07	−0.36	−4.24 ***		

*** $p < 0.001$; eGFR, estimated glomerular filtration rate; FEUA, fractional excretion of uric acid; and PTH, parathyroid hormone.

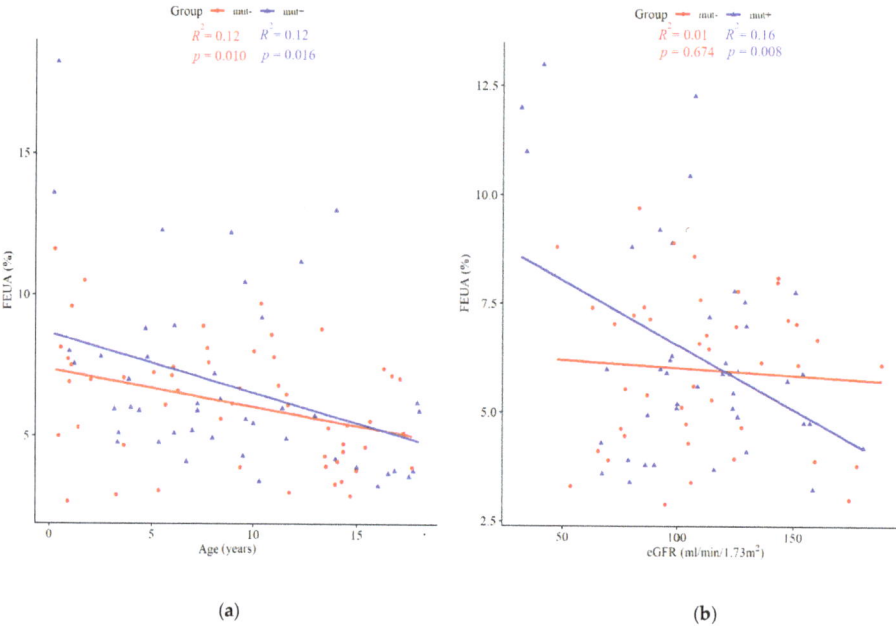

Figure 3. Fractional excretion of uric acid (FEUA) according to age (**a**) versus estimated glomerular filtration rate (eGFR) (**b**) in the *HNF1B* positive cohort (mut+, blue triangles) and *HNF1B* negative cohort (mut-, red dots).

3.5. Hyperuricemia as a Predictor of HNF1B Mutation

The potential of hyperuricemia for mutation prediction was tested in a model with all parameters that were significantly greater in the mut+ group compared with the mut- group of patients. A model including hypomagnesemia and hyperparathyroidism showed an accuracy of 85% (sensitivity: 83%, specificity: 86%). Adding hyperuricemia to the model did not increase the accuracy (79%; sensitivity: 77%, specificity: 82%). Information gain, which represents the selective potential of each parameter, was the lowest for hyperuricemia (0.34 compared with 0.99 and 0.63 for hyperparathyroidism and hypomagnesemia, respectively).

4. Discussion

This is the first study to comprehensively assess uric acid handling in a large cohort of pediatric patients with renal anomalies. We show that hyperuricemia is a relatively common feature in patients with *HNF1B*-related kidney disease, already present in early childhood. The age of manifestation of hyperuricemia is in line with previous observations [7,12]. Importantly, the frequency of hyperuricemia was compared to that present in counterparts who are negative for *HNF1B* mutations. Here, we showed a significant difference, which cannot be due to the effects of age, renal function and phenotype, body mass, gender, or hypertension, as the two cohorts we analyzed were comparable with respect to these parameters. Furthermore, a sensitivity analysis, which excluded individuals with glucose metabolism disorders, retained the difference. This result is in concordance with the findings of Bingham et al. [15], and this suggests that hyperuricemia is not just secondary to hyperglycemia/diabetes. Based on our findings, we can conclude that elevated sUA is causally related to *HNF1B* defect.

Although plenty of data exist on the presence of this abnormality in *HNF1B* patients, there has been a lack of good evidence on this association to date. For example, to exclude the effect of renal dysfunction, in a study by Bingham et al. [15], a comparison of sUA levels was made between *HNF1B* subjects ($n = 8$) with gender-matched subjects with renal impairment of other causes ($n = 32$). Notably, the analysis did not show significance. Although the authors claimed hyperuricemia is a feature of *HNF1B* mutation, the conclusions are vague due to the small sample size. In other studies, the frequency of hyperuricemia was not significantly different compared to *HNF1B* negative patients [10,11]. The lack of differences could possibly be explained by some differences in patient age and severity of CKD. For these reasons, our analysis was restricted only to children, who are free of co-morbidities and characterized by no alcohol consumption or multidrug use. Unfortunately, in our study we cannot exclude other variables that may impact sUA, with these three parameters explaining 85% of the total model variance. Lack of information about diet, physical activity, and blood lipids is a limitation of our study.

It is well known that elevated sUA is attributed to renal dysfunction. sUA is cleared by the kidney, and its level rises with declining kidney function [28]. Our data reflect this in that eGFR was a strong independent predictor of sUA along with FEUA and PTH. Unlike renal dysfunction, an independent relationship between sUA and PTH was quite unexpected. However, a literature search showed that there are several studies, which indicate hyperuricemia is more common among patients with primary hyperparathyroidism [29,30]. An evidence supporting the effect of PTH on sUA was delivered by Hui et al. in a large national population of adults from the USA [31]. By using data from 8316 participants, authors proved that serum PTH levels are independently associated with sUA levels and the frequency of hyperuricemia at the population level. This association is independent of renal function. Elevated PTH is thought to reduce renal uric acid excretion, but the exact mechanism is not known [32]. Our finding provides further evidence on this relationship. Given our observations, one has to take into consideration not only GFR, but also PTH when assessing hyperuricemia. This, however, might be a limitation when considering hyperuricemia as a reliable predictor of *HNF1B* nephropathy.

As we have shown, appropriate norms are instrumental in the assessment of hypomagnesemia in children with *HNF1B* mutations [18]. In this respect, applying the most recent reference limits for sUA could be regarded as a strength of the study. We used age- and gender-specific upper limits for sUA, as norms change when the body grows. A comprehensive review article by Kubota [33] shows that there are many conditions leading to hyperuricemia in children and adolescents. Among these, a range of both congenital and acute diseases, as well as lifestyle-related disorders, are listed as strongly associated with elevated sUA. Hyperuricemia may be encountered across the entire age spectrum of pediatric patients, and appropriate reference values should therefore be applied. Ridefelt et al. [17] defined these by calculating 2.5th and 97.5th percentiles of sUA in a group of 1998 healthy children and adolescents from Sweden and Denmark. Three age subgroups were distinguished, however differences between boys and girls were only observed in children > 10 years of age.

Importantly, in our study hyperuricemia was present in 42.5% of *HNF1B* mutation carriers. Notably, the cohort was characterized by a mild stage of CKD, which excludes a significant effect of renal insufficiency from impacting the results. In this context, the hyperuricemia prevalence is within the expected range; a literature review shows that, to date, prevalence has been recorded in the range of 11–71%. This variation could be mostly due to differences in age or renal function (Table 5). Unfortunately, some authors do not provide reference values and/or the data are not presented separately for children and adults (i.e., one cut-off value is applied for the mixed cohort) or the number of patients with available data on hyperuricemia is too small to draw conclusions from. The above limitations might have resulted in under-recognition of this parameter for predicting *HNF1B* mutation. Indeed, the screening tool to select patients eligible for genetic analysis of the *HNF1B* gene (HNF1B score) does not recognize hyperuricemia as a weighted parameter [20]. Instead, only gout is considered an important symptom [20], which in fact does not usually present until adulthood. In this respect, we provide the evidence that hyperuricemia is not an accurate predictor and, consequently, its application in HNF1B score might be of little value. In comparison to hypomagnesemia and hyperparathyroidism, both of which were significantly higher in the mut+ versus mut- group, the information gain, which describes the power of a variable, was rather low and did not significantly improve the model fit. One could expect that additional assessment of FEUA could improve the prediction. However, we demonstrated no difference in FEUA between the two groups (Figure 3a), which is concordant with the findings from the study by Bingham et al. [15]. Furthermore, FEUA values in patients with mutations in the uromodulin gene overlap slightly with those obtained from controls with normal kidney function [34], which confirms it is unreliable measure, and eliminates FEUA as a discriminative marker.

Table 5. Literature overview of the frequency of hyperuricemia in different patient cohorts.

Study Group	Hyperuricemia				Renal Function in Hyperuricemic Patients (Number of Cases)	Reference Values for Hyperuricemia
	HNF1B+		HNF1B-			
	Children	Adults	Children	Adults		
Ulinski et al. (2006) [6]	7/23 [a] (30%)	-	-	-	not specified	not given
Decramer et al. (2007) [7]	11/18 (61%)	-	-	-	CKD I (3), CKD II (2), CKD III (5), CKD 5 (1)	not given
Adalat et al. (2009) [8]	10/14 (71%)	-	7/15 (47%)	-	CKD ≤ III only for both HNF1B+ and HNF1B-	age-dependent reference limits
Heidet et al. (2010) [9]	12/75 (16%) [b]		-		CKD I (3), CKD II (1), CKD III (1), CKD V (1), no data on remaining 6 cases	not given
Raaijmakers et.al (2014) [10]	4/20 (20%)		41/185 (22.2%)		CKD I–III (in all HNF1B+ cohort), no data on renal function in HNF1B-	>5.7 mg/dL in females, >7 mg/dL in males, irrespective of age
Madariaga et al. (2018) [11]	6/17 (27%)	0/4	12/36 (33%)	-	CKD I (1), CKD II (1), CKD III (2), CKD V (2) in HNF1B+, no data on renal function in HNF1B-	not given
Okorn et al. (2019) [12]	19/52 (37%)	-	-	-	CKD I (10), CKD II (5), CKD IV (2), CKD V (2)	age-dependent reference limits
Nagano et al. (2019) [13]	2/18 (11%)	4/13 (31%)	-	-	CKD III (5), CKD IV (1)	sUA > 7 mg/dL, irrespective of age and sex
Lim et al. (2020) [14]	8/11 (73%)	3/3 (100%)	-	-	CKD I (2), CKD II (4), CKD III (4), CKD V (1)	sUA > 7 mg/dL, irrespective of age and sex
Our study (2021)	17/40 (42.5%)	-	10/65 (15.4%)	-	CKD I (7), CKD II (8), CKD III (2)	age- and sex-appropriate norms

CKD, chronic kidney disease; HNF1B+, HNF1B positive patients; HNF1B-, HNF1B negative patients; and sUA, serum uric acid. [a] moderately elevated level of serum uric acid (<1.5 times the upper normal level). [b] gout and/or hyperuricemia.

Among other laboratory observations that could be used as predictors of HNF1B, hypomagnesemia seems to be particularly valuable, as confirmed by our study. Notably, when we utilized age- and gender-dependent norms for sMg [17], hypomagnesemia was present in 65% of mut+ patients, which sharply contrasted with 4.8% in the mut- group. Here, we demonstrated for the first time that applying the appropriate reference lower limits for sMg instead of one cut-off value (sMg < 0.7 mmol/L) for the entire cohort we achieved a good discrimination between mut+ and mut- cohorts. Despite this, it is highly reasonable to use a combination of easily available laboratory markers instead of one in creation of a HNF1B score, which could be used as a tool for HNF1B mutation prediction in children. Interestingly, we showed that hyperparathyroidism, already described by others as a feature of *HNF1B* nephropathy [35], could also be instrumental, but probably only in those with good renal function. There is a concern that in a more severe CKD population, secondary hyperparathyroidism will distort this relationship. Importantly, the HNF1B score by Faguer et al. [20] was developed for both adults and children, which makes this score imperfect, especially in young children, wrongly predicting the absence of a mutation [14]. In this respect, there is a need for revision of the existing score or creation of a new HNF1B score or a diagnostic algorithm that could be applicable specifically in children. Based on our findings, hyperuricemia should not be highly valued.

We are aware of some limitations relating to the retrospective nature of this study. For some patients, the data were not complete, and parameters were obtained at unequal time points. As the patients were recruited from different centers, the method of sUA assessment was non-uniform, and extra-renal abnormalities were not studied formally. On the other hand, there are some strengths that need to be stressed. These are: a relatively large patient cohort free of co-morbidities and with only few patients requiring pharmacological treatment, and a well-matched control group of patients with urinary tract malformations and negative for *HNF1B* mutations. As mentioned before, our study was performed in a cohort with mildly affected renal function, which eliminates to some extent a confounding effect of renal dysfunction. Finally, the application of the most recent reference data for sUA is of great value. On the other hand, due to lack of local sUA reference values, we applied those derived from a Nordic population. This could impact our results on the frequency of hyperuricemia, as sUA levels may differ between populations and ethnicities. Thus, our findings should be validated in an international cohort.

5. Conclusions

We demonstrated that hyperuricemia is an early and prevalent feature in children with *HNF1B* nephropathy when compared to well-matched mutation negative patients. Thus, we provide evidence that this abnormality is causally related to *HNF1B* defect. A strong association of sUA with renal function and PTH limits a clinical assessment of hyperuricemia. Although our results derive from pediatric population, it especially applies to adults who are at a greater risk of CKD. As we showed, the utility of hyperuricemia as a predictor of *HNF1B*-related disease is limited, and should not be relied upon when selecting patients for genetic testing. We also propose that assessment of FEUA would not be helpful. The presence of hyperparathyroidism seems to be discriminative, however further studies are needed to prove this observation.

Supplementary Materials: The following are available online at https://www.mdpi.com/article/10.3390/jcm10153265/s1, Table S1: Results of univariate regression analysis performed in the entire cohort of patients.

Author Contributions: Conception and design: M.K. and M.Z.; data analysis: M.K., M.F.K., B.B.B. and M.Z.; data interpretation: M.K., B.B., S.H., M.F.K., M.S., K.K.-P., A.W., P.A., R.M., M.T., P.S., B.B.B. and M.Z.; drafting manuscript: M.K. and M.Z. All authors have read and agreed to the published version of the manuscript.

Funding: This research received no external funding.

Institutional Review Board Statement: Ethical approval for this study has been waived by the Institutional Ethics Committee due to the retrospective nature of the study. No patient identifiable data was recorded. The study was conducted in accordance with the 1964 Helsinki declaration.

Informed Consent Statement: Informed consent was obtained from all subjects involved in the study.

Data Availability Statement: The data presented in this study are available on request from the corresponding author.

Acknowledgments: The authors thank the patients and their families for their participation, and their referring doctors for providing data and making this study possible. These include: Monika Pawlak-Bratkowska, Maria Kniażewska, Aleksandra Krzemień, Katarzyna Zachwieja, Omar Bjanid, and Tomasz Jarmoliński.

Conflicts of Interest: The authors declare no conflict of interest.

References

1. Adalat, S.; Bockenhauer, D.; Ledermann, S.E.; Hennekam, R.C.; Woolf, A.S. Renal malformations associated with mutations of developmental genes: Messages from the clinic. *Pediatr. Nephrol.* **2010**, *25*, 2247–2255. [CrossRef]
2. Bingham, C.; Hattersley, A.T. Renal cysts and diabetes syndrome resulting from mutations in hepatocyte nuclear factor-1beta. *Nephrol. Dial. Transplant.* **2004**, *19*, 2703–2708. [CrossRef] [PubMed]
3. Ferrè, S.; Igarashi, P. New insights into the role of HNF-1β in kidney (patho)physiology. *Pediatr. Nephrol.* **2019**, *34*, 1325–1335. [CrossRef] [PubMed]
4. Bockenhauer, D.; Jaureguiberry, G. HNF1B-associated clinical phenotypes: The kidney and beyond. *Pediatr. Nephrol.* **2016**, *31*, 707–714. [CrossRef]
5. Clissold, R.L.; Hamilton, A.J.; Hattersley, A.T.; Ellard, S.; Bingham, C. HNF1B-associated renal and extra-renal disease-an expanding clinical spectrum. *Nat. Rev. Nephrol.* **2015**, *11*, 102–112. [CrossRef]
6. Ulinski, T.; Lescure, S.; Beaufils, S.; Guigonis, V.; Decramer, S.; Morin, D.; Clauin, S.; Deschênes, G.; Bouissou, F.; Bensman, A.; et al. Renal phenotypes related to hepatocyte nuclear factor-1beta (TCF2) mutations in a pediatric cohort. *J. Am. Soc. Nephrol.* **2006**, *17*, 497–503. [CrossRef] [PubMed]
7. Decramer, S.; Parant, O.; Beaufils, S.; Clauin, S.; Guillou, C.; Kessler, S.; Aziza, J.; Bandin, F.; Schanstra, J.P.; Bellanné-Chantelot, C. Anomalies of the TCF2 gene are the main cause of fetal bilateral hyperechogenic kidneys. *J. Am. Soc. Nephrol.* **2007**, *18*, 923–933. [CrossRef] [PubMed]
8. Adalat, S.; Woolf, A.S.; Johnstone, K.A.; Wirsing, A.; Harries, L.W.; Long, D.A.; Hennekam, R.C.; Ledermann, S.E.; Rees, L.; van't Hoff, W.; et al. HNF1B mutations associate with hypomagnesemia and renal magnesium wasting. *J. Am. Soc. Nephrol.* **2009**, *20*, 1123–1131. [CrossRef]
9. Heidet, L.; Decramer, S.; Pawtowski, A.; Morinière, V.; Bandin, F.; Knebelmann, B.; Lebre, A.-S.; Faguer, S.; Guigonis, V.; Antignac, C.; et al. Spectrum of HNF1B mutations in a large cohort of patients who harbor renal diseases. *Clin. J. Am. Soc. Nephrol.* **2010**, *5*, 1079–1090. [CrossRef]
10. Raaijmakers, A.; Corveleyn, A.; Devriendt, K.; van Tienoven, T.P.; Allegaert, K.; Van Dyck, M.; van den Heuvel, L.; Kuypers, D.; Claes, K.; Mekahli, D.; et al. Criteria for HNF1B analysis in patients with congenital abnormalities of kidney and urinary tract. *Nephrol. Dial. Transplant.* **2015**, *30*, 835–842. [CrossRef]
11. Madariaga, L.; García-Castaño, A.; Ariceta, G.; Martínez-Salazar, R.; Aguayo, A.; Castaño, L. Variable phenotype in HNF1B mutations: Extrarenal manifestations distinguish affected individuals from the population with congenital anomalies of the kidney and urinary tract. *Clin. Kidney J.* **2019**, *12*, 373–379. [CrossRef] [PubMed]
12. Okorn, C.; Goertz, A.; Vester, U.; Beck, B.B.; Bergmann, C.; Habbig, S.; König, J.; Konrad, M.; Müller, D.; Oh, J.; et al. HNF1B nephropathy has a slow-progressive phenotype in childhood-with the exception of very early onset cases: Results of the German Multicenter HNF1B Childhood Registry. *Pediatr. Nephrol.* **2019**, *34*, 1065–1075. [CrossRef] [PubMed]
13. Nagano, C.; Morisada, N.; Nozu, K.; Kamei, K.; Tanaka, R.; Kanda, S.; Shiona, S.; Araki, Y.; Ohara, S.; Matsumura, C.; et al. Clinical characteristics of HNF1B-related disorders in a Japanese population. *Clin. Exp. Nephrol.* **2019**, *23*, 1119–1129. [CrossRef] [PubMed]
14. Lim, S.H.; Kim, J.H.; Han, K.H.; Ahn, Y.H.; Kang, H.G.; Ha, I.-S.; Cheong, H. Il Genotype and Phenotype Analyses in Pediatric Patients with HNF1B Mutations. *J. Clin. Med.* **2020**, *9*, 2320. [CrossRef] [PubMed]
15. Bingham, C.; Ellard, S.; van't Hoff, W.G.; Simmonds, H.A.; Marinaki, A.M.; Badman, M.K.; Winocour, P.H.; Stride, A.; Lockwood, C.R.; Nicholls, A.J.; et al. Atypical familial juvenile hyperuricemic nephropathy associated with a hepatocyte nuclear factor-1beta gene mutation. *Kidney Int.* **2003**, *63*, 1645–1651. [CrossRef]
16. Baldree, L.A.; Stapleton, F.B. Uric acid metabolism in children. *Pediatr. Clin. N. Am.* **1990**, *37*, 391–418. [CrossRef]
17. Ridefelt, P.; Hilsted, L.; Juul, A.; Hellberg, D.; Rustad, P. Pediatric reference intervals for general clinical chemistry components— Merging of studies from Denmark and Sweden. *Scand. J. Clin. Lab. Investig.* **2018**, *78*, 365–372. [CrossRef]
18. Kołbuc, M.; Leßmeier, L.; Salamon-Słowińska, D.; Małecka, I.; Pawlaczyk, K.; Walkowiak, J.; Wysocki, J.; Beck, B.B.; Zaniew, M. Hypomagnesemia is underestimated in children with HNF1B mutations. *Pediatr. Nephrol.* **2020**, *35*, 1877–1886. [CrossRef]
19. Motyka, R.; Kołbuc, M.; Wierzchołowski, W.; Beck, B.B.; Towpik, I.E.; Zaniew, M. Four Cases of Maturity Onset Diabetes of the Young (MODY) Type 5 Associated with Mutations in the Hepatocyte Nuclear Factor 1 Beta (HNF1B) Gene Presenting in a 13-Year-Old Boy and in Adult Men Aged 33, 34, and 35 Years in Poland. *Am. J. Case Rep.* **2020**, *22*, e928994. [CrossRef]
20. Faguer, S.; Chassaing, N.; Bandin, F.; Prouheze, C.; Garnier, A.; Casemayou, A.; Huart, A.; Schanstra, J.P.; Calvas, P.; Decramer, S.; et al. The HNF1B score is a simple tool to select patients for HNF1B gene analysis. *Kidney Int.* **2014**, *86*, 1007–1015. [CrossRef]
21. Schwartz, G.J.; Brion, L.P.; Spitzer, A. The use of plasma creatinine concentration for estimating glomerular filtration rate in infants, children, and adolescents. *Pediatr. Clin. N. Am.* **1987**, *34*, 571–590. [CrossRef]

22. Schwartz, G.J.; Muñoz, A.; Schneider, M.F.; Mak, R.H.; Kaskel, F.; Warady, B.A.; Furth, S.L. New equations to estimate GFR in children with CKD. *J. Am. Soc. Nephrol.* **2009**, *20*, 629–637. [CrossRef]
23. Levey, A.S.; Coresh, J.; Bolton, K.; Culleton, B.; Harvey, K.S.; Ikizler, T.A.; Johnson, C.A.; Kausz, A.; Kimmel, P.L.; Kusek, J.; et al. K/DOQI clinical practice guidelines for chronic kidney disease: Evaluation, classification, and stratification. *Am. J. Kidney Dis.* **2002**, *39*, S1–S266.
24. Mayer-Davis, E.J.; Kahkoska, A.R.; Jefferies, C.; Dabelea, D.; Balde, N.; Gong, C.X.; Aschner, P.; Craig, M.E. ISPAD Clinical Practice Consensus Guidelines 2018: Definition, epidemiology, and classification of diabetes in children and adolescents. *Pediatr. Diabetes* **2018**, *19* (Suppl. 27), 7–19. [CrossRef] [PubMed]
25. Grajda, A.; Kułaga, Z.; Gurzkowska, B.; Wojtyło, M.; Góźdź, M.; Litwin, M. Preschool children blood pressure percentiles by age and height. *J. Hum. Hypertens.* **2017**, *31*, 400–408. [CrossRef]
26. Kułaga, Z.; Litwin, M.; Grajda, A.; Kułaga, K.; Gurzkowska, B.; Góźdź, M.; Pan, H. OLAF Study Group. Oscillometric blood pressure percentiles for Polish normal-weight school-aged children and adolescents. *J. Hypertens.* **2012**, *30*, 1942–1954. [CrossRef] [PubMed]
27. National High Blood Pressure Education Program Working Group on High Blood Pressure in Children and Adolescents. The fourth report on the diagnosis, evaluation, and treatment of high blood pressure in children and adolescents. *Pediatrics* **2004**, *114* (Suppl. S2), 555–576. [CrossRef]
28. Fathallah-Shaykh, S.A.; Cramer, M.T. Uric acid and the kidney. *Pediatr. Nephrol.* **2014**, *29*, 999–1008. [CrossRef] [PubMed]
29. Mintz, D.H.; Canary, J.J.; Carreon, G.; Kyle, L.H. Hyperuricemia in hyperparathyroidism. *N. Engl. J. Med.* **1961**, *265*, 112–115. [CrossRef]
30. Christensson, T. Serum urate in subjects with hypercalcaemic hyperparathyroidism. *Clin. Chim. Acta* **1977**, *80*, 529–533. [CrossRef]
31. Hui, J.Y.; Choi, J.W.J.; Mount, D.B.; Zhu, Y.; Zhang, Y.; Choi, H.K. The independent association between parathyroid hormone levels and hyperuricemia: A national population study. *Arthritis Res. Ther.* **2012**, *14*, R56. [CrossRef] [PubMed]
32. Hisatome, I.; Ishimura, M.; Sasaki, N.; Yamakawa, M.; Kosaka, H.; Tanaka, Y.; Kouchi, T.; Mitani, Y.; Yoshida, A.; Kotake, H. Renal handling of urate in two patients with hyperuricemia and primary hyperparathyroidism. *Intern. Med.* **1992**, *31*, 807–811. [CrossRef] [PubMed]
33. Kubota, M. Hyperuricemia in Children and Adolescents: Present Knowledge and Future Directions. *J. Nutr. Metab.* **2019**, *2019*, 3480718. [CrossRef]
34. Stiburkova, B.; Bleyer, A.J. Changes in serum urate and urate excretion with age. *Adv. Chronic Kidney Dis.* **2012**, *19*, 372–376. [CrossRef] [PubMed]
35. Ferrè, S.; Bongers, E.M.H.F.; Sonneveld, R.; Cornelissen, E.A.M.; van der Vlag, J.; van Boekel, G.A.J.; Wetzels, J.F.M.; Hoenderop, J.G.J.; Bindels, R.J.M.; Nijenhuis, T. Early development of hyperparathyroidism due to loss of PTH transcriptional repression in patients with HNF1β mutations? *J. Clin. Endocrinol. Metab.* **2013**, *98*, 4089–4096. [CrossRef] [PubMed]

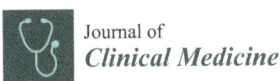

Article

Involvement of Hemopexin in the Pathogenesis of Proteinuria in Children with Idiopathic Nephrotic Syndrome

Agnieszka Pukajło-Marczyk * and Danuta Zwolińska

Department of Pediatric Nephrology, Wroclaw Medical University, Borowska 213, 50-556 Wroclaw, Poland; danuta.zwolinska@umed.wroc.pl
* Correspondence: pukajlo-marczyk@umed.wroc.pl

Abstract: Hemopexin (Hpx) is considered a factor in the pathogenesis of idiopathic nephrotic syndrome (INS). The aim of the study was to evaluate the serum and urine values of Hpx (sHpx and uHpx) in children with INS, analyze the role of Hpx, and assess its usefulness as a marker of the disease course. 51 children with INS and 18 age-matched controls were examined. Patients were divided into subgroups depending on the number of relapses (group IA—the first episode of INS, group IB—with relapses) and according to method of treatment (group IIA treated with gluco-corticosteroids (GCS), group IIB treated with GCS and other immunosuppressants). Hpx concentrations were determined by enzyme-linked immunosorbent assay (ELISA). sHpx and uHpx values in relapse were elevated in the whole INS group versus controls ($p < 0.000$). In remission their levels decreased, but still remained higher than in the control group ($p < 0.000$). In group IB uHpx levels were increased during remission as compared to group IA ($p < 0.006$). No significant impact of immuno-suppressants on sHpx was observed, but uHpx excretion in group IIA was higher in relapse ($p < 0.026$) and lower in remission ($p < 0.0017$) as compared to group IIB. The results suggest the role of Hpx in the pathogenesis of INS. Hpx may be a useful indicator for continuation of treatment, but it requires confirmation by further controlled studies.

Keywords: hemopexin; nephrotic syndrome; children

1. Introduction

Various factors can damage the glomerular filtration barrier and trigger nephrotic proteinuria. The child's age at the time of the manifestation of symptoms allows the diagnostic process to be directed in search of the disease etiology. Up to 1 year of age, nephrotic syndrome is the result of mutations in genes encoding podocyte proteins or may be associated with congenital infections such as syphilis or toxoplasmosis [1]. Podocyte function may also be impaired in the course of lysosomal diseases, which should be considered in the diagnostic procedure, especially in the case of the development of nephropathy in young children [2]. In older children, nephrotic syndrome may develop in the course of autoimmune inflammatory diseases, such as lupus erythematosus, acute poststreptococcal glomerulonephritis, IgAN (IgA Nephropathy) or IgAVN (Immunoglobulin (Ig)A vasculitis nephritis) [3–5].

Idiopathic nephrotic syndrome (INS) is the most common form of podocytopathy in children. It accounts for over 90% of cases in the group between 1 and 10 years of age and about 50% in the group of children over 10 years of age. The incidence is estimated at about 16 cases per 100,000 of the pediatric population and at two–seven new cases per 100,000 children under 15 years of age. The diagnostic criteria are massive proteinuria above 50 mg/kg/day, hypoalbuminemia (<2.5 g/L) and edema [6,7]. These symptoms are accompanied by hyperlipidemia. Minimal change disease (MCD) is the most common morphologic feature of this syndrome (approximately 85% of cases), followed by focal segmental glomerulosclerosis (FSGS) and mesangial proliferative glomerulonephritis (MPGN). In each of these forms, there is the effacement of podocyte foot processes and structural

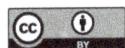

disorganization of the glomerular filtration barrier (GFB). While the vast majority of patients (80–90%) respond well to gluco-corticosteroids (GCS), primary steroid resistance is observed in approximately 10%, mainly in FSGS patients, with a poorer prognosis for renal survival [8,9]. The course of INS is characterized by periods of remissions and relapses, usually induced by upper respiratory tract infections.

The pathogenesis of nephrotic proteinuria in MCD is complex and still not fully elucidated, as evidenced by the emergence of new hypotheses [10]. The earliest, from the 1970s, suggested that circulating protein permeability factors released by dysfunctional T lymphocytes were responsible for the development of proteinuria in MCD [11]. Various candidate cytokines, whose elevated levels were observed in the serum and urine of children with recurrent MCD, were considered. Out of these, IL-8 and IL-13 were found to be the most likely pathogenic factors. However, it should be emphasized that the reported results of many studies were inconclusive [12–14].

A more recent theory, the "two-hit" theory, posits that the process of podocyte damage is more complex and partially combines the earlier hypotheses [15,16]. The first hit is the stimulation of podocytes by T-linked cytokines, bacterial or viral fragments, allergens or other factors, resulting in increased expression of CD80 (B7-1). Induction of CD80 leads to podocyte damage and increased permeability to proteins. If normal podocyte autoregulation is maintained, T-regulatory cells (T-reg) prevent this phenomenon, with the involvement of the CTLA-4 molecule, IL-10 and TGF-beta [17]. If these mechanisms fail, permanent overexpression of CD80 occurs, resulting in the full-blown MCD. In contrast, achieving remission after rituximab, a monoclonal antibody directed against CD-20, points to the involvement of B lymphocytes in INS development [18]. The role of circulating factors in the pathogenesis of proteinuria in INS remains of interest [19–23].

Hemopexin (Hpx) is a circulating plasma β-1 glycoprotein with a molecular weight of 60 kDa, encoded by a gene located on chromosome 11 (pp. 15.4–15.5) [24–26]. It is synthesized mainly in hepatocytes as a single polypeptide chain. Its spatial structure is determined by two disulfide bonds connecting structurally related domains (C- and N-terminal) and binding the heme moiety [27]. Hpx plays a role in iron homeostasis by binding heme released into serum and then transporting it to the liver where it is disintegrated [28,29]. The half-life of Hpx in serum is 7 days. Low concentrations may be a marker of hemolysis severity, whereas its absence may indicate either insufficient synthesis in the course of chronic liver diseases or severe malnutrition. Under physiological conditions, the mean urinary Hpx concentration is 2 mg/L, and its increase has been observed in diabetes, when glomerular proteinuria develops [30,31]. Increased levels of Hpx have also been shown in inflammatory psychiatric disorders, cancer, and neuromuscular diseases [32–34].

Hpx has serine protease activity. It exhibits anti- and pro-inflammatory effects and inhibits multinuclear granulocyte necrosis and cell adhesion [23]. In recent years, the effect of Hpx as a circulating factor on GFB permeability and the development of proteinuria has been postulated.

2. Aim of the Study

The aim of the study was to evaluate the serum and urine Hpx concentration in children with INS as a pathogenic factor and to determine its usefulness as a predictor of disease severity.

3. Material and Methods

The study group consisted of 69 children, including 51 children with INS (INS group), 19 girls and 32 boys, ranging in age from 1.25–18 years (mean age 8.86 ± 5.2 years). The diagnosis of INS was established according to ISKDC criteria [35]. Steroid sensitivity was defined as the achievement of remission during the first 4 weeks of GCS treatment, and steroid dependence as the occurrence of at least two relapses during the period of steroid dose reduction or within 2 weeks after GCS cessation. Remission was defined as the absence of protein in urine for at least 3 consecutive days.

The group of patients with INS was further divided into subgroups: group IA consisted of 20 children (5 girls, 15 boys; mean age 5.90 ± 4.91 years), with the first occurrence of INS, and group IB consisted of 31 children (14 girls, 17 boys; mean age 10.31 ± 4.81 years), with relapses (from 2–16 relapses, mean 11.8).

Additionally, in order to assess the severity of the course of INS, a second division was made according to the applied treatment. Group IIA included 26 children (7 girls, 19 boys; mean age 5.59 ± 4.04 years), treated only with GCS. In relapse standard doses of prednisone (2 mg/kg/day) were used, and in individual cases pulses of methylprednisolone 0.5 g/dose were also required. Group II B included 22 children (9 girls, 13 boys; mean age 12.31 ± 4.06 years) treated with GCS and corticosteroid-sparing agents: cyclosporin (CsA), mycophenolate mofetil (MMF), and azathioprine (AZA). The distribution of administered immunosuppressive drugs in this subgroup was as follows: 17 children—CsA + GCS, 2 children—MMF + GCS, 2 children—CsA + AZA + GCS, 1 child—CsA + MMF + GCS.

The control group consisted of 18 healthy children (12 girls, 6 boys; mean age 8.40 ± 3.87 years), diagnosed for primary nocturnal enuresis or suspected urinary tract abnormalities, which were finally excluded.

Blood and urine were collected once in the control group and twice in the children with INS: at disease onset and immediately after remission was achieved. Blood samples were drawn from cubital vein after an overnight fast, during routinely performed laboratory tests. Samples were clotted for 30 min and then centrifuged at room temperature for 15 min. Urine samples were collected on the same day as blood samples. After centrifuging them for 15 min, sediment was removed. Biological material was stored frozen at −70 °C until assayed. Serum and urine Hpx, serum creatinine, albumin, total cholesterol and CRP (C-reactive protein) levels, and urine creatinine and protein concentrations were determined in all children. In all enrolled patients, inflammatory parameters were negative and renal function was normal (creatinine was determined by enzymatic method, the estimated GFR calculated according to the Schwartz formula [36]). Proteinuria was assessed by the urinary protein creatinine ratio (uPCR) on a first morning urine sample. A uPCR > 2 (2 mg/mg) was assumed as the value defining nephrotic proteinuria [2]. Other biochemical tests were determined by standard laboratory methods using an Olympus 5800 analyzer.

Hemopexin concentrations in serum (sHpx) and urine (uHpx) were determined by ELISA using commercial assays according to the manufacturer's instructions (AssayPro, St. Charles, MO, USA, kit catalog number for serum assays: EH1001-1, for urine assays: EH2001-1). The evaluations were performed twice and then the average of obtained results was calculated. Hpx values were expressed in ng/mL. The sensitivity of the method was 50 ng/mL and 4 ng/mL for sHpx and uHpx, respectively.

Kidney biopsy was performed in 18 children with INS with frequent relapses: MCD was diagnosed in 3 children, FSGS in 7, and MGN in 8. In the remaining patients with a good therapeutic response to GCS, MCD was diagnosed empirically, which is in line with the current recommendations. Histopathological examinations of kidney biopsies were carried out and assessed at the Department of Patho-morphology and Oncological Cytology of the Medical University in Wroclaw. Histopathological analysis included light microscopy, histochemical and immunohistochemical examinations.

The study was conducted according to the guidelines of the Declaration of Helsinki, and approved by the Bioethics Committee of the Wroclaw Medical University (No. KB—199/2009). Informed consent was obtained from the parents and subjects above 16 years old.

4. Statistical Analysis

The results are expressed as median values and interquartile ranges. Due to the small number of patients, verification of the hypothesis of median value equality in regard to studied parameters in individual groups was carried out using the non-parametric Kruskal-Wallis rank sum test. Verification of the hypothesis of median value equality in regard to the studied parameters in individual dependent samples (e.g., relapse–remission) was conducted using non-parametric Wilcoxon pair sequence test. Relations between parameters were defined by Pearson's correlation coefficient r. A p value < 0.05 was considered statistically significant. The statistical analysis was performed using a software package EPIINFO Ver. 7.1.1.14 Centers for Disease Control and Prevention (CDC), Atlanta, GA, USA (dated 2 July 2013). The results are presented in the tables and figure.

5. Results

All examined parameters in controls were within the normal range.

The data of basic biochemical parameters in children with INS are shown in the table below (Table 1). A significantly higher level of proteinuria during relapse was shown in children requiring additional immunosuppressive treatment compared to the group treated only with GCS.

Table 1. Selected biochemical parameters in all children with INS and in examined subgroups according to the number of relapses and treatment modality. Data are presented as median values and interquartile ranges.

Parameter Group	Serum Albumin [g/dL]	Total Cholesterol [mg/dL]	Protein/Creatinine Ratio [g Protein/g Creatinine]	CRP [mg/L]
Total INS N = 51	1.90 (1.05–2.55)	363.0 (268.0–475.0)	6.2 (3.0–10.6)	2.90 (0.80–3.60)
Group IA N = 20	1.70 (1.40–2.20)	372.0 (297.0–464.0)	4.85 (2.40–7.90)	1.75 (0.40–3.60)
Group IB N = 31	2.40 (1.00–3.10)	329.5 (238.0–601.0)	7.0 (3.9–10.7)	3.10 (1.65–3.69)
Group IIA N = 26	1.90 (1.10–2.50)	366.5 (286.5–442.5)	4.71 (2.5–7.76) [a]	3.30 (1.40–3.60)
Group IIB N = 22	2.0 (1.00–2.50)	329.5 (264.0–636.0)	9.6 (6.2–19.2)	2.56 (1.60–4.20)

[a]—group IIA versus group IIB, $p = 0.023$, Kruskal-Wallis test. INS, idiopathic nephrotic syndrome; CRP, C-reactive protein; Group IA- children with the first occurrence of INS; Group IB- children with relapses of INS; Group IIA- children treated only with GCS, gluco-corticosteroids; Group IIB- children treated with GCS and corticosteroid-sparing agents.

sHpx and uHpx levels in the whole INS group were significantly higher, both in relapse and remission, compared to the controls. Additionally, sHpx and uHpx values in relapse were increased compared to those in remission (Table 2, Figure 1).

Table 2. Serum and urine Hpx levels in the whole group of INS children, depending on disease clinical phase compared to the control group. Data are presented as median values and interquartile ranges.

Group Parameter	Relapse	Remission	Control
sHpx [ng/mL]	107.6 (97.2–114.0) [a,b]	51.2 (46.4–55.6) [a]	32.2 (30.8–33.6)
uHpx [ng/mL]	62.8 (55.3–128.0) [a,b]	27.5 (22.9–31.1) [a]	15.8 (14.4–17.5)

[a]—relapse INS versus control group and remission INS vs. control group (sHpx, uHpx), $p = 0.0000$, Kruskal-Wallis test. [b]—relapse INS versus remission INS (sHpx, uHpx), $p = 0.00000$, Wilcoxon test. Hpx, hemopexin.

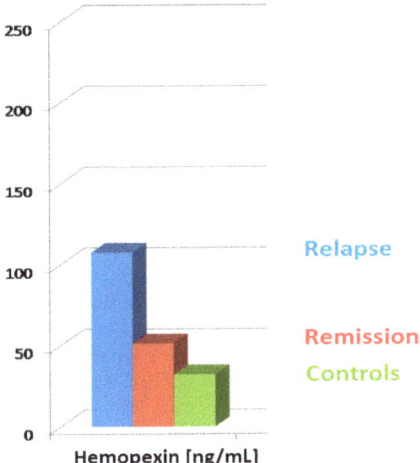

Figure 1. sHpx levels according to clinical phase of the disease, compared to control group. sHpx, serum hemopexin.

Analyzing the group of children with the first manifestation of the disease and the group of children with subsequent relapses, we did not show a significant difference in the concentration of sHpx, both in relapse and in remission. uHpx excretion was comparable in the acute phase of the disease in both groups.

On the other hand, children with the first onset of the disease shortly after reaching remission demonstrated lower uHpx values than those with subsequent remission (Table 3).

Table 3. sHpx and uHpx levels in INS subgroups according to the number of relapses (group IA—the onset of disease, IB—subsequent relapses). Data are presented as median values and interquartile ranges.

Group Parameter	IA Relapse N = 20	IB Relapse N = 31	IA Remission N = 9	IB Remission N = 26
sHpx [ng/mL]	108.8 (104.0–115.8)	105.2 (96.0–114.0)	46.4 (42.0–58.0)	51.2 (49.2–53.6)
uHpx [ng/mL]	61.8 (57.1–148.0)	71.4 (55.2–121.4)	24.2 (21.7–26.0) [a]	28.2 (24.8–33.2)

[a]—group IA versus group IB, $p = 0.006$.

There was no difference in sHpx levels between the group receiving only GCS (group IIA) and children receiving GCS and additional immunosuppressants (group IIB), both in the relapse and in the remission. However, there was a difference in uHpx values between these groups. During the relapse uHpx was significantly higher, and then in the remission—lower in children receiving only GCS (Table 4).

Table 4. sHpx and uHpx levels in the patient groups according to the treatment modality (group IIA—only GCS, IIB—GCS with immunosuppressive sparing agents). Data are presented as median values and interquartile ranges.

Group Parameter	IIA Relapse N = 26	IIB Relapse N = 22	IIA Remission N = 17	IIB Remission N = 17
sHpx [ng/mL]	108.2 (97.2–123.6)	103.4 (95.6–108.8)	51.2 (42.0–55.6)	51.2 (49.2–53.6)
uHpx [ng/mL]	103.0 (57.2–158.0) [a]	61.1 (55.2–81.4)	24.8 (22.1–27.5) [b]	31.1 (27.5–35.0)

[a]—group IIA vs. IIB, $p = 0.026$; [b]—group IIA vs. IIB, $p = 0.0017$.

Correlation analysis performed in the whole group of INS children in relapse did not show any relationship between the sHpx and uHpx levels and CRP, albumin, total cholesterol or proteinuria.

The analysis of sHpx and uHpx concentrations in the acute phase of the disease did not show any significant statistical difference between the groups depending on the histopathological diagnosis. However, in remission, a statistically significant lower median concentration of uHpx was demonstrated in the group of children diagnosed with MCD compared to the group with MGN ($p = 0.01$). However, due to the small number of patients in the analyzed subgroups, the above observations have not been fully presented in our current study.

6. Discussion

The involvement of circulating factors in the pathogenesis of nephrotic syndrome in children, not associated with mutation of genes encoding podocyte or basement membrane proteins, has long been discussed [37–39]. Experimental results have suggested that one of these factors may be hemopexin, existing in plasma in an inactive form. The active form of Hpx exhibits serine protease properties and can affect podocyte function and structure [40]. Studies in rats have shown, among other facts, that administration of recombinant Hpx to one kidney results in a reversible, massive proteinuria and morphological changes, similar to those observed in MCD, with a loss of negative charge of the glomerular filtration barrier [41]. Lennon et al. demonstrated that Hpx induces nephrin-dependent reorganization of the cytoskeleton of podocytes by rearranging the actin in their cytoskeleton and reducing the glycocalyx [42]. The authors also found that preincubation of podocytes with plasma from healthy humans significantly reduced the degree of cytoskeletal reorganization after Hpx administration, suggesting that, in patients with MCD lesions, protective plasma factors may be lost, rendering podocytes vulnerable to active Hpx. The aim of our study was to show whether the Hpx levels in serum and urine change in children with INS, which would indirectly indicate their role in the induction of nephrotic proteinuria. In this study, the whole INS group showed significantly increased levels of sHpx and uHpx in the relapse, compared to the control group. In remission, the sHpx and uHpx values decreased, but they were still significantly higher than in healthy children, which may suggest the influence of Hpx on the induction of proteinuria. In our study, we also attempted to measure Hpx in children with nephrotic proteinuria in the course of other glomerulopathies. Our preliminary research showed increased sHpx and uHpx concentrations during the relapse and the remission, and these values were not statistically different from those in the group of children diagnosed with INS (results not published). However, it was a very heterogeneous and small group (10 children) and for this reason, we did not include this group in this study. Despite the fact that our observation is based on a small group of children, it seems interesting in the context of further research on the role of Hpx in the development of proteinuria, not only in INS but also in children with other glomerulopathies.

In the literature, data on this subject are scarce. The results of the only study are not entirely consistent with our observations. Bakker et al., who studied nephrotic syndrome due to MCD in children, showed reduced plasma Hpx levels compared to controls [38]. The lowest values were noted in the relapse [43]. These discrepancies are probably due to the use of different methods for Hpx determination and, in addition, the control group was numerically small and differed in age from the study group. The rocket electrophoresis method was used to determine the plasma Hpx titer using anti-Hx IgG. The authors emphasized that plasma titers could be underestimated due to changed Hpx configurations. On the other hand, the control group of 10 subjects consisted of adults up to 35 years of age, whose Hpx titers did not differ from two control samples of children, whose age was not given. It is worth reminding that serum Hpx level changes with age: in neonates this value constitutes about 20% and in children about 80% of the adult value (i.e., 0.4–1.5 g/L) [44–46]. The fact that children in remission constituted a different group than those in relapse, as well as a lack of data concerning the time when the samples were taken from the moment of achieving remission, also raises doubts. The methods of statistical analysis were not provided either. Regarding urinary Hpx levels, the authors only report that their values in patients in the relapse were higher than in remission, which is consistent with our results, but lower compared to the controls. However, the lack of data on the statistical significance of the differences does not allow us to interpret the results or to compare them with our results. The authors explain the decrease in plasma Hpx levels in the acute phase of MCD by a possible change in the configuration of the Hpx molecule into an isoform exhibiting protease activity. In fact, they found a marked increase in it by examining the expression of ecto-apyrase, an indicator of glomerular extracellular matrix damage, after prior incubation of kidney sections in plasma from children with nephrotic range proteinuria. In contrast, protease activity was not demonstrated after using plasma from patients with MCD in remission and plasma from healthy subjects. What is the explanation for the increase of Hpx concentration in MCD? Hpx is mainly produced by the liver as an acute phase protein after stimulation with post-inflammatory cytokines, including IL-1 and IL-6, and reflects activation of the inflammatory cascade [47]. In this study no correlation between Hpx and CRP was found, which does not exclude its hepatic synthesis by other inflammatory factors. Indeed, IL-6 levels have been shown to increase in MCD relapse, both in adults and children [48,49].

Hpx can also be partially released into the circulation from glomerular mesangial cells, as evidenced by the observations of Kapajos et al. [50]. Indeed, they demonstrated the presence of Hpx in the supernatant of glomerular mesangial cells collected from healthy individuals after prior incubation with TNF-alpha. It is likely that the local production of Hpx by these cells also acts directly on the glomerular filtration barrier, including podocytes. In our study, the fact that shortly after reaching remission Hpx levels, although lower than in relapse, do not normalize, indicates that pathological processes have not been fully silenced.

This is a premise for the continuation of treatment. From the previously presented experimental studies, it is clear that Hpx affects the permeability of the glomerular filtration barrier and leads to proteinuria. Therefore, one would expect a relationship between the tested glycoprotein and proteinuria. However, no such correlation was demonstrated. This may be due to the small size of the study group. The relationship between serum Hpx and proteinuria was demonstrated by Krikken et al. in their study of 557 renal transplant recipients at risk of graft loss. They demonstrated significantly higher proteinuria in patients with higher plasma Hpx levels and more rapid dysfunction of the transplanted kidney compared with patients with lower Hpx values. Although multivariate analysis showed that this glycoprotein is also an independent risk factor for kidney allograft loss, according to the authors increased permeability of glomerular filtration barrier to proteins is important; proteinuria is a recognized modifiable factor in the progression of chronic kidney disease [51].

Considering the division of patients according to the number of relapses (first occurrence of INS vs. subsequent relapses of INS, treated with GCS), it was shown that serum Hpx levels in relapse and remission are similar, whereas urinary Hpx levels in remission are significantly higher in children with subsequent relapses compared to patients with first episode of INS. To the best of our knowledge, this is the first observation of this kind, probably related to shorter intervals between relapses, which are not sufficient to silence the disorganization of the glomerular filtration barrier. Similar observations were made by Pukajło and Zwolińska, who studied the same groups of children with INS in relation to IL-13—a circulating factor considered a significant enhancer of glomerular permeability in MCD [52].

Taking into account the division according to a more or less intensive therapy, it was demonstrated that serum Hpx concentration, both in relapse and remission, is similar in both groups, contrary to its urinary values. Urinary Hpx excretion was significantly higher in relapse than in remission in children treated only with GCS. This is also the first observation of this kind. Perhaps, during relapse in the group receiving additional immunosuppressive drugs, it is related to a greater suppression of immunocompetent cells with a subsequent decrease in the production of cytokines involved in the pathogenesis of MCD, according to the "two-hit" theory. In turn, increased uHpx in remission could be explained by the persistence of higher local levels of these cytokines in children receiving combination therapy. This hypothesis is supported, among other factors, by the higher urinary IL-13 levels in this group of patients during remission; however, it should be emphasized that they are significantly lower in relation to the values in relapse [52].

Correlation studies on Hpx and biochemical markers of nephrotic syndrome did not show significant associations in the whole group of patients.

As mentioned above, the expected correlation between proteinuria and Hpx was not found in any of the study groups. The explanation of this fact may be, apart from the small number of patients, the influence of other circulating factors, including cytokines, which interact leading to one goal. The link between Hpx and the cytokine network is supported by the results of numerous studies, concerning inflammatory processes, including sepsis [53,54], as well as the aforementioned observations presented by Kapajos et al. [45].

This study has several limitations. Firstly, it is a single center study and the group size is limited. We are aware that the number of children in the control group is relatively small. However, it should be noted that small differences in values of Hpx, both in the serum and urine, between the healthy subjects were shown. Secondly, the subgroup receiving combination therapy is rather heterogenic. However, pediatric nephrologists are familiar with the difficulty of selecting a homogeneous group among children with steroid-dependent and frequent-relapsing INS, requiring alternative treatment. Third, our study is a retrospective study. A long-term prospective study would be necessary to confirm our suggestion concerning the role of Hpx as a disease predictor. It would be very valuable to compare the dynamics of Hpx concentrations at the first onset of the disease and at each subsequent relapse in a single patient, and then to analyze the results in groups depending on the number of relapses. We hope that our current results will encourage the programming of further research in this area.

7. Conclusions

The increased sHpx and uHpx levels in relapse of INS, as well as their significant decrease in remission, suggest the role of this circulating factor in the pathogenesis of nephrotic range proteinuria. Maintenance of elevated sHpx and uHpx values just after reaching remission speak to the persistence of immune system activation and the need for further treatment. Increased uHpx concentration in children with subsequent relapses, when compared to patients with the first INS episode, may be a useful prognostic marker of the course of INS and an indicator for continuation of immunosuppressive treatment.

Further prospective studies are needed to confirm our results and to concern Hpx as a target for alternative therapy. We are aware that the pathogenesis of INS is complex and that new factors involved in this process are constantly being sought. Our work is part of the research on new pathogenetic links that may enrich therapeutic solutions in the future.

Author Contributions: A.P.-M.: conception, study design, collection and interpretation of data, and manuscript writing; D.Z.: conception, interpretation of data, revision of the manuscript. All authors have read and agreed to the published version of the manuscript.

Funding: This work was financed by a grant from the Wroclaw Medical University, Poland (grant number: Pbmn35).

Institutional Review Board Statement: Not applicable.

Informed Consent Statement: Informed consent was obtained from all subjects (≥ 16 years) and their representatives involved in the study.

Data Availability Statement: Not applicable.

Conflicts of Interest: All the authors declared no conflict of interest.

References

1. Lipska-Ziętkiewicz, B.S.; Ozaltin, F.; Hölttä, T.; Bockenhauer, D.; Bérody, S.; Levtchenko, E.; Vivarelli, M.; Webb, H.; Haffner, D.; Schaefer, F.; et al. Genetic aspects of congenital nephrotic syndrome: A consensus statement from the ERKNet-ESPN inherited glomerulopathy working group. *Eur. J. Hum. Genet.* **2020**, *28*, 1368–1378. [CrossRef]
2. Giliberti, M.; Mitrotti, A.; Gesualdo, L. Podocytes: The Role of Lysosomes in the Development of Nephrotic Syndrome. *Am. J. Pathol.* **2020**, *190*, 1172–1174. [CrossRef]
3. Shima, Y.; Nakanishi, K.; Sato, M.; Hama, T.; Mukaiyama, H.; Togawa, H.; Tanaka, R.; Nozu, K.; Sako, M.; Iijima, K.; et al. IgA nephropathy with presentation of nephrotic syndrome at onset in children. *Pediatr. Nephrol.* **2016**, *32*, 457–465. [CrossRef]
4. Peruzzi, L.; Coppo, R. IgA vasculitis nephritis in children and adults: One or different entities? *Pediatr. Nephrol.* **2020**, *20*. [CrossRef]
5. Pinheiro, S.V.B.; Dias, R.; Fabiano, R.C.G.; Araujo, S.D.A.; e Silva, A.C.S. Pediatric lupus nephritis. *Braz. J. Nephrol.* **2019**, *41*, 252–265. [CrossRef]
6. Nephrotic syndrome in children: Prediction of histopathology from clinical and laboratory characteristics at time of diagnosis. A report of the International Study of Kidney Disease in Children. Available online: https://pubmed.ncbi.nlm.nih.gov/713276/ (accessed on 30 May 2021).
7. KDIGO Clinical Practice Guideline for Glomerulonephritis. Available online: https://kdigo.org/wp-content/uploads/2017/02/KDIGO-2012-GN-Guideline-English.pdf (accessed on 30 May 2021).
8. Lombel, R.M.; Gipson, D.; Hodson, E.M. Treatment of steroid-sensitive nephrotic syndrome: New guidelines from KDIGO. *Pediatr. Nephrol.* **2013**, *28*, 415–426. [CrossRef] [PubMed]
9. Mendonça, A.C.Q.; Oliveira, E.A.; Fróes, B.P.; Faria, L.D.C.; Pinto, J.S.; Nogueira, M.M.I.; Lima, G.O.; Resende, P.I.; Assis, N.S.; e Silva, A.C.S.; et al. A predictive model of progressive chronic kidney disease in idiopathic nephrotic syndrome. *Pediatr. Nephrol.* **2015**, *30*, 2011–2020. [CrossRef] [PubMed]
10. Chen, J.; Qiao, X.-H.; Mao, J.-H. Immunopathogenesis of idiopathic nephrotic syndrome in children: Two sides of the coin. *World J. Pediatr.* **2021**, *17*, 115–122. [CrossRef] [PubMed]
11. Shalhoub, R. PATHOGENESIS OF LIPOID NEPHROSIS: A DISORDER OF T-CELL FUNCTION. *Lancet* **1974**, *304*, 556–560. [CrossRef]
12. Garin, E.H.; West, L.; Zheng, W. Effect of interleukin-8 on glomerular sulfated compounds and albuminuria. *Pediatr. Nephrol.* **1997**, *11*, 274–279. [CrossRef] [PubMed]
13. Souto, M.F.O.; Teixeira, A.L.; Russo, R.C.; Penido, M.-G.M.G.; Silveira, K.D.; Teixeira, M.M.; e Silva, A.C.S. Immune Mediators in Idiopathic Nephrotic Syndrome: Evidence for a Relation Between Interleukin 8 and Proteinuria. *Pediatr. Res.* **2008**, *64*, 637–642. [CrossRef] [PubMed]
14. Lai, K.-W.; Wei, C.-L.; Tan, L.-K.; Tan, P.-H.; Chiang, G.S.; Lee, C.; Jordan, S.C.; Yap, H.K. Overexpression of Interleukin-13 Induces Minimal-Change–Like Nephropathy in Rats. *J. Am. Soc. Nephrol.* **2007**, *18*, 1476–1485. [CrossRef]
15. Reiser, J.; Mundel, P. Danger signaling by glomerular podocytes defines a novel function of inducible B7-1 in the pathogenesis of nephrotic syndrome. *J. Am. Soc. Nephrol.* **2004**, *15*, 2246–2248. [CrossRef]
16. Shimada, M.; Araya, C.; Rivard, C.; Ishimoto, T.; Johnson, R.J.; Garin, E.H. Minimal change disease: A "two-hit" podocyte immune disorder? *Pediatr. Nephrol.* **2011**, *26*, 645–649. [CrossRef] [PubMed]
17. Cara-Fuentes, G.; Wasserfall, C.H.; Wang, H.; Johnson, R.J.; Garin, E.H. Minimal change disease: A dysregulation of the podocyte CD80–CTLA-4 axis? *Pediatr. Nephrol.* **2014**, *29*, 2333–2340. [CrossRef]
18. Kim, J.E.; Park, S.J.; Ha, T.S.; Shin, J.I. Effect of rituximab in MCNS: A role for IL-13 suppression? *Nat. Rev. Nephrol.* **2013**, *9*, 551. [CrossRef] [PubMed]
19. Davin, J.-C. The glomerular permeability factors in idiopathic nephrotic syndrome. *Pediatr. Nephrol.* **2015**, *31*, 207–215. [CrossRef]
20. Wei, C.; Trachtman, H.; Li, J.; Dong, C.; Friedman, A.L.; Gassman, J.J.; McMahan, J.L.; Radeva, M.; Heil, K.M.; Trautmann, A.; et al. PodoNet and FSGS CT Study Consortia. Circulating suPAR in Two Cohorts of Primary FSGS. *J. Am. Soc. Nephrol.* **2012**, *23*, 2051–2059. [CrossRef]

21. Li, F.; Zheng, C.; Zhong, Y.; Zeng, C.; Xu, F.; Yin, R.; Jiang, Q.; Zhou, M.; Liu, Z.-H. Relationship between Serum Soluble Urokinase Plasminogen Activator Receptor Level and Steroid Responsiveness in FSGS. *Clin. J. Am. Soc. Nephrol.* **2014**, *9*, 1903–1911. [CrossRef]
22. Wada, T.; Nangaku, M. A circulating permeability factor in focal segmental glomerulosclerosis: The hunt continues. *Clin. Kidney J.* **2015**, *8*, 708–715. [CrossRef]
23. Cara-Fuentes, G.; Wei, C.; Segarra, A.; Ishimoto, T.; Rivard, C.; Johnson, R.J.; Reiser, J.; Garin, E.H. CD80 and suPAR in patients with minimal change disease and focal segmental glomerulosclerosis: Diagnostic and pathogenic significance. *Pediatr. Nephrol.* **2014**, *29*, 1363–1371. [CrossRef]
24. Muller-Eberhard, U. Hemopexin. *Methods Enzymol.* **1998**, *163*, 536–568. [CrossRef] [PubMed]
25. Naylor, S.L.; Altruda, F.; Marshall, A.; Silengo, L.; Bowman, B.H. Hemopexin is localized to human chromosome 11. *Somat. Cell Mol. Genet.* **1987**, *13*, 355–358. [CrossRef] [PubMed]
26. Altruda, F.; Poli, V.; Restagno, G.; Silengo, L. Structure of the human hemopexin gene and evidence for intron-mediated evolution. *J. Mol. Evol.* **1988**, *27*, 102–108. [CrossRef] [PubMed]
27. Takahasi, N.; Takahashi, Y.; Putnam, F.W. Complete aminoacid sequence of human hemopexin, the heme-binding protein of serum. *Proc. Natl. Acid. Sci. USA* **1985**, *82*, 73–77. [CrossRef] [PubMed]
28. Smith, A. Role of Redox-Reactive Metals in the Regulation of Metallothionein and Hemeoxygenase Genes by Heme and Hemopexin. In *Iron Metabolism*; Ferreira, G.C., Moura, J.J.G., Franco, R., Eds.; Wiley-VCH: Weinheim, Germany, 1999; pp. 65–92.
29. Delanghe, J.R.; Langlois, M.R. Hemopexin: A review of biological aspects and the role in laboratory medicine. *Clin. Chim. Acta* **2001**, *312*, 13–23. [CrossRef]
30. Bernard, A.; Amor, A.O.; Goemare-Vanneste, J.; Antoine, J.-L.; Lauwerys, R.; Colin, I.; Vandeleene, B.; Lambert, A. Urinary proteins and red blood cell membrane negative charges in diabetes mellitus. *Clin. Chim. Acta* **1990**, *190*, 249–262. [CrossRef]
31. Chen, C.-C.; Lu, Y.-C.; Chen, Y.-W.; Lee, W.-L.; Lu, C.-H.; Chen, Y.-H.; Lee, Y.-C.; Lin, S.-T.; Timms, J.; Lee, Y.-R.; et al. Hemopexin is up-regulated in plasma from type 1 diabetes mellitus patients: Role of glucose-induced ROS. *J. Proteom.* **2012**, *75*, 3760–3777. [CrossRef]
32. Maes, M.; Delange, J.; Ranjan, R.; Meltzer, H.Y.; Desnyder, R.; Cooremans, W.; Scharpé, S. Acute phase proteins in schizophrenia, mania and major depression: Modulation by psychotropic drugs. *Psychiatry Res.* **1997**, *66*, 1–11. [CrossRef]
33. Manuel, Y.; Defontaine, M.; Bourgoin, J.; Dargent, M.; Sonneck, J. Serum haemopexin levels in patients with malignant melanoma. *Clin. Chim. Acta* **1971**, *31*, 485–486. [CrossRef]
34. Percy, M.E.; Pichora, G.A.; Chang, L.S.; Manchester, K.E.; Andrews, D.F.; Opitz, J.M. Serum myoglobin in Duchenne muscular dystrophy carrier detection: A comparison with creatine kinase and hemopexin using logistic discrimination. *Am. J. Med. Genet.* **1984**, *18*, 279–287. [CrossRef]
35. International Study of Kidney Disease in Children. Primary nephrotic syndrome in children: Clinical significance of histopathologic variants of minimal change and of diffuse mesangial hypercellularity. A Report of the International Study of Kidney Disease in Children. *Kidney Int.* **1981**, *20*, 765–771. [CrossRef]
36. Schwartz, G.J.; Muñoz, A.; Schneider, M.F.; Mak, R.H.; Kaskel, F.; Warady, B.A.; Furth, S.L. New Equations to Estimate GFR in Children with CKD. *J. Am. Soc. Nephrol.* **2009**, *20*, 629–637. [CrossRef] [PubMed]
37. Cheung, P.K.; Boes, A.; Dijkhuis, F.W.J.; Klok, P.A.; Bakker, W.W. Enhanced glomerular permeability andminimal change disease like alterations of the rat kidney indced by a vasoactive human plasma factor. *Kidney Int.* **1995**, *47*, 1218.
38. Cheung, P.K.; Klok, P.A.; Bakker, W.W. Induction of experimental proteinuria in vivo following infusion of a human stain factor associated with minimal change disease. *Kidney Int.* **1997**, *52*, 562.
39. Cheung, P.K.; Klok, P.A.; Bakker, W.W. Minimal change-like glomerular alterations induced by a human plasma factor. *Nephron* **1996**, *74*, 586–593. [CrossRef]
40. Cheung, P.K.; Stulp, B.; Immenschuh, S.; Borghuis, T.; Baller, J.F.W.; Bakker, W.W. Is 100KF an Isoform of Hemopexin? Immunochemical Characterization of the Vasoactive Plasma Factor 100KF. *J. Am. Soc. Nephrol.* **1999**, *10*, 1700–1708. [CrossRef] [PubMed]
41. Bakker, W.W.; Borghuis, T.; Harmsen, M.; Berg, A.V.D.; Kema, I.P.; Niezen, K.E.; Kapojos, J.J. Protease activity of plasma hemopexin. *Kidney Int.* **2005**, *68*, 603–610. [CrossRef]
42. Lennon, R.; Singh, A.; Welsh, G.I.; Coward, R.; Satchell, S.; Ni, L.; Mathieson, P.W.; Bakker, W.W.; Saleem, M.A. Hemopexin Induces Nephrin-Dependent Reorganization of the Actin Cytoskeleton in Podocytes. *J. Am. Soc. Nephrol.* **2008**, *19*, 2140–2149. [CrossRef] [PubMed]
43. Bakker, W.W.; Van Dael, C.M.L.; Pierik, L.J.W.M.; Van Wijk, J.A.E.; Nauta, J.; Borghuis, T.; Kapojos, J.J. Altered activity of plasma hemopexin in patients with minimal change disease in relapse. *Pediatr. Nephrol.* **2005**, *20*, 1410–1415. [CrossRef]
44. Thomas, L. Haptoglobin/Hemopexin. In *Clinical Laboratory Diagnostics*; Thomas, L., Ed.; TH-Books: Frankfurt/Main, Germany, 1998; pp. 663–667.
45. Kanakoudi, F.; Drossou, V.; Tzimouli, V.; Diamanti, E.; Konstantinidis, T.; Germenis, A.; Kremenopoulos, G. Serum concentrations of 10 acute-phase proteins in healthy term and preterm infants from birth to age 6 months. *Clin. Chem.* **1995**, *41*, 605–608. [CrossRef]
46. Weeke, B.; Krasilnikoff, P.A. The concentration of 21 serum proteins in normal children and adults. *Acta Med. Scand.* **2009**, *192*, 149–155. [CrossRef]

47. Tolosano, E.; Altruda, F. Hemopexin: Structure, Function, and Regulation. *DNA Cell Biol.* **2002**, *21*, 297–306. [CrossRef] [PubMed]
48. Oniszczuk, J.; Beldi-Ferchiou, A.; Audureau, E.; Azzaoui, I.; Molinier-Frenkel, V.; Frontera, V.; Karras, A.; Moktefi, A.; Pillebout, E.; Zaidan, M.; et al. Circulating plasmablasts and high level of BAFF are hallmarks of minimal change nephrotic syndrome in adults. *Nephrol. Dial. Transplant.* **2021**, *36*, 609–617. [CrossRef]
49. Nickavar, A.; Valavi, E.; Safaeian, B.; Amoori, P.; Moosavian, M. Predictive Value of Serum Interleukins in Children with Idiopathic Nephrotic Syndrome. *Iran. J. Allergy Asthma Immunol.* **2020**, *19*, 632–639. [CrossRef]
50. Kapojos, J.J.; Berg, A.V.D.; van Goor, H.; Loo, M.W.T.; Poelstra, K.; Borghuis, T.; Bakker, W.W. Production of hemopexin by TNF-α stimulated human mesangial cells. *Kidney Int.* **2003**, *63*, 1681–1686. [CrossRef] [PubMed]
51. Krikken, J.A.; Van Ree, R.M.; Klooster, A.; Seelen, M.A.; Borghuis, T.; Lems, S.P.M.; Schouten, J.P.; Bakker, W.W.; Gans, R.; Navis, G.; et al. High plasma hemopexin activity is an independent risk factor for late graft failure in renal transplant recipients. *Transpl. Int.* **2010**, *23*, 805–812. [CrossRef] [PubMed]
52. Pukajło-Marczyk, A.; Zwolińska, D. The role of IL-13 in the pathogenesis of idiopathic nephrotic syndrome (INS) in children. *Fam. Med. Prim. Care Rev.* **2016**, *2*, 149–154. [CrossRef]
53. Liang, X.; Lin, T.; Sun, G.; Beasley-Topliffe, L.; Cavaillon, J.-M.; Warren, H.S. Hemopexin down-regulates LPS-induced proinflammatory cytokines from macrophages. *J. Leukoc. Biol.* **2009**, *86*, 229–235. [CrossRef] [PubMed]
54. Lin, T.; Kwak, Y.H.; Sammy, F.; He, P.; Thundivalappil, S.; Sun, G.; Chao, W.; Warren, H.S. Synergistic Inflammation Is Induced by Blood Degradation Products with Microbial Toll-Like Receptor Agonists and Is Blocked by Hemopexin. *J. Infect. Dis.* **2010**, *202*, 624–632. [CrossRef]

Article

An Examination of the Relationship between Urinary Neurotrophin Concentrations and Transcutaneous Electrical Nerve Stimulation (TENS) Used in Pediatric Overactive Bladder Therapy

Joanna Bagińska *, Edyta Sadowska and Agata Korzeniecka-Kozerska

Department of Pediatrics and Nephrology, Medical University of Białystok, 17 Waszyngtona Str., 15-274 Białystok, Poland; iklinped@umb.edu.pl (E.S.); agatakozerska@poczta.onet.pl (A.K.-K.)
* Correspondence: joasiabaginska14@wp.pl

Abstract: This article aims to explore changes in urinary concentrations of selected neurotrophins in the course of TENS therapy in children with overactive bladder (OAB). A two-group open-label prospective study was conducted. The intervention group comprised 30 children aged between 5 and 12 years old with OAB refractory to conservative therapy. They received 12 weeks of TENS therapy in a home setting. The urinary neurotrophins, NGF, BDNF, NT3, NT4, were measured by ELISA at baseline and at the end of the TENS therapy. Total urinary neurotrophins levels were standardized to mg of creatinine (Cr). We compared the results with the reference group of 30 participants with no symptoms of bladder overactivity. The results revealed that children with OAB both before and after TENS therapy had higher NGF, BDNF, and NT4 concentrations in total and after normalization to Cr than the reference group in contrast to NT3. The response to the therapy expressed as a decrease of urinary neurotrophins after TENS depended on the age and the presenting symptoms. In conclusion, children older than 8 years of age with complaints of daytime incontinence responded better to TENS.

Keywords: neurotrophins; transcutaneous electrical nerve stimulation; overactive bladder

1. Introduction

Urinary incontinence is a frequent problem in pediatrics with increasing evidence that this is the second most common chronic condition of childhood after the atopy/allergy complex with a great impact on quality of life [1]. Overactive bladder (OAB) is the main cause of wetting in children defined by the International Children's Continence Society (ICCS) as urinary urgency usually accompanied by frequency and nocturia, with or without urinary incontinence, in the absence of a urinary tract infection or other obvious pathology [2]. Although OAB is a widespread problem, the pathophysiology is still unclear. It is likely multifactorial but increasing recent evidence supports a central role of disturbed brain and bladder connection [3,4]. Previously, everything was concentrated only around the bladder. It has become apparent that the management of this problem should be based on the foundation that this is a delay in the children's nervous system maturation. The available data indicate that pediatric OAB syndrome and many voiding dysfunctions may be part of a more generalized problem that affects multiple systems, notably, the bladder, bowels, and nervous system [5]. Several neurotransmitters have been identified in afferent nerves, including the family of neurotrophins: nerve growth factor receptors (NGF), brain derived neurotrophic factor (BDNF), neurotrophin-3 (NT3), and neurotrophin-4 (NT4). They play an important role in the plasticity of afferent nerves and spinal micturition pathways controlling bladder function [6], but the relationships between them and OAB have not been thoroughly investigated.

Most studies have compared urinary neurotrophin levels in OAB before and after pharmacological treatment. Antimuscarinic agents are currently the mainstay of OAB therapy. The reported rate of response is high and equals 70% to 80%, but the rate of complete symptom resolution is much lower and ranges from 14% to 35%. Urinary NGF and BDNF constitute the most well-studied neurotrophins as predictive biomarkers to assess the therapeutic outcome of antimuscarinic treatment. In the last decade, several studies on NGF were conducted in the adult population [7–9] with the same conclusions that urinary NGF levels are higher in patients with OAB when compared with a reference group, and decreased in response to anticholinergics. Antunes-Lopes et al. [10] found that urinary BDNF was increased in OAB patients at the baseline and were highly sensitive to OAB treatment with antimuscarinic agents. In addition, a strong correlation was found between the decrease of urinary BDNF concentration and the reduction in the number of urgency episodes per week. Several papers [11–13] on the pediatric population have appeared in recent years confirming previous observations that urinary NGF and BDNF could not only be potential biomarkers for children with OAB but also predictors of therapeutic efficacy. Interestingly, urinary levels of NGF and BDNF decreased upon OAB management, including not only pharmacological treatment but also lifestyle interventions [10] and detrusor injection of botulinum toxin A [14].

With the progress of medicine, novel efficacious options have emerged in the last decade in the management of OAB. Transcutaneous electrical nerve stimulation (TENS) is one of them and has become a subject of great interest [15]. TENS is based on neuromodulation, a process which regulates nervous system activity by controlling the physiological levels of neurotransmitters. Surprisingly, to the best of our knowledge, the relationship between neurotrophins and TENS efficacy in OAB has not been described. TENS has been used for pain control for several decades and provides relief to a remarkable number of patients affected by chronic pain. However, its value has been expanding in recent times due to rapid improvements in neuromodulation technologies, as well as research revealing more potential uses for this form of treatment. TENS has shown to be efficacious and has become a new tool in lower urinary tract dysfunction therapies [16]. According to the ICCS guidelines, the main indication for TENS in pediatrics is OAB refractory to the first line of treatment.

The exact mechanism of TENS action is unknown. There is a clear need to fill this knowledge gap. We aimed to pursue investigations of the changes in urinary concentrations of neurotrophins in pediatric patients with refractory OAB during TENS therapy. Based on the evidence available, we are not able to completely understand the pathophysiology of OAB as well as the exact mechanism of TENS action. The objective of this paper was to find a relationship between neurotrophins and TENS, which may help us to better understand the role of the nervous system in the pathophysiologic mechanisms responsible for OAB in childhood and the neurochemical pathways connecting the brain and bladder.

To the best of our knowledge, our study represents the first investigation of the relationships between TENS therapy and neurotrophins. The role of neurotransmitters excreted in the urine as biomarkers of the effectiveness of TENS therapy in children reporting OAB symptoms has not been described. The research at hand aimed to systematically describing how TENS influences the concentrations of neurotrophins and the clinical outcome in children with OAB. The detailed research goals included:

Research Objective 1. To compare urinary neurotrophin concentrations between children with OAB and healthy participants.

Hypothesis 1 (H1). *The urinary level of neurotrophins will be elevated in children with OAB compared with healthy participants.*

Research Objective 2. To establish the effects of TENS therapy on urinary concentrations of neurotrophins in the management of refractory OAB in children.

Hypothesis 2 (H2). *TENS therapy will result in decreasing urinary concentration of neurotrophins in children with refractory OAB.*

2. Materials and Methods

2.1. Participants

The open-label prospective study was conducted in 60 children (30 with OAB and 30 controls) aged between 5 and 17 years old between September 2020 and May 2021. To be eligible to enter the study, participants met the inclusion criteria presented in detail in Table 1. All 30 children with OAB had discontinued medical treatment with anticholinergics due to side effects or inefficacy and were off medical treatment for at least three months. Participants to the reference group were recruited to the study as children-volunteers of the hospital staff.

Table 1. Criteria for enrollment to the study.

	Inclusion Criteria	Exclusion Criteria
Study group	- Age 5–18 years old with a clinical diagnosis of OAB with urodynamically proven detrusor overactivity - Refractory to standard urotherapy and pharmacotherapy with anticholinergics for at least 3 months - Normal physical examination and unremarkable urinary tract ultrasound	- Neurogenic bladder dysfunction - Anatomical abnormalities of the urinary or gastrointestinal track - Prior urinary tract surgery - Constipation according to Rome III criteria - Recurrent UTI within the last 3 months - High bladder capacity (>150% of expected bladder capacity) - Pacemakers or implantable defibrillators - Current urinary tract or vaginal infection - Lack of child's cooperation
Reference group	- Age 5–18 years old with no urinary and nervous system problems - Normal physical examination and unremarkable urinary tract ultrasound	- Anatomical abnormalities of the urinary or gastrointestinal track - Recurrent UTI within the last 3 months - Current urinary tract or vaginal infection

2.2. Intervention—TENS Treatment and Follow-Up Assessment

The intervention group received 12 weeks of TENS therapy in a home setting with a control visit after 4 and 8 weeks. Prior to starting the TENS therapy, the children in collaboration with their caregivers provided their medical history and underwent physical examination. Then they were thoroughly instructed on how to handle the TENS stimulator at home. A double-channel stimulator (Premier Stim Plus DIGITAL EM-6300) was used with 50×50 mm adhesive electrodes placed on the skin at the level of S2 to S3. A 2 Hz frequency was used with a 150 s pulse duration. The children were instructed to use the highest tolerable intensity up to a maximum of 40 mA. Sessions were performed once a day, every day for 2 h. During each follow-up, bladder diary, 48 h volume, and frequency charts were analyzed. After 12 weeks of treatment, TENS was discontinued in all patients. Throughout the study, the treatment was well-tolerated and no adverse events were reported.

2.3. Biochemistry

Urine samples of 10 mL were obtained as free-voided samples at the beginning and at the end of the TENS therapy in the intervention group and once in the reference group. Voided urine was put on ice immediately and transferred to the laboratory for preparation. The samples were centrifuged at 4000 rpm for 10 min at 4 °C. The supernatant was separated into aliquots in 2 mL tubes and preserved at −80 °C until measurements. Another 2 mL urine was stored separately to measure creatinine (Cr) levels.

NGF, BDNF, NT3, NT4 concentrations were determined using the immunoassay system for NGF (SEA105Hu, Cloud-Clone Corp., Wuhan, China), BDNF (SEA011Hu,

Cloud-Clone Corp., Wuhan, China), NT3 (SEA106Hu, Cloud-Clone Corp., Wuhan, China), NT4 (SEA107Hu, Cloud-Clone Corp., Wuhan, China) with a specific and highly sensitive ELISA kit, which had a minimum sensitivity of 5.4 pg/mL for NGF, 11.6 pg/mL for BDNF, 5.7 pg/mL for NT3, and 6.0 pg/mL for NT4. Assays were performed according to the manufacturer's instructions. All kit components and samples were brought to room temperature. Then, 100 µL of NGF/BDNF/NT3/NT4 standards, blank and urine was added to the appropriate wells, covered, and incubated for 1 h at 37 °C. Next, 100 µL of biotin antibody was added to each well, covered, and incubated for 1 h at 37 °C. After incubation, plates was washed three times and 100 µL of streptavidin solution was added to each well. The plate was incubated for 30 min at 37 °C and after incubation was washed five times. Then, tetra methyl benzidine (TMB) reactive substrate was added to the wells and incubated for about 30 min until the color development was visualized. Then, a stop solution was added and the plates were read at 450 nm with an ELISA reader.

The concentration of urinary Cr was measured using the calorimetric method by Jaffe (Cobas 6000 C501). The results were expressed as the total concentration of measured urine markers in pg/mL and were also divided by urinary Cr (mg/mL) for standardization as NGF/Cr, BDNF/Cr, NT3/Cr, NT4/Cr ratios.

2.4. Statistics

The data were collected in a Microsoft Excel database. Statistical analysis was performed using Statistica 13.0 (StatSoft Inc, Tulsa, OK, USA). Continuous variables were expressed as median and range, unless stated otherwise. All studied parameters were analyzed using nonparametric tests: Mann–Whitney, Kruskal–Wallis and chi-squared test. Correlations were assessed with the Spearman test. Values of $p < 0.05$ were considered significant.

2.5. Ethical Issues

This study was approved by the Ethics Committee of the Medical University of Bialystok (R-I-002/602/2019) which complies with the World Medical Association Declaration of Helsinki regarding ethical conduct of research involving human subjects and/or animals. All participants were given detailed information about the content of the study and all caregivers signed an informed consent form before initiation of the study.

3. Results

A detailed outline of the organization of the study is presented in Figure 1. We screened 70 participants: 40 to the study group and 30 to the reference group. We excluded 10 patients because they did not have OAB proven by urodynamic study, the diagnosis was made only on the basis of the patient's symptoms.

The patients' clinical characteristics are presented in Table 2. There were no differences in the age, weight, height, or sex between the study and the reference group.

In comparison between the groups before and after TENS therapy, statistically significant differences were observed in the parameters obtained from bladder diaries and volume/frequency charts including the number of wet nights during a 30-day period with a median of 8 (0–30) before TENS in contrast to 3.5 (0–30) after TENS, the voiding frequency from 7.5 (5–23) to 5 (4–9) and minimum voided volume from 50 mL (15–130) to 80 mL (25–250) ($p = 0.041$, $p = 0.029$, $p = 0.022$, respectively; $p < 0.05$). No statistically significant differences were noted in maximal voided volume with a median of 195 mL (95–500 mL) before TENS and 190 mL (90–370 mL) after therapy ($p = 0.53$; $p < 0.05$).

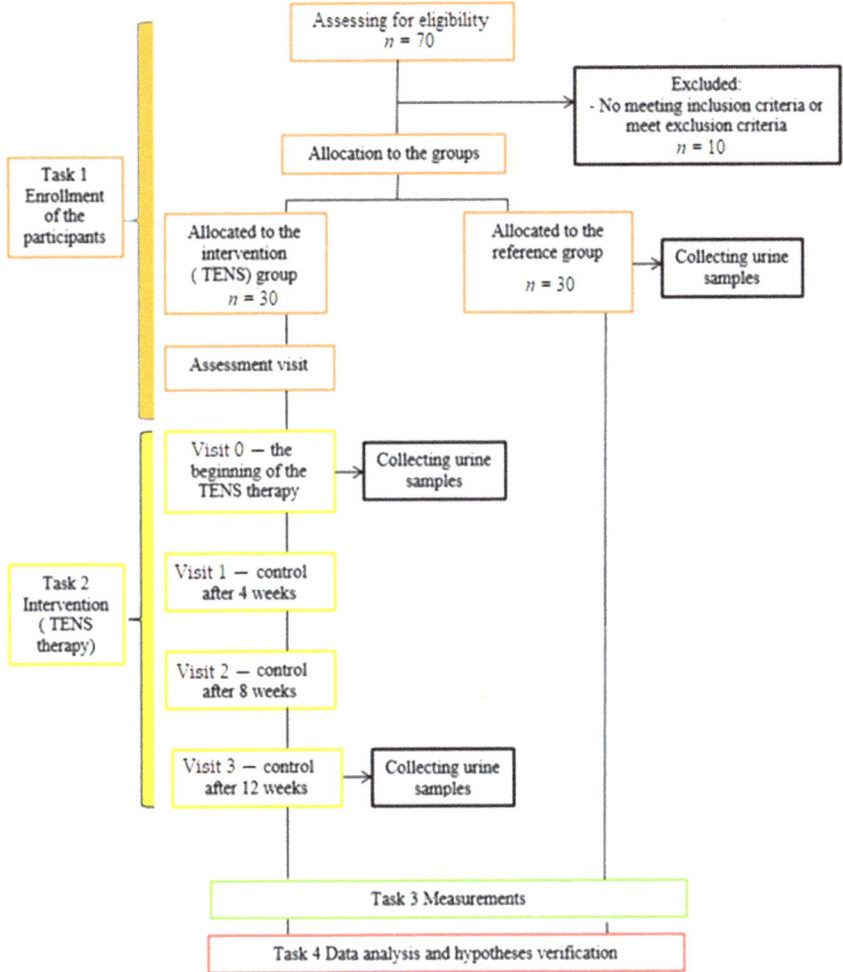

Figure 1. Outline of the organization of the study.

The comparison of urinary neurotrophins revealed that children with OAB both before and after TENS therapy had higher NGF, BDNF, and NT4 concentrations in total and after normalization to Cr than the reference group, in contrast to NT3, which in total was lower in the study group but after normalization to Cr showed the same tendency. The differences are graphically presented in Figure 2. Additionally, a statistically significant difference was observed in urinary Cr.

To establish the effects of TENS therapy on urinary concentrations of neurotrophins, we calculated the "delta" values (Δ) for each neurotrophin. The Δ was considered as the changes in the absolute and ratios values of neurotrophins (subtracting the absolute value at baseline from the value at the end of TENS therapy). A Δ > 0 was considered a response to the therapy, while Δ ≤ 0 indicated the failure of the therapy. The Δ values are presented in detail in Table 3.

Table 2. Characteristics of studied patients and comparison between groups.

	OAB Patients		Group C: Reference Group	p-Value		
	Group A: Before TENS	Group B: After TENS		A&B	A&C	B&C
	Median, Range					
Girls/boys (n)	15/15		19/11	-	0.39	0.39
Age (years)	8.7 (5.25–12.3)	8.83 (5.5–12.6)	8.4 (5–17)	0.55	0.85	0.6
Body weight (kg)	29.5 (17–62)		31.5 (15.5–70)	-	0.55	0.55
Height (cm)	134 (110–158)		135 (104–174)	-	0.81	0.81
NGF (pg/mL)	16.7 (5.4–101.3)	17.9 (6.33–103)	12.7 (6.3–73.7)	0.98	0.14	0.04 *
BDNF (pg/mL)	12.7 (11.3–189.9)	24.6 (11.3–515.3)	12.7 (11.3–40.8)	0.03 *	0.01 *	<0.001 *
NT4 (pg/mL)	107.9 (6–1245)	107.9 (6–2095)	79.4 (6.0–1096)	0.71	0.94	0.52
NT3 (pg/mL)	87 (5.7–1854)	72 (15.9–2934)	216 (17.9–4483)	0.81	0.03 *	0.04 *
Urinary Cr (mg/mL)	0.39 (0.04–2.4)	0.13 (0.04–1.5)	1.29 (0.49–3.32)	0.049 *	<0.001 *	<0.001 *
NGF/Cr (pg/mg)	55.9 (3.3–894.6)	126.5 (5.6–802.5)	7.8 (2.4–68.7)	0.36	<0.001 *	<0.001 *
BDNF/Cr (pg/mg)	49.7 (4.7–536.7)	217.7 (8.7–5725)	11.2 (3.8–44.9)	0.004 *	<0.001 *	<0.001 *
NT4/Cr (pg/mg)	171.8 (11.2–6316)	748.6 (5.7–3958)	52.8 (2.2–664)	0.11	<0.001 *	<0.001 *
NT3/Cr (pg/mg)	379.6 (3.5–3387)	687.5 (10.9–3532)	132.6 (10.8–2312)	0.18	0.36	0.03 *

OAB—overactive bladder, Cr—creatinine, * $p < 0.05$.

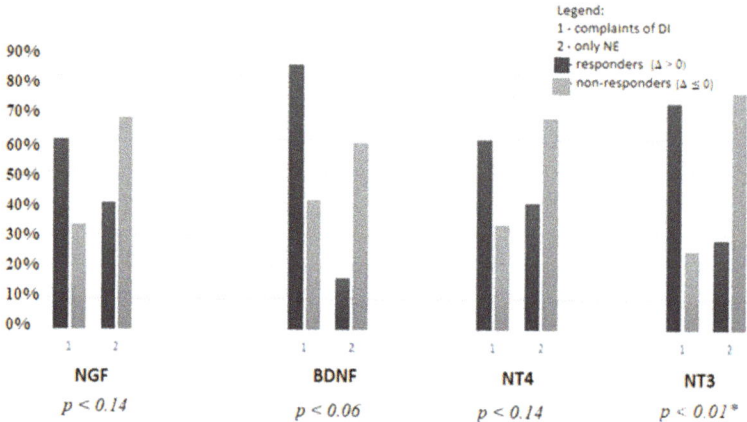

Figure 2. The comparison between response to the TENS therapy expressed as the change of urinary concentrations of neurotrophins in terms of urinary incontinence complaints. DI, daytime incontinence; NE, nocturnal enuresis, * $p < 0.05$.

Table 3. The delta values for each neurotrophin.

The Δ Values (Mean; Median, Range)		Responders/Non-Responders n (%)
NGF	4.38; 0.16 (−97.6–78.2)	15 (50)/15 (50)
BDNF	−45.8; −3.26 (−502–177.3)	7 (23)/23 (77)
NT4	−5.7; 2.63 (−2084–1201)	15 (50)/15 (50)
NT3	−6.97; −1.22 (−2840–1639)	14 (47)/16 (53)
NGF/Cr	30.7; 7.04 (−797–820)	12 (40)/18 (60)
BDNF/Cr	−567; −99 (−5693–219)	7 (23)/23 (77)
NT4/Cr	−173; −158 (−3939–5516)	11 (37)/19 (63)
NT3/Cr	−273; −59 (−2486–2293)	10 (33)/20 (67)

Only in the case of NGF the median Δ was higher than 0. Statistically significant differences were observed in urinary NGF according to age. The median age in children with Δ > 0 was 10.1 years (5.5–12.3) in contrast to 7.8 years (5.3–11) in children with Δ ≤ 0. We divided the cases into two subgroups—children older than 8 years at baseline and children aged 8 years or younger—and compared the response to TENS therapy. Twelve out of 18 (66.7%) children older than 8 years old responded well to the TENS therapy in contrast to 3/12 (25%) children younger than 8 years old. The differences were statistically significant ($\chi^2 = 5.0$, $p = 0.025$; $p < 0.05$).

Moreover, children with complaints of daytime incontinence (DI) had a better response to TENS therapy in contrast to those presenting only with nocturnal enuresis (NE). Differences were noted in the urinary concentrations of all neurotrophins: NGF, BDNF, NT4, and NT3, but only in the case of the last one they were statistically significant ($\chi^2 = 2.14$, $p = 0.14$; $\chi^2 = 3.39$, $p = 0.06$; $\chi^2 = 2.14$, $p = 0.14$; $\chi^2 = 6.47$, $p = 0.01$, respectively), presented in detail in Figure 2.

4. Discussion

To the best of our knowledge, this is the first prospective study evaluating the efficacy of TENS in pediatric OAB with measurement of urinary neurotrophins. A homogeneous sample was chosen, comprising of patients only with confirmed detrusor overactivity in urodynamic examination without pharmacological treatment for at least three months before the intervention.

The literature on the efficacy of neuromodulation techniques in pediatric OAB shows a variety of approaches. At the beginning of the 2000s, the first studies of TENS in the treatment of urinary incontinence in children were done [17–19]. The pilot study was performed by Hoebeke et al. [17] in a group of children with urodynamically proven detrusor overactivity presenting with only DI with promising results, including an increase in cystometric bladder capacity, decrease in urge and incontinence episodes. Similar results were obtained by Bower et al. [18] with the first attempt to assess TENS therapy performed in a home setting. Malm-Buatsi et al. [19] reported a 73% urinary incontinence improvement after TENS therapy in OAB. A key limitation of all the above-mentioned research was that TENS was not the single therapy, the majority of participants continued taking anticholinergics. In the last decade, several controlled studies [20–22] have been conducted. Hagstroem et al. [20] conducted a study in which 27 children with refractory OAB were treated with TENS or sham stimulation for 4 weeks, with the conclusion that TENS had a superior effect to sham treatment, although the percent of responders in the active group was lower than reported previously in uncontrolled research. On the other hand, the results obtained from other controlled research suggested that the effect of neuromodulation in patients receiving urotherapy is marginal [21] and may give a high placebo effect based on the attention given to the child's problem by the caregivers and physicians [22]. Such contradictory results show a need to find a better tool to answer the question of whether TENS is effective or not.

Our observations showed a reduction in the number of wet nights and frequency after TENS therapy. Additionally, an increase of minimum voided volume was recorded. However, the minimum storage after neuromodulation continued to be significantly lower than would be expected for children with no urinary problems. In contrast to some reports [17,18,23], we did not find statistically significant differences in maximal voided volume. It has been hypothesized that an increase in the bladder reservoir is the main mechanism of TENS action. Studies that evaluated the urodynamic parameters immediately after the first session of TENS as well as at the end of the therapeutic period demonstrated that the only urodynamic finding that showed improvement was bladder capacity [24]. Further studies [20,21] provided contradictory results, suggesting that the positive effect of TENS is the result of improved bladder sensation signals. Therefore, a new, reliable, and objective tool for evaluating TENS efficacy and relevant therapeutic outcomes is needed. It is well-described that the electric current stimulates the release of a wide range of neurotransmitters [6,25]. We wanted to take into account a novel theory and check changes in neurotrophins as a potential explanation for the TENS mechanism of action.

4.1. Neurotrophins at Baseline

NGF is the most studied and the best characterized neurotrophin in OAB, especially in the adult population [26]. Nonetheless, few studies have focused on the association between urinary NGF concentrations and OAB symptoms in children. According to the latest systemic review about the role of urinary NGF in pediatric OAB, three case-control studies were published between 2012 and 2017, which included 99 patients and 61 controls [27]. Children with OAB had a significantly higher baseline urinary NGF/Cr compared with controls, which is in accordance with our observations. However, the selected samples were heterogeneous. In 2012, Oktar et al. [11], as one of the first authors to do so, performed a study about the relation between pediatric OAB and NGF in the course of the anticholinergic treatment. However, not all participants had urodynamically confirmed detrusor overactivity. Additionally, the study group comprised patients with primarily diagnosed OAB but also those who had failed antimuscarinic treatment. The results indicated that, following antimuscarinic treatment, urinary NGF/Cr levels were significantly reduced at 6 months but not at 3 months. In 2015, a second study in the pediatric population was conducted in our Department by Korzeniecka-Kozerska et al. [12], with the inclusion criteria of primary diagnosed OAB proven in urodynamics before pharmacological treatment. Our actual study in contrast to the above-mentioned one analyzed NGF concentrations in children with refractory OAB after pharmacological treatment with persistent urinary symptoms. In 2016, another modification was made by adding BDNF as a potential biomarker and the combination of two urinary neurotrophins was measured in 24 patients with newly diagnosed OAB confirmed by urodynamics [13]. In the course of pharmacological treatment, BDNF showed a statistically significant decrease at 3 and 6 months of therapy in contrast to NGF. The authors suggested the use of urinary NGF/Cr as a marker for OAB diagnosis, and BDNF/Cr to evaluate treatment efficacy. The sensitivity and specificity of urinary BDNF levels for OAB patients was significantly higher than for NGF.

In our study we also observed elevated levels of NGF and BDNF in OAB compared with the control group at baseline. On the basis of previous reports [28] we could speculate that the overexpression of neurotrophins in OAB may be due to its extensive production by the urothelium, suburothelium, and the smooth muscle of the urinary tract. It was proven that especially NGF plays a key role in the pathophysiology of OAB, most probably by changing the threshold for bladder sensory neuron response. The increased amount of neurotransmitters substance being released by the urothelium leads to sensory urgency, and ultimately reflex bladder hyperactivity, causing OAB symptoms. Local release of NGF and BDNF by the urothelium was widely proven. The originality of our findings lies in the fact that we also measured two novel members of the neurotrophin family: NT3 and NT4. To our knowledge, an eventual relationship between them and OAB is totally unknown. They were scarcely investigated only from the theoretical point of view. They represent master modulators of neural plasticity, both in the peripheral and central nervous system, comparably to the better-described NGF and BDNF [29]. The role of NT3 and NT4 in the bladder dysfunction has not been described. NGF and BDNF have been identified in the peripheral tissues of the bladder, including the urothelium and detrusor muscles [30]. It has been suggested that NT3 and NT4 might also be expressed in the bladder, although their exact role and location are unclear [31].

In this paper, we proposed measurements of urinary NT3 and NT4 as potential markers of OAB and/or efficacy of TENS therapy. Interestingly, NT4 levels showed the same tendency as NGF and BDNF. At baseline, the total concentration was higher in OAB children than in the controls, but the differences were not statistically significant. After normalization to Cr, the differences were much more noticeable. Interestingly, NT3 acted differently to the others neurotrophins. Total concentrations of NT3 before TENS therapy were lower in the intervention group compared with the controls; whereas, after normalization to Cr, they showed an inverse relation. With a lack of studies on NT3 and urinary dysfunction we may only speculate about the reason. We found data suggesting a role of NT3 in the pathophysiology of nerve functions in diabetic animals with the conclusion that it may play a role in underactive bladder as a consequence of diabetic cystopathy [32,33]. Other studies on neurogenic underactive bladder stressed the role of decreased levels of NGF and NT3 in bladder compartments and afferent nerves as the most important changes leading to detrusor underactivity [34].

We observed statistically significant differences in urinary Cr between the studied groups. Cr differences could not be explained by variations in age and sex distributions across groups. Typically, Cr is thought to be excreted at a normal and constant rate in healthy children, so it is mostly used as a factor for normalization. However, in some studies it was found that the concentration of urinary Cr was highly variable in the adult population with OAB [35]. We decided to concentrate mostly on total levels of neurotrophins in formulating our conclusions.

4.2. Neurotrophins after TENS Therapy

In the whole study group we did not record statistically significant differences in urinary neurotrophins after TENS treatment, except for BDNF concentration, which surprisingly increased. Similarly to previous research on neurotrophins in the course of anticholinergic treatment, we assumed that increases in urinary markers at baseline would significantly diminish following TENS. Nevertheless, the general tendency was that the median levels of neurotrophins increased after the 12 weeks of therapy, but in particular cases, we observed a variation of neurotrophin concentrations. Some of the participants responded well to the therapy in contrast to those who completely failed the treatment. We attempted to identify those who were more likely to benefit from TENS by calculating delta values for each.

Interestingly, a good response to therapy expressed as a decrease of urinary levels of neurotrophins after TENS was observed in children presenting with DI. This result is in accordance with previous studies [36]. In this paper, while we refer to earlier work, measurement of the primary outcome is different. Previously, a reduction of urinary incontinence episodes was considered to be the main effect parameter. We used urinary biomarkers as a more objective tool.

In our study, all children had confirmed detrusor overactivity in urodynamic studies. In the clinical manifestation, the majority of patients (54%) complained only about NE. We observed the clinical response to TENS as a reduction of wet nights after therapy. However, this was not supported by a significant decrease in urinary neurotrophins in all cases. In our observations, NE may be a predictor of a worse response to TENS therapy. This may be a possible explanation for the lack of significant differences in urinary neurotrophins after TENS in the whole group. Additionally, modification of the time of day for TENS therapy may be a potential issue. In our study, we allowed patients to use TENS at any convenient time. It is possible that TENS performed before going to sleep or during the night in children with NE may be more effective. To prove such a statement, controlled studies are needed in the future.

Several studies about TENS in enuresis were performed. In 2010, Lorento et al. [37] evaluated the effectiveness of TENS in the treatment of non-monosymptomatic NE with 43% of cases cured, but 32% showed no improvement at all. In 2013, a prospective randomized clinical trial was performed in a group of children with primary monosymptomatic enuresis [38] treated with behavioral therapy and/or TENS. A statistically significant reduction in wet nights was observed (49.5 and 31.2%, respectively, at the end of treatment), but no patient had complete resolution of symptoms. A randomized, double-blind, placebo-controlled study was performed by Jørgensen et al. [39] on a group of 47 children with monosymptomatic NE demonstrating that TENS did not lead to significant changes in nocturnal urine production on wet or dry nights, voided volumes, or voiding frequency. Recently, a study on predictors of outcome in children and adolescents with OAB treated with TENS was performed. The results suggest that NE was the only symptom associated with poor outcome. The authors also assessed age as a potential predictor of response to

TENS therapy but no statistically significant differences were observed [40]. In our study, children who were older than 8 years of age responded better to therapy when the effect of TENS was expressed as a decrease in NGF concentration after therapy. By contrast, the effectiveness rate in children younger than 8 years of age was much lower. The most likely explanation is the fact that older children may be more determined and motivated to use TENS, as well as follow the instruction more accurately. However, it cannot be excluded that it may be due to the maturation of nervous system control of micturition in older children.

The present study should be considered a preliminary one, because the main limitation of the experimental results is the small study sample. It should also be added that the optimum number of sessions, ideal time of the day, and TENS duration, as well as its settings, have not been established yet.

5. Conclusions

To the best of our knowledge, this is the first study in which four urinary neurotrophins were used as potential predictors of TENS efficacy in pediatric OAB. To conclude, we would like to highlight the following facts:

1. Urinary NGF, BDNF, and NT4 were increased in OAB refractory to the standard treatment in contrast to NT3;
2. The variation of urinary neurotrophins in the course of TENS depended on the age and clinical manifestation of OAB.

Author Contributions: J.B. conceived the study, collected and analyzed data, acquired funds; E.S. performed laboratory analysis; A.K.-K. supervised the study. All authors have read and agreed to the published version of the manuscript.

Funding: This research was funded by the National Science Centre, Poland, under research project 'Preludium-17': the grant No. 2019/33/N/NZ5/02132.

Institutional Review Board Statement: The study was conducted according to the guidelines of the Declaration of Helsinki, and approved by the Ethics Committee of the Medical University of Bialystok (protocol code R-I-002/602/2019, date of the approval 19 December 2019).

Informed Consent Statement: Informed consent was obtained from all subjects involved in the study.

Data Availability Statement: The data presented in this study are available on request from the corresponding author. The data are not publicly available for ethical and privacy reasons.

Conflicts of Interest: The authors declare no conflict of interest.

References

1. Nieuwhof-Leppink, A.J.; Schroeder, R.P.J.; van de Putte, E.M.; de Jong, T.P.V.M.; Schappin, R. Daytime urinary incontinence in children and adolescents. *Lancet Child. Adolesc.* **2019**, *3*, 492–501. [CrossRef]
2. Austin, P.F.; Bauer, S.B.; Bower, W.; Chase, J.; Franco, I.; Hoebeke, P.; Rittig, S.; Walle, J.V.; von Gontard, A.; Wright, A.; et al. The standardization of terminology of lower urinary tract function in children and adolescents: Update report from the standardization committee of the International Children's Continence Society. *Neurourol. Urodyn.* **2016**, *35*, 471–481. [CrossRef]
3. Smith, A.L. Understanding overactive bladder and urgency incontinence: What does the brain have to do with it? *F1000Research* **2018**, *7*, F1000. [CrossRef] [PubMed]
4. Apostolidis, A.; Wagg, A.; Rahnama'i, M.S.; Panicker, J.N.; Vrijens, D.; von Gontard, A. Is there "brain OAB" and how can we recognize it? International Consultation on Incontinence-Research Society (ICI-RS) 2017. *Neurourol. Urodyn.* **2018**, *37*, S38–S45. [CrossRef] [PubMed]
5. Franco, I. Overactive bladder in children. *Nat. Rev. Urol.* **2016**, *13*, 520–532. [CrossRef] [PubMed]
6. Cruz, C.D. Neurotrophins in bladder function: What do we know and where do we go from here? *Neurourol. Urodyn.* **2014**, *33*, 39–45. [CrossRef]
7. Liu, H.T.; Kuo, H.C. Urinary nerve growth factor levels are increased in patients with bladder outlet obstruction with overactive bladder symptoms and reduced after successful medical treatment. *J. Urol.* **2008**, *72*, 104–108. [CrossRef] [PubMed]
8. Liu, H.T.; Chancellor, M.B.; Kuo, H.C. Decrease of urinary nerve growth factor levels after antimuscarinic therapy in patients with overactive bladder. *BJU Int.* **2009**, *103*, 1668–1672. [CrossRef]

9. Cho, K.J.; Kim, H.S.; Koh, J.S.; Kim, J.C. Changes in urinary nerve growth factor and prostaglandin E2 in women with overactive bladder after anticholinergics. *Int. Urogynecol. J.* **2013**, *24*, 325–330. [CrossRef]
10. Antunes-Lopes, T.; Pinto, R.; Barros, S.C.; Botelho, F.; Silva, C.M.; Cruz, C.D.; Cruz, F. Urinary neurotrophic factors in healthy individuals and patients with overactive bladder. *J. Urol.* **2013**, *189*, 359–365. [CrossRef]
11. Oktar, T.; Kocak, T.; Oner-Iyidogan, Y. Urinary nerve growth factor in children with overactive bladder: A promising, non-invasive and objective biomarker. *J. Pediatr. Urol.* **2013**, *9*, 617–621. [CrossRef]
12. Korzeniecka-Kozerska, A.; Wasilewska, A. Urinary nerve growth factor in patients with detrusor overactivity. *Ir. J. Med. Sci.* **2015**, *184*, 737–743. [CrossRef]
13. Özdemir, K.; Dinçel, N.; Berdeli, A.; Mir, S. Can Urinary Nerve Growth Factor and Brain-Derived Neurotrophic Factor be used in the Diagnosis and Follow-Up of Voiding Dysfunction in Children? *Urol. J.* **2016**, *13*, 2690–2696.
14. Liu, H.T.; Chancellor, M.B.; Kuo, H.C. Urinary nerve growth factor levels are elevated in patients with detrusor overactivity and decreased in responders to detrusor botulinum toxin-A injection. *Eur. Urol.* **2009**, *56*, 700–706. [CrossRef]
15. Wright, A.J.; Haddad, M. Electroneurostimulation for the management of bladder bowel dysfunction in childhood. *Eur. J. Paediatr. Neurol.* **2017**, *21*, 67–74. [CrossRef] [PubMed]
16. Barroso, U., Jr. Superficial stimulation therapy for the treatment of functional voiding problems. In *Pediatric Incontinence: Evaluation and Clinical Management*, 1st ed.; Franco, I., Austin, P.F., Bauer, S.B., von Gontard, A., Homsy, Y., Eds.; John Wiley & Sons: Hoboken, NJ, USA, 2015; pp. 183–188. [CrossRef]
17. Hoebeke, P.; Van Laecke, E.; Everaert, K.; Renson, C.; De Paepe, H.; Raes, A.; Vande Walle, J. Transcutaneous neuromodulation for the urge syndrome in children: A pilot study. *J. Urol.* **2001**, *166*, 2416–2419. [CrossRef]
18. Bower, W.F.; Moore, K.H.; Adams, R.D. A pilot study of the home application of transcutaneous neuromodulation in children with urgency or urge incontinence. *J. Urol.* **2001**, *166*, 2420–2422. [CrossRef]
19. Malm-Buatsi, E.; Nepple, K.G.; Boyt, M.A.; Austin, J.C.; Cooper, C.S. Efficacy of trancutaneous electrical nerve stimulation in children with overactive bladder refractory to pharmacotherapy. *Urology* **2007**, *70*, 980–983. [CrossRef] [PubMed]
20. Hagstroem, S.; Mahler, B.; Madsen, B.; Djurhuus, J.C.; Rittig, S. Transcutaneous electrical nerve stimulation for refractory daytime urinary urge incontinence. *J. Urol.* **2009**, *182*, 2072–2078. [CrossRef] [PubMed]
21. Sillén, U.; Arwidsson, C.; Doroszkiewicz, M.; Antonsson, H.; Jansson, I.; Stålklint, M.; Abrahamsson, K.; Sjöström, S. Effects of transcutaneous neuromodulation (TENS) on overactive bladder symptoms in children: A randomized controlled trial. *J. Pediatr. Urol.* **2014**, *10*, 1100–1105. [CrossRef] [PubMed]
22. Boudaoud, N.; Binet, A.; Line, A.; Chaouadi, D.; Jolly, C.; Fiquet, C.F.; Ripert, T.; Merol, M.L. Management of refractory overactive bladder in children by transcutaneous posterior tibial nerve stimulation: A controlled study. *J. Pediatr. Urol.* **2015**, *11*, 138.e1–138.e10. [CrossRef] [PubMed]
23. Lordelo, P.; Teles, A.; Veiga, M.L.; Correia, L.C.; Barroso, U., Jr. Transcutaneous electrical nerve stimulation in children with overactive bladder: A randomized clinical trial. *J. Urol.* **2010**, *184*, 683–689. [CrossRef] [PubMed]
24. Barroso, U., Jr.; Carvalho, M.T.; Veiga, M.L.; Moraes, M.M.; Cunha, C.C.; Lordêlo, P. Urodynamic outcome of parasacral transcutaneous electrical neural stimulation for overactive bladder in children. *Int. Braz. J. Urol.* **2015**, *41*, 739–743. [CrossRef] [PubMed]
25. Bower, W.F.; Yeung, C.K. A review of non-invasive electro neuromodulation as an intervention for non-neurogenic bladder dysfunction in children. *Neurourol. Urodyn.* **2004**, *23*, 63–67. [CrossRef] [PubMed]
26. Suh, Y.S.; Ko, K.J.; Kim, T.H.; Lee, H.S.; Sung, H.H.; Cho, W.J.; Lee, K.S. Urinary Nerve Growth Factor as a Potential Biomarker of Treatment Outcomes in Overactive Bladder Patients. *Int. Neurourol. J.* **2017**, *21*, 270–281. [CrossRef]
27. Deng, C.; Zhang, W.; Peng, Q.; Hu, X.; Li, M.; Gao, L.; Xu, J.; Su, J.; Xia, X. Urinary nerve growth factor: A biomarker for overactive bladder in children? A meta-analysis and trail sequential analysis. *Pediatr. Surg. Int.* **2019**, *35*, 1027–1032. [CrossRef]
28. Antunes-Lopes, T.; Cruz, F. Urinary Biomarkers in Overactive Bladder: Revisiting the Evidence in 2019. *Eur. Urol. Focus* **2019**, *5*, 329–336. [CrossRef]
29. Ochodnicky, P.; Cruz, C.D.; Yoshimura, N.; Cruz, F. Neurotrophins as regulators of urinary bladder function. *Nat. Rev. Urol.* **2012**, *9*, 628–637. [CrossRef]
30. Pinto, R.; Frias, B.; Allen, S.; Dawbarn, D.; McMahon, S.B.; Cruz, F.; Cruz, C.D. Sequestration of brain derived nerve factor by intravenous delivery of TrkB-Ig2 reduces bladder overactivity and noxious input in animals with chronic cystitis. *Neuroscience* **2010**, *166*, 907–916. [CrossRef]
31. Vizzard, M.A.; Wu, K.H.; Jewett, I.T. Developmental expression of urinary bladder neurotrophic factor mRNA and protein in the neonatal rat. *Brain Res. Dev. Brain Res.* **2000**, *119*, 217–224. [CrossRef]
32. Pradat, P.F.; Kennel, P.; Naimi-Sadaoui, S.; Finiels, F.; Orsini, C.; Revah, F.; Delaere, P.; Mallet, J. Continuous delivery of neurotrophin 3 by gene therapy has a neuroprotective effect in experimental models of diabetic and acrylamide neuropathies. *Hum. Gene Ther.* **2001**, *12*, 2237–2249. [CrossRef] [PubMed]
33. Miyazato, M.; Yoshimura, N.; Chancellor, M.B. The other bladder syndrome: Underactive bladder. *Rev. Urol.* **2013**, *15*, 11–22. [PubMed]
34. Corcos, J.; Przydacz, M. Neurogenic Bladder Pathophysiology. In *Consultation in Neurourology*, 1st ed.; Corcos, J., Przydacz, M., Eds.; Springer: Cham, Switzerland, 2018; pp. 7–16. [CrossRef]

35. Ognenovska, S.; Cheng, Y.; Li, A.; Mansfield, K.J.; Moore, K.H. What's normal? Should urinary creatinine or osmolarity be used to normalise urinary protein measurements? In Proceedings of the International Continence Society, Philadelphia, PA, USA, 28–31 August 2018; p. 138.
36. Barroso, U., Jr.; Tourinho, R.; Lordêlo, P.; Hoebeke, P.; Chase, J. Electrical stimulation for lower urinary tract dysfunction in children: A systematic review of the literature. *Neurourol. Urodyn.* **2011**, *30*, 1429–1436. [CrossRef] [PubMed]
37. Lordêlo, P.; Benevides, I.; Kerner, E.G.; Teles, A.; Lordêlo, M.; Barroso, U., Jr. Treatment of non-monosymptomatic nocturnal enuresis by transcutaneous parasacral electrical nerve stimulation. *J. Pediatr. Urol.* **2010**, *6*, 486–489. [CrossRef] [PubMed]
38. de Oliveira, L.F.; de Oliveira, D.M.; da Silva de Paula, L.I.; de Figueiredo, A.A.; de Bessa, J., Jr.; de Sá, C.A.; Bastos Netto, J.M. Transcutaneous parasacral electrical neural stimulation in children with primary monosymptomatic enuresis: A prospective randomized clinical trial. *J. Urol.* **2013**, *190*, 1359–1363. [CrossRef] [PubMed]
39. Jørgensen, C.S.; Kamperis, K.; Borch, L.; Borg, B.; Rittig, S. Transcutaneous Electrical Nerve Stimulation in Children with Monosymptomatic Nocturnal Enuresis: A Randomized, Double-Blind, Placebo Controlled Study. *J. Urol.* **2017**, *198*, 687–693. [CrossRef] [PubMed]
40. Hoffmann, A.; Sampaio, C.; Nascimento, A.A.; Veiga, M.L.; Barroso, U. Predictors of outcome in children and adolescents with overactive bladder treated with parasacral transcutaneous electrical nerve stimulation. *J. Pediatr. Urol.* **2018**, *14*, 54.e1–54.e6. [CrossRef]

Article

Are Tubular Injury Markers NGAL and KIM-1 Useful in Pediatric Neurogenic Bladder?

Joanna Bagińska * and Agata Korzeniecka-Kozerska

Department of Pediatrics and Nephrology, Medical University of Białystok, 17 Waszyngtona Str, 15-274 Białystok, Poland; iklinped@umb.edu.pl
* Correspondence: joasiabaginska14@wp.pl

Abstract: The lack of early biomarkers of renal damage in children with neurogenic bladder (NB) prompts us to investigate the role of promising proteins: neutrophil gelatinase-associated lipocalin (NGAL) and kidney injury molecule-1 (KIM-1). This prospective analysis was conducted on 58 children with NB and 25 healthy children. We assessed urinary levels of NGAL and KIM-1 in both groups. Age, sex, anthropometric measurements, activity assessment, renal function, and urodynamics parameters were analyzed. The differences between the median uNGAL and uKIM-1 in the NB group compared to control were recorded. However, only uNGAL levels were statistically significantly higher. Statistically significant correlation was found between gender, recurrent urinary tract infections, bladder trabeculation, its compliance, activity assessment, and uNGAL. To conclude, elevated levels of uNGAL may be considered a biomarker of tubular injury in children with NB due to MMC in contrast to uKIM-1.

Keywords: neurogenic bladder; myelomeningocele; markers

1. Introduction

Neurogenic bladder (NB) due to myelomeningocele (MMC), with an estimated prevalence of 1/700 live births, is a condition strongly associated with multiple disturbances which, untreated, can result in progressive renal damage. This process may occur silently, and eventually leads to chronic renal failure [1]. Hence, NB patients require close monitoring to evaluate the evolution of glomerular and tubular renal function in order to rapidly diagnose and treat the worsening of renal outcome. Identifying the biomarkers that are capable of early detection of renal damage would represent a tremendous advance in the care of NB children. Recently, several biomarkers related to inflammation and tubular injury have been identified as potent predictors of renal outcome, including neutrophil gelatinase-associated lipocalin (NGAL) and kidney injury molecule-1 (KIM-1).

NGAL belongs to the lipocalin proteins, is expressed at very low levels in human tissues, including kidney, lungs or stomach, and its expression increases in inflammation and injured epithelia [2,3]. KIM-1 is a transmembrane glycoprotein highly expressed in regenerating proximal tubular cells [4,5]. Due to their small molecular size, NGAL and KIM-1 are freely filtered and can be easily detected in urine. Urinary NGAL (uNGAL) and urinary KIM-1 (uKIM-1) are rapidly released in response to tubular damage. Therefore, they are very sensitive biomarkers of acute kidney injury (AKI) [4–6]. However, it is now increasingly recognized that the inflammatory process and tubular injury have an important role in the pathogenesis and progression of chronic processes, and the severity of tubulointerstitial lesions has a significant impact on renal outcome in, e.g., diabetic nephropathy [7] or chronic kidney disease (CKD) [8–12]. Little is known about tubular injury with regards to pediatric NB. To the best of our knowledge, our study represents the first investigation of uNGAL and uKIM-1 in NB as potential markers in detecting tubular damage.

2. Materials and Methods

2.1. Patients

This prospective analysis was conducted on 83 children divided into two groups. The study group included 58 children with congenital NB after MMC. We assessed all participants' medical charts to determine age, sex, anthropometric measurements, and standard deviation scores (WHO z-scores). The presence of urinary tract infection was excluded on the basis of urinary testing and urine culture. A negative C-reactive protein (CRP) excluded current infection. Nonetheless, the history of recurrent urinary tract infections (rUTIs) was recorded. We defined rUTIs as two or more episodes of pyelonephritis, or one episode of pyelonephritis plus one or more episodes of cystitis, or three or more episodes of cystitis, in accordance with the Polish Society of Pediatric Nephrology Guidelines published in 2015 concerning the management of UTI in children.

Renal function parameters included: urinary and serum creatinine (Cr), serum cystatin C (Cys), and glomerular filtration rate (eGFR). Two pediatric equations espoused by the National Kidney Foundation were used to calculate eGFR, incorporating Cr-only (based on the new Schwartz formula: eGFR = 41.3 × (height/Cr)) and Cys-only (eGFR = 70.69 × $Cys^{-0.931}$). The assessment of Cys was not performed in four children younger than two years of age due to the fact that it is not validated for this age group. The inclusion criterion for the study group was eGFR > 90 mL/min/1.73 m^2 (in both above-mentioned formulas) to choose NB patients without the biochemical signs of glomerular impairment.

The presence of abnormalities in the upper urinary tract system was assessed by abdominal ultrasound and voiding cystourethrogram. The following ultrasound parameters were evaluated: length and width of the kidneys, bladder wall thickness, hydronephrosis, parenchymal echogenicity, corticomedullary differentiation, and the presence of trabeculation. In the voiding cystourethrogram, we analyzed the presence of vesicoureteral reflux, its grade, laterality, and activity. We divided NB children into three groups: 1—Without VUR, 2—With present VUR, and 3—With a history of VUR in the past.

The assessment of the lower urinary tract system included urodynamic study where the measurements of bladder wall compliance (comp), detrusor pressure at urgency (Pdet urg), cystometric capacity (CC), and maximum detrusor pressure on voiding phase (max p det) were recorded. Patients with high-pressure bladders were included in the study after the appropriate treatment with anticholinergics. The urine samples were collected from them when the bladder pressures had decreased. In this way, we aimed to avoid the influence of high bladder pressures on biomarkers concentrations.

The ambulatory function of MMC patients was defined according to Hoffer's scale (HS) using the four categories of community: 1HS—Nonambulator, 2HS—Nonfunctional ambulator, 3HS—Household walkers, and 4HS—Community walkers [13]. The lesion level in MMC patients was reported intraoperatively and radiologically and scored from 1 to 3 (1—Thoracolumbar, 2—Lumbosacral, 3—Sacral lesion).

The control group consisted of 25 healthy children who visited a pediatrician for balance tests and had no abnormalities in the urinary or nervous systems.

2.2. Biochemistry

First, morning void spot urine samples were collected for measurement of KIM-1 and NGAL. The levels of biomarkers were measured for KIM 1 using BioAssay Human KIM-1 ELISA) and for NGAL using BioVendor Human Lipocalin-2/NGAL ELISA, according to the manufacturer's instructions. The urinary Cr concentration was used to normalize NGAL and KIM-1 measurements to account for the influence of urinary dilution on concentration. Urinary levels of the biomarkers were expressed as uNGAL/Cr and uKIM-1/Cr ratios (ng/mg Cr).

2.3. Statistics

The data were collected in a Microsoft Excel database. Statistical analysis was performed using Statistica 13.0 (StatSoft Inc, Tulsa, OK, USA). Continuous variables were expressed as the median and range, unless stated otherwise. All studied parameters were analyzed using nonparametric tests: Mann–Whitney, Kruskal–Wallis and Chi2 analysis. Correlations were assessed with the Spearman test. Values of $p < 0.05$ were considered significant.

2.4. Ethical Issues

This study was approved by the Ethics Committee of the Medical University of Bialystok (R-I-002/105/2018) which complies with the World Medical Association Declaration of Helsinki regarding ethical conduct of research involving human subjects and/or animals. Patients and their caregivers were enrolled in the study after obtaining informed consent.

3. Results

The characteristics of the studied children are presented in Table 1. The median age of the enrolled patients was 10 (0.58–17.7) years. There were no differences in age, sex, weight-to-age z-scores, and BMI-to-age z-scores, excluding height-to-age z-scores. This resulted from shorter vertebral dimensions and malformations of the bone structure due to MMC in NB group. We found statistically significant differences in the urinary and serum Cr concentrations and eGFR Schwartz between the studied groups.

Table 1. Demographic characteristics of patients with NB and control participants.

Variables	NB Patients $n = 58$	Control Participants $n = 25$	p Value
Gender: female/male n (%)	32 (55)/26 (45)	17 (68)/8 (32)	0.36
	Median (minimum–maximum)		
Age (years)	9.2 (0.58–17.7)	12 (1–17)	0.07
Z-score: height-to-age	−0.9 (−5.1–3.1)	0.25 (−3.3–2.7)	0.01 *
Z-score: weight-to-age	−0.7 (−6–2.8)	−0.15 (−2.4–2.2)	0.08
Z-score: BMI (kg/m^2)	−0.2 (−6–2.8)	−0.35 (−2.1–3)	0.95
Serum creatinine (mg/dL)	0.31 (0.18–0.88)	0.52 (0.2–0.85)	<0.001 *
Urinary creatinine (mg/dL)	52.1 (12.6–234.7)	129.5 (51–244)	<0.001 *
eGFR Schwartz (mL/min/1.73 m^2)	157.5 (90–268)	117 (90–247)	<0.001 *

NB, neurogenic bladder; * $p < 0.05$.

Additionally, in the NB children we assessed the serum Cys, with a median concentration of 0.63 (0.18–0.85) mg/L. The eGFR formula with the use of Cys was equal to 105 (90–162) mL/min/1.73 m^2.

A comparison of the biochemical indices is presented in Table 2. As shown, children with NB have significantly elevated urinary NGAL levels in contrast to healthy participants. We recorded differences in the levels of urinary KIM-1 between the studied groups, but they were not statistically significant.

Table 2. Biochemical parameters in patients with NB after MMC and control participants.

Variables	NB Patients $n = 58$	Control Group $n = 25$	p Value
Urinary KIM-1 (ng/mL)	0.46 (0–1.93)	0.62 (0–3.8)	0.1
Urinary KIM-1/Cr ratio (ng/mg)	0.76 (0–3.01)	0.54 (0–1.46)	0.08
Urinary NGAL (ng/mL)	10.3 (0.55–73)	1.32 (0–62)	<0.001 *
Urinary NGAL/Cr ratio (ng/mg)	27.1 (1.08–240.1)	0.98 (0–93)	<0.001 *

* $p < 0.05$.

There were no statistically significant differences between girls and boys participating in the study, excluding the uNGAL/Cr ratio ($p = 0.02$; $p < 0.05$). In both studied groups, a higher uNGAL/Cr ratio was observed in girls. In NB girls, a median of 45 (3.0–240) ng/mg in the uNGAL/Cr ratio was recorded in contrast to 18 (1.07–213.39) ng/mg in the NB boys. In the control group, a median uNGAL/Cr ratio in girls equaled 1.63 (0–93) ng/mL in comparison to 0 (0–3.95) ng/mL in boys.

3.1. NB Children

3.1.1. History of Urinary Tract Infections

The majority of NB patients (38/58 (65%)) had no history of rUTIs in contrast to 20/62 (35%) with rUTIs in the past. A comparison of the studied parameters revealed statistically significant differences between NB children with and without rUTIs ($p = 0.014$; $p < 0.05$). The active UTI was an exclusion criterion. However, children who had rUTIs tended to have a higher uNGAL/Cr ratio with a median of 45.13 (7.06–240.1) ng/mg in contrast to children without rUTI history with a median of 19.05 (1.08–213.4) ng/mg.

3.1.2. Assessment of Urinary Tract

Children without VUR constituted 72% (42/58) of the NB group. VUR was present in 9/58 (15%) children, and 7/58 (13%) patients had a history of VUR in the past. The comparison of KIM-1 and NGAL in the above-mentioned groups did not reveal statistically significant differences (Chi2 = 3, $p = 0.214$; Chi2 = 2.22, $p = 0.327$, respectively).

The increase in uNGAL concentrations was associated with bladder trabeculation ($p = 0.014$; $p < 0.05$). In children with trabeculated bladder, the median of NGAL concentration was 32.13 (3.43–73) ng/mL in contrast to children without the trabeculation with a median of 4.93 (0.55–5.11) ng/mL. Additionally, the uNGAL/Cr ratio positively correlated with the bladder wall thickness ($r = 0.57$, $p < 0.05$, Figure 1).

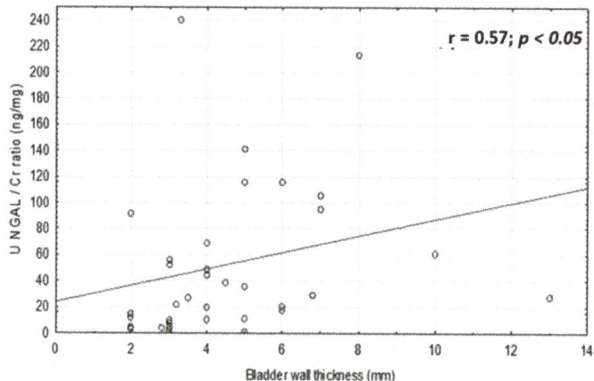

Figure 1. Correlation between uNGAL/Cr ratio and bladder wall thickness.

In urodynamics, we evaluated Pdet urg (median 20 (5–60) cm H_2O), CC (median 155 (20–300) mL), comp (median 9 (1–40) mL/cm H_2O) and max p det (median 12 (1–58) cm H_2O). No correlation was observed between bladder pressures and the investigated biomarkers. However, the uNGAL/Cr ratio negatively correlated with compl ($r = -0.52$, $p < 0.05$, Figure 2).

3.1.3. Level of Spinal Lesion/Mobility

The majority of NB patients (35/58 (61%)) had lumbosacral spinal lesion, 15/58 (25%) had thoracolumbar and 8/58 (14%) sacral lesion level. We did not find statistically significant differences in NGAL and KIM-1 between the abovementioned groups. However, statistically significant differences were recorded in height-to-age z-score, serum and urinary Cr, eGFR Schwartz, and NGAL between the HS groups. More detailed data are shown in Table 3. Children from the 4HS group, described as community walkers, had the lowest urinary NGAL levels and uNGAL/Cr ratio in contrast to children with different stages of walking impairment from the remaining HS groups. In our studies, no significant difference was found among the HS groups for KIM-1 (Chi2 = 5.69, $p = 0.13$).

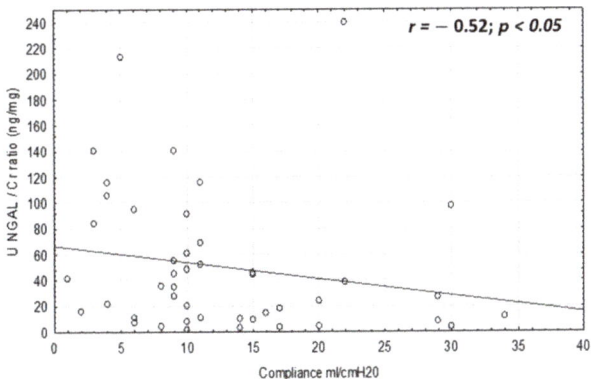

Figure 2. Correlation between uNGAL/Cr ratio and bladder compliance.

Table 3. Comparison between HS groups.

Variables	HS1 Wheelchair Dependent	HS2 Walking Only in Therapy	HS3 Household Walkers	HS4 Community Walkers	Chi 2	p Value
n (%)	29 (50)	9 (16)	7 (12)	13 (22)		
z-score: height-to-age	−1.8(−5.1–3.1)	−1 (−4.3–1.4)	0.1 (−2–1.5)	−0.7 (−2.5–2)	9.48	0.02 *
Serum creatinine (mg/dL)	0.27 (0.18–0.73)	0.35 (0.2–0.64)	0.33 (0.24–0.88)	0.4 (0.23–0.76)	11.28	0.01 *
Urinary creatinine (mg/dL)	42 (12.6–114.1)	61.5 (24.3–234.7)	65.3 (32.6–75.81)	58.1 (19–182.1)	7.93	0.04 *
eGFR Schwartz (mL/min/1.73 m^2)	178.5 (91.4–268.4)	167.6 (100–239.5)	146.55 (90–178.97)	123 (92.4–175.6)	9.28	0.02 *
Cystatin C (mg/L)	0.66 (0.18–0.83)	0.69 (0.54–0.85)	0.63 (0.59–0.83)	0.61 (0.4–0.75)	2.79	0.42
eGFR with cystatinC (mL/min/1.73 m^2)	104 (84–278)	99 (90–123)	108 (90–116)	112 (91–162)	2.95	0.39
Urinary NGAL (ng/mL)	27.6 (1.28–73)	12.14 (4.87–51.75)	31.6 (1.87–51.14)	4.68 (0.55–28.82)	11.17	0.01 *
Urinary NGAL/Cr ratio (ng/mg)	37.14 (4.57–240.1)	26.61 (3.19–140.6)	58.03 (3.37–96.9)	9.2 (1.08–45.7)	10.63	0.01 *

* $p < 0.05$.

4. Discussion

To the best of our knowledge, this study is the first to focus on urinary biomarkers, KIM-1 and NGAL, as potential predictors of renal tubular injury in children with NB after MMC. Owing to adequate nephro-urological management in the last decade, the prognosis of MMC children has greatly improved, but the prompt recognition of renal damage in NB still remains a challenge. It is a largely asymptomatic process, and establishing the diagnosis currently depends on clinical tests, including elevated serum Cr and decreasing eGFR. Unfortunately, they are delayed and unreliable biomarkers of the future course of the disease for a variety of reasons. Cr depends on body muscle mass. In children with MMC, muscle wasting due to denervation is observed. What is more, MMC children often have impaired linear growth [14]. In these cases, Cr and precise estimation of eGFR may be impossible. There may be substantial inaccuracy when we compare eGFR between NB patients and the general population [1,15]. Recently, Cys has been shown to be a reliable marker in detecting renal deterioration in patients with NB [16,17]. It is not influenced by age, gender or muscle mass, consistent with our results. Additionally, it is not dependent on the patient's level of physical activity assessed by HS. In our study, we do not reveal the differences in Cys and Cys-based eGFR between HS groups in contrast to Cr and eGFR Schwartz.

Our findings also reveal that the Schwartz equation gave a higher median eGFR compared to the Cys-based eGFR, likely due to the higher inaccuracy of Cr and height. These results are in good agreement with other studies [17] which have shown that lower eGFR in NB were observed when calculated using Cys than Cr, with the conclusion that Cys-based eGFR is a more sensitive parameter. However, serum Cr is still more popular, available and less expensive than Cyc in daily clinical practice. A clinical decision in the management of NB children made only with Cr and its associated eGFR may give the impression that overall kidney function is in the normal range, when in fact the opposite may be true. Moreover, they are primarily markers of glomerular disease and do not necessarily detect tubular dysfunction.

The presented study aimed to investigate early indicators of tubular damage in MMC patients. One of the inclusion criteria for our project was eGFR > 90 mL/min/1.73 m^2 to choose NB patients without the biochemical signs of glomerular impairment assessed by common and widespread used renal parameters. Other objective methods of renal damage include image testing and urodynamic studies. Much research on risk factors of renal damage in patients with MMC has been conducted. The proposed risk factors included the identification of urinary tract abnormalities in, e.g., voiding cystourethrograms, ultrasonography, renal scintigraphy, or the presence of high-pressure bladder in urodynamics. However, the above-mentioned diagnostic tools can only identify upper tract abnormalities once they have already occurred. In our paper, the focus of our attention was on NGAL and KIM as markers that appear before the damage is present.

In our study, children with NB had significantly elevated uNGAL levels in comparison with healthy participants in contrast to uKIM-1. Additionally, girls have higher uNGAL levels compared to boys. This result is consistent with the observation by Pennemans et al. [18] who reported that in the group of healthy children, uNGAL levels were positively correlated with female gender in young children.

There are plenty of other factors that may influence the urinary levels of NGAL. Children with NB require clean intermittent catheterization which predisposes them to rUTIs. All patients from the study group were catheterized several times per day. In our study, higher uNGAL concentrations were observed in NB children with rUTI history. The most likely explanation of this result may be the greater expression of uNGAL by tubular epithelial cells in response to chronic inflammatory processes. There are several surveys conducted on the general pediatric population that show that uNGAL is higher in UTIs [19,20]. Only one study, performed by Foster et al. [21], focused on children with NB and indicated that uNGAL has a high predictive value for UTI in this population. However, it is not comparable to our research because the study group comprised NB children with active UTI or bacterial colonization of the urinary tract. In our study, the active UTI was an exclusion criterion. However, chronic inflammation may be the cause of fibroproliferative changes in the bladder wall including smooth muscle cell proliferation and hypertrophy. According to our results, uNGAL was increased in trabeculated, non-compliant bladder with a thickened wall. These factors may lead to high intravesical pressures during urine storage that impair its drainage into the bladder. High pressure requires more aggressive treatment to avoid further wall hypertrophy and potential deterioration of the bladder and upper urinary tract. The management must start before consequences of bladder dysfunction become apparent. On the basis of our results, we deduce that uNGAL may increase before the upper urinary tract damage is present or before the markers of glomerular function are able to detect it. uNGAL is released in response to tubular injury. Quite recently, considerable attention has been paid to the relation between tubulointerstitial damage and renal function decline. Several publications have documented that tubular dysfunction correlates better with renal deterioration than glomerular injury and may be a separate aspect of kidney pathology not fully reflected by glomerular biomarkers [22]. It is possible that in NB children with detected trabeculation and poor bladder compliance, tubular injury has occurred and is present but is not detectable because of the lack of tubular markers. This is the reason why uNGAL may become the potential tubular biomarker for predicting early renal dysfunction in NB.

An additional risk factor associated with rUTIs in the NB population is the presence of VUR. Several publications have appeared in recent years documenting the relationship between uNGAL and VUR but these results are not conclusive. Parmaksız [23] and Nickavar [24] indicate that uNGAL may be considered as a noninvasive diagnostic biomarker of primary VUR, especially of its long-term consequences such as renal scarring. However, our results are in good agreement with other studies which showed that presence of VUR did not change the uNGAL concentrations [25].

According to our results, the patient's level of mobility is another factor affecting uNGAL. Wheelchair-dependent children had higher uNGAL levels than walkers. This finding suggests that children who are wheelchair-dependent have a higher risk of tubular dysfunction than others. Surprisingly, the parameters of glomerular function also differed but the median serum concentration of creatinine was the lowest and the creatinine-based eGFR was the highest in HS1 compared to other HS groups. The most likely explanation of this result is the fact that wheelchair-dependent patients have the most impaired linear growth and muscle atrophy. Especially in this group, the precise estimation of renal function with available parameters is impossible, so uNGAL may be the promising marker of renal function in this population of patients. On the basis of the promising findings presented in this paper, work on the remaining issues is still warranted to gain further insight on uNGAL and NB.

5. Conclusions

To conclude, we would like to highlight that:

1. Elevated levels of uNGAL could be considered a biomarker of tubular damage in children with NB due to MMC in contrast to uKIM-1.
2. Cystatin C is a more sensitive parameter of glomerular function in NB than creatinine.
3. Gender, history of recurrent UTIs, bladder trabeculation, wall thickening, and compliance may be factors influencing uNGAL concentration.

Author Contributions: J.B. conceived the study and collected and analyzed data; A.K.-K. supervised the study. Both authors have read and agreed to the published version of the manuscript.

Funding: This research was funded by Medical University of Białystok grant number [N/ST/MN/18/001/1141].

Institutional Review Board Statement: The study was conducted according to the guidelines of the Declaration of Helsinki, and approved by the Ethics Committee of the Medical University of Bialystok (protocol code R-I-002/105/2018, date of the approval 22 March 2018).

Informed Consent Statement: Informed consent was obtained from all subjects involved in the study.

Data Availability Statement: The data presented in this study are available on request from the corresponding author. The data are not publicly available for ethical and privacy reasons.

Conflicts of Interest: The authors declare no conflict of interest.

References

1. Sung, B.M.; Oh, D.J.; Choi, M.H.; Choi, H.M. Chronic kidney disease in neurogenic bladder. *Nephrology* **2018**, *23*, 231–236. [CrossRef]
2. Buonafine, M.; Martinez-Martinez, E.; Jaisser, F. More than a simple biomarker: The role of NGAL in cardiovascular and renal diseases. *Clin. Sci.* **2018**, *132*, 909–923. [CrossRef] [PubMed]
3. Zhou, F.; Luo, Q.; Wang, L.; Han, L. Diagnostic value of neutrophil gelatinase-associated lipocalin for early diagnosis of cardiac surgery-associated acute kidney injury: A meta-analysis. *Eur. J. Cardiothorac. Surg.* **2016**, *49*, 746–755. [CrossRef] [PubMed]

4. Sinkala, M.; Zulu, M.; Kaile, T.; Simakando, M.; Chileshe Ch Kafita, D.; Nkhoma, P. Performance Characteristics of Kidney Injury Molecule-1 In Relation to Creatinine, Urea, and Microalbuminuria in the Diagnosis of Kidney Disease. *Int. J. Basic Med. Res.* **2017**, *7*, 94–99. [CrossRef]
5. Moresco, R.N.; Bochi, G.V.; Stein, C.S.; De Carvalho, J.A.M.; Cembranel, B.M.; Bollick, Y.S. Urinary kidney injury molecule-1 in renal disease. *Clin. Chim. Acta* **2018**, *487*, 15–21. [CrossRef] [PubMed]
6. Malhotra, R.; Siew, E.D. Biomarkers for the Early Detection and Prognosis of Acute Kidney Injury. *Clin. J. Am. Soc. Nephrol.* **2017**, *12*, 149–173. [CrossRef]
7. Duan, S.; Chen, J.; Wu, L.; Nie, G.; Sun, L.; Zhang, C.; Huang, Z.; Xing, C.; Zhang, B.; Yuan, Y. Assessment of urinary NGAL for differential diagnosis and progression of diabetic kidney disease. *J. Diabetes Complicat.* **2020**, *34*, 107665. [CrossRef] [PubMed]
8. Bolignano, D.; Lacquaniti, A.; Coppolino, G.; Donato, V.; Campo, S.; Fazio, M.R.; Nicocia, G.; Buemi, M. Neutrophil gelatinase-associated lipocalin (NGAL) and progression of chronic kidney disease. *Clin. J. Am. Soc. Nephrol.* **2009**, *4*, 337–344. [CrossRef]
9. Patel, M.L.; Sachan, R.; Misra, R.; Kamal, R.; Shyam, R.; Sachan, P. Prognostic significance of urinary NGAL in chronic kidney disease. *Int. J. Nephrol. Renovasc. Dis.* **2015**, *8*, 139–144. [CrossRef]
10. Holzscheiter, L.; Beck, C.; Rutz, S.; Manuilova, E.; Domke, I.; Guder, W.G.; Hofmann, W. NGAL, L-FABP, and KIM-1 in comparison to established markers of renal dysfunction. *Clin. Chem. Lab. Med.* **2014**, *52*, 537–546. [CrossRef]
11. Uwaezuoke, S.N.; Ayuk, A.C.; Muoneke, V.U.; Mbanefo, N.R. Chronic kidney disease in children: Using novel biomarkers as predictors of disease. *Saudi J. Kidney Dis. Transpl.* **2018**, *29*, 775–784. [CrossRef] [PubMed]
12. Seibert, F.S.; Sitz, M.; Passfall, J.; Haesner, M.; Laschinski, P.; Buhl, M.; Bauer, F.; Babel, N.; Pagonas, N.; Westhoff, T.H. Prognostic Value of Urinary Calprotectin, NGAL and KIM-1 in Chronic Kidney Disease. *Kidney Blood Press Res.* **2018**, *43*, 1255–1262. [CrossRef] [PubMed]
13. Hoffer, M.M.; Feiwell, E.; Perry, R.; Perry, J.; Bonnettet, C. Functional ambulation in patients with myelomeningocele. *J. Bone Jt. Surg. Am.* **1973**, *55*, 137–148. [CrossRef]
14. Satin-Smith, M.S.; Katz, L.L.; Thornton, P.; Gruccio, D.; Moshang, T. Arm span as measurement of response to growth hormone (GH) treatment in a group of children with meningomyelocele and GH deficiency. *J. Clin. Endocrinol. Metab.* **1996**, *81*, 1654–1656. [CrossRef] [PubMed]
15. Fox, J.A.; Dudley, A.G.; Bates, C.; Cannon, G.M., Jr. Cystatin C as a marker of early renal insufficiency in children with congenital neuropathic bladder. *J. Urol.* **2014**, *191*, 1602–1607. [CrossRef] [PubMed]
16. Dangle, P.P.; Ayyash, O.; Kang, A.; Bates, C.; Fox, J.; Stephany, H.; Cannon, G., Jr. Cystatin C-calculated Glomerular Filtration Rate-A Marker of Early Renal Dysfunction in Patients With Neuropathic Bladder. *Urology* **2017**, *100*, 213–217. [CrossRef]
17. Chu, D.I.; Balmert, L.C.; Arkin, C.M.; Meyer, T.; Rosoklija, I.; Li, B.; Hodgkins, K.S.; Furth, S.L.; Cheng, E.Y.; Yerkes, E.B.; et al. Estimated kidney function in children and young adults with spina bifida: A retrospective cohort study. *Neurourol. Urodyn.* **2019**, *38*, 1907–1914. [CrossRef] [PubMed]
18. Pennemans, V.; Rigo, J.M.; Faes, C.; Reynders, C.; Penders, J.; Swennen, Q. Establishment of reference values for novel urinary biomarkers for renal damage in the healthy population: Are age and gender an issue? *Clin. Chem. Lab. Med.* **2013**, *51*, 1795–1802. [CrossRef]
19. Valdimarsson, S.; Jodal, U.; Barregård, L.; Hansson, S. Urine neutrophil gelatinase-associated lipocalin and other biomarkers in infants with urinary tract infection and in febrile controls. *Pediatr. Nephrol.* **2017**, *32*, 2079–2087. [CrossRef]
20. Lee, H.E.; Kim, D.K.; Kang, H.K.; Park, K. The diagnosis of febrile urinary tract infection in children may be facilitated by urinary biomarkers. *Pediatr. Nephrol.* **2015**, *30*, 123–130. [CrossRef]
21. Forster, C.S.; Jackson, E.; Ma, Q.; Bennett, M.; Shah, S.S.; Goldstein, S.L. Predictive ability of NGAL in identifying urinary tract infection in children with neurogenic bladders. *Pediatr. Nephrol.* **2018**, *33*, 1365–1374. [CrossRef] [PubMed]
22. Liu, B.C.; Tang, T.T.; Lv, L.L.; Lan, H.Y. Renal tubule injury: A driving force toward chronic kidney disease. *Kidney Int.* **2018**, *93*, 568–579. [CrossRef] [PubMed]
23. Parmaksız, G.; Noyan, A.; Dursun, H.; İnce, E.; Anarat, R.; Cengiz, N. Role of new biomarkers for predicting renal scarring in vesicoureteral reflux: NGAL, KIM-1, and L-FABP. *Pediatr. Nephrol.* **2016**, *31*, 97–103. [CrossRef] [PubMed]
24. Nickavar, A.; Valavi, E.; Safaeian, B.; Moosavian, M. Validity of urine neutrophile gelatinase-associated lipocalin in children with primary vesicoureteral reflux. *Int. Urol. Nephrol.* **2020**, *52*, 599–602. [CrossRef]
25. Kitao, T.; Kimata, T.; Yamanouchi, S.; Kato, S.; Tsuji, S.; Kaneko, K. Urinary Biomarkers for Screening for Renal Scarring in Children with Febrile Urinary Tract Infection: Pilot Study. *J. Urol.* **2015**, *194*, 766–771. [CrossRef] [PubMed]

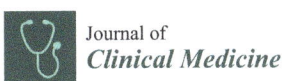

Article

Serum Periostin as a Potential Biomarker in Pediatric Patients with Primary Hypertension

Michał Szyszka [1], Piotr Skrzypczyk [2,*], Anna Stelmaszczyk-Emmel [3] and Małgorzata Pańczyk-Tomaszewska [2]

[1] Department of Pediatrics and Nephrology, Doctoral School, Medical University of Warsaw, 02-091 Warsaw, Poland; michalszyszkaa@gmail.com
[2] Department of Pediatrics and Nephrology, Medical University of Warsaw, 02-091 Warsaw, Poland; mpanczyk1@wum.edu.pl
[3] Department of Laboratory Diagnostics and Clinical Immunology of Developmental Age, Medical University of Warsaw, 02-091 Warsaw, Poland; anna.stelmaszczyk-emmel@wum.edu.pl
* Correspondence: pskrzypczyk@wum.edu.pl; Tel.: +48-22-317-96-53; Fax: +48-22-317-99-54

Abstract: Experimental studies suggest that periostin is involved in tissue repair and remodeling. The study aimed to evaluate serum periostin concentration as potential biomarker in pediatric patients with primary hypertension (PH). We measured serum periostin, blood pressure, arterial damage, biochemical, and clinical data in 50 children with PH and 20 age-matched healthy controls. In univariate analysis, children with PH had significantly lower serum periostin compared to healthy peers (35.42 ± 10.43 vs. 42.16 ± 12.82 [ng/mL], $p = 0.038$). In the entire group of 70 children serum periostin concentration correlated negatively with peripheral, central, and ambulatory blood pressure, as well as with aortic pulse wave velocity (aPWV). In multivariate analysis, periostin level significantly correlated with age ($\beta = -0.614$, [95% confidence interval (CI), -0.831–-0.398]), uric acid ($\beta = 0.328$, [95%CI, 0.124–0.533]), body mass index (BMI) Z-score ($\beta = -0.293$, [95%CI, -0.492–-0.095]), high-density lipoprotein (HDL)-cholesterol ($\beta = 0.235$, [95%CI, 0.054–0.416]), and triglycerides ($\beta = -0.198$, [95%CI, -0.394–-0.002]). Neither the presence of hypertension nor blood pressure and aPWV influenced periostin level. To conclude, the role of serum periostin as a biomarker of elevated blood pressure and arterial damage in pediatric patients with primary hypertension is yet to be unmasked. Age, body mass index, uric acid, and lipid concentrations are key factors influencing periostin level in pediatric patients.

Keywords: periostin; primary hypertension; children; adolescents; arterial damage; blood pressure

Citation: Szyszka, M.; Skrzypczyk, P.; Stelmaszczyk-Emmel, A.; Pańczyk-Tomaszewska, M. Serum Periostin as a Potential Biomarker in Pediatric Patients with Primary Hypertension. *J. Clin. Med.* **2021**, *10*, 2138. https://doi.org/10.3390/jcm10102138

Academic Editors: Katarzyna Taranta-Janusz and Kinga Musiał

Received: 5 April 2021
Accepted: 11 May 2021
Published: 15 May 2021

Publisher's Note: MDPI stays neutral with regard to jurisdictional claims in published maps and institutional affiliations.

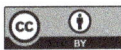

Copyright: © 2021 by the authors. Licensee MDPI, Basel, Switzerland. This article is an open access article distributed under the terms and conditions of the Creative Commons Attribution (CC BY) license (https://creativecommons.org/licenses/by/4.0/).

1. Introduction

Arterial hypertension (AH), one of the most common diseases worldwide, is a recognized risk factor for renal and cardiovascular diseases [1]. Its prevalence is constantly increasing, not only among adults, but also in the pediatric population. The increasingly common sedentary lifestyle, especially during the coronavirus disease 2019 (COVID-19) pandemic, as well as excessive salt intake accelerated the prevalence of AH. As recent studies show, AH is found in approximately 3–5% of all children [2]. Although in early childhood the majority of hypertension cases are secondary to other disorders, according to some new data, primary hypertension (PH) is taking the lead as the most common form of hypertension in children over 7 years of age [3]. PH emerges from the complex interactions of genetic and environmental factors. One of them is dysregulation of the renin–angiotensin–aldosterone system (RAAS), which plays a pivotal role in PH development [4].

Evaluation of arterial stiffness and common carotid artery intima-media thickness (cIMT) are included in the assessment of hypertension-mediated organ damage in children [5,6]. Increased cIMT and excessive arterial stiffness are common among pediatric patients with PH [7]. Furthermore, current observations and reviews point out that not only reduction of systolic and diastolic blood pressure (BP) should be taken into consideration as an aim in PH therapy, but also lowering pulse pressure and arterial stiffness are important independent treatment goals [8,9]. Oxidative stress, endothelial dysfunction, calcification, high collagen concentrations, and subclinical inflammation are linked to arterial wall dysfunction and its stiffening [10,11].

Periostin is a matricellular protein, a member of the fasciclin family [12]. It is produced mostly in utero and in differentiated connective tissues exposed to mechanical load such as aorta, heart valves, stomach, skin, tendons, and bones [13]. Periostin can also be upregulated after injury, and during remodeling and wound healing [14]. Experimental studies suggested a significant role of periostin in the development of arterial hypertension and hypertension-mediated organ damage. Firstly, periostin was found to interact with RAAS [15–17]; secondly, its expression in the arterial wall was elevated in a mice model of arterial hypertension [18]. Finally, periostin was found to be a promising marker of hypertension-induced cardiac remodeling [17] and hypertensive nephropathy [19]. Of note, treatment with RAAS-inhibiting agents led to significant down-regulation of tissue periostin level and reversal of kidney [19] and heart failure [20]. In addition, few human adult studies point to the role of periostin as a biomarker in cardiovascular and renal diseases. Periostin was revealed as a promising marker of diabetic kidney disease [21] and chronic allograft nephropathy [22] and increased periostin expression was found in patients with glomerulopathies [23]. Ling revealed that high serum periostin not only correlated with left ventricular ejection fraction but was also a marker of poor prognosis in patients with acute myocardial infarction (AMI) [24]. Nonetheless, little is known about the significance of the evaluation of periostin level in hypertensive patients.

We hypothesize that serum periostin could serve as a useful biomarker in hypertensive pediatric patients. Hence, the aims of our study were: 1. to compare serum periostin level in pediatric patients with primary hypertension and their healthy peers; 2. to reveal the relation between blood pressure (including central and 24-h ambulatory blood pressure), arterial damage (cIMT and increased arterial stiffness) and serum periostin 3. to reveal other significant determinants of serum periostin 4. to test serum periostin as a potential biomarker of subclinical arterial damage in children and adolescents with PH.

2. Materials and Methods

2.1. Study Group

Sample size was estimated based on available literature on periostin with statistical power 0.8, $p = 0.05$, and effect size 0.55 should be ~50 [25–35]. Fifty pediatric patients with PH were recruited to this single-center cross-sectional study from patients hospitalized in a pediatric nephrology center between February 2018 and March 2019. Participants' age varied from 5.58 to 17.92 years. The inclusion criterion was arterial hypertension diagnosed according to current European guidelines [5]. The exclusion criteria were secondary hypertension, clinically significant or laboratory confirmed allergic disease, known heart, renal, vascular, or other serious pathology, and acute inflammatory infections (temporary exclusion—4 weeks). 20 age-, and sex-matched healthy subjects were included in the control group. Their age varied from 8.33 to 17.83 years. The flow diagram of recruited patients is shown in Figure 1.

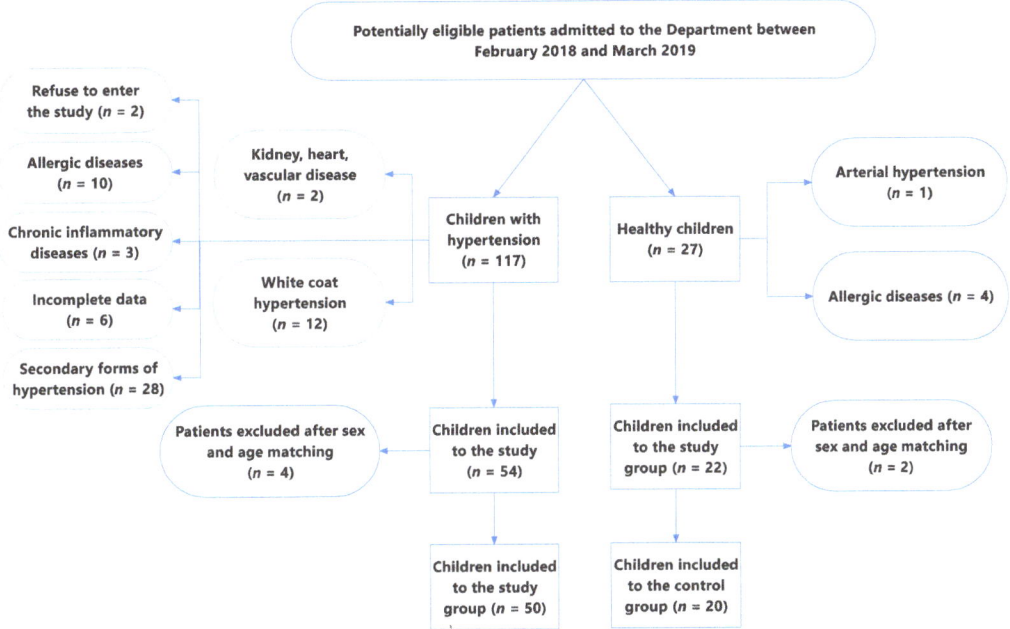

Figure 1. Flow diagram of the patients' recruitment.

2.2. Ethical Issues

Approval of the Bioethical Committee of the Medical University of Warsaw was obtained before the initiation of the research (approval no. KB/58/2016, 15 March 2016). All procedures involving human participants were in accordance with the highest ethical standards of the institutional research committee and were performed in accordance with the Declaration of Helsinki on the treatment of human subjects and its later amendments. Informed consent was obtained from all participants (≥16 years) and their representatives included in the study.

2.3. Clinical Parameters

In all patients upon admission, we assessed basic anthropometric parameters including height (cm), weight (kg), and body mass index (BMI) (kg/m^2). These measurements were compared with Polish normative data and expressed as Z-score [36]. In accordance with the World Health Organization definition, children with BMI Z-score values >1 and >2 were regarded as overweight and obese, respectively [37].

2.4. Serum Periostin

Venous peripheral blood was collected after overnight fasting. Next, blood was centrifuged to obtain serum, and stored at −80 °C until further analysis. Periostin levels were measured in serum samples by enzyme-linked immunosorbent assay (ELISA) (Human ELISA kit, Cat. No. RAG019R (ng/mL), Biovendor, Brno, Czech Republic) and the results were read using Biochrom Asys UVM 340 Scanning Microplate Reader (Biochrom Ltd., Cambridge, UK).

2.5. Other Laboratory Tests

Other parameters measured from peripheral blood in all children included: number of neutrophils (NEU; 1000/µL), lymphocytes (LYM; 1000/µL), platelets (PLT; 1000/µL), mean platelet volume (MPV; fL), and neutrophil-to-lymphocyte as well as platelet-to-lymphocyte ratios (NLR and PLR, respectively), serum creatinine (mg/dL), uric acid (mg/dL), total, low density lipoprotein (LDL), high-density lipoprotein (HDL) cholesterol (mg/dL), and triglycerides (mg/dL), calcium (mg/dL), phosphate (mg/dL), parathormone (PTH; pg/mL), alkaline phosphatase (IU/L), and vitamin D concentration (25(OH)D) (ng/mL). Glomerular filtration rate was estimated according to the revised Schwartz formula (eGFR) (mL/min/1.73 m^2) [38].

2.6. Blood Pressure and Arterial Damage Parameters

In all patients with PH, the duration of hypertension was estimated based on medical records and in those receiving pharmacological treatment antihypertensive medications were analyzed. The BP measurement methodology and arterial damage assessment were described in detail in our previous manuscripts [39–42]. In short, peripheral office BP was evaluated oscillometrically by Welch Allyn VSM Patient Monitor 300 (Welch Allyn Inc., Skaneateles Falls, NY, USA) ((mmHg) and Z-scores) [43]. We performed 24 h ambulatory blood pressure monitoring (ABPM) with SUNTECH OSCAR 2 oscillometric device (SunTech Medical, Inc., Morrisville, NC, USA) and interpreted according to pediatric recommendations [44] with the following parameters included in the final analysis: systolic, diastolic, and mean arterial pressure (SBP, DBP, MAP, respectively) during 24 h (mm Hg), MAP 24 h Z-score, pulse pressure (mm Hg), heart rate (beats per minute), SBP and DBP load during 24 h (%), and nocturnal blood pressure dip (%) [44]. Central (aortic) blood pressure (AoBP) (mm Hg), augmentation index normalized to heart rate of 75 beats per minute (Aix75HR) (%), subendocardial viability ratio (SEVR) (%), and aortic pulse wave velocity (aPWV) (m/s) were measured using the Sphygmocor device (AtCor Medical Pty Ltd., Sydney, Australia) and applanation tonometry. Aloka Prosound Alpha 6 (Hitachi Aloka Medical, Mitaka, Japan) equipped with a 13 MHz linear transducer was used to measure common carotid intima media thickness (cIMT) (mm) and elasticity parameters of the right common carotid artery (ECHO-tracking (ET) preset): beta (stiffness index), Ep (pressure strain elasticity modulus) (kPa), AC (arterial compliance) (mm^2/kPa), AIx (augmentation index) (%), PWVbeta (pulse wave velocity beta) (m/s), D_max (mm), D_min (mm) (maximal and minimal diameter of the artery), DATmax (acceleration time to artery maximal diameter) (ms). aPWV and cIMT were presented as numeric values and Z-scores [45,46].

2.7. Statistical Analysis

Statistical data were analyzed using Dell Statistica 13.0 PL software (TIBCO Software Inc., Palo Alto, CA, USA). All data were reported as absolute numbers, mean ± standard deviation (SD), and interquartile range (IQR). Normality of data distribution was analyzed with the Shapiro–Wilk test. The following tests were used (depending upon variables' distribution): Student *t*-test, U Mann–Whitney test, Spearman rank correlation, chi-square test, and Fisher's exact test. Multivariate analysis was performed using a general regression model. Parameters that correlated with each other with r >0.600 were excluded from the regression model to avoid collinearity. A *p*-value below 0.05 was considered as statistically significant.

3. Results

3.1. Periostin, Clinical and Laboratory Parameters

Both groups' basic clinical parameters and results of key laboratory tests, including periostin levels, were depicted in Table 1. PH and healthy children did not differ in terms of age, sex, height, height Z-score, eGFR, and total-, and LDL- cholesterol. Periostin levels were significantly lower in hypertensive children compared to healthy ones ($p = 0.038$). Children with PH were characterized also by significantly higher weight, BMI, concentrations of uric acid, and triglycerides. HDL-cholesterol levels were significantly lower in the study group compared to healthy children. In the PH group 21 (42%) of all patients were overweight and 7 (14%) were obese. The duration of hypertension in the study group was 18.14 ± 20.86 (4–24) (months). At the moment of evaluation, 27 (54.0%) children received pharmacological antihypertensive treatment—23 were on monotherapy, 3 were treated with 2 medications, and one child received 3 medications. Most commonly used agents were as follows: calcium channel blockers (17 children), angiotensin-converting enzyme inhibitors (9 children), and beta-adrenolytics (3 children). In addition, 3 children were treated with doxazosin, valsartan, and hydrochlorothiazide. Parameters of complete blood count and calcium-phosphate metabolism were presented in Supplementary Table S1.

Table 1. Clinical and biochemical parameters of the study and the control group (data presented as numbers or mean ± standard deviation and interquartile range).

Parameter	Study Group	Control Group	p
Number of patients (n)	50	20	NA
Age (years)	14.76 ± 3.08 (14.42–16.75)	14.11 ± 2.99 (13.00–16.38)	0.261
Boys/Girls	29/21 (58%/42%)	11/9 (55%/45%)	0.819
Height (cm)	166.7 ± 16.51 (160.5–178.5)	161.9 ± 15.26 (151.5–171.5)	0.259
Height Z-score	0.54 ± 0.99 (−0.45–1.16)	0.69 ± 1.23 (0.13–1.22)	0.589
Weight (kg)	70.29 ± 19.6 (61.5–85.0)	55.2 ± 16.55 (46.0–61.0)	0.003
Weight Z-score	1.23 ± 0.80 (0.49–1.83)	0.61 ± 0.98 (−0.26–1.25)	0.009
BMI	24.78 ± 4.63 (21.27–28.89)	20.67 ± 3.59 (18.30–22.03)	0.001
BMI Z-score	1.09 ± 0.82 (0.5–1.78)	0.35 ± 0.94 (−0.43–1.12)	0.004
Periostin (ng/mL)	35.42 ± 10.43 (27.73–39.02)	42.16 ± 12.82 (32.21–51.45)	0.038
eGFR acc. to Schwartz (L/min/1.73 m^2)	100.12 ± 21.16 (86.73–115.64)	108.12 ± 18.48 (95.42–121.9)	0.100
Uric acid (mg/dL)	5.56 ± 1.34 (4.7–6.4)	4.56 ± 1.10 (3.95–5.35)	0.004
Total cholesterol (mg/dL)	153.98 ± 33.92 (132.0–168.0)	154.75 ± 30.71 (135.0–179.5)	0.927
LDL-cholesterol (mg/dL)	85.63 ± 30.38 (64.0–95.8)	81.2 ± 24.19 (63.8–103.6)	0.654
HDL-cholesterol (mg/dL)	49.5 ± 10.28 (43.0–53.0)	61.05 ± 13.05 (52.5–69.5)	0.001
Triglycerides (mg/dL)	95.24 ± 43.18 (64.0–120.0)	64.5 ± 23.86 (49.5–71.5)	0.002

NA: not applicable; BMI: body mass index; eGFR: estimated glomerular filtration rate; LDL: low-density lipoprotein; HDL: high-density lipoprotein.

3.2. Blood Pressure and Parameters of Arterial Damage

The comparison of peripheral and central blood pressure, arterial stiffness, and intima media thickness in the study and control group are shown in Supplementary Tables S2 and S3.

Children and adolescents with PH had higher office peripheral and central blood pressures, as well as blood pressure measured with ABPM. There was no difference in 24 h ABPM heart rate and pulse pressure (PP), and aortic pulse pressure (AoPP) and both systolic and diastolic nocturnal BP dipping between both groups. Patients with PH were characterized by faster aortic pulse wave velocity (5.17 ± 0.93 vs. 4.49 ± 0.72 (m/s), $p = 0.004$), thicker common carotid artery intima media layer (0.45 ± 0.07 vs. 0.39 ± 0.03 (mm), $p < 0.001$), and larger common carotid artery (maximal and minimal) diameters. No differences were found in aortic augmentation index, subendocardial viability ratio, and local stiffness parameters.

3.3. Determinants of Serum Periostin Level

Periostin level did not differ between PH patients either on or off antihypertensive drugs (34.89 ± 9.86 (28.80–37.89) vs. 36.00 ± 11.36 (27.22–41.10) (ng/mL), $p = 0.954$) and between 10 PH patients not treated and 40 patients not treated with renin-angiotensin-aldosterone system inhibitors (34.96 ± 6.47 (30.77–37.41) vs. 35.54 ± 11.27 (27.42–40.20) (ng/mL), $p = 0.602$). Additionally, no difference between hypertensive boys and girls was found (34.89 ± 9.86 (28.80–37.89) vs. 36.00 ± 11.36 (27.22–41.10) (ng/mL), $p = 0.954$).

The correlations of periostin with clinical and laboratory parameters in the whole group of 70 children are shown in Table 2. We found positive correlations of periostin concentration with HDL-cholesterol and phosphate, calcium-phosphate product, and alkaline phosphatase activity. Negative correlations of periostin with age, height, weight, BMI, NLR, and concentrations of creatinine, uric acid, and triglycerides were observed. Furthermore, periostin level correlated negatively with numerous indices of blood pressure, aortic pulse wave velocity, and common carotid artery diameters. The correlations of periostin with the studied parameters in separate groups are shown in Tables 3 and 4 for the study and the control group, respectively. In 50 children with PH periostin correlated positively with height Z-score, number of lymphocytes, calcium, phosphate, calcium-phosphate product, and alkaline phosphatase, and negatively with age, weight, and BMI. These three anthropometrical parameters as well as serum creatinine, PWV, PWV Z-score, office SBP, AoSBP (aortic systolic blood pressure) were also negatively correlated with periostin in 20 healthy children. In the control group periostin also correlated positively with HDL-cholesterol, phosphate, alkaline phosphatase, and AIx75HR. No significant correlation between serum periostin and eGFR in the whole group, and in patients with primary hypertension, and control group were found.

Table 2. Correlations of periostin concentration with clinical, biochemical parameters, blood pressure, and arterial damage parameters in 70 studied children.

Analyzed Parameter	R	p
Periostin (ng/mL) vs. age (years)	−0.561	<0.001
Periostin (ng/mL) vs. height Z-score	−0.278	0.020
Periostin (ng/mL) vs. weight (kg)	−0.505	<0.001
Periostin (ng/mL) vs. BMI (kg/m^2)	−0.585	<0.001
Periostin (ng/mL) vs. BMI Z-score	−0.298	0.012
Periostin (ng/mL) vs. NLR	−0.270	0.024
Periostin (ng/mL) vs. creatinine (mg/dL)	−0.301	0.011
Periostin (ng/mL) vs. uric acid (mg/dL)	−0.240	0.045
Periostin (ng/mL) vs. HDL-cholesterol (mg/dL)	0.397	<0.001
Periostin (ng/mL) vs. triglycerides (mg/dL)	−0.245	0.041
Periostin (ng/mL) vs. phosphate (mg/dL)	0.421	<0.001
Periostin (ng/mL) vs. Ca * P (mg^2/dL^2)	0.423	<0.001
Periostin (ng/mL) vs. alkaline phosphatase (IU/L)	0.694	<0.001
Periostin (ng/mL) vs. SBP (mm Hg)	−0.370	0.004
Periostin (ng/mL) vs. SBP Z-score	−0.269	0.024
Periostin (ng/mL) vs. DBP (mm Hg)	−0.303	0.011
Periostin (ng/mL) vs. DBP Z-score	−0.323	0.006
Periostin (ng/mL) vs. MAP (mm Hg)	−0.320	0.007
Periostin (ng/mL) vs. ABPM SBP 24 h (mm Hg)	−0.285	0.017
Periostin (ng/mL) vs. ABPM MAP 24 h (mm Hg)	−0.251	0.036
Periostin (ng/mL) vs. ABPM PP 24 h (mm Hg)	−0.243	0.043
Periostin (ng/mL) vs. AoSBP (mm Hg)	−0.340	0.004
Periostin (ng/mL) vs. AoDBP (mm Hg)	−0.333	0.005
Periostin (ng/mL) vs. AoMAP (mm Hg)	−0.334	0.005
Periostin (ng/mL) vs. aPWV (m/s)	−0.342	0.004

Table 2. Cont.

Analyzed Parameter	R	p
Periostin (ng/mL) vs. aPWV Z-score	−0.306	0.010
Periostin (ng/mL) vs. ET D max (mm)	−0.379	0.001
Periostin (ng/mL) vs. ET D min (mm)	−0.353	0.003

BMI: body mass index; NLR: neutrophil-to-lymphocyte ratio; HDL: high-density lipoprotein; Ca * P: calcium phosphate product; SBP: systolic blood pressure; DBP: diastolic blood pressure; MAP: mean arterial pressure; PP: pulse pressure; ABPM: ambulatory blood pressure; HR: heart rate; bpm: beats per minute; SBPL: systolic blood pressure load; DBPL: diastolic blood pressure load; AoSBP: aortic (central) systolic blood pressure; AoDBP: aortic (central) diastolic blood pressure; AoMAP: aortic (central) mean blood pressure; aPWV: aortic pulse wave velocity; ET: ECHO-tracking; beta: stiffness index; D max: maximal diameter of the right common carotid artery; D min: minimal diameter of the right common carotid artery.

Table 3. Correlations of periostin concentration with clinical, biochemical parameters, blood pressure, and arterial damage parameters in 50 children with primary hypertension.

Analyzed Parameter	R	p
Periostin (ng/mL) vs. Age (years)	−0.554	<0.001
Periostin (ng/mL) vs. Height Z-score	0.325	0.021
Periostin (ng/mL) vs. Weight (kg)	−0.388	0.005
Periostin (ng/mL) vs. BMI (kg/m^2)	−0.471	0.001
Periostin (ng/mL) vs. BMI Z-score	−0.194	0.177
Periostin (ng/mL) vs. NLR	−0.181	0.209
Periostin (ng/mL) vs. Creatinine (mg/dL)	−0.138	0.341
Periostin (ng/mL) vs. Uric acid (mg/dL)	−0.103	0.477
Periostin (ng/mL) vs. HDL-cholesterol (mg/dL)	0.239	0.094
Periostin (ng/mL) vs. Triglycerides (mg/dL)	−0.092	0.524
Periostin (ng/mL) vs. Phosphate (mg/dL)	0.369	0.008
Periostin (ng/mL) vs. Ca * P (mg^2/dL^2)	0.447	0.001
Periostin (ng/mL) vs. Alkaline Phosphatase (IU/L)	0.651	<0.001
Periostin (ng/mL) vs. SBP (mm Hg)	−0.208	0.148
Periostin (ng/mL) vs. SBP Z-score	−0.031	0.832
Periostin (ng/mL) vs. DBP (mm Hg)	−0.207	0.149
Periostin (ng/mL) vs. DBP Z-score	−0.205	0.153
Periostin (ng/mL) vs. MAP (mm Hg)	−0.208	0.147
Periostin (ng/mL) vs. ABPM SBP 24 h (mm Hg)	−0.182	0.205
Periostin (ng/mL) vs. ABPM MAP 24 h (mm Hg)	−0.134	0.352
Periostin (ng/mL) vs. ABPM PP 24 h (mm Hg)	−0.138	0.340
Periostin (ng/mL) vs. AoSBP (mm Hg)	−0.182	0.205
Periostin (ng/mL) vs. AoDBP (mm Hg)	−0.255	0.074
Periostin (ng/mL) vs. AoMAP (mm Hg)	−0.220	0.125
Periostin (ng/mL) vs. aPWV (m/s)	−0.226	0.115
Periostin (ng/mL) vs. aPWV Z-score	−0.172	0.233
Periostin (ng/mL) vs. ET D max (mm)	−0.276	0.053
Periostin (ng/mL) vs. ET D min (mm)	−0.244	0.088

BMI: body mass index; NLR: neutrophil-to-lymphocyte ratio; HDL: high-density lipoprotein; Ca * P: calcium phosphate product; SBP: systolic blood pressure; DBP: diastolic blood pressure; MAP: mean arterial pressure; PP: pulse pressure; ABPM: ambulatory blood pressure; HR: heart rate; bpm: beats per minute; SBPL: systolic blood pressure load; DBPL: diastolic blood pressure load; AoSBP: aortic (central) systolic blood pressure; AoDBP: aortic (central) diastolic blood pressure; AoMAP: aortic (central) mean blood pressure; aPWV: pulse wave velocity; ET: ECHO-tracking; beta: stiffness index; D max: maximal diameter of right common carotid artery; D min: minimal diameter of right common carotid artery.

Table 4. Correlations of periostin concentration with clinical, biochemical parameters, blood pressure, and arterial damage parameters in 20 healthy children.

Analyzed Parameter	R	p
Periostin (ng/mL) vs. Age (years)	−0.570	0.009
Periostin (ng/mL) vs. Height Z-score	0.198	0.403
Periostin (ng/mL) vs. Weight (kg)	−0.633	0.003

Table 4. Cont.

Analyzed Parameter	R	p
Periostin (ng/mL) vs. BMI (kg/m^2)	−0.734	<0.001
Periostin (ng/mL) vs. BMI Z-score	−0.324	0.163
Periostin (ng/mL) vs. NLR	−0.277	0.238
Periostin (ng/mL) vs. Creatinine (mg/dL)	−0.474	0.035
Periostin (ng/mL) vs. Uric acid (mg/dL)	−0.108	0.651
Periostin (ng/mL) vs. HDL-cholesterol (mg/dL)	0.514	0.021
Periostin (ng/mL) vs. Triglycerides (mg/dL)	−0.351	0.130
Periostin (ng/mL) vs. Phosphate (mg/dL)	0.552	0.012
Periostin (ng/mL) vs. Ca * P (mg^2/dL^2)	0.416	0.068
Periostin (ng/mL) vs. Alkaline Phosphatase (IU/L)	0.693	0.001
Periostin (ng/mL) vs. SBP (mm Hg)	−0.454	0.044
Periostin (ng/mL) vs. SBP Z-score	−0.444	0.050
Periostin (ng/mL) vs. DBP (mm Hg)	−0.369	0.110
Periostin (ng/mL) vs. DBP Z-score	−0.277	0.238
Periostin (ng/mL) vs. MAP (mm Hg)	−0.361	0.118
Periostin (ng/mL) vs. ABPM SBP 24 h (mm Hg)	−0.078	0.742
Periostin (ng/mL) vs. ABPM MAP 24 h (mm Hg)	−0.156	0.512
Periostin (ng/mL) vs. ABPM PP 24 h (mm Hg)	0.018	0.939
Periostin (ng/mL) vs. AoSBP (mm Hg)	−0.477	0.034
Periostin (ng/mL) vs. AoDBP (mm Hg)	−0.328	0.158
Periostin (ng/mL) vs. AoMAP (mm Hg)	−0.361	0.118
Periostin (ng/mL) vs. PWV (m/s)	−0.462	0.040
Periostin (ng/mL) vs. PWV Z-score	−0.448	0.048
Periostin (ng/mL) vs. ET D max (mm)	−0.350	0.130
Periostin (ng/mL) vs. ET D min (mm)	−0.341	0.141

BMI: body mass index; NLR: neutrophil-to-lymphocyte ratio; HDL: high-density lipoprotein; Ca * P: calcium phosphate product; SBP: systolic blood pressure; DBP: diastolic blood pressure; MAP: mean arterial pressure; PP: pulse pressure; ABPM: ambulatory blood pressure; HR: heart rate; bpm: beats per minute; SBPL: systolic blood pressure load; DBPL: diastolic blood pressure load; AoSBP: aortic (central) systolic blood pressure; AoDBP: aortic (central) diastolic blood pressure; AoMAP: aortic (central) mean blood pressure; PWV: pulse wave velocity; ET: ECHO-tracking; beta: stiffness index; D max: maximal diameter of right common carotid artery; D min: minimal diameter of right common carotid artery.

To verify independent associations between periostin, blood pressure, and arterial stiffness, multivariate analysis was performed (Table 5). As shown in Table 5, age, BMI Z-score, uric acid, HDL-cholesterol, and triglycerides were the significant independent determinants of periostin concentration in children.

Table 5. Multivariate analysis of periostin determinants in children.

Parameter	Beta	95% Confidence Interval	p
Age (years)	−0.614	−0.831–(−0.398)	<0.001
Uric acid (mg/dL)	0.328	0.124–0.533	0.002
BMI Z-score	−0.293	−0.492–(−0.095)	0.005
HDL-cholesterol (mg/dL)	0.235	0.054–0.416	0.012
Triglycerides (mg/dL)	−0.198	−0.394–(−0.002)	0.048
DBP Z-score	−0.205	−0.434–0.025	0.079
Presence of hypertension (yes/no)	0.219	−0.032–0.469	0.087
ET D max (mm)	−0.149	−0.330–0.031	0.104
AoSBP (mm Hg)	−0.142	−0.381–0.097	0.240
Ca * P (mg^2/dL^2)	0.066	−0.119–0.251	0.478
NLR	−0.062	−0.245–0.121	0.499
Height Z-score	0.052	−0.124–0.229	0.555
aPWV Z-score	0.024	−0.162–0.210	0.795

BMI: body mass index; HDL: high-density lipoprotein; DBP: diastolic blood pressure; ET: ECHO-tracking; beta: stiffness index; D max: maximal diameter of the right common carotid artery; AoSBP: aortic (central) systolic blood pressure; Ca * P: calcium phosphate product; NLR: neutrophil-to-lymphocyte ratio; aPWV: aortic pulse wave velocity.

4. Discussion

Our cross-sectional study analyzed periostin as a possible biomarker of blood pressure and subclinical arterial damage in pediatric patients with primary hypertension. Univariate analysis showed that periostin level was lower in hypertensive individuals as compared to the control group. Moreover, it revealed numerous negative correlations between periostin level, blood pressure, and arterial damage parameters. Nevertheless, these relations disappeared in multivariate analysis leaving only the following significant predictors of periostin: age, BMI Z-score, uric acid, HDL-cholesterol, and triglycerides. In multivariate analysis, neither the presence of hypertension nor blood pressure significantly influenced periostin level.

Periostin was found to be involved in tissue repair after vascular injury, e.g., in acute rheumatic fever [28], hypertensive nephropathy [19], myocardial infarction [47], and subarachnoid hemorrhage [48]. Periostin plays a critical role in the interaction with signaling proteins such as NF-kB (nuclear factor kappa B) or STAT3 (signal transducer and activator of transcription) to modulate the response of the extracellular matrix in various tissue pathologies [28]. It is hypothesized that after injury periostin expression increases and thus facilitates tissue repair and remodeling. A cross-talk between periostin and transforming growth factor beta (TGFβ) signals in different tissues and pathological conditions was described [49]. This mutual, reciprocal relation was revealed e.g., in scleroderma and allergic diseases [50]. Periostin augments adhesion and TGFβ release in immune cells. Reciprocally, TGFβ induces periostin production in fibroblasts [50]. Similar interplay was revealed in kidney tissue, where periostin can induce cell dedifferentiation, increase in TGFβ expression and extracellular matrix deposition. In addition, TGFβ can also promote the expression of periostin, which, in turn, induces the loss of renal tubular epithelial phenotype (epithelial-mesenchymal transition) and ultimately leads to fibrosis [51].

It is noteworthy that elevated expression of periostin in the arterial wall was found in a hypoxia-induced model of pulmonary hypertension [52]. Moreover, periostin played a pivotal role in aortic thickening in hypertensive rats [18]. Hence, one would expect a higher periostin level in hypertensive patients and its positive correlation with arterial damage parameters. Unintuitively, in our hypertensive patients periostin level was lower and correlated negatively with both blood pressure and aortic pulse wave velocity. Notably, these relations disappeared in multivariate analysis. It is possible that periostin is not released yet in the subclinical damage found in our patients or serum periostin concentrations do not correspond with tissue (arterial wall) periostin expression. Further studies are needed to elucidate the role of periostin in the development of early stages of hypertensive diseases and vascular damage in these patients.

Interleukins (ILs) 3, 4, 6, 13, tumor necrosis factor alpha (TNFα), TGFβ, and vascular endothelial growth factor (VEGF) are the best known inducers of periostin expression and release [53]. In particular, increased IL-4 and IL-13 were found to be responsible for high periostin levels in allergic children [26] and TNFα and IL-6 in obese adults [33]. That is why the patients with chronic inflammatory diseases, allergies, and acute infections were excluded from the analysis to avoid the impact of these comorbidities on the periostin level. However, nowadays arterial hypertension is considered a state of subclinical inflammation with numerous inflammatory markers elevated that may link PH with dysregulation of periostin level [54]. Our PH children had higher neutrophil count, lower platelet volume, and a trend towards a higher neutrophil-to-lymphocyte ratio as compared to healthy peers. Univariate analysis showed a negative correlation between NLR and periostin level, but this relation was excluded in the multivariate analysis. Based on these results, no definite statement on the mutual relation between subclinical inflammation and periostin level in PH patients can be made. Analysis of the relation between periostin and more precise markers of inflammation (e.g., high-sensitivity C-reactive protein or interleukin levels) in patients with PH would be of special interest.

Activation of the renin–angiotensin–aldosterone system could be a link between periostin and cardiovascular system regulation. One study showed increased periostin levels in rats in response to chronic infusion of angiotensin II [16]. Other paper points out that periostin can contribute to oxidative stress and is upregulated by angiotensin II via the reactive oxygen species signaling pathway in fibroblasts of hypertensive rats [17]. The mutual relation between RAAS and periostin may be more complex as periostin downregulation attenuated 5/6 nephrectomy-induced intrarenal RAAS activation and renal tissue fibrosis [15]. We did not measure plasma renin activity or aldosterone levels in the studied subjects. Twenty percent of our hypertensive patients were on RAAS blockade and no difference was found between those treated and not treated with angiotensin receptor blockers and angiotensin converting enzyme inhibitors.

Age was the strongest predictor of periostin level in our cohort. Limited studies showed decrease in periostin levels with age [34,35]. Similarly to our observations, O'Connell at al. found a negative relation between periostin level and age. Of note, these authors analyzed only children aged less than two years [34]. Elevated periostin levels seen in younger children may reflect the accelerated cell turnover and growth in the first few years of life and which would naturally increase periostin expression. Negative correlations of periostin, blood pressure, and pulse wave velocity were absent in multivariate analysis, as these parameters are strongly related to age and BMI in the pediatric population [36,43,45].

Epidemiological studies show an association between cardiovascular diseases, hypertension, metabolic syndrome, and high levels of uric acid. In addition, some data suggest that high uric acid levels can predict the development of hypertension [55]. Animal studies revealed positive correlations between uric acid concentration, inflammation, and decreased expression of neuronal nitric oxide synthase, which results in blood vessel contraction [56]. Additionally, in our cohort almost half of hypertensive subjects presented with hyperuricemia. Our multivariate analysis revealed a positive correlation between uric acid and periostin levels. A similar positive relation was found in Chinese adult women with polycystic ovary syndrome [29]. It is possible that periostin is released in response to subclinical damage caused by uric acid elevation.

In univariate analysis, serum periostin inversely correlated with serum creatinine, which could seemingly indicate the dependence of this marker on renal function. However, it should be noted that patients in both groups had normal renal function (eGFR > 60 mL/min/1.73 m^2 according to Schwartz's formula, which is known to underestimate glomerular filtration rate in adolescents [38,57]). Serum creatinine concentration is dependent on weight and age, hence this apparent relationship disappeared in the multivariate analysis. We did not observe any relationship between periostin and eGFR in the children studied. Published data on mutual relation between kidney function and serum periostin level are scarce. A trend towards positive correlation between creatinine and serum periostin was found in adults with diabetic kidney disease [58]. On the other hand, urinary periostin was negatively correlated with eGFR in adult patients with diabetic kidney disease [21] and chronic allograft nephropathy [22]. Also, increased glomerular periostin staining was related to low eGFR in different glomerulopathies [23].

The results of our multivariate analysis demonstrated that periostin level is positively correlated with HDL-cholesterol and negatively with triglyceride concentration as well as with BMI Z-score. HDLs are characterized by a well-established protective effect on the arterial wall and their negative correlations with cardiovascular incidents are well documented [59]. There is conflicting data concerning the role of periostin in lipid metabolism. By contrast with our results, in two Chinese studies involving young women with polycystic ovary syndrome [29] and adult obese patients with type 2 diabetes [33], periostin concentration was directly correlated with BMI and triglycerides and inversely correlated with HDL-cholesterol. Lu et al. found that overexpression of periostin in obese rats resulted in liver steatosis and hypertriglyceridemia via activation of c-Jun N-terminal kinase (JNK) signaling pathway and downregulation of peroxisome proliferator-activated receptor alpha (PPARα) [60]. On the other hand, a recent interventional study in rats after myocardial infarction showed a beneficial effect of periostin supply on HDL-cholesterol [47]. These experimental results suggest the positive impact of the studied particle on the regulation of cholesterol and triglycerides levels.

The cross-sectional nature of the study that precludes drawing final casual relationships between the measured parameters is a major limitation of our study. A low number of patients in the control group is another disadvantage. The large heterogeneity in age and BMI of the patients resulted in the demonstration of numerous correlations in univariate analysis that proved to be statistically insignificant in multivariate analysis (e.g., creatinine). Of note, our analysis of immune system activation was limited only to low-precision parameters derived from peripheral complete blood count. In addition, we have not evaluated concentrations of other key players in pathogenesis of tissue damage and repair e.g., TGFβ. Finally, neither urine nor tissue (vascular wall) periostin levels were analyzed in the studied children. Of note, deep analysis of blood pressure and general and local (carotid artery) vascular damage are particular strengths of the study.

5. Conclusions

The role of serum periostin as a biomarker of elevated blood pressure and arterial damage in pediatric patients with primary hypertension is yet to be unmasked. More clinical studies are needed to reveal the changes of periostin in hypertensive patients' serum and urine, and to clarify its role in this population. Age seems to be the strongest predictor of serum periostin level in pediatric population. We have not found any significant dependences of serum periostin with blood pressure and arterial damage analyzed according to different aspects. On the other hand, there was a significant relation of serum periostin with well-established cardiovascular risk factors. Considering young age of our patients and relatively short duration of PH as compared to adults, it is possible that these correlations have not markedly influenced blood pressure and target organs in children with PH yet.

Supplementary Materials: The following are available online at https://www.mdpi.com/article/10.3390/jcm10102138/s1, Table S1: Parameters of complete blood count and parameters of calcium-phosphate metabolism of the study and the control group (data presented as mean ± standard deviation and interquartile range)., Table S2: Blood pressure in the study and the control group (data presented as numbers or mean ± standard deviation and interquartile range), Table S3: Parameters of arterial structure and function in the study and the control group (data presented as numbers or mean ± standard deviation and interquartile range). Table S4: Patient data (patient_data.xlsx).

Author Contributions: Conceptualization, M.S., P.S. and M.P.-T.; methodology, P.S.; validation, P.S., M.P.-T.; formal analysis, M.S. and P.S.; investigation, M.S., P.S., A.S.-E.; resources, A.S.-E. and M.P.-T.; data curation, M.S. and P.S.; writing—original draft preparation, M.S. and P.S.; writing—review and editing, A.S.-E. and M.P.-T.; visualization, M.S. and P.S.; supervision, M.P.-T.; project administration, P.S. and M.P.-T.; funding acquisition, M.P.-T. All authors have read and agreed to the published version of the manuscript.

Funding: This research was funded from the statutory funds of the Department of Pediatrics and Nephrology, Medical University of Warsaw.

Institutional Review Board Statement: The study was conducted according to the guidelines of the Declaration of Helsinki, and approved by the Local Bioethics Committee of the Medical University of Warsaw (approval no. KB/58/2016, 15 March 2016).

Informed Consent Statement: Informed consent was obtained from all subjects (≥ 16 years) and their representatives involved in the study.

Data Availability Statement: Data used to support the findings of this study are included within the supplementary information files, Supplementary Table S4 (patient_data.xlsx).

Conflicts of Interest: The authors declare no conflict of interest.

References

1. Williams, B.; Mancia, G.; Spiering, W.; Agabiti Rosei, E.; Azizi, M.; Burnier, M.; Clement, D.L.; Coca, A.; de Simone, G.; Dominiczak, A.; et al. 2018 ESC/ESH Guidelines for the management of arterial hypertension. *Eur. Heart J.* **2018**, *39*, 3021–3104. [CrossRef] [PubMed]
2. Song, P.; Zhang, Y.; Yu, J.; Zha, M.; Zhu, Y.; Rahimi, K.; Rudan, I. Global Prevalence of Hypertension in Children: A Systematic Review and Meta-analysis. *JAMA Pediatr.* **2019**, 1–10. [CrossRef] [PubMed]
3. Gupta-Malhotra, M.; Banker, A.; Shete, S.; Hashmi, S.S.; Tyson, J.E.; Barratt, M.S.; Hecht, J.T.; Milewicz, D.M.; Boerwinkle, E. Essential hypertension vs. secondary hypertension among children. *Am. J. Hypertens.* **2015**, *28*, 73–80. [CrossRef] [PubMed]
4. Abdel Ghafar, M.T. An overview of the classical and tissue-derived renin-angiotensin-aldosterone system and its genetic polymorphisms in essential hypertension. *Steroids* **2020**, *163*, 108701. [CrossRef]
5. Lurbe, E.; Agabiti-Rosei, E.; Cruickshank, J.K.; Dominiczak, A.; Erdine, S.; Hirth, A.; Invitti, C.; Litwin, M.; Mancia, G.; Pall, D.; et al. 2016 European Society of Hypertension guidelines for the management of high blood pressure in children and adolescents. *J. Hypertens.* **2016**, *34*, 1887–1920. [CrossRef]
6. Urbina, E.M.; Lande, M.B.; Hooper, S.R.; Daniels, S.R. Target Organ Abnormalities in Pediatric Hypertension. *J. Pediatr.* **2018**, *202*, 14–22. [CrossRef]
7. Litwin, M.; Trelewicz, J.; Wawer, Z.; Antoniewicz, J.; Wierzbicka, A.; Rajszys, P.; Grenda, R. Intima-media thickness and arterial elasticity in hypertensive children: Controlled study. *Pediatr. Nephrol.* **2004**, *19*, 767–774. [CrossRef]
8. Hvidt, K.N.; Olsen, M.H.; Ibsen, H.; Holm, J.C. Weight reduction and aortic stiffness in obese children and adolescents: A 1-year follow-up study. *J. Hum. Hypertens.* **2015**, *29*, 535–540. [CrossRef]
9. Son, W.M.; Sung, K.D.; Bharath, L.P.; Choi, K.J.; Park, S.Y. Combined exercise training reduces blood pressure, arterial stiffness, and insulin resistance in obese prehypertensive adolescent girls. *Clin. Exp. Hypertens.* **2017**, *39*, 546–552. [CrossRef]
10. Sun, Z. Aging, arterial stiffness, and hypertension. *Hypertension* **2015**, *65*, 252–256. [CrossRef]
11. Durham, A.L.; Speer, M.Y.; Scatena, M.; Giachelli, C.M.; Shanahan, C.M. Role of smooth muscle cells in vascular calcification: Implications in atherosclerosis and arterial stiffness. *Cardiovasc. Res.* **2018**, *114*, 590–600. [CrossRef] [PubMed]
12. Kudo, A. Introductory review: Periostin-gene and protein structure. *Cell Mol. Life Sci.* **2017**, *74*, 4259–4268. [CrossRef]
13. Idolazzi, L.; Ridolo, E.; Fassio, A.; Gatti, D.; Montagni, M.; Caminati, M.; Martignago, I.; Incorvaia, C.; Senna, G. Periostin: The bone and beyond. *Eur. J. Intern. Med.* **2017**, *38*, 12–16. [CrossRef] [PubMed]
14. Prakoura, N.; Chatziantoniou, C. Matricellular Proteins and Organ Fibrosis. *Current. Pathobiol. Rep.* **2017**, *5*, 111–121. [CrossRef]
15. Bian, X.; Bai, Y.; Su, X.; Zhao, G.; Sun, G.; Li, D. Knockdown of periostin attenuates 5/6 nephrectomy-induced intrarenal renin-angiotensin system activation, fibrosis, and inflammation in rats. *J. Cell Physiol.* **2019**, *234*, 22857–22873. [CrossRef] [PubMed]
16. Li, L.; Fan, D.; Wang, C.; Wang, J.Y.; Cui, X.B.; Wu, D.; Zhou, Y.; Wu, L.L. Angiotensin II increases periostin expression via Ras/p38 MAPK/CREB and ERK1/2/TGF-β1 pathways in cardiac fibroblasts. *Cardiovasc. Res.* **2011**, *91*, 80–89. [CrossRef]
17. Wu, H.; Chen, L.; Xie, J.; Li, R.; Li, G.N.; Chen, Q.H.; Zhang, X.L.; Kang, L.N.; Xu, B. Periostin expression induced by oxidative stress contributes to myocardial fibrosis in a rat model of high salt-induced hypertension. *Mol. Med. Rep.* **2016**, *14*, 776–782. [CrossRef]
18. Zempo, H.; Suzuki, J.I.; Ogawa, M.; Watanabe, R.; Fujiu, K.; Manabe, I.; Conway, S.J.; Taniyama, Y.; Morishita, R.; Hirata, Y.; et al. Influence of periostin-positive cell-specific Klf5 deletion on aortic thickening in DOCA-salt hypertensive mice. *Hypertens. Res.* **2016**, *39*, 764–768. [CrossRef]
19. Guerrot, D.; Dussaule, J.C.; Mael-Ainin, M.; Xu-Dubois, Y.C.; Rondeau, E.; Chatziantoniou, C.; Placier, S. Identification of periostin as a critical marker of progression/reversal of hypertensive nephropathy. *PLoS ONE* **2012**, *7*, e31974. [CrossRef]
20. Muñoz-Pacheco, P.; Ortega-Hernández, A.; Caro-Vadillo, A.; Casanueva-Eliceiry, S.; Aragoncillo, P.; Egido, J.; Fernández-Cruz, A.; Gómez-Garre, D. Eplerenone enhances cardioprotective effects of standard heart failure therapy through matricellular proteins in hypertensive heart failure. *J. Hypertens.* **2013**, *31*, 2309–2318. [CrossRef]
21. Satirapoj, B.; Tassanasorn, S.; Charoenpitakchai, M.; Supasyndh, O. Periostin as a tissue and urinary biomarker of renal injury in type 2 diabetes mellitus. *PLoS ONE* **2015**, *10*, e0124055. [CrossRef] [PubMed]
22. Satirapoj, B.; Witoon, R.; Ruangkanchanasetr, P.; Wantanasiri, P.; Charoenpitakchai, M.; Choovichian, P. Urine periostin as a biomarker of renal injury in chronic allograft nephropathy. *Transplant. Proc.* **2014**, *46*, 135–140. [CrossRef]
23. Sen, K.; Lindenmeyer, M.T.; Gaspert, A.; Eichinger, F.; Neusser, M.A.; Kretzler, M.; Segerer, S.; Cohen, C.D. Periostin is induced in glomerular injury and expressed de novo in interstitial renal fibrosis. *Am. J. Pathol.* **2011**, *179*, 1756–1767. [CrossRef] [PubMed]
24. Ling, L.; Cheng, Y.; Ding, L.; Yang, X. Association of serum periostin with cardiac function and short-term prognosis in acute myocardial infarction patients. *PLoS ONE* **2014**, *9*, e88755. [CrossRef] [PubMed]
25. Cho, J.H.; Kim, K.; Yoon, J.W.; Choi, S.H.; Sheen, Y.H.; Han, M.; Ono, J.; Izuhara, K.; Baek, H. Serum levels of periostin and exercise-induced bronchoconstriction in asthmatic children. *World Allergy Organ. J.* **2019**, *12*, 100004. [CrossRef]
26. Nejman-Gryz, P.; Gorska, K.; Krenke, K.; Peradzynska, J.; Paplinska-Goryca, M.; Kulus, M.; Krenke, R. Periostin concentration in exhaled breath condensate in children with mild asthma. *J. Asthma.* **2019**, 1–9. [CrossRef] [PubMed]
27. Ozceker, D.; Yucel, E.; Sipahi, S.; Dilek, F.; Ozkaya, E.; Guler, E.M.; Kocyigit, A.; Guler, N.; Tamay, Z. Evaluation of periostin level for predicting severity and chronicity of childhood atopic dermatitis. *Postepy. Dermatol. Alergol.* **2019**, *36*, 616–619. [CrossRef] [PubMed]

28. Epcacan, S.; Yucel, E. Serum periostin levels in acute rheumatic fever: Is it useful as a new biomarker? *Paediatr. Int. Child. Health* **2020**, *40*, 111–116. [CrossRef]
29. Chen, X.; Huo, L.; Ren, L.; Li, Y.; Sun, Y.; Li, Y.; Zhang, P.; Chen, S.; Song, G.Y. Polycystic Ovary Syndrome is Associated with Elevated Periostin Levels. *Exp. Clin. Endocrinol. Diabetes* **2019**, *127*, 571–577. [CrossRef]
30. Fujitani, H.; Kasuga, S.; Ishihara, T.; Higa, Y.; Fujikawa, S.; Ohta, N.; Ono, J.; Izuhara, K.; Shintaku, H. Age-related changes in serum periostin level in allergic and non-allergic children. *Allergol. Int.* **2019**, *68*, 285–286. [CrossRef] [PubMed]
31. Heinks, K.; De Schutter-Nusse, C.; Boekhoff, S.; Bogusz, A.; Zhu, J.; Peng, J.; Muller, H.L. Periostin concentrations in childhood-onset craniopharyngioma patients. *J. Endocrinol. Investig.* **2019**, *42*, 815–824. [CrossRef]
32. Konstantelou, E.; Papaioannou, A.I.; Loukides, S.; Bartziokas, K.; Papaporfyriou, A.; Papatheodorou, G.; Bakakos, P.; Papiris, S.; Koulouris, N.; Kostikas, K. Serum periostin in patients hospitalized for COPD exacerbations. *Cytokine* **2017**, *93*, 51–56. [CrossRef]
33. Luo, Y.; Qu, H.; Wang, H.; Wei, H.; Wu, J.; Duan, Y.; Liu, D.; Deng, H. Plasma Periostin Levels Are Increased in Chinese Subjects with Obesity and Type 2 Diabetes and Are Positively Correlated with Glucose and Lipid Parameters. *Mediat. Inflamm.* **2016**, *2016*, 6423637. [CrossRef]
34. O'Connell, P.; Gaston, B.; Bonfield, T.; Grabski, T.; Fletcher, D.; Shein, S.L. Periostin levels in children without respiratory disease. *Pediatr. Pulmonol.* **2019**, *54*, 200–204. [CrossRef] [PubMed]
35. Walsh, J.S.; Gossiel, F.; Scott, J.R.; Paggiosi, M.A.; Eastell, R. Effect of age and gender on serum periostin: Relationship to cortical measures, bone turnover and hormones. *Bone* **2017**, *99*, 8–13. [CrossRef] [PubMed]
36. Kułaga, Z.; Litwin, M.; Tkaczyk, M.; Palczewska, I.; Zajączkowska, M.; Zwolińska, D.; Krynicki, T.; Wasilewska, A.; Moczulska, A.; Morawiec-Knysak, A.; et al. Polish 2010 growth references for school-aged children and adolescents. *Eur. J. Pediatr.* **2011**, *170*, 599–609. [CrossRef] [PubMed]
37. De Onis, M.; Onyango, A.W.; Borghi, E.; Siyam, A.; Nishida, C.; Siekmann, J. Development of a WHO growth reference for school-aged children and adolescents. *Bull. World Health Organ.* **2007**, *85*, 660–667. [CrossRef]
38. Schwartz, G.J.; Muñoz, A.; Schneider, M.F.; Mak, R.H.; Kaskel, F.; Warady, B.A.; Furth, S.L. New equations to estimate GFR in children with CKD. *J. Am. Soc. Nephrol.* **2009**, *20*, 629–637. [CrossRef]
39. Skrzypczyk, P.; Ofiara, A.; Szyszka, M.; Dziedzic-Jankowska, K.; Sołtyski, J.; Pańczyk-Tomaszewska, M. Vitamin D in children with primary hypertension. *Arter. Hypertens.* **2018**, *22*, 127–134. [CrossRef]
40. Skrzypczyk, P.; Ozimek, A.; Ofiara, A.; Szyszka, M.; Sołtyski, J.; Stelmaszczyk-Emmel, A.; Górska, E.; Pańczyk-Tomaszewska, M. Markers of endothelial injury and subclinical inflammation in children and adolescents with primary hypertension. *Cent. Eur. J. Immunol.* **2019**, *44*, 253–261. [CrossRef]
41. Skrzypczyk, P.; Przychodzień, J.; Mizerska-Wasiak, M.; Kuźma-Mroczkowska, E.; Okarska-Napierała, M.; Górska, E.; Stelmaszczyk-Emmel, A.; Demkow, U.; Pańczyk-Tomaszewska, M. Renalase in Children with Glomerular Kidney Diseases. *Adv. Exp. Med. Biol.* **2017**, *1021*, 81–92. [CrossRef]
42. Skrzypczyk, P.; Przychodzień, J.; Mizerska-Wasiak, M.; Kuźma-Mroczkowska, E.; Stelmaszczyk-Emmel, A.; GóRska, E.; Pańczyk-Tomaszewska, M. Asymmetric dimethylarginine is not a marker of arterial damage in children with glomerular kidney diseases. *Cent. Eur. J. Immunol.* **2019**, *44*, 370–379. [CrossRef] [PubMed]
43. Kułaga, Z.; Litwin, M.; Grajda, A.; Kułaga, K.; Gurzkowska, B.; Góźdź, M.; Pan, H. Oscillometric blood pressure percentiles for Polish normal-weight school-aged children and adolescents. *J. Hypertens.* **2012**, *30*, 1942–1954. [CrossRef]
44. Flynn, J.T.; Daniels, S.R.; Hayman, L.L.; Maahs, D.M.; McCrindle, B.W.; Mitsnefes, M.; Zachariah, J.P.; Urbina, E.M. Update: Ambulatory blood pressure monitoring in children and adolescents: A scientific statement from the American Heart Association. *Hypertension* **2014**, *63*, 1116–1135. [CrossRef]
45. Reusz, G.S.; Cseprekal, O.; Temmar, M.; Kis, E.; Cherif, A.B.; Thaleb, A.; Fekete, A.; Szabó, A.J.; Benetos, A.; Salvi, P. Reference values of pulse wave velocity in healthy children and teenagers. *Hypertension* **2010**, *56*, 217–224. [CrossRef] [PubMed]
46. Doyon, A.; Kracht, D.; Bayazit, A.K.; Deveci, M.; Duzova, A.; Krmar, R.T.; Litwin, M.; Niemirska, A.; Oguz, B.; Schmidt, B.M.; et al. Carotid artery intima-media thickness and distensibility in children and adolescents: Reference values and role of body dimensions. *Hypertension* **2013**, *62*, 550–556. [CrossRef]
47. Devrim, A.K.; Sozmen, M.; Devrim, T.; Sudagidan, M.; Cinar, M.; Kabak, Y.B. Periostin normalizes levels of cardiac markers in rats with experimental isoproterenol cardiotoxicity. *Bratisl. Lek. Listy.* **2017**, *118*, 705–709. [CrossRef]
48. Luo, W.; Wang, H.; Hu, J. Increased concentration of serum periostin is associated with poor outcome of patients with aneurysmal subarachnoid hemorrhage. *J. Clin. Lab. Anal.* **2018**, *32*, e22389. [CrossRef] [PubMed]
49. Nanri, Y.; Nunomura, S.; Terasaki, Y.; Yoshihara, T.; Hirano, Y.; Yokosaki, Y.; Yamaguchi, Y.; Feghali-Bostwick, C.; Ajito, K.; Murakami, S.; et al. Cross-Talk between Transforming Growth Factor-β and Periostin Can Be Targeted for Pulmonary Fibrosis. *Am. J. Respir. Cell Mol. Biol* **2020**, *62*, 204–216. [CrossRef]
50. Izuhara, K.; Nunomura, S.; Nanri, Y.; Ogawa, M.; Ono, J.; Mitamura, Y.; Yoshihara, T. Periostin in inflammation and allergy. *Cell Mol. Life Sci.* **2017**, *74*, 4293–4303. [CrossRef] [PubMed]
51. Mael-Ainin, M.; Abed, A.; Conway, S.J.; Dussaule, J.C.; Chatziantoniou, C. Inhibition of periostin expression protects against the development of renal inflammation and fibrosis. *J. Am. Soc. Nephrol.* **2014**, *25*, 1724–1736. [CrossRef]
52. Seki, M.; Furukawa, N.; Koitabashi, N.; Obokata, M.; Conway, S.J.; Arakawa, H.; Kurabayashi, M. Periostin-expressing cell-specific transforming growth factor-β inhibition in pulmonary artery prevents pulmonary arterial hypertension. *PLoS ONE* **2019**, *14*, e0220795. [CrossRef] [PubMed]

53. Norris, R.A.; Moreno-Rodriguez, R.; Hoffman, S.; Markwald, R.R. The many facets of the matricelluar protein periostin during cardiac development, remodeling, and pathophysiology. *J. Cell Commun. Signal.* **2009**, *3*, 275–286. [CrossRef] [PubMed]
54. Litwin, M.; Feber, J.; Niemirska, A.; Michałkiewicz, J. Primary hypertension is a disease of premature vascular aging associated with neuro-immuno-metabolic abnormalities. *Pediatr. Nephrol.* **2016**, *31*, 185–194. [CrossRef]
55. Johnson, R.J.; Kang, D.H.; Feig, D.; Kivlighn, S.; Kanellis, J.; Watanabe, S.; Tuttle, K.R.; Rodriguez-Iturbe, B.; Herrera-Acosta, J.; Mazzali, M. Is there a pathogenetic role for uric acid in hypertension and cardiovascular and renal disease? *Hypertension* **2003**, *41*, 1183–1190. [CrossRef] [PubMed]
56. Mazzali, M.; Hughes, J.; Kim, Y.G.; Jefferson, J.A.; Kang, D.H.; Gordon, K.L.; Lan, H.Y.; Kivlighn, S.; Johnson, R.J. Elevated uric acid increases blood pressure in the rat by a novel crystal-independent mechanism. *Hypertension* **2001**, *38*, 1101–1106. [CrossRef]
57. Zachwieja, K.; Korohoda, P.; Kwinta-Rybicka, J.; Miklaszewska, M.; Moczulska, A.; Bugajska, J.; Berska, J.; Drożdż, D.; Pietrzyk, J.A. Which equations should and which should not be employed in calculating eGFR in children? *Adv. Med. Sci.* **2015**, *60*, 31–40. [CrossRef] [PubMed]
58. El-Dawla, N.M.Q.; Sallam, A.M.; El-Hefnawy, M.H.; El-Mesallamy, H.O. E-cadherin and periostin in early detection and progression of diabetic nephropathy: Epithelial-to-mesenchymal transition. *Clin. Exp. Nephrol.* **2019**, *23*, 1050–1057. [CrossRef]
59. Mathieu, P.; Pibarot, P.; Larose, É.; Poirier, P.; Marette, A.; Després, J.-P. Visceral obesity and the heart. *Int. J. Biochem. Cell Biol.* **2008**, *40*, 821–836. [CrossRef]
60. Lu, Y.; Liu, X.; Jiao, Y.; Xiong, X.; Wang, E.; Wang, X.; Zhang, Z.; Zhang, H.; Pan, L.; Guan, Y.; et al. Periostin promotes liver steatosis and hypertriglyceridemia through downregulation of PPARα. *J. Clin. Investig.* **2014**, *124*, 3501–3513. [CrossRef]

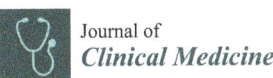

Article

Galectin-3—A New Player of Kidney Damage or an Innocent Bystander in Children with a Single Kidney?

Eryk Latoch [1], Katarzyna Konończuk [1], Anna Jander [2], Elżbieta Trembecka-Dubel [3], Anna Wasilewska [4] and Katarzyna Taranta-Janusz [4,*]

[1] Department of Pediatric Oncology and Hematology, Medical University of Bialystok, 15-274 Białystok, Poland; eryklatoch@gmail.com (E.L.); kononczukk@gmail.com (K.K.)
[2] Department of Pediatrics, Immunology and Nephrology, Polish Mother's Memorial Hospital Research Institute, 93-338 Łódź, Poland; ajander@wp.pl
[3] Department of Pediatrics, Faculty of Medical Sciences in Zabrze, Medical University of Silesia in Katowice, 41-800 Zabrze, Poland; etdubel@interia.pl
[4] Department of Pediatrics and Nephrology, Medical University of Bialystok, 15-274 Białystok, Poland; annwasil@interia.pl
* Correspondence: katarzyna.taranta@wp.pl; Tel.: +48-85-745-0651

Citation: Latoch, E.; Konończuk, K.; Jander, A.; Trembecka-Dubel, E.; Wasilewska, A.; Taranta-Janusz, K. Galectin-3—A New Player of Kidney Damage or an Innocent Bystander in Children with a Single Kidney? *J. Clin. Med.* **2021**, *10*, 2012. https://doi.org/10.3390/jcm10092012

Academic Editor: Bruno Vogt

Received: 14 March 2021
Accepted: 5 May 2021
Published: 8 May 2021

Publisher's Note: MDPI stays neutral with regard to jurisdictional claims in published maps and institutional affiliations.

Copyright: © 2021 by the authors. Licensee MDPI, Basel, Switzerland. This article is an open access article distributed under the terms and conditions of the Creative Commons Attribution (CC BY) license (https://creativecommons.org/licenses/by/4.0/).

Abstract: The aim of this study was to evaluate the galectin-3 (Gal-3) level in children with a congenital solitary functioning kidney (cSFK) and determine its association with common renal function parameters. The study consisted of 68 children (49 males) with cSFK. We demonstrated that children with cSFK had a lower level of galectin-3 than that of healthy subjects ($p < 0.001$). No significant differences in serum cystatin C (Cys C) levels between the cSFK children and the reference group were found. The subjects with cSFK and reduced estimated glomerular filtration rate (eGFR) had significantly higher levels of Gal-3 and Cys C compared to those with normal eGFR ($p < 0.05$). Children with eGFR <60 mL/min/1.73 m^2 showed significant statistical differences between the values of area under ROC curve (AUC) for Gal-3 (AUC 0.91) and Cys C (AUC 0.96) compared to that for creatinine level (AUC 0.76). Similar analyses carried out among cSFK children with eGFR <90 mL/min/1.73 m^2 revealed an AUC value of 0.69 for Gal-3, 0.74 for Cys C, and 0.64 for creatinine; however, no significant superiority was shown for any of them. The receiver operating characteristic (ROC) analyses for identifying the SFK children among all participants based on the serum levels of Gal-3 and Cys C did not show any diagnostic profile (AUCs for Gal-3 and Cys C were 0.22 and 0.59, respectively). A positive correlation between the Gal-3 and Cys C concentrations was found ($r = 0.39$, $p = 0.001$). We demonstrated for the first time that Gal-3 might play an important role in the subtle kidney damage in children with cSFK. However, further prospective studies are required to confirm the potential applicability of Gal-3 as an early biomarker for kidney injury and possible progression to CKD.

Keywords: children; chronic kidney disease; cystatin C; galectin-3; solitary functioning kidney

1. Introduction

A solitary functioning kidney (SFK) is a common abnormality in the spectrum of congenital anomalies of the kidney and urinary tract (CAKUT). It may cause chronic kidney disease (CKD) in approximately 50% of cases [1,2]. Children diagnosed with congenital SFK (cSFK) are at higher risk of kidney diseases and hypertension later in life. The slightly progressive deterioration of renal function over time is mainly due to reduced nephron endowment resulting in glomerular hyperfiltration and subsequent hyperperfusion injury of glomeruli [3,4]. However, in recent years, the influence of other factors in renal function decline in individuals with SFK has also been emphasized [5,6]. Currently, the available methods, including estimated glomerular filtration rate (eGFR), renal nuclear scans, or ultrasonography, do not allow for early detection of renal impairment, and these are not good predictors of the future course of kidney disease. Since the mechanisms that result in renal function decline in children born with SFK are only partly understood, there is a need for new biomarkers to distinguish those at higher risk.

Galectin-3 (Gal-3) is a β-galactoside-binding lectin protein coded by a single gene (LGALS3) located on chromosome 14. It is widely expressed in human tissues, including many types of cells, such as epithelial and endothelial cells; neurons; and many types of immune cells. The contribution of Gal-3 to various cellular functions depends on its locations (intra- or extra-cellular) and plays an important role in cell-to-matrix and cell-to-cell interactions [7]. Hence, it is involved in numerous physiological pathways, including embryogenesis, cell differentiation and proliferation, inflammation, fibrosis, and angio- and onco-genesis [8]. Interestingly, the expression of galectin-3 is substantially upregulated during embryogenesis and in the first years of development. It is more specific to particular organ tissues, such as kidney, bone, or liver, compared to adults [9]. Upregulation of Gal-3 in the ureteric bud and its derivations is crucial for the formation of ureteric bud branching [10–12]. Moreover, Henderson et al. demonstrated that Gal-3 expression was upregulated in a mouse model of progressive renal fibrosis in unilateral ureteric obstruction. The absence of Gal-3 protected against renal myofibroblast accumulation and activation in fibrosis [13]. Available experimental and clinical data support the hypothesis that Gal-3 may be both a biomarker and a biotarget. As a biomarker, increased or increasing Gal-3 may identify patients with excessive risk for poor outcomes. As a biotarget, possibly according to the galectin level, it would be plausible to estimate which patients could benefit from intensified therapy with Gal-3 inhibition [14]. Studies in humans have demonstrated that Gal-3 may be used as a useful diagnostic and prognostic biomarker in kidney diseases, cardiovascular diseases, and certain types of cancer [9].

To date, there is a limited number of studies on the role of Gal-3 in children with cSFK. Serum creatinine (cr.) is widely used to estimate glomerular filtration rate; however, due to its vulnerability to many factors, such as diet, lean mass, age, sex, and hydration status, it is a poor marker of early renal damage with many limitations. Moreover, a significant increase in creatinine level occurs long after the onset of deterioration of renal function. Cystatin C (Cys C) plays important pleiotropic roles in, among other things, cellular protein catabolism and vascular pathophysiology, in particular, regulating cathepsins S and K. In recent years, it has been postulated that Cys C may be a better biomarker of kidney function compared to traditional diagnostic measures; however, there is still no widespread recommendations for its use [15–18]. In this regard, new biomarkers of early kidney damage are sought.

The aims of this multicenter preliminary study were to evaluate the galectin-3 level in children with a congenital SFK and to determine whether there is a relationship between the tested marker and commonly used methods of accessing renal function.

2. Materials and Methods

Sixty-eight children (49 males) with a congenital solitary functioning kidney were enrolled in the study. The participants were recruited from three Polish units (the Department of Pediatrics and Nephrology, Medical University of Bialystok; the Department of Pediatrics, Immunology and Nephrology, Polish Mother's Memorial Hospital Research Institute, Łódź; and the Department of Pediatrics, Faculty of Medical Sciences in Zabrze, Medical University of Silesia in Katowice) between 2018 and 2020. The study's inclusion criteria were congenital unilateral kidney agenesis diagnosed under the age of 18 and availability of clinical data. Since the levels of the proteins studied can be affected by many diseases, children with any comorbidities or current infection were excluded from the survey. Written informed consent to the release of medical record information was obtained from parents or guardians and children aged 16 or older. The study was conducted according to the guidelines of the Declaration of Helsinki and was approved by the Institutional Review Board of the Medical University of Bialystok (APK.002.73.2020). The reference group consisted of 20 healthy peers (14 males), who were children of the

Department of Pediatrics and Nephrology employees. They were full-term, normal birth weight children, and they were not receiving any medication at the time of the study.

At the follow-up visit, all participants underwent a clinical examination and anthropometric measurements using standard techniques. Body mass index (BMI) was calculated using the following formula: weight (kg)/height^2 (m^2). Systolic (SBP) and diastolic (DBP) blood pressure were measured with a standardized sphygmomanometer. Hypertension was defined as a mean SBP and/or DBP level ≥95th percentile adjusted for age, sex, and height (based on the mean of the three measurements with two-minute intervals). Glomerular filtration rate was assessed by the updated Schwartz formula (eGFR = 0.413 × (height in cm/serum creatinine in mg/dL)). Excretion of urinary albumin (albuminuria) was determined in the urine collected during a 24 h period. In younger children, due to the difficulty in collecting 24 h urine, the albumin/creatinine ratio in the morning urine sample (UACR) was assessed. Albuminuria was defined as a daily excretion in the range of 30–300 mg/24 h and UACR 30–300 mg/g creatinine. For all children, the clinical history was collected from the medical records or patient database. On ultrasound examination of the abdominal cavity, a solitary functioning kidney was identified and confirmed on dynamic renoscintigraphy.

The collected blood samples were stored frozen at −80 °C after a 12 h overnight fast. The serum creatinine level (cr.) was determined by the Jaffe reaction. The serum galectin-3 expressed as picograms per milliliter (pg/mL) was measured with a commercial immunoassay kit (Wuhan EIAab® Science CO, Wuhan, Hubei, China) in accordance with instructions for the ELISA kit. The serum cystatin C level (expressed in milligrams/liter—mg/L) was determined by the nephelometric immunoassay (PENIA) method on the Dade Behring nephelometer systems (BNA, BN II).

According to Kidney Disease: Improving Global Outcomes (KDIGO) guidelines, CKD is diagnosed based on structural or functional impairment of renal function and/or reduction of GFR to less than 60 mL/min/1.73 m^2, lasting more than three months [19].

Statistical analyses were performed using the STATA 12.1 version (StataCorp, College Station, TX, USA). Variable distribution was tested with the Shapiro–Wilk tests. The normally distributed data were presented as mean ± SD and the skewed data as the median and interquartile range (IQR). After the examination of distribution and skew, correlations were assessed using Spearman's rank correlation for non-parametric data and Pearson's correlation for parametric data. In the analysis of the categorical variables, the chi-square test or Fisher exact test was used. The *t*-Student test or Mann–Whitney U test was used to compare the continuous variables. Univariable and multivariable logistic regression analyses between the galectin-3 and cystatin C levels and reduced eGFR (<90 mL/min/1.73 m^2) were performed. The receiver operating characteristic (ROC) curve was used to determine the diagnostic value of the examined markers and the optimum cut-off values. The statistical significance was determined at 0.05.

3. Results

The demographic characteristics of the study and the reference group are presented in Table 1. The median time at the study was 7.26 years (range: 3 months–18.1 years). Age, gender, and anthropometric measurements did not differ between the children with a cSFK and the reference group. In the study group, cSFK on the left side predominated, and boys outnumbered the girls. Six (8.8%) hypertensive children in the cSFK group were identified.

As shown in Table 2, there were no significant differences in the serum creatinine level and eGFR between the analyzed groups. Higher levels of serum urea and uric acid were found in the cSFK children. Only galectin-3 differed significantly between the groups, and its lower concentrations were observed in cSFK patients compared to healthy controls (302.8 vs. 475.9 pg/mL, $p < 0.001$) (Figure 1). Five of all children presented albuminuria (7%). There was no correlation between albuminuria and galectin-3 level among children with cSFK ($p < 0.05$).

Table 1. Clinical characteristics of patients with a solitary functioning kidney and the reference group.

	Congenital Solitary Functioning Kidney	Reference Group	p
Patients (n)	68 (100%)	20 (100%)	-
Male (n)	49 (72%)	14 (70%)	1.000
Female (n)	19 (28%)	6 (30%)	
Age at diagnosis (years)	0.08 (0.00–4.69)	-	-
Age at study (years)	7.26 (4.16–11.78)	5.1 (0.63–11.71)	0.120
Laterality (left/right)	45/23	-	-
BMI (Z-score)	0.35 (−0.41–0.96)	−0.91 (−1.15–1.13)	0.427
SBP (mmHg)	109 (100–117)	99 (94–110)	0.241
DBP (mmHg)	65 (60–73.5)	65 (56–68)	0.540

BMI, body mass index; SBP, systolic blood pressure; DBP, diastolic blood pressure. Data are presented as median and interquartile range; categorical variables are presented as numbers (%).

Table 2. Summary of the biochemical parameters in children with a congenital solitary functioning kidney and the reference group.

	Congenital Solitary Functioning Kidney	Reference Group	p
Total	68	20	
Galectin-3 (pg/mL)	302.8 (200.7–401.6)	475.9 (329.8–700.0)	<0.001
Cystatin C (mg/L)	0.98 (0.79–1.18)	0.91 (0.83–0.95)	0.202
Urea (mg/dL)	28.0 (21.9–33.5)	19.0 (16.5–23.2)	0.011
Uric acid (mg/dL)	4.7 (4.0–5.3)	3.35 (3.1–4.1)	0.014
Serum creatinine (mg/dL)	0.4 (0.4–0.6)	0.4 (0.3–0.5)	0.070
eGFR (mL/min/1.73 m^2)	106.0 (87.6–128.3)	112.6 (102.9–131.4)	0.583

eGFR, estimated glomerular filtration rate. Data are given as the median (Me) with interquartile range (IQR).

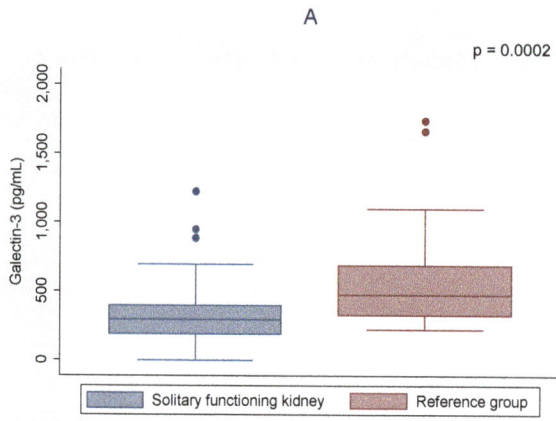

Figure 1. Cont.

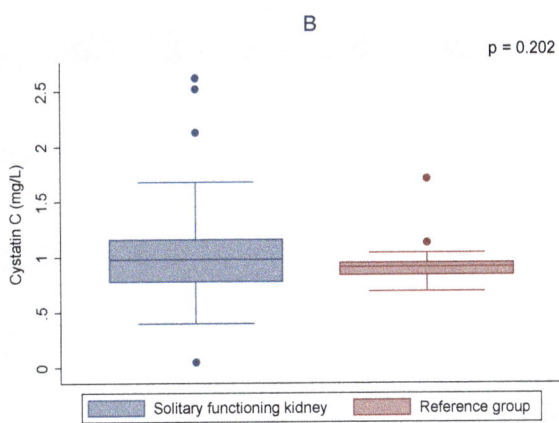

Figure 1. Comparison of the galectin-3 (**A**) and cystatin C (**B**) levels between the children with solitary functioning kidney and the reference group.

Of all children with cSFK, 13 (19%) had a decreased eGFR—10 (14.7%) in the range of 90 and 60 mL/min/1.73 m² and 3 (4.4%) between 59 and 30 mL/min/1.73 m². As shown in Table 3, the mean levels of both Gal-3 and Cys C were significantly higher in the subset of patients with a reduced eGFR compared to those cSFK patients who had a normal eGFR (412.1 ± 275.0 vs. 293.3 ± 202.3 pg/mL, $p = 0.049$ and 1.41 ± 0.62 vs. 0.95 ± 0.29, $p = 0.012$, respectively). In contrast, the Spearman correlations showed no correlation between eGFR and Gal-3 level ($r = -0.06$, $p = 0.65$), whereas a negative correlation between Cys C and eGFR was observed ($r = -0.43$, $p = 0.001$)—Figure 2. Moreover, the higher odds ratio of a reduced eGFR (<90 mL/min/1.73 m²) among cSFK children and a high cystatin C level was observed (OR 15.29, $p = 0.012$).

Table 3. Summary of the biochemical parameters in children with a congenital solitary functioning kidney according to estimated glomerular filtration rate.

	eGFR		
	<90 mL/min/1.73 m²	>90 mL/min/1.73 m²	p
	$n = 13$	$n = 55$	
Urea (mg/dL)	19.3 (7.25–42.9)	28.0 (25.0–34.0)	0.213
Uric acid (mg/dL)	5.2 (7.25–42.9)	4.6 (4.0–4.9)	0.359
Galectin-3 (pg/mL)	378.9 (284.2–444.9)	270.9 (163.5–362.2)	0.049
Cystatin C (mg/L)	1.13 (0.98–1.88)	0.94 (0.77–1.14)	0.012

Data are given as the median (Me) with interquartile range (IQR).

Univariable linear regression analysis showed significant correlations between the levels of Gal-3 and age at study (coefficient (coeff.) -15.9, $p = 0.002$). Other independent variables, such as BMI Z-score (coeff. 25.45, $p = 0.261$), SBP (coeff. 0.41, $p = 0.771$), DBP (coeff. 1.41, $p = 0.451$), eGFR (coeff. -0.44, $p = 0.654$), serum levels of urea (coeff. -7.15, $p = 0.001$), or uric acid (coeff. -62.6, $p = 0.289$), did not significantly affect the Gal-3 concentration. Univariate analysis between the cystatin C level and potentially confounding factors showed an association with eGFR (coeff. -0.006, $p = 0.001$), but not with BMI Z-score (coeff. 0.024, $p = 0.604$), SBP (coeff. -0.002, $p = 0.615$), DBP (coeff. -0.004, $p = 0.434$), serum levels of urea (coeff. 0.54, $p = 0.784$), or uric acid (coeff. 0.13, $p = 0.347$). A positive correlation between the levels of Gal-3 and Cys C was found ($r = 0.39$, $p = 0.001$)—Figure 3.

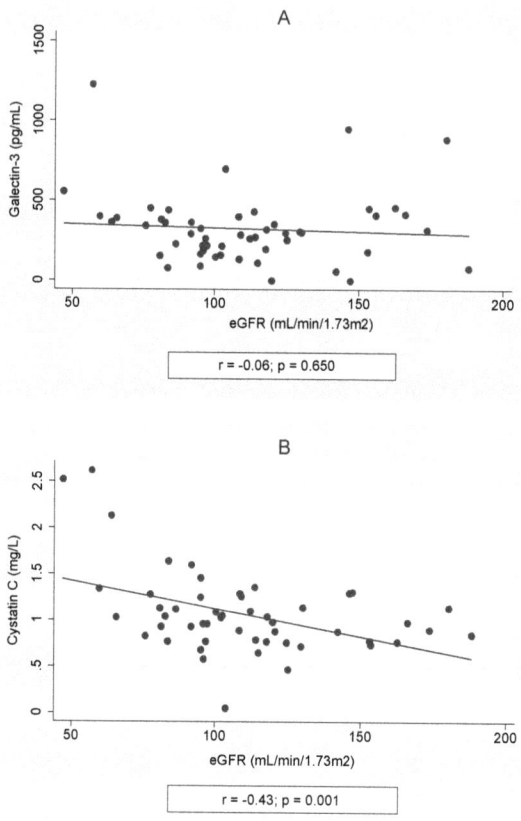

Figure 2. Spearman correlations of galectin-3 (**A**) and cystatin C (**B**) according to estimated glomerular filtration rate (eGFR).

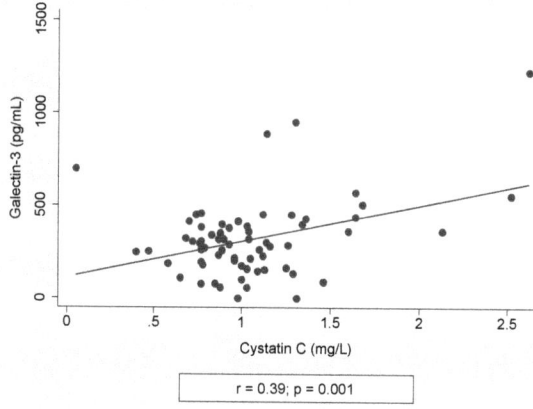

Figure 3. Spearman correlation of galectin-3 and cystatin C levels.

As shown in Figure 4, receiving operating curve analyses in cSFK subjects were conducted in order to define the diagnostic profile of Gal-3 level in identifying children with decreased eGFR (Figure 4A) below 90 mL/min/1.73 m² and (Figure 4B) below 60 mL/min/1.73 m²) compared to the Cys C and creatinine levels. In the first subset of patients (Figure 4A), the AUC for the Gal-3 level was 0.69 with the best cut-off value of 227.2 pg/mL (sensitivity: 84.6%; specificity: 41.1%), whilst Cys C and cr. showed a diagnostic profile describing the AUC of 0.74 and 0.78, respectively ($p = 0.643$). The AUCs for the group with an eGFR below 60 mL/min/1.73 m² were 0.91 for Gal-3, 0.96 for Cys C, and 0.76 for creatinine ($p = 0.029$). The ROC analyses for identifying the SFK children among all participants based on the serum levels of Gal-3 and Cys C were performed. However, they did not show any diagnostic profile (AUCs for Gal-3, Cys C, and creatinine were 0.22, 0.59, and 0.64, respectively).

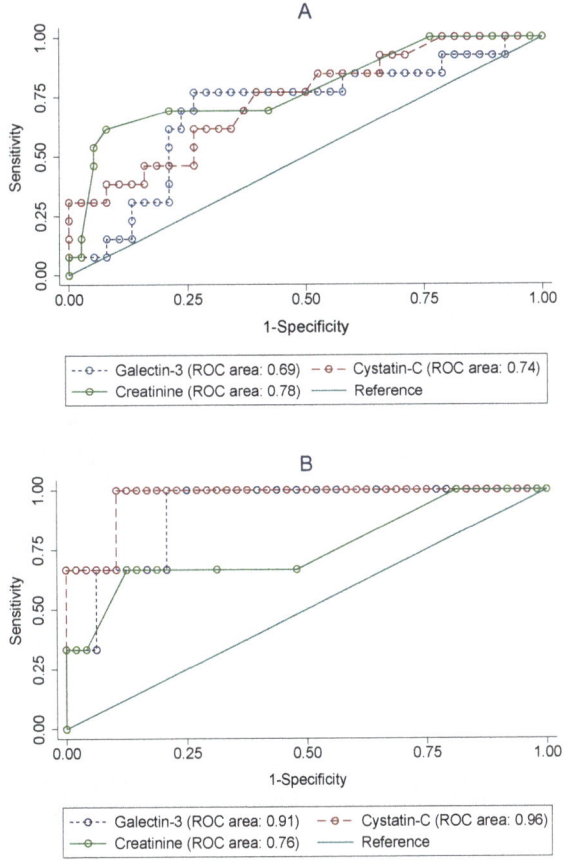

Figure 4. Receiver operating characteristic (ROC) analyses for prediction of decreased eGFR below 90 mL/min/m² (**A**) and below 60 mL/min/m² (**B**) based on the serum levels of galectin-3, cystatin C, and creatinine in congenital solitary functioning kidney children.

4. Discussion

In recent years, the number of patients with chronic kidney disease has increased due to many nephropathies. Currently, the greatest challenge is to distinguish individuals who may be at increased risk of CKD before the onset of overt disease. Data from the literature indicate that children with ipsilateral CAKUT had higher proportions of renal injury (48.3% versus 24.6%), while longitudinal models showed a decrease in glomerular filtration rate from the beginning of puberty onwards [20]. It was initially thought that children with SFK, despite compensatory renal hypertrophy, did not experience serious medical conditions. This hypothesis was supported, among others, by a study of adult kidney donors who lived for more than 20 years after donation. The authors showed no serious complications regarding impaired renal function, the incidence of hypertension, or proteinuria [21,22]. However, the studies in the subsequent years showed that kidney donors had an increased risk of end-stage renal diseases compared with matched healthy non-donors [23]. Moreover, the studies in patients with cSFK revealed that this particular population is at higher risk of hypertension, deterioration in kidney function, and proteinuria [24,25].

Due to the fact that current methods assessing kidney function do not reflect an early kidney injury, new biomarkers that distinguish children at an increased risk of kidney damage are needed. This necessity is also attributed to the fact that the mechanisms leading to nephron damage have not been fully elucidated. Some of the candidate biomarkers include galectin-3.

In this multicenter, preliminary study, we aimed to investigate a potential biomarker of kidney injury, galectin-3, in children with a congenital SFK and to determine its relationship with commonly used methods, the levels of creatinine, and eGFR.

To our best knowledge, this is the first clinical study of the association between Gal-3 and cSFK in children. We demonstrated herein that children with unilateral congenital agenesis had a significantly lower level of Gal-3 than that of a healthy reference group. The normal range of Gal-3 may differ in individuals with normal kidneys from those with cSFK. No data were found on the Gal-3 level according to the unilateral absence of kidney when reviewing the literature. However, Gal-3 is known to play an important role in nephrogenesis, and its concentration in different renal structures varies with the period of embryogenesis. In the mature kidneys, Gal-3 is only poorly found in the distal tubules and in a subset of collecting duct cells. On the other hand, during development, it is highly expressed in ureteric bud brunches of the metanephros [8,26]. Therefore, we cannot exclude the dependency of Gal-3 concentration on renal mass. The absence of galectin-3 might also be related to protection against renal fibrosis and consequently better renal outcomes among children with cSFK. Many types of cells expressed Gal-3 at different times, pointing to a specific role at different times. It has been demonstrated that the Gal-3 knockout mouse has a smaller number of glomeruli than the wild type with kidney hypertrophy. Lesser tissue damage was observed in the knockout mouse, which may reflect a reduced extent of renal injury [27]. Moreover, the univariable analysis showed a significant negative correlation between Gal-3 and age at study in children with cSFK, which suggests decreasing Gal-3 levels with age during childhood. However, conclusions from this analysis should be drawn with caution, as the level of Gal-3 may depend on many factors, and further longitudinal studies on a large cohort of participants need to be conducted. In our opinion, the presented data on decreased galectin-3 in SFK children could lead to new insights into the complex pathogenesis of SFK.

Interestingly, despite the fact that children with cSFK had a lower level of Gal-3 compared to controls in this study, further analysis of children with cSFK in relation to eGFR values (below and over 90 mL/min/1.73 m^2 as well as below and over 60 mL/min/1.73 m^2) showed that individuals with reduced eGFR had a significantly higher Gal-3 level compared to those who had normal eGFR. This finding suggests that Gal-3 may play an important role in the subtle kidney damage in children with SFK, which was also confirmed in previous studies [28–32]. There are many studies highlighting the role of an elevated level of Gal-3 in various kidney diseases, including acute kidney disease (AKI), CKD, diabetic nephropathy, cardiorenal syndrome, polycystic kidney diseases, renal cell carcinoma, and glomerulonephritis [8]. An elevated serum level of Gal-3 has been associated with a higher risk of CKD and renal dysfunction, suggesting that Gal-3 can predict renal damage years before CKD is detected clinically, facilitating targeted treatment and disease. To date, among many diseases, the relationship between Gal-3 and cardiovascular disease has been best understood. It is well known that patients with CKD are at a much higher risk of mortality due to cardiovascular disease, and these two conditions are strongly interrelated. Furthermore, Gal-3 inhibition is considered a therapeutic pathway to prevent cardiac inflammation and fibrosis [7,33]. Similar investigations of Gal-3 inhibition in animal models with experimental kidney diseases have been conducted to date [8].

There is a well-established linkage between the level of Cys C and renal damage. Therefore, we set out to additionally refer the results of Gal-3 to Cys C level. Our previous study demonstrated that increased serum of Cys C concentration in patients with unilateral cSFK occurs after 12 years of age and correlates with compensatory overgrowth of the kidney [34].

As previously mentioned, some authors emphasize that the use of a combination of different biomarkers may be beneficial in detecting kidney injury. Ji et al. showed that the joint analysis of Gal-3, Cys C, and creatinine may distinctly improve the diagnostic accuracy in CKD patients [32]. The present study has demonstrated a positive correlation between Gal-3 and Cys C as well as elevated levels of both biomarkers in individuals with reduced eGFR, which may suggest their common role in the pathomechanisms of renal tissue damage in children with cSFK.

Moreover, the ROC analyses carried out among cSFK children to identify subjects with eGFR < 90 mL/min/1.73 m^2 revealed an AUC value of 0.69 for Gal-3, 0.74 for Cys C, and 0.64 for creatinine. However, no significant superiority was shown for any of them. Further analysis in the subset of participants with eGFR <60 mL/min/1.73 m^2 showed significant statistical differences between AUC values for Gal-3 (AUC 0.91) and Cys C (AUC 0.96) compared to that of creatinine level (AUC 0.76). All of these findings may suggest a valuable role of Gal-3 in predicting renal impairment. Yet, it may be hazardous to draw definitive conclusions from the comparison of galectin-3 levels according to eGFR groups, as the galectin-3 level was decreased compared to healthy peers. We have to temper our conclusions, as this is just a preliminary study, and assessment of children with GFR <90 mL/min/1.73 m^2 showed only an increasing tendency in comparison with the reference group, which requires confirmation in further studies on a larger group of patients. Similar analyses for identifying the cSFK children among all participants based on the serum levels of Gal-3, Cys C, and cr. did not show any diagnostic profile (AUCs were 0.22, 0.59, and 0.64, respectively). It seems that galectin-3 may be a useful marker for identifying individuals at high risk of developing new-onset CKD, and it could be a relevant target for pharmacotherapy for the prevention of CKD incidence and progression.

In our analysis, the prevalence of hypertension was 8.8%, while in previous studies in children with SFK, the number of hypertensive patients ranged from 13 to 26% [25,35]. In the KIMONO study by Westland et al., the authors concluded that an SFK from childhood implies a substantial risk for hypertension [20]. The relatively small number of hypertensive patients in our study may be due to the fact that most of the enrolled participants were prepubertal, as well as the small group size.

There are several limitations to this study. Firstly, the number of patients included in this study was small, which may influence the final results. Secondly, the cross-sectional study should be interpreted in a context of possible bias that may occur, and the diagnostic value of estimated markers can only be speculated upon. Finally, the study group consisted of children of different ages and pubertal status. There is still no unanimity among investigators regarding the best estimation of GFR in prepubertal children and which formula reliably reflects kidney function in this group of children. Another limitation of the present study is that GFR was only estimated from creatinine values instead of being measured by standard techniques, e.g., iohexol plasma clearance. However, this is a rapid, precise, and accurate measurement of kidney function essential for daily workup with children. The strengths of our study include a homogeneous group of children with unilateral congenital agenesis, the multi-center design, and the lack of ethnic diversity.

Pooling all data, we demonstrated that children with congenital SFK had a lower level of galectin-3 than that of healthy subjects. We provided new data that children with cSFK and reduced eGFR had significantly higher levels of Gal-3 compared to those with normal eGFR. Moreover, a positive correlation between Gal-3 and Cys C concentrations was found. All these findings suggest that Gal-3 may be a new player of the subtle kidney damage in children with cSFK. However, further prospective studies are required to confirm the potential applicability of Gal-3 as an early biomarker for kidney injury and progression of CKD. There are still several questions that need to be answered. Among other things, it has not yet been established whether age affects estimated biomarker concentrations. Another issue that needs clarification is the relationship between Gal-3 levels and renal mass.

Considering all of the above limitations of the study, we believe that these results have important diagnostic potential, which, however, requires further verification in prospective, longitudinal studies.

Author Contributions: E.L. and K.T.-J. designed the study and wrote the manuscript. A.W., K.T.-J., K.K., A.J., and E.T.-D. contributed to the collection and interpretation of data and assisted in the preparation of the manuscript. E.L. and K.T.-J. performed statistical analysis. All authors have read and agreed to the published version of the manuscript.

Funding: This work was financed by a grant from the Medical University of Bialystok, Poland (grant number: SUB/1/DN/20/004/1141).

Institutional Review Board Statement: The study was conducted according to the guidelines of the Declaration of Helsinki and approved by the Institutional Review Board of the Medical University of Bialystok (APK.002.73.2020).

Informed Consent Statement: Informed consent was obtained from all subjects involved in the study.

Conflicts of Interest: All authors declare no conflicts of interest.

References

1. Becherucci, F.; Roperto, R.M.; Materassi, M.; Romagnani, P. Chronic Kidney Disease in Children. *Clin. Kidney J.* **2016**, *9*, 583–591. [CrossRef]
2. McArdle, Z.; Schreuder, M.F.; Moritz, K.M.; Denton, K.M.; Singh, R.R. Physiology and Pathophysiology of Compensatory Adaptations of a Solitary Functioning Kidney. *Front. Physiol.* **2020**, *11*. [CrossRef]
3. Brenner, B.M.; Mackenzie, H.S. Nephron Mass as a Risk Factor for Progression of Renal Disease. *Kidney Int. Suppl.* **1997**, *63*, S124–S127.
4. Sanna-Cherchi, S.; Ravani, P.; Corbani, V.; Parodi, S.; Haupt, R.; Piaggio, G.; Innocenti, M.L.D.; Somenzi, D.; Trivelli, A.; Caridi, G.; et al. Renal Outcome in Patients with Congenital Anomalies of the Kidney and Urinary Tract. *Kidney Int.* **2009**, *76*, 528–533. [CrossRef]
5. Cachat, F.; Combescure, C.; Chehade, H.; Zeier, G.; Mosig, D.; Meyrat, B.; Frey, P.; Girardin, E. Microalbuminuria and Hyperfiltration in Subjects with Nephro-Urological Disorders. *Nephrol. Dial. Transplant.* **2013**, *28*, 386–391. [CrossRef] [PubMed]
6. Taranta-Janusz, K.; Moczulska, A.; Nosek, H.; Michaluk-Skutnik, J.; Klukowski, M.; Wasilewska, A. Urinary Procollagen III Aminoterminal Propeptide and β-Catenin—New Diagnostic Biomarkers in Solitary Functioning Kidney? *Adv. Med. Sci.* **2019**, *64*, 189–194. [CrossRef] [PubMed]
7. Hara, A.; Niwa, M.; Noguchi, K.; Kanayama, T.; Niwa, A.; Matsuo, M.; Hatano, Y.; Tomita, H. Galectin-3 as a Next-Generation Biomarker for Detecting Early Stage of Various Diseases. *Biomolecules* **2020**, *10*, 389. [CrossRef] [PubMed]
8. Desmedt, V.; Desmedt, S.; Delanghe, J.R.; Speeckaert, R.; Speeckaert, M.M. Galectin-3 in Renal Pathology: More than Just an Innocent Bystander. *Am. J. Nephrol.* **2016**, *43*, 305–317. [CrossRef]
9. Dong, R.; Zhang, M.; Hu, Q.; Zheng, S.; Soh, A.; Zheng, Y.; Yuan, H. Galectin-3 as a Novel Biomarker for Disease Diagnosis and a Target for Therapy (Review). *Int. J. Mol. Med.* **2018**, *41*, 599–614. [CrossRef]
10. Chiu, M.G.; Johnson, T.M.; Woolf, A.S.; Dahm-Vicker, E.M.; Long, D.A.; Guay-Woodford, L.; Hillman, K.A.; Bawumia, S.; Venner, K.; Hughes, R.C.; et al. Galectin-3 Associates with the Primary Cilium and Modulates Cyst Growth in Congenital Polycystic Kidney Disease. *Am. J. Pathol.* **2006**, *169*, 1925–1938. [CrossRef]
11. Bichara, M.; Attmane-Elakeb, A.; Brown, D.; Essig, M.; Karim, Z.; Muffat-Joly, M.; Micheli, L.; Eude-Le Parco, I.; Cluzeaud, F.; Peuchmaur, M.; et al. Exploring the Role of Galectin 3 in Kidney Function: A Genetic Approach. *Glycobiology* **2006**, *16*, 36–45. [CrossRef]
12. Saccon, F.; Gatto, M.; Ghirardello, A.; Iaccarino, L.; Punzi, L.; Doria, A. Role of Galectin-3 in Autoimmune and Non-Autoimmune Nephropathies. *Autoimmun. Rev.* **2017**, *16*, 34–47. [CrossRef]

13. Henderson, N.C.; Mackinnon, A.C.; Farnworth, S.L.; Kipari, T.; Haslett, C.; Iredale, J.P.; Liu, F.T.; Hughes, J.; Sethi, T. Galectin-3 Expression and Secretion Links Macrophages to the Promotion of Renal Fibrosis. *Am. J. Pathol.* **2008**, *172*, 288–298. [CrossRef] [PubMed]
14. De Boer, R.A.; van der Velde, A.R.; Mueller, C.; van Veldhuisen, D.J.; Anker, S.D.; Peacock, W.F.; Adams, K.F.; Maisel, A. Galectin-3: A Modifiable Risk Factor in Heart Failure. *Cardiovasc. Drugs Ther.* **2014**, *28*, 237–246. [CrossRef]
15. Dharnidharka, V.R.; Kwon, C.; Stevens, G. Serum Cystatin C Is Superior to Serum Creatinine as a Marker of Kidney Function: A Meta-Analysis. *Am. J. Kidney Dis.* **2002**, *40*, 221–226. [CrossRef]
16. Roos, J.F.; Doust, J.; Tett, S.E.; Kirkpatrick, C.M.J. Diagnostic Accuracy of Cystatin C Compared to Serum Creatinine for the Estimation of Renal Dysfunction in Adults and Children—A Meta-Analysis. *Clin. Biochem.* **2007**, *40*, 383–391. [CrossRef] [PubMed]
17. van der Laan, S.W.; Fall, T.; Soumaré, A.; Teumer, A.; Sedaghat, S.; Baumert, J.; Zabaneh, D.; van Setten, J.; Isgum, I.; Galesloot, T.E.; et al. Cystatin C and Cardiovascular Disease: A Mendelian Randomization Study. *J. Am. Coll. Cardiol.* **2016**, *68*, 934–945. [CrossRef] [PubMed]
18. Nakhjavan-Shahraki, B.; Yousefifard, M.; Ataei, N.; Baikpour, M.; Ataei, F.; Bazargani, B.; Abbasi, A.; Ghelichkhani, P.; Javidilarijani, F.; Hosseini, M. Accuracy of Cystatin C in Prediction of Acute Kidney Injury in Children; Serum or Urine Levels: Which One Works Better? A Systematic Review and Meta-Analysis. *BMC Nephrol.* **2017**, *18*, 120. [CrossRef]
19. Levin, A.; Stevens, P.E. Summary of KDIGO 2012 CKD Guideline: Behind the Scenes, Need for Guidance, and a Framework for Moving Forward. *Kidney Int.* **2014**, *85*, 49–61. [CrossRef] [PubMed]
20. Westland, R.; Schreuder, M.F.; van Goudoever, J.B.; Sanna-Cherchi, S.; van Wijk, J.A.E. Clinical Implications of the Solitary Functioning Kidney. *Clin. J. Am. Soc. Nephrol.* **2014**, *9*, 978–986. [CrossRef]
21. Goldfarb, D.A.; Matin, S.F.; Braun, W.E.; Schreiber, M.J.; Mastroianni, B.; Papajcik, D.; Rolin, H.A.; Flechner, S.; Goormastic, M.; Novick, A.C. Renal Outcome 25 Years after Donor Nephrectomy. *J. Urol.* **2001**, *166*, 2043–2047. [CrossRef]
22. Gai, M.; Giunti, S.; Lanfranco, G.; Segoloni, G.P. Potential Risks of Living Kidney Donation–a Review. *Nephrol. Dial. Transplant.* **2007**, *22*, 3122–3127. [CrossRef]
23. Muzaale, A.D.; Massie, A.B.; Wang, M.C.; Montgomery, R.A.; McBride, M.A.; Wainright, J.L.; Segev, D.L. Risk of End-Stage Renal Disease Following Live Kidney Donation. *JAMA* **2014**, *311*, 579–586. [CrossRef] [PubMed]
24. Seeman, T.; Patzer, L.; John, U.; Dusek, J.; Vondrák, K.; Janda, J.; Misselwitz, J. Blood Pressure, Renal Function, and Proteinuria in Children with Unilateral Renal Agenesis. *Kidney Blood Press Res.* **2006**, *29*, 210–215. [CrossRef]
25. Dursun, H.; Bayazit, A.K.; Cengiz, N.; Seydaoglu, G.; Buyukcelik, M.; Soran, M.; Noyan, A.; Anarat, A. Ambulatory Blood Pressure Monitoring and Renal Functions in Children with a Solitary Kidney. *Pediatr Nephrol.* **2007**, *22*, 559–564. [CrossRef] [PubMed]
26. Winyard, P.J.; Bao, Q.; Hughes, R.C.; Woolf, A.S. Epithelial Galectin-3 during Human Nephrogenesis and Childhood Cystic Diseases. *J. Am. Soc. Nephrol.* **1997**, *8*, 1647–1657. [CrossRef] [PubMed]
27. Fernandes Bertocchi, A.P.; Campanhole, G.; Wang, P.H.M.; Gonçalves, G.M.; Damião, M.J.; Cenedeze, M.A.; Beraldo, F.C.; de Paula Antunes Teixeira, V.; Dos Reis, M.A.; Mazzali, M.; et al. A Role for Galectin-3 in Renal Tissue Damage Triggered by Ischemia and Reperfusion Injury. *Transpl. Int.* **2008**, *21*, 999–1007. [CrossRef]
28. O'Seaghdha, C.M.; Hwang, S.J.; Ho, J.E.; Vasan, R.S.; Levy, D.; Fox, C.S. Elevated Galectin-3 Precedes the Development of CKD. *J. Am. Soc. Nephrol.* **2013**, *24*, 1470–1477. [CrossRef]
29. Drechsler, C.; Delgado, G.; Wanner, C.; Blouin, K.; Pilz, S.; Tomaschitz, A.; Kleber, M.E.; Dressel, A.; Willmes, C.; Krane, V.; et al. Galectin-3, Renal Function, and Clinical Outcomes: Results from the LURIC and 4D Studies. *J. Am. Soc. Nephrol.* **2015**, *26*, 2213–2221. [CrossRef]
30. Gurel, O.M.; Yilmaz, H.; Celik, T.H.; Cakmak, M.; Namuslu, M.; Bilgiç, A.M.; Bavbek, N.; Akcay, A.; Eryonucu, B. Galectin-3 as a New Biomarker of Diastolic Dysfunction in Hemodialysis Patients. *Herz* **2015**, *40*, 788–794. [CrossRef]
31. Bansal, N.; Katz, R.; Seliger, S.; DeFilippi, C.; Sarnak, M.J.; Delaney, J.A.; Christenson, R.; de Boer, I.H.; Kestenbaum, B.; Robinson-Cohen, C.; et al. Galectin-3 and Soluble ST2 and Kidney Function Decline in Older Adults: The Cardiovascular Health Study. *Am. J. Kidney Dis.* **2016**, *67*, 994–996. [CrossRef]
32. Ji, F.; Zhang, S.; Jiang, X.; Xu, Y.; Chen, Z.; Fan, Y.; Wang, W. Diagnostic and Prognostic Value of Galectin-3, Serum Creatinine, and Cystatin C in Chronic Kidney Diseases. *J. Clin. Lab. Anal.* **2017**, *31*. [CrossRef]
33. Blanda, V.; Bracale, U.M.; Di Taranto, M.D.; Fortunato, G. Galectin-3 in Cardiovascular Diseases. *Int. J. Mol. Sci.* **2020**, *21*, 9232. [CrossRef] [PubMed]
34. Wasilewska, A.; Zoch-Zwierz, W.; Jadeszko, I.; Porowski, T.; Biernacka, A.; Niewiarowska, A.; Korzeniecka-Kozerska, A. Assessment of Serum Cystatin C in Children with Congenital Solitary Kidney. *Pediatr. Nephrol.* **2006**, *21*, 688–693. [CrossRef] [PubMed]
35. Nosek, H.; Jankowska, D.; Brzozowska, K.; Kazberuk, K.; Wasilewska, A.; Taranta-Janusz, K. Tumor Necrosis Factor-Like Weak Inducer of Apoptosis and Selected Cytokines-Potential Biomarkers in Children with Solitary Functioning Kidney. *J. Clin. Med.* **2021**, *10*, 497. [CrossRef] [PubMed]

Article

Is Urinary Netrin-1 a Good Marker of Tubular Damage in Preterm Newborns?

Monika Kamianowska [1,*], Marek Szczepański [1], Natalia Chomontowska [1], Justyna Trochim [2] and Anna Wasilewska [3]

[1] Department of Neonatology and Neonatal Intensive Care, Medical University of Bialystok, 15-276 Bialystok, Poland; szczepanski5@gazeta.pl (M.S.); natkachom@tlen.pl (N.C.)
[2] Department of Pediatric Laboratory Diagnostics, Medical University of Bialystok, 15-276 Bialystok, Poland; justynatrochim@wp.pl
[3] Department of Pediatrics and Nephrology, Medical University of Bialystok, 15-276 Bialystok, Poland; annwasil@interia.pl
* Correspondence: monikakamm@wp.pl; Tel.: +48-85-746-84-98; Fax: +48-85-746-86-63

Abstract: There is a lack of a good marker for early kidney injury in premature newborns. In recent publications, netrin-1 seems to be a promising biomarker of kidney damage in different pathological states. The study aimed to measure the urinary level of netrin-1 depending on gestational age. A prospective study involved 88 newborns (I-60 premature newborns, II-28 healthy term newborns). Additionally, premature babies were divided for 2 groups: IA-28 babies born between 30–34 weeks of gestation and IB-32 born at 35–36 weeks. The median urinary concentration of netrin-1 was: IA-(median, Q1–Q3) 63.65 (56.57–79.92) pg/dL, IB-61.90 (58.84–67.17) pg/dL, and II-60.37 (53.77–68.75) pg/dL, respectively. However urinary netrin-1 normalized by urinary concentration of creatinine were IA-547.9 (360.2–687.5) ng/mg cr., IB-163.64 (119.15–295.96) ng/mg cr., and II-81.37 (56.84–138.58) ng/mg cr., respectively and differ significantly between the examined groups ($p = 0.00$). The netrin-1/creatinine ratio is increased in premature babies. Further studies examining the potential factors influencing kidney function are necessary to confirm its potential value in the diagnosis of subclinical kidney damage in premature newborns.

Keywords: netrin-1; renal tubular damage; premature newborns

1. Key Notes

Premature babies are exposed to kidney dysfunction. There is a lack of a good marker for early kidney injury in this group of children. In recent publications, netrin-1 seems to be a promising biomarker of kidney damage in different pathological states. We showed that the netrin-1/creatinine ratio is increased in premature babies which may have potential diagnostic value in the diagnosis of subclinical kidney damage in premature newborns.

2. Introduction

Worldwide data show that about 15 million premature babies are born each year [1]. The significant improvement in intensive care of newborns has led to increased survival rate of premature babies [1,2]. Unfortunately, although the survival of the smallest children has improved, long-term morbidity remains high [3]. It is believed that renal dysfunction in preterm babies promises poor short- and long-term results, regardless of concomitant diseases and interventions, both in children and adults [4,5]. This is because the nephrogenesis lasts from 6 to 36 weeks of gestation, and almost 60% of nephrons are formed only in the third trimester of pregnancy [6].

It is known that the primary cause of complications of early and late prematurity is immaturity. However, early detection and implementation of treatment in the event of perinatal problems can significantly reduce late multi-organ damage [7]. Owing to the fact that the traditional markers of kidney damage (filtration marker-creatinine and markers of kidney damage, such as urine sediment abnormalities and albuminuria) are not very precise (they increase with delay after the operation of the damage, are not specific to determine the site of damage, depend on factors not related to kidney damage), new, more effective biomarkers are being sought [8,9].

Netrin-1 a 72 KDa laminin-related secreted protein, initially found in the central nervous system during neurogenesis is expressed in many tissues, including renal tissues. It is shown that netrin-1 promotes cell migration, angiogenesis, tissue morphogenesis, and takes a significant part in the regulation of the inflammatory process [10]. It is unlikely that netrin-1 is filtered by the glomerulus under basic conditions due to its molecular weight, however, in acute and chronic kidney damage, netrin-1 is highly induced and excreted to the urine of both animals and humans [11,12]. This property caused recognition of netrin-1 as an early diagnostic marker of kidney damage [13].

In this study, we analyzed whether prematurity affects the function of renal tubules assessed by the tubular damage marker-netrin-1.

3. Patients and Methods

3.1. Patient Recruitment and Sample Collection

This prospective study included 88 neonates hospitalized at the Department of Neonatology and Intensive Neonatal Care, Medical University of Bialystok, Poland between December 2017 and December 2018. Sixty newborns were born prematurely between 30–36 weeks of gestation. All these newborns were appropriate for gestational age (AGA) with the weight between the 10th and 90th percentile of birth weight for their gestational age using normalized growth curves [14]. Their clinical condition was assessed as good or fair. Since the premature babies born between 30–36 weeks of gestation constitute a very diverse group of children, in terms of both body weight and clinical status we identified two groups: IA-28 newborns born between 30–34 weeks and IB-32 newborns born between 35–36 weeks of gestation. Twenty-eight healthy newborns (reference group) were the result of normal pregnancies without any prenatal and perinatal complications. Subjects enrolled in this study met the following criteria: normal prenatal and postnatal ultrasound examination of the kidney, and good or average clinical condition. The exclusion criteria from the study included Apgar (Appearance, Pulse, Grimace, Activity, Respiration) score lower than 4 in the 1st minute after birth, any congenital anomaly, severe clinical condition, inborn error of metabolism, kidney damage, heart disease, abnormal ultrasound examination of the kidney, abnormal to a large extent the image of the central nervous system (accepted hyperechoic zones around the lateral ventricles of the brain and intraventricular hemorrhage grade I and II), elevated inflammatory markers, abnormal laboratory tests, use of mechanical ventilation or drugs (antibiotics, diuretics, catecholamines). The children of mothers with a burdened medical history were excluded from the study too.

In the study group, urine samples were collected using single-use sterile bags (Medres, Zabrze, Poland). Urine was collected once in the first or second day of life. The blood samples were collected during routine practice in the Unit during the first or second day of life. We used S-Monovette 1.2 mL, Clotting Activator/Serum test tubes (Sarstedt AG & Co, Nümbrecht, Germany) to venous blood sampling. Blood cell morphology tests and blood biochemistry tests were performed immediately after taking blood samples. The urine samples obtained after centrifugation were kept in the fridge (4 °C) for maximum of 2 h and then frozen at −80 °C. We did not use repeated freeze-thaw cycles.

3.2. Determination of Urinary Netrin-1

The levels of urinary netrin-1 were measured using a commercially available ELISA kit (Cloud—Clone Corp. R&D Systems, Katy, TX, USA) according to manufacturer's instructions and were expressed in picograms per milliliter. According to specifications of this kit the detection range was 31.2–2000 pg/mL, the minimum detectable dose of netrin-1 was typically less than 12.4 pg/mL. The mean intra-assay coefficients of variation (CV) for urine netrin-1 were <10%, and inter-assay coefficients were <12%.

The urinary concentrations of netrin-1 were normalized for the urinary concentrations of creatinine determined with Jaffé's method to account for the potential confounding effects of urinary dilution and expressed in nanograms per milligram creatinine (ng/mg cr).

The morphology and serum biochemistry tests were performed in the Department of Laboratory Diagnostics University Clinical Hospital in Bialystok.

Estimated GFR (glomerular filtration rate) was calculated according to Schwartz formula for the term babies (eGFR = 0.45 × L/Scr., and preterm babies eGFR = 0.33 × L/Scr where L is the length in centimeters, and Scr is serum creatinine in milligrams per deciliter).

4. Statistical Analysis

The results were analyzed with Statistica 13.3 package (StatSoft, Cracow, Poland). Discrete variables were expressed as counts (percentage), continuous variables as median and quartiles (Q1–Q3). The Shapiro-Wilk test was used to determine normal distribution. Because the data were not normally distributed, Mann-Whitney U-test was used for intergroup comparisons of continuous variables. Spearman's rank correlation coefficients were used to determine the direction and power of association between the urinary netrin-1/cr. ratio and other variables. The results were considered significant at $p < 0.05$.

5. Results

The study included 88 neonates: sixty babies born prematurely between 30–36 weeks of pregnancy and twenty-eight healthy newborns. Both groups were sex-matched ($p > 0.05$). Table 1 shows the characteristics of the premature babies.

Table 1. Characteristics of premature newborn.

Parameters	Premature (I) (30–36 wk) (n = 60)	Premature (IA) (30–34 wk) (n = 28)	Premature (IB) (35–36 wk) (n = 32)	p
	Median (Q1–Q3)			
Gender (boys/girls)	33/27	16/12	17/15	NS
Gestational age (weeks)	35 (33–36)	33 (32–34)	36 (35–36)	<0.001
Vaginal delivery/Caesarean delivery	16/44	10/22	6/22	NS
Birth weight (g)	2450 (2195–2740)	2295 (1720–2450)	2620 (2415–2800)	<0.001
Birth weight (10–50 percentile/ 51–90 percentile)	17/43	7/21	10/22	NS
Length (cm)	50 (47–52)	48.00 (45–50)	52 (49.5–53)	<0.001
Head circuit (cm)	32 (31–33.5)	31 (29–32)	33 (32–34)	<0.001
Chest circuit (cm)	30 (28–31)	28.5 (26.5–30)	31 (30–32)	<0.001
1 min Apgar score (8–10/4–7)	39/21	13/15	26/6	0.02
3 min Apgar score (8–10/4–7)	47/13	18/10	29/3	0.01
5 min Apgar score (8–10/4–7)	60/0	28/0	32/0	NS
10 min Apgar score (8–10/4–7)	60/0	28/0	32/0	NS
nCPAP	18	17	1	<0.001
Oxygen therapy	24	19	5	<0.001
Parenteral nutrition	29	24	5	<0.001
Prenatal steroid therapy	12	12	0	<0.001

p-30–34 wk and 35–36 wk; NS non statistical.

In younger babies, parameters of physical development (birth weight, length, head and chest circuit) were significantly lower than in term newborns. All these newborns, however, were appropriate for gestational age and there were no statistically significant differences, even if the children were divided into 10–50 percentile and 51–90 percentile subgroups. Younger babies had lower Apgar scores at 1st and 3rd minute. All newborns had Apgar scores ≥ 8 at a 5th and 10th minute. No statistically significant differences were found in the delivery of premature babies in both examined groups.

Blood morphology and biochemical tests did not show any deviations from the norm in both groups of preterm children. Younger newborns had statistically significantly higher leukocytosis, urea and alanine aminotransferase concentrations (Table 2).

Table 2. The results of basic laboratory tests of premature newborns.

Parameters	Premature (I) (30–36 wk) (n = 60)	Premature (IA) (30–34 wk) (n = 28)	Premature (IB) (35–36 wk) (n = 32)	p
Leukocytes $\times 10^3/\mu L$	14.65 (11.57–17.2)	11.57 (10.04–15.58)	16.53 (14.02–18.92)	0.001
Hemoglobin (g/dL)	17.95 (16.7–18.95)	17.75 (15.6–19.05)	18.11 (16.9–18.95)	NS
Hematocrite (%)	49.95 (46.6–52.51)	49.20 (42.55–52.75)	50.1 (47.4–52.4)	NS
Platelets $\times 10^3/\mu L$	258 (210–293.5)	267 (232–300.5)	247.5 (204–290.5)	NS
Urea (mg/dL)	25.5 (18–32)	29.50 (22–45.5)	22.5 (15–29.5)	<0.001
Aspartate aminotransferase (IU/L)	48.5 (38–59.5)	40.50 (34.5–59)	22.5 (15–29.5)	NS
Alanine aminotransferase (IU/L)	10 (7–13)	8.00 (6–11)	11.5 (9–14.5)	0.001
Bilirubin (mg/dL)	5.19 (4.05–6.2)	5.45 (3.9–6.25)	4.8 (4.1–6.13)	NS
Protein (mg/dL)	4.85 (4.4–5.2)	4.85 (4.55–5.2)	4.85 (4.3–5.2)	NS
Sodium (mmol/L)	141.5 (139–143)	141 (138–143)	141 (140–143)	NS
Potassium (mmol/L)	4.97 (4.5–5.48)	4.89 (4.5–5.47)	5.07 (4.47–5.48)	NS
Calcium (mmol/L)	2.12 (2.02–2.20)	2.14 (2.03–2.22)	2.12 (2.01–2.18)	NS
Magnesium (mmol/L)	0.86 (0.81–0.92)	0.86 (0.81–0.96)	0.84 (0.81–0.91)	NS
Phosphorus (mmol/L)	2.01 (1.64–2.28)	0.86 (0.81–0.96)	0.84 (0.81–0.91)	NS

p-30–34 wk and 35–36 wk.

Renal function parameters such as serum and urinary concentration of creatinine, estimated GFR and urine output were normal in all babies. There was no statistically significant difference in serum concentration of creatinine between all children. The urine concentration of creatinine was significantly higher in older premature newborns and highest in term newborns ($p < 0.001$). The eGFR was similar in premature babies and statistically significantly higher in term newborns (Table 3).

The urinary concentration of netrin-1 did not differ between all babies. However, urinary netrin-1 normalized by urinary creatinine differed significantly between all the groups. The highest levels of netrin-1/cr. were observed in babies born between 30–34 weeks of gestation. Also, in babies born between 35–36 weeks of gestation, urinary level of netrin-1/cr. was higher comparing to the reference group ($p < 0.001$; $p < 0.001$), respectively (Table 3).

Table 3. Median values and interquartile range (IQR) of examined parameters in premature newborns and the reference group.

Parameters	Premature (I) (30–36wk) (n = 60)	Premature (IA) (30–34 wk) (n = 28)	Premature (IB) (35–36wk) (n = 32)	Reference group (II) (n = 28)	p_1	p_2	p_3	p_4
	Median (Q1–Q3)							
Netrin-1 (pg/mL)	62.68 (57.70–75.19)	63.65 (56.57–79.92)	61.90 (58.84–67.17)	60.37 (53.77–68.75)	NS	NS	NS	NS
Netrin-1/creatinine (ng/mg cr.)	285.41 (142.55–543.71)	543.71 (294.38–682.78)	163.64 (119.15–295.96)	81.37 (56.84–138.58)	<0.001	<0.001	<0.001	<0.001
Urine creatinine (mg/dL)	23.88 (3.43–43.58)	14.95 (9.47–25.05)	35.26 (21.38–57.73)	82.315 (38.99–118.66)	<0.001	<0.001	<0.001	<0.001
Serum creatinine (mg/dL)	0.66 (0.61–0.75)	0.635 (0.59–0.68)	0.7 (0.63–0.76)	0.68 (0.55–0.80)	NS	NS	NS	NS
eGFR (mL/min/1.73 m^2)	24.58 (21.71–27.11)	24.38 (21.45–27.82)	24.86 (21.99–26.60)	37.62 (33.75–47.97)	<0.001	<0.001	<0.001	NS

p_1-30–36 wk and reference group; p_2-30–34 wk and reference group; p_3-35–36 wk and reference group; p_4-30–34 wk and 35–36 wk creatinine; eGFR estimated glomerular filtration rate.

We did not find any relationship between the concentration of urinary netrin-1 and also urinary netrin-1/cr. and gender, way of delivery, Apgar score, prenatal steroid therapy, respiratory disorders (use of nasal continuous positive airway pressure (nCPAP), oxygen therapy), parenteral nutrition.

6. Discussion

Detecting kidney damage early and with the precise location is currently a priority in the diagnosis of kidney diseases. It allows to quickly implement the appropriate treatment, monitor its effectiveness and prognosis, and due to that increase, the chance for cure [8]. Netrin-1 can be an early marker of tubular kidney damage [13,15,16]. Ramesh et al. showed that urinary netrin-1 excretion in children increased at 2 h after cardiopulmonary bypass (CPB), peaked at 6 h and remained elevated up to 48 h after CPB. The 6-h urine netrin-1 measurement strongly correlated with duration and severity of AKI (acute kidney injury), as well as length of hospital stay (all $p < 0.05$) [15]. Higher concentrations of urinary netrin-1 have been found by Jayakumar et al. in normoalbuminuric diabetic patients than in the healthy groups and even more elevated in patients diagnosed with microalbuminuria or overt nephropathy [13]. There are only a few published studies on the determination of netrin-1 in newborns [8,17,18].

This prospective study was the first conducted to determine the values of urinary netrin-1 in premature newborns in good or stable clinical condition. In this study, we hypothesized that the prematurity could lead to renal tubular injury and urinary netrin-1 could be used as an early marker of tubular damage. It is known that there are several factors that can lead to tubular damage. We have therefore identified a group of 60 newborns with birth weight appropriate for gestational age and in clinical condition assessed as good or stable. None of the children required mechanical ventilation and drugs. They all had normal prenatal and postnatal ultrasound examination of the kidney and did not have any deviation in laboratory tests and parameters of renal function (Tables 2 and 3). In our studied groups, eGFR was comparable in premature babies and statistically significantly higher in term newborns, which is in agreement with the literature [19]. The urine concentration of creatinine was the lowest in the babies from the group born between 30–34 weeks of pregnancy. This is in line with the results of Al-Dahhan et al. who similarly showed that urinary excretion of creatinine positively correlates with body weight and gestational age [20].

We showed that the median of urinary netrin-1 level did not differ between the examined groups. However, it is well-known that the values of urine parameters closely depend on water content or urinary concentration throughout the day, we used urine creatinine concentration to normalize the results [8]. It turned out that we found the highest urinary level of netrin-1/cr. in babies born between 30–34 weeks of gestation and it differs significantly from the other two groups. Also, in babies born between 35-36 weeks of gestation, urinary level of netrin-1/cr. was higher when compared to the reference group ($p = 0.00$; $p = 0.00$), respectively (Table 3). Al Morsy et al. in their study showed higher netrin level-1 in premature babies with AKI-880.10 ± 69.12 pg/mL than in premature babies without AKI-693.10 ± 47.15 pg/mL. They did not normalize netrin-1 concentration by urine creatinine. The results they obtained were higher than those obtained by us. However, the sample size in this study was limited (20), children were younger (32.2 ± 1.24 wk), born with definitely lower Apgar score (6 (6–7), at 5th minutes), all required mechanical ventilation or nCPAP respiratory support [17]. To the best of our knowledge, there are very few studies reporting urinary netrin-1 concentrations in newborns or children [16,18,21]. In the study by Oncel et al. the concentrations of urinary netrin-1 on the first postnatal day were higher in newborns with perinatal asphyxia (848 ± 239 pg/mL; mean ± SD) compared to controls (592 ± 181 pg/mL mean ± SD) [21]. Unfortunately, urinary netrin-1 was not normalized by urinary creatinine in this study. Cao et al. show that the newborns with asphyxia had significantly higher urinary levels of netrin-1 within 48 h after birth ($p < 0.05$) [18]. Övünç Hacıhamdioğlu et al. found that obese patients had significantly higher netrin-1 excretion than the controls (841.68 ± 673.17 vs. 228.94 ± 137.25 pg/mg cr., $p = 0.000$; mean ± SD) [16].

In the further analysis, we paid attention to other factors that might affect the function of the renal tubules. We did not find any relationship between the concentration of urinary netrin-1 or urinary netrin-1/cr. and gender, delivery, birth weight, percentile of birth weight, Apgar score, prenatal steroid therapy, respiratory disorders (use of nCPAP, oxygen therapy), parenteral nutrition.

Considering the results of a study by Dakouane-Giudicelli et al. and Kang et al. who confirmed that netrin-1 plays a significant role in neurogenesis and angiogenesis, being a significant factor into the establishment of neurovascular networks in the developing kidney we suggest that the results of our study also show on the rule of netrin-1 as a marker of maturation of the kidneys in premature babies [22,23].

To the best of our knowledge, this is the first work suggesting that urinary netrin-1 normalized by urinary creatinine is a good marker of subclinical tubular damage in preterm newborns. It should be noted that this is a preliminary observation that should be confirmed in a multicenter study. Besides, it would be worthwhile to conduct a long-term study to analyze the netrin-1/cr value, especially in correlation with eGFR, in further stages of life. Because we are unable to exclude the influence of the kidney maturation process on netrin-1/cr value, it seems necessary to also analyze this value in premature babies in serious clinical condition.

Author Contributions: Conceptualization, M.K., A.W.; Data curation, M.S.; Formal analysis, M.K., M.S.; Investigation, M.K., N.C. and J.T.; Methodology, M.K., A.W.; Resources, M.K., N.C.; Software, A.W., M.K.; Supervision, A.W.; Validation, M.K.; Visualization, M.K.; Writing—original draft, M.K.; Writing—reviewing and editing, M.K., A.W.; Project Administration, M.K. All authors have read and agreed to the published version of the manuscript.

Funding: This study was funded by the grant of the Medical University of Białystok.

Institutional Review Board Statement: The protocol of the study was approved by the Local Bioethics Committee at the Medical University of Bialystok (R-I-002/443/2017). All the procedures were conducted by following the Helsinki Declaration. Informed consent was obtained from all parents of the neonates involved in the study.

Acknowledgments: This research was made possible as the result of a funding grant by the Medical University of Bialystok. This work has been prepared only by the authors and is not endorsed or guaranteed by the funder.

Conflicts of Interest: The authors have no conflict of interest to declare.

References

1. Starr, M.C.; Hingorani, S.R. Prematurity and future kidney health: The growing risk of chronic kidney disease. *Curr. Opin. Pediatr.* **2018**, *30*, 228–235. [CrossRef] [PubMed]
2. Horbar, J.D.; Carpenter, J.H.; Badger, G.J.; Kenny, M.J.; Soll, R.F.; Morrow, K.A.; Buzas, J.S. Mortality and neonatal morbidity among infants 501 to 1500 grams from 2000 to 2009. *Pediatrics* **2012**, *129*, 1019–1026. [CrossRef]
3. Wilson-Costello, D.; Friedman, H.; Minich, N.; Fanaroff, A.A.; Hack, M. Improved Survival Rates with Increased Neurodevelopmental Disability for Extremely Low Birth Weight Infants in the 1990s. *Pediatrics* **2005**, *115*, 997–1003. [CrossRef] [PubMed]
4. Kaddourah, A.; Basu, R.K.; Bagshaw, S.M.; Goldstein, S.L. Epidemiology of Acute Kidney Injury in Critically Ill Children and Young Adults. *N. Engl. J. Med.* **2017**, *376*, 11–20. [CrossRef] [PubMed]
5. Bagshaw, S.M.; George, C.; Bellomo, R. Changes in the incidence and outcome for early acute kidney injury in a cohort of Australian intensive care units. *Crit. Care* **2007**, *11*, R68. [CrossRef]
6. Rodríguez, M.M.; Gómez, A.H.; Abitbol, C.L.; Abitbol, C.L.; Chandar, J.J.; Duara, S.; Zilleruelo, G.E. Histomorphometric analysis of postnatal glomerulogenesis in extremely preterm infants. *Pediatr. Dev. Pathol.* **2004**, *7*, 17–25. [CrossRef]
7. McMahon, G.M.; Waikar, S.S. Biomarkers in Nephrology. *Am. J. Kidney Dis.* **2013**, *62*, 165–178. [CrossRef]
8. Greenberg, J.H.; Parikh, C.R. Biomarkers for Diagnosis and Prognosis of AKI in Children: One Size Does Not Fit All. *Clin. J. Am. Soc. Nephrol.* **2017**, *12*, 1551–1557. [CrossRef]
9. Kamianowska, M.; Szczepański, M.; Wasilewska, A. Tubular and Glomerular Biomarkers of Acute Kidney Injury in Newborns. *Curr. Drug Metab.* **2019**, *20*, 332–349. [CrossRef]
10. Ramesh, G. Role of netrin-1 Beyond the Brain: From Biomarker of Tissue Injury to Therapy for Inflammatory Diseases. *Recent. Pat. Biomark* **2012**, *2*, 202–208. [CrossRef]
11. Wang, W.; Reeves, W.; Ramesh, G. Netrin-1 and kidney injury. I. Netrin-1 protects against ischemia-reperfusion injury of the kidney. *Am. J. Physiol. Renal Physiol.* **2008**, *294*, F739–F747. [CrossRef]
12. White, J.J.; Mohamed, R.; Jayakumar, C.; Ramesh, G. Tubular injury marker netrin-1 is elevated early in experimental diabetes. *J. Nephrol.* **2013**, *26*, 1055–1064. [CrossRef] [PubMed]
13. Jayakumar, C.; Nauta, F.L.; Bakker, S.J.; Bilo, H.; Gansevoort, R.T.; Johnson, M.H.; Ramesh, G. Netrin-1, a urinary proximal tubular injury marker, is elevated early in the time course of human diabetes. *J. Nephrol* **2014**, *27*, 151–157. [CrossRef]
14. Fenton, T.R.; Kim, J.H. A systematic review and meta-analysis to revise the Fenton growth chart for preterm infant. *BMC Pediatrics.* **2013**, *13*, 59. [CrossRef]
15. Ramesh, G.; Krawczeski, C.D.; Woo, J.G.; Wang, Y.; Devarajan, P. Urinary netrin-1 is an early predictive biomarker of acute kidney injury after cardiac surgery. *Clin. J. Am. Soc. Nephrol.* **2010**, *5*, 395–401. [CrossRef]
16. Övünç Hacıhamdioğlu, D.; Hacıhamdioğlu, B.; Altun, D.; Müftüoğlu, T.; Karademir, F.; Süleymanoğlu, S. Urinary Netrin-1: A New Biomarker for the Early Diagnosis of Renal Damage in Obese Children. *J. Clin. Res. Pediatr. Endocrinol.* **2016**, *8*, 282–287. [CrossRef] [PubMed]
17. Al Morsy, E.A.; Mokhtar, E.R.; Ibrahim, G.E.; El-Nasser, A.M.; Ebrahem, E.E.; Elattar, S. Urinary metabolomic profiles and netrin-1 as diagnostics and predictors of acute kidney injury in preterm neonates. *Am. J. Med. Med. Sci.* **2018**, *8*, 79–90.
18. Cao, X.Y.; Zhang, H.R.; Zhang, W.; Chen, B. Diagnostic values of urinary netrin-1 and kidney injury molecule-1 for acute kidney injury induced by neonatal asphyxia. *Zhongguo Dang Dai Er Ke Za Zhi.* **2016**, *18*, 24–28.
19. Vogt, B.A.; Dell, K.M. The kidney and urinary tract. In *Fanaroff and Martin's Neonatal Perinatal Medicine*, 9th ed.; Martin, R., Fanaroff, A., Walsh, M., Eds.; Elsevier: Amsterdam, The Netherlands, 2008; pp. 1660–1670.
20. Al-Dahhan, J.; Stimmler, L.; Chantler, C.; Haycock, G.B. Urinary creatinine excretion in the newborn. *Arch. Dis. Child.* **1988**, *63*, 398–402. [CrossRef] [PubMed]
21. Oncel, M.Y.; Canpolat, F.E.; Arayici, S.; Alyamac Dizdar, E.; Uras, N.; Oguz, S.S. Urinary markers of acute kidney injury in newborns with perinatal asphyxia. *Ren. Fail.* **2016**, *38*, 882–888. [CrossRef]
22. Dakouane-Giudicelli, M.; Alfaidy, N.; de Mazancourt, P. Netrins and Their Roles in Placental Angiogenesis. *Biomed. Res. Int.* **2014**, *2014*, 901941. [CrossRef] [PubMed]
23. Kang, D.-S.; Yang, Y.R.; Lee, C.; Park, B.; Park, K.I.; Seo, J.K.; Cho, H.; Lucio, C.; Suh, P.-G. Netrin-1/DCC-mediated PLCγ1 activation is required for axon guidance and brain structure development. *EMBO Rep.* **2018**, *19*, e46250. [CrossRef] [PubMed]

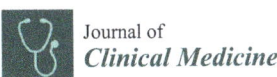

Article

Tumor Necrosis Factor-Like Weak Inducer of Apoptosis and Selected Cytokines—Potential Biomarkers in Children with Solitary Functioning Kidney

Hanna Nosek [1], Dorota Jankowska [2], Karolina Brzozowska [3], Katarzyna Kazberuk [3], Anna Wasilewska [3] and Katarzyna Taranta-Janusz [3,*]

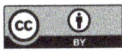

Citation: Nosek, H.; Jankowska, D.; Brzozowska, K.; Kazberuk, K.; Wasilewska, A.; Taranta-Janusz, K. Tumor Necrosis Factor-Like Weak Inducer of Apoptosis and Selected Cytokines—Potential Biomarkers in Children with Solitary Functioning Kidney. *J. Clin. Med.* **2021**, *10*, 497. https://doi.org/10.3390/jcm10030497

Academic Editor: Madhav C. Menon
Received: 24 December 2020
Accepted: 23 January 2021
Published: 1 February 2021

Publisher's Note: MDPI stays neutral with regard to jurisdictional claims in published maps and institutional affiliations.

Copyright: © 2021 by the authors. Licensee MDPI, Basel, Switzerland. This article is an open access article distributed under the terms and conditions of the Creative Commons Attribution (CC BY) license (https://creativecommons.org/licenses/by/4.0/).

[1] Department of Pediatrics, Gastroenterology and Nutrition, University of Warmia and Mazury, 10-719 Olsztyn, Poland; hanna.nosek@wp.pl
[2] Department of Statistics and Medical Informatics, Medical University of Bialystok, 15-295 Białystok, Poland; dorota.jankowska@umb.edu.pl
[3] Department of Paediatrics and Nephrology, Medical University of Bialystok, Kilinskiego 1 st., 15-089 Białystok, Poland; karolina.brzozowska@udsk.pl (K.B.); katarzyna.kazberuk@udsk.pl (K.K.); annwasil@interia.pl (A.W.)
* Correspondence: katarzyna.taranta@wp.pl; Tel.: +48-85-745-06-51; Fax: +48-85-742-18-38

Abstract: This study was performed to explore serum tumor necrosis factor-like weak inducer of apoptosis (TWEAK) and its dependent cytokines urinary excretion: monocyte chemoattractant protein-1 (MCP-1) and regulated on activation, normal T cell expressed and secreted chemokine (RANTES) with their relation to the kidney function parameters in children with solitary functioning kidney (SFK). The study included 80 children and adolescents (median age 9.75 year) with congenital and acquired (after surgical removal) SFK. Serum TWEAK and urinary MCP-1 and RANTES levels were significantly higher in SFK patients ($p < 0.05$). The serum TWEAK was positively related to serum creatinine ($r = 0.356$; $p < 0.001$). Moreover, in SFK the receiver operating characteristic analyses revealed good diagnostic profile for serum TWEAK with AUC (Area Under The Curve)—0.853, uRANTES—0.757, and for RANTES/cr.: AUC—0.816. Analysis carried out to identify children with impaired renal function (albuminuria and/or decreased estimated glomerular filtration rate < 90 mL/min/1.73 m^2 and/or hypertension) showed good profile for TWEAK (AUC—0.79) and quite good profile for uRANTES and RANTES/cr. (AUC 0.66 and 0.631, respectively). This is the first study investigating serum TWEAK and urinary excretion of MCP-1 and RANTES together in children with SFK. Obtained results indicate that TWEAK and RANTES may serve as potential markers of renal impairment.

Keywords: chronic kidney disease; cytokines; solitary functioning kidney; tumor necrosis factor-like weak inducer of apoptosis

1. Introduction

Congenital anomalies of kidney and urinary tract (CAKUT) are one of the most common defects seen in newborns, with occurrence from 1:500 to 1:2000 births [1,2]. Currently, due to the high availability of ultrasound, the initial suspicion of solitary functioning kidney (SFK), is diagnosed in about 60–80% of cases prenatally.

People with congenital absence of one kidney (unilateral renal agenesis) or loss due to disease or kidney donation have decreased renal mass which is associated with compensatory increase in glomerular filtration rate (GFR) of the other kidney. The clinical significance of the reduced number of nephrons was described over thirty years ago by Brenner et al. [3] in the theory of hyperfiltration. Persistent hyperfiltration and glomerular hypertension caused glomerular sclerosis, as a result of which the number of normal nephrons continued to decline. Kidney biopsy in adult patients with unilateral renal agenesis showed features of glomerular sclerosis and interstitial fibrosis. The reasons for the development of nephropathy occurring in some patients with a solitary functioning kidney have not been confirmed. The factors determining the degree of compensatory hypertrophy of a solitary functioning kidney and the severity of hyperfiltration have not been explained either.

The importance of the problem is evidenced by the fact that main causes of chronic kidney disease (CKD) in the pediatric population are congenital anomalies of the kidneys and urinary system, which account for approximately 50% of all cases. Due to the improvement of perinatal care and more effective treatment of children with CAKUT, more and more patients survive to adulthood and develop symptoms of CKD.

The tests assessing kidney function (GFR, endogenous creatinine clearance, serum creatinine concentration) available in routine diagnostics are still not perfect, and most importantly, they do not detect subclinical changes. Proper biochemical assessment of patients with kidney disease is extremely important from the clinician's point of view. Progressive kidney damage is often asymptomatic or mildly symptomatic for a very long time. Therefore, only the early detection of this damage on the basis of laboratory tests can help to reduce the risk of chronic complications and slow down the progression of the disease. That is why the search for new biomarkers with high sensitivity and specificity for the assessment of early renal impairment is ongoing.

Recent years, there has been a growing interest in the role of a protein important in the diagnosis of inflammatory and systemic diseases with multi-organ involvement, such as the tumor necrosis factor-like weak inducer of apoptosis (TWEAK). TWEAK belongs to the tumor necrosis factor superfamily of cytokines [4]. It is a type II transmembrane glycoprotein composed of 249 amino acids (mTWEAK—TWEAK anchored in the membrane). In the kidneys, TWEAK is expressed both on the proper cells of the kidney (renal tubular cells, and mesangial cells) and cells of the immune system infiltrating the kidneys, for example some leukocytes (monocytes, T lymphocytes). Fn14 expression in healthy kidneys is low, but increases with its damage. Pro-inflammatory cytokines increase the expression of TWEAK receptor within two hours. The presence of Fn14 can be found on mesangial cells, renal tubular cells, and podocytes [5]. Stimulating the Fn14 receptors, the TWEAK cytokine induces an inflammatory reaction in the glomeruli and interstitium, leading to mesangial cell proliferation and chronic fibrosis, and consequently to the development and progression of chronic kidney disease.

In studies carried out on a mouse model, TWEAK, apart from causing a direct inflammatory reaction, also stimulated mesangial cells, endothelial cells and podocytes to secrete cytokines, including the monocyte chemoattractant protein-1 (MCP-1, CCL2) and regulated on activation, normal T cell expressed and secreted chemokine (RANTES, CCL5). TWEAK was also confirmed to be a promoter of non-inflammatory compensatory hypertrophy of the kidney after unilateral nephrectomy in mice [6].

Hence, the question whether, similarly to the mouse model, also in children with a solitary functioning kidney, the concentrations of the above-mentioned markers increase and whether there is a relationship between their levels and the progression of chronic kidney disease.

The aim of this study was to 1. Assess and compare serum TWEAK concentration and urinary excretion of MCP-1 and RANTES in patients with congenital and acquired solitary functioning kidney; 2. Test TWEAK and the cytokines MCP-1 and RANTES potential usefulness as biomarkers of renal impairment in children with solitary functioning kidney; 3. Determine probable cut-off points, which may be used in clinical practice in differentiation of SFK children with impaired renal function.

2. Material and Methods

The study included 120 children and adolescents with congenital and acquired SFK and healthy peers diagnosed and treated at the Department of Pediatrics and Nephrology, Medical University of Bialystok and the Department of Pediatrics, Gastroenterology, and Nutrition, University of Warmia and Mazury, Poland.

The study group (B group) was divided into 2 subgroups. The A group consisted of 54 children (33 males, 21 females) with congenital unilateral renal agenesis; N group—26 children (15 males, 11 females) with acquired (after surgical removal) SFK. Additionally, patients from the study group (group B) were divided into those with features of impaired renal function (albuminuria and/or decreased eGFR < 90 mL/min/1.73 m^2 and/or hypertension)—this subgroup consisted of 52 children (65% of studied patients; 32 males, 20 females) and those whose kidney function was normal (normoalbuminuria, eGFR > 90 mL/min/1.73 m^2, without hypertension)—28 children (35% of studied patients; 18 males, 10 females).

Inclusion criteria for the study group were: aged 1 month—18 years with confirmed single functioning kidney (kidney ultrasound examination, dynamic renoscintigraphy). The group N included children whose nephrectomy was a consequence of a congenital kidney defect or trauma.

Exclusion criteria were: presence of other organs chronic diseases, a recent (within 4 weeks) acute illness of any kind, as well as clinical or laboratory signs of infection (elevated C-reactive protein, procalcitonin, normal urinalysis), use of drugs that may affect kidney function, other abnormalities in kidney ultrasound.

The exclusion criterion in the N group was nephrectomy due to a kidney tumor, in order to exclude the influence of chemotherapy on the obtained results.

The reference group (K) consisted of 40 children (median age 6.54 year; 21 males, 19 females), appropriately matched according to sex and age. Subjects in the reference group were recruited among medical staff children, and among participants from the OLAF study [7].

Inclusion criteria for the reference group: children and adolescents aged 1 month to 18 years, born at term, with normal birth weight, in whom physical examination, blood and urine laboratory tests, and kidney ultrasound were normal. Children were in good overall health, without history of a recent (within 4 weeks) acute illness of any kind, and any history of chronic diseases. They were not taking any medications relevant to kidney disease. No data relating the risk of hypertension and other cardiovascular diseases, diabetes or gout were found.

Demographic and clinical data were assessed. In all children, careful clinical history, underlying comorbidities and physical examination were estimated. Blood pressure (BP) was measured using either a manual auscultatory or an automatic oscillometric device. High BP was defined as systolic BP (SBP) and/or diastolic BP (DBP) values above the 95th percentile adjusted for age, gender, and height. SBP and DBP load was calculated as the percentage of readings exceeding the 95th percentile for age, sex, and height percentile during each period. BP load analyses were conducted using 25% as the cut-off value [7].

Venous blood for biochemical tests (creatinine, urea, uric acid, TWEAK) was collected in the morning after an overnight fast. Laboratory tests in all patients were performed during routine diagnostics.

The estimated glomerular filtration rate according to Schwartz (eGFR) was calculated with use of the formula: eGFR = 0.413 × height in cm/serum creatinine in mg/dL [8].

Excretion of urinary albumin (albuminuria) was determined in the urine collected during a 24 h period. In younger children, due to the difficulty in collecting 24 h urine, the albumin/creatinine ratio in the morning urine sample (UACR) was assessed. Albuminuria was defined as a daily excretion in the range of 30–300 mg/24 h and UACR 30–300 mg/g creatinine.

TWEAK concentration was determined by commercially available sandwich ELISA immunoassay kit from MyBioSource Inc., San Diego, CA, USA.

Urinary levels of MCP-1 and RANTES (uMCP-1 and uRANTES) were determined using a commercially available immunoassay kits from Wuhan Fine Biotech Co., Ltd., Wuhan, Hubei, China.

The urine for the determination of the tested markers levels (uMCP-1, uRANTES) was collected from the first morning urine sample into a disposable container. The urine was centrifuged and specimens were stored at <−80 °C for up to 6 months. Urine samples were gradually thawed at room temperature prior to testing.

The study was approved by the Bioethics Committee of the Medical University of Bialystok (RI-002/137/2018) and the Bioethics Committee at the Faculty of Medical Sciences of the University of Warmia and Mazury in Olsztyn (No. 27/2017).

The statistical analysis was performed using the Statistica 12.0 PL computer program (StatSoft, Tulsa, OK, USA). The significance level of $p < 0.05$ was used in all tests.

The relation between estimated markers and baseline characteristics was assessed using the Spearman or Pearson correlation analyses.

A receiver operating characteristic (ROC) curve analysis was performed to determine the predictive value of estimated biomarkers as well as to define their optimal cut-off values.

Additionally, to search for the optimal cut-off point to differentiate patients with impaired renal function from those with normal renal function the method of Classification and Regression Trees (CART) was used.

3. Results

The demographic, anthropometric, biochemical parameters and estimated biomarkers in patients and control subjects are shown in Table 1.

Table 1. Demographic, anthropometric, biochemical parameters, and estimated biomarkers in patients with solitary functioning kidney (groups A and N) and healthy peers; comparisons between estimated groups.

	A n = 54 M/F: 33/21	N n = 26 M/F: 15/11	K n = 40 M/F: 21/19	p (A vs. N)	p (A vs. K)	p (N vs. K)
	Median (Q1–Q3)					
Age (years)	9.37 (4.75–13.25)	10.16 (3.25–15.16)	6.54 (3.50–11.20)	NS	NS	NS
Body weight (kg)	33.0 (24.0–55.8)	27.0 (14.9–61.2)	24.5 (14.50–52.0)	NS	NS	NS
Height (cm)	142.0 (115.0–163.0)	145.5 (99.0–168.0)	139.0 (105.0–154.5)	NS	NS	NS
SBP (mmHg)	111.5 (102.0–120.0)	106.50 (99.00—114.0)	100.0 (88.0–113.0)	NS	0.022	NS
Serum creatinine (mg/dL)	0.52 (0.39–0.63)	0.50 (0.32–0.85)	0.40 (0.30–0.60)	NS	0.041	NS
Serum urea (mg/dL)	27.0 (22.0–30.0)	26.0 (20.0–28.0)	29.0 (19.0–30.0)	NS	NS	NS
eGFR by Schwartz (mL/min/1.73 m^2)	112.19 (96.81–125.37)	105.83 (89.56–128.32)	112.49 (101.12–143.92)	NS	NS	NS
Creatinine clearance (mL/min)	86.0 (62.73–115.81)	92.9 (72.26–112.0)	101.01 (119.22–152.97)	NS	NS	NS
Albuminuria (mg/day)	34.45 (8.47–92.65)	18.87 (3.26–89.21)	-	NS	-	-
UACR (mg/g cr.)	96.15 (0.0–214.66)	84.61 (0.0—825.0)	-	NS	-	-
TWEAK (pg/mL)	486.09 (363.65–631.0)	577.18 (356.26–603.25)	164.94 (78.1–278.53)	NS	*<0.0001*	*<0.0001*

Table 1. Cont.

	A n = 54 M/F: 33/21	N n = 26 M/F: 15/11	K n = 40 M/F: 21/19	p (A vs. N)	p (A vs. K)	p (N vs. K)
		Median (Q1–Q3)				
uMCP-1 (pg/mL)	50.84 (12.29–118.28)	16.61 (8.28–81.33)	12.55 (3.9–36.23)	NS	0.01	NS
MCP-1/cr. (pg/mg cr.)	61.14 (14.26–205.79)	61.91 (10.18–145.22)	14.52 (6.37–35.11)	NS	0.014	NS
uRANTES (pg/mL)	8.58 (7.23–14.07)	8.31 (7.77–9.66)	6.96 (6.42–7.50)	NS	0.001	0.0004
RANTES/cr. (pg/mg cr.)	11.90 (7.28–26.30)	15.11 (13.13–22.45)	6.49 (3.4–8.20)	NS	0.006	0.004

A—congenital unilateral renal agenesis; N—acquired SFK (after surgical removal); Q1—lower quartile; Q3—upper quartile, NS—not significant, M—males, F—females.

The demographic and anthropometric parameters (age, weight, height) did not significantly differ among the groups (B vs. K). Higher values of systolic blood pressure were found in the group of children with SFK (group B) compared to the reference group ($p < 0.05$). Congenital unilateral renal agenesis was diagnosed at the median age 3.67 years (Q1: 0.58; Q3: 9.50); the median age at which the nephrectomy was performed was 0.91 years (Q1: 0.6; Q3: 2.0). Comparison of patients between groups with congenital and acquired SFK showed significantly higher values of systolic blood pressure in manual measurements in the group of children with unilateral renal agenesis ($p < 0.05$). No differences were found between A and N groups ($p > 0.05$).

Both, in the group with unilateral renal agenesis (A), as well as in patients after nephrectomy (N), there were no significant differences between female and male patients in the assessed demographic and anthropometric parameters (age, weight, height), laboratory parameters (creatinine, urea, albuminuria levels), and blood pressure ($p > 0.05$).

Serum creatinine levels differed between the congenital SFK (group A) and healthy subjects (K), but not between the nephrectomy (N) and the reference (K) groups.

Moreover in the group of patients with unilateral renal agenesis (A) and after nephrectomy (N), albuminuria was found, without significant differences between these groups ($p > 0.05$).

The serum concentrations of TWEAK in the study group (B) were much higher than in the reference group ($p < 0.0001$). Urinary excretion of MCP-1 and RANTES in B group, both presented in pg/mL and in values adjusted to creatinine (pg/mg cr.), showed significant increase in comparison to healthy peers ($p < 0.05$).

Comparisons of all assessed biomarkers between studied patients with congenital and acquired solitary functioning kidney and healthy peers are presented in Figure 1.

The median serum concentration of TWEAK in patients from group A was 486.09 pg/mL, and in group N it was 577.18 pg/mL. These values did not differ significantly between SFK groups ($p > 0.05$). The median serum TWEAK in the reference group was 164.94 pg/mL, and revealed significant difference between groups A vs. K, and N vs. K ($p < 0.0001$). Higher excretion of uMCP-1 (pg/mL) was demonstrated only in patients with unilateral renal agenesis (A) compared to the reference group (K) ($p < 0.05$). MCP-1 urinary excretion adjusted to creatinine (MCP-1/cr.) showed similar pattern between A vs. K groups ($p < 0.05$).

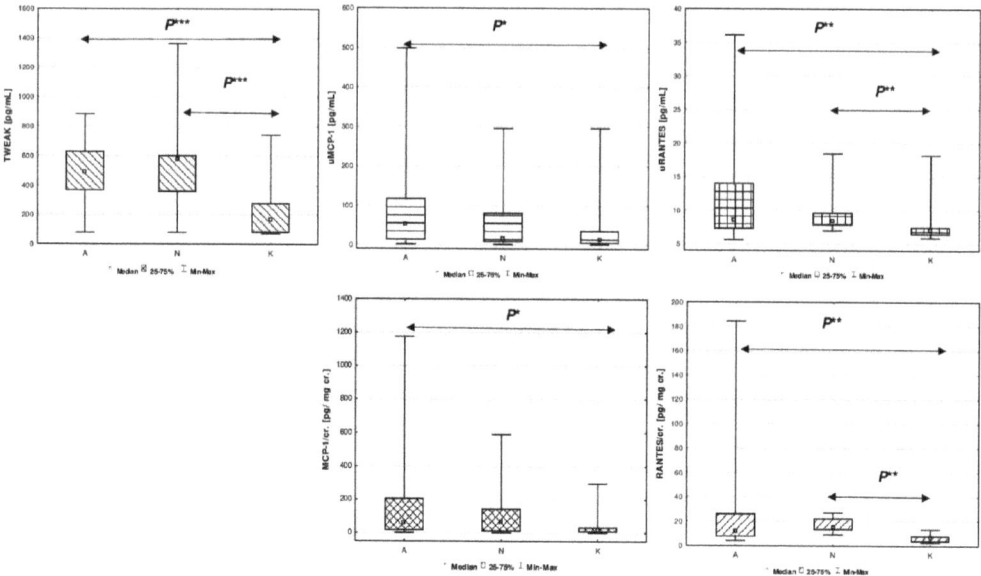

Figure 1. Comparison of estimated biomarkers between studied children with congenital A, acquired solitary functioning kidney N and the reference K groups. Figure legend: P* $p < 0.05$, P** $p < 0.01$, P*** $p < 0.0001$. (**A**) TWEAK [pg/mL]; (**B**) uMCP-1 [pg/mL]; (**C**) uRANTES [pg/mL]; (**D**) MCP-1/cr. [pg/mg cr.]; (**E**) RANTES/cr. [pg/mg cr.].

Increase in urinary RANTES (pg/mL) was found in patients with congenital SFK patients (A) compared to the reference group (K) ($p < 0.01$). Higher values of uRANTES were also found in the group of patients after nephrectomy (N) compared to the reference group (K) ($p < 0.01$). Similarly, the ratio of urinary RANTES to creatinine concentration (RANTES/cr.) was much higher in children with congenital (A) and acquired solitary functioning kidney (N) compared to the reference group (K) ($p < 0.01$).

Further tests were carried out to identify correlations of estimated markers with parameters of renal function. As shown in Figure 2, in univariate analysis, serum TWEAK was positively correlated with serum creatinine ($r = 0.356$; $p < 0.001$).

In additional evaluation we found that 52 patients (65%) from the study group (B) showed renal impairment defined with albuminuria and/or decreased eGFR <90 mL/min/1.73 m^2 and/or hypertension. The presence of albuminuria was found in 47.5% of patients from the study group, (51.8% of patients with unilateral renal agenesis and 38.5% of patients after unilateral nephrectomy). In total, 55% of all patients in the study group had eGFR <90 mL/min/1.73 m^2, including 50% in the A group, and 65.4% in the group with acquired SFK. Hypertension was found in 15% of children from the study group (14.8% of children with congenital and 15.4% of children with the acquired SFK). Interestingly, higher TWEAK serum concentrations were observed in studied children with albuminuria and normal eGFR in comparison to control individuals with comparable eGFR and non-albuminuria (median 512.23 pg/mL, Q1–Q3: 389.09–731.51 pg/mL, $p < 0.001$).

ROC analyses were performed in order to assess the diagnostic efficiency of evaluated biomarkers (TWEAK, MCP-1, RANTES) in identifying children with SFK among all examined children (Table 2A), which revealed good diagnostic profile for serum TWEAK with AUC—0.853, uRANTES—0,757, and for RANTES/cr.: AUC—0.816. Analysis carried out to identify children with impaired renal function (albuminuria and/or decreased eGFR <90 mL/min/1.73 m^2 and/or hypertension) among studied patients (Table 2B), showed good profile for TWEAK (AUC—0.79) and quite good profile for uRANTES and RANTES/cr. (AUC 0.66 and 0.631, respectively).

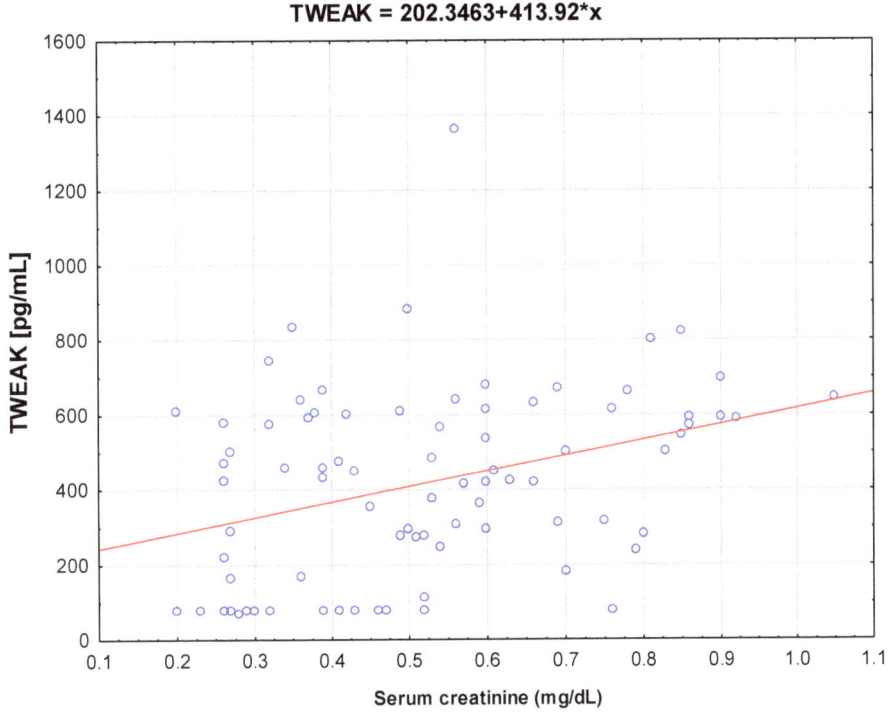

Figure 2. Correlations between serum tumor necrosis factor-like weak inducer of apoptosis (TWEAK) and serum creatinine levels in the study group (B).

Table 2. Receiver Operating Characteristic (ROC) analyses for TWEAK, uMCP-1, MCP-1/cr., uRANTES, RANTES/cr. levels in (**A**) children with SFK among all examined children, and (**B**) in children with impaired renal function (albuminuria and/or decreased eGFR <90 mL/min/1.73 m^2 and/or hypertension) among all SFK children.

(A)								
Cut-Off Values	AUC	SE	−95% CI	+95% CI	p Value	Sensitivity	Specificity
TWEAK ≥ 288.24	0.853	0.049	0.758	0.948	<0.001	80%	91.3%
uMCP-1 ≥ 5.053	0.656	0.066	0.527	0.784	<0.05	89.2%	60.9%
MCP-1/cr. ≥ 8.907	0.670	0.062	0.549	0.791	<0.01	60%	78.3%
uRANTES ≥ 7.236	0.757	0.057	0.645	0.868	<0.001	81.5%	56.5%
RANTES/cr. ≥ 4.049	0.816	0.072	0.675	0.958	<0.001	63.8%	87.5%
(B)								
Cut-Off Values	AUC	SE	−95% CI	+95% CI	p Value	Sensitivity	Specificity
TWEAK ≥ 421.934	0.790	0.050	0.691	0.889	<0.001	79.1%	76.7%
uMCP-1 ≥ 36.717	0.594	0.063	0.471	0.717	NS	57.4%	67.7%
MCP-1/cr. ≥ 48.606	0.599	0.063	0.477	0.722	NS	61.7%	67.6%
uRANTES ≥ 10.734	0.660	0.060	0.542	0.777	<0.01	34%	86.5%
RANTES/cr. ≥ 15.801	0.631	0.080	0.473	0.788	NS	40.5%	83.3%

AUC—Area Under Curve, SE—Standard Error.

Furthermore the CART classification tree method was used for the differentiation of patients with impaired renal function from those with normal renal function.

Figure 3: The *CART* showed that the most optimal cut-off point of the serum TWEAK was value of 395.628 pg/mL. Patients with measurements above this value can be classified as participants with impaired kidney function, as in the study group (B) 76.6% of patients with TWEAK levels above 395.628 pg/mL presented with features of impaired kidney function (albuminuria and/or decreased eGFR < 90 mL/min/1.73 m^2 and/or hypertension). It should be noted that when analyzing with ROC curve, a cut-off point of 421.934 pg/mL was determined (Table 2B); which is similar to the cut-off point proposed by the Classification and Regression Trees analysis.

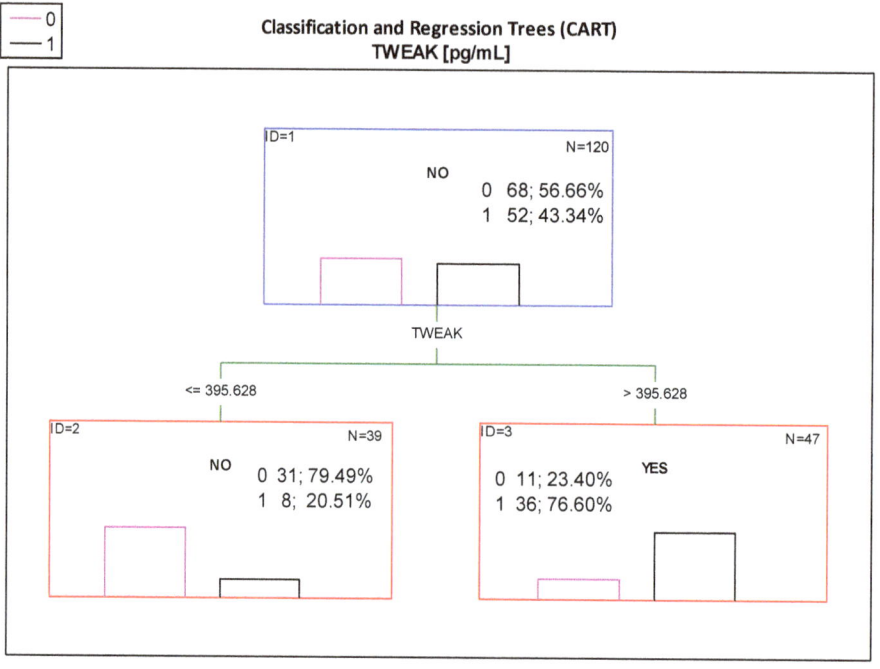

Figure 3. Classification tree for impaired renal function (albuminuria and/or decreased eGFR < 90 mL/min/1.73 m^2 and/or hypertension) created by analysis taking into account the TWEAK serum concentration. Figure legend: 0—normal kidney function (pink column), 1—impaired renal function (albuminuria and/ or decreased eGFR < 90 mL/min/1.73 m^2 and/ or hypertension) (black column).

In the case of uMCP-1, the process of creating a classification tree and searching for homogeneous classes leads to a large fragmentation of the study group. Therefore, it was not possible to emerge a clear division rule that could be applied in practice.

The optimal cut-off point for uRANTES excretion was 6.826 pg/mL. However, the diagram presented in Figure 4 showed that patients with uRANTES levels above 10.332 pg/mL were at risk of developing impaired renal function, and presented 80.95% of children with impaired renal function.

Importantly, according the ROC curve analysis the best cut-off value for uRANTES excretion was 10.734 pg/mL (Table 2B); in the analysis using the CART method, the proposed cut-off point is almost the same—10.332 pg/mL.

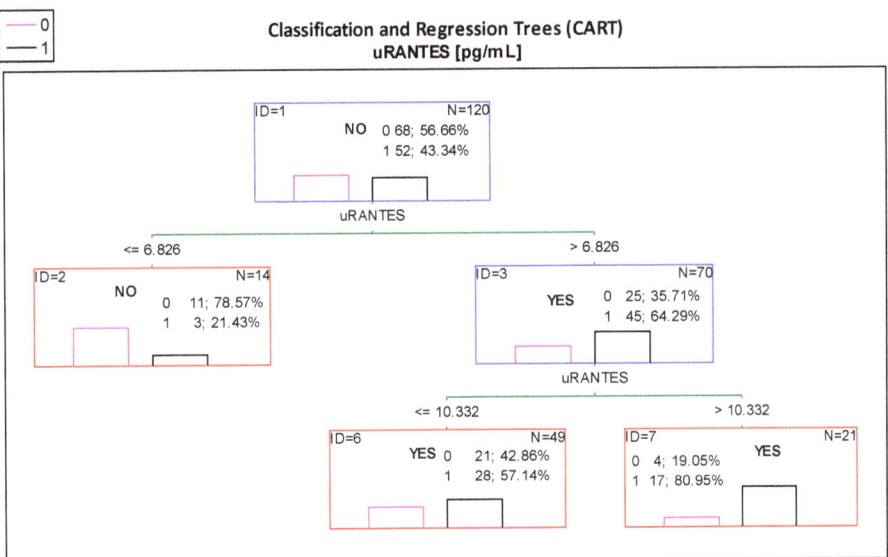

Figure 4. Classification tree for impaired renal function (albuminuria and/or decreased eGFR < 90 mL/min/1.73 m² and/or hypertension) created by analysis taking into account the uRANTES urinary excretion. Figure legend: 0—normal kidney function (pink column), 1—impaired renal function (albuminuria and/or decreased eGFR < 90 mL/min/1.73 m² and/or hypertension) (black column).

4. Discussion

Due to the increasing number of patients with chronic kidney disease, apart from tests aimed at detecting pathogenetic factors influencing the development of CKD, it is important to develop specific and sensitive diagnostic methods that will allow the detection of kidney damage very early, before the onset of clinical symptoms.

We can divide patients with solitary functioning kidney into two groups. The primary SFK results from congenital disorders of nephrogenesis, i.e., unilateral renal agenesis. The second group is called acquired SFK, resulting from postnatal renal loss due to trauma or as a result of therapeutic nephrectomy, for example, in patients with obstructive or reflux nephropathy.

For many years it has been believed that the absence of one kidney is a benign condition with no sequelae of proteinuria, hypertension or chronic kidney disease. This was due to the observation of adult living kidney donors, who, as assessed by Goldfarb et al. [9], 20–25 years after the donation of the kidney for transplantation, showed no significant sequelae in the form of proteinuria, deterioration of single kidney function, and hypertension. This was also confirmed by Gai et al. [10] in a literature review on living kidney donors. However, the study of Seeman et al. [11] showed that hypertension, proteinuria, and renal impairment were more frequent in children with unilateral renal agenesis than in the population of healthy children. In the group of children with SFK, both with congenital defects and after nephrectomy, Dursun et al. [12] demonstrated significantly higher serum creatinine concentration and lower eGFR compared to the reference group.

It is known that creatinine concentration depends on many external factors, such as gender, body structure, muscle mass, and diet. Importantly, increase in creatinine appears relatively late, when renal impairment is already severe. Furthermore, the presence of albuminuria and high blood pressure usually indicates advanced kidney damage. It was found that the loss of nephron mass (in the case of congenital or acquired SFK) leads to hyperfiltration of a single nephron and nephron hyperplasia. Hence, for a long time, we may not see an increase in creatinine concentration or observe albuminuria in the presence of SFK. Overload of individual nephrons leads to focal glomerulosclerosis and interstitial fibrosis what was confirmed in kidney biopsy of patients with unilateral renal agenesis [13,14].

Over the years, the search for markers of impaired renal function has been carried out, which would have a much greater sensitivity and specificity than creatinine, and would allow for subclinical kidney damage detection, differentiation between patients with mild to severe impaired renal function, and earlier implementation of therapies slowing the progression of the disease.

The discovered representative of the tumor necrosis factor superfamily—TWEAK seems to be a good candidate for the role of such a marker. It is still the subject of many studies, and its role, and importance in the course of various diseases in humans is still not fully understood.

It has been shown that TWEAK, by stimulating Fn14 receptors, directly induces an inflammatory response within the glomeruli and interstitium with the expression of various pro-inflammatory molecules, including MCP-1 and RANTES cytokines. It may stimulate angiogenesis and initiate the process of fibrosis [15,16]. In vitro, TWEAK has also been shown to have a proliferative effect on renal tubular epithelial cells growth and to influence on compensatory renal hypertrophy in mice undergoing unilateral nephrectomy [6]. TWEAK involvement in non-inflammatory kidney hyperplasia in an animal model raised the question whether similar changes occur in humans, and more specifically in children with solitary functioning kidney.

In the present study, we undertook the assessment of TWEAK and selected markers of fibrosis (MCP-1 and RANTES) in children with SFK, and their correlation with the parameters of kidney function. We tried to answer the question whether they might serve as potential indicators of early renal impairment.

Initially, the analysis included a comparison of biochemical parameters in studied children. Study by Schreuder et al. [17] conducted in 66 children with SFK showed similarly to our results significantly higher serum creatinine in comparison to participants with two normal kidneys. The presence of albuminuria (>20 µg/min) was found in 23% of patients, what is in disagreement with our results, but 17% of these patients had hypertension, which is consistent with the results of the current study. The prevalence of hypertension in our study was 15%. Hypertension was noted in 13% of cases by Westland et al. [1], 17% by Schreuder [17], and 26% by Dursun et al. [12]. In Radhakrishna et al. [18] study 91% of their study group had at least one of the markers of renal injury such as albuminuria, reduced eGFR, or hypertension. We also found that the major part of the study group had features of kidney damage (65% of the study population), which is more than found in other studies such as by Sanna-Cherchi et al. [19] (29.5%) and Akl (20%) [20].

In the largest retrospective KIMONO study [1,21], which included 407 children with congenital or acquired solitary functioning kidneys, 37% of respondents showed features of kidney damage (31% with congenital SFK and 45% with acquired kidney). These differences are probably due to different criteria for including patients in the group with decreased eGFR (our study eGFR < 90 mL/min/1.73 m^2; in the KIMONO study eGFR < 60 mL/min/1.73 m^2).

Then we analyzed the concentrations of the tested markers. In the available literature, we have not found data on the assessment of TWEAK concentration in children with SFK. Our study revealed higher serum TWEAK in the study group than in the reference group, and these differences were significant. Further, a separate analysis of TWEAK concentrations in group A and group N showed significant increase in TWEAK in group A compared to group K and in group N vs. K. However, there were no significant differences in the serum TWEAK between patient groups A and N. These results may indicate that an assessment of serum TWEAK levels could be useful in distinguishing patients with reduced nephron mass from those who have both normal kidneys. However, based on the evaluation of TWEAK values, it is not possible to differentiate the cause of the reduced presence of a solitary functioning kidney—congenital or acquired. Obtained results also raised the question if this molecule is accumulating due to eGFR decline? All of evidence suggests that TWEAK is involved in the pathological processes that occur locally in the kidneys. Indeed, it is unknown whether a relevant increase in the production of TWEAK or a severe reduction in renal filtration of TWEAK may increase their serum concentrations. Currently it is thought that TWEAK levels increase in patients with impaired renal function. However, up to now, very few data are available on the precise relationship between TWEAK and the level of GFR. In fact, in patients with severe decline in eGFR serum concentrations of different proteins are definitely increased, and as a consequence, the filtered load of these proteins to the residual nephrons may become higher than single-nephron maximal tubular reabsorptive capacity, increasing its urinary excretion. Interestingly, the urinary excretion of molecules begins from different threshold values of GFR and at different levels of serum concentrations, indicating that proximal tubular cells probably have a different reabsorptive capacity for the different proteins.

The largest amount of data from the literature regarding TWEAK levels concerns adult patients with lupus nephropathy. In 2007, Schwartz et al. in a cross-sectional, multicenter study [22] found that patients with lupus nephritis have significantly higher urinary TWEAK excretion than patients without renal involvement. The concentration of TWEAK in urine was already rising 4–6 months before the disease presentation. Many authors [23–26] have shown that urinary TWEAK excretion mirrors disease activity and correlates with other potential biomarkers such as MCP-1. This finding confirmed previous in vitro observations that TWEAK induces inflammatory mediators, known to be involved in the pathogenesis of lupus nephritis (MCP-1, RANTES) by stimulating murine mesangial cells [27].

Further results were obtained in terms of MCP-1 and RANTES urinary excretion (both in pg/mL as well as in pg/mg of creatinine). The couple of tested cytokines showed significantly higher values in the study group than in the reference group. A detailed analysis comparing the urinary excretion of the tested biomarkers in studied subgroups did not show significant differences in the urinary MCP-1 and RANTES between the unilateral renal agenesis group and the nephrectomy group. MCP-1 levels, both in pg/mL and expressed as pg/mg cr., were significantly higher in group A compared to the reference group. There was no difference in MCP-1 excretion between N and K groups. The analysis of RANTES revealed significant differences both between patients with unilateral renal agenesis and the reference group; as well as between nephrectomized patients and the healthy peers. Thus, it seems that the determination of RANTES concentrations in urine could be used to differentiate patients with SFK from those with two normal kidneys.

There is a little data in available literature on the assessment of MCP-1 concentration in the urine of children with a single kidney.

In study conducted in adults living kidney donors the authors concluded that MCP-1 concentration in urine may detect early tubulointerstitial fibrosis in adults with normal renal function determined with normal creatinine levels and absence of albuminuria, and can therefore be considered a non-invasive marker of renal fibrosis [28]. In another prospective study published by Bartoli et al. [29] in a group of 80 children with CAKUT (hypoplastic, agenetic, and nephrectomized due to CAKUT) increased levels of MCP-1 were demonstrated only in SFK groups. Above-mentioned results, in opinion of authors, are due to chronic renal inflammation.

Promising results of studies of this marker in adults with various kidney diseases, but also in children with urinary tract defects, suggest that MCP-1 could be a potential biomarker for the assessment of early kidney damage also in children with a single functioning kidney. Our study confirmed higher values of MCP-1 in SFK group, but there was no possibility to differentiate with its use between agenetic and nephrectomized patient.

The RANTES cytokine was also assessed as a potential biomarker of kidney damage in patients with systemic lupus erythematosus. In the group of 88 adult patients, Chan et al. [30] found a significantly higher urinary levels of RANTES. In another Chinese study, patients with lupus nephritis showed higher urinary RANTES and MCP-1 levels, however, only increased urinary RANTES levels seemed to be independent predictor of lupus nephritis [31]. We did not find reports regarding the use of urinary RANTES levels as a biomarker of kidney damage in children with a solitary functioning kidney.

Finally we tried to determine the cut-off points of the studied markers by analyses with the use of ROC curve and CART classification trees, which would allow us classifying children with SFK group with normal and impaired kidney function on the basis of the studied markers levels.

The ROC analysis determined the cut-off point for TWEAK equal to 421.934 pg/mL. Patients with a TWEAK levels above this value showed evidence of renal impairment, and the test specificity was 76.7%, and sensitivity 79.1%.

The analysis of CART classification trees showed that the most optimal cut-off point of patient differentiation is the TWEAK value of 395.628 pg/mL. Patients with serum TWEAK concentration above this value can be classified as impaired kidney function, because in the group with TWEAK > 395.628 pg/mL 77.60% of patients showed signs of renal impairment (albuminuria and/or decreased eGFR < 90 mL/min/1.73 m^2 and/or hypertension). It should be noted that in both analyses the proposed cut-off point was similar.

For uMCP-1 concentrations, on the basis of the performed analyses, it was not possible to obtain the optimal concentration that would clearly indicate the presence of impaired renal function in patients with SFK.

In the case of uRANTES, the ROC analysis determined the cut-off point equal to 10.734 pg/mL. Patients with uRANTES above this value showed renal impairment, and the test specificity was 86.5%.

Based on the CART classification trees analysis, it was possible to determine the optimal division point—6.826 pg/mL. Among the patients with uRANTES levels above this value, 64.29% had impaired renal function. Further analysis with CART trees allowed the determine even more optimal level of uRANTES. The value of 10.332 pg/mL definitely differentiates patients into those with normal and impaired renal function, as 80.95% of patients with uRANTES concentration above 10.332 pg/mL showed features of impaired renal function. It is also very important that both the cut-off points in the ROC curve and CART trees are almost identical.

The results presented in this study confirm that in patients with unilateral renal agenesis and acquired SFK, increased serum levels of TWEAK as well as increased urinary RANTES excretion are observed in comparison to the reference group. Increased excretion of uMCP-1 occurs only in patients with congenital SFK. Unfortunately, no significant correlations between serum TWEAK concentration and urinary excretion of tested chemokines could be established. However, it was possible to confirm a significant positive correlation between serum TWEAK and creatinine concentrations.

All assessed markers achieved significantly higher concentrations in patients with SFK and features of impaired renal function, compared to those who did not show impaired function. Therefore, it is possible to use their determination to differentiate patients with a solitary functioning kidney with features of impaired renal function from those with normal kidney function. It should be mentioned that our study failed in differentiation between unilateral renal agenesis and acquired SFK with use of estimated markers.

We are fully aware of the limitations of the study, being small, single center and cross-sectional. Moreover, most of our patients were young children, an appropriate measurement of blood pressure in children is difficult because of "white coat" anxiety, widely varying arm size, and occasional poor cooperation. Furthermore, in prepubertal and younger children no formula of GFR estimation gives acceptable results. It is still controversial, whether in this population a correct estimation of GFR could be obtained from serum creatinine concentration. We still do not know which formula is the least misleading in younger children.

Further work is necessary to better define obtained results. For example, better standardization of methods for its measurement in serum and urine, evaluation of MCP-1, RANTES activity in serum, assessment of its protective role in renal injuries once damage has already occurred. Additional efforts comparing serum TWEAK concentration with its urinary excretion would be helpful for detailed answer the question of molecules accumulation due to eGFR decline.

In conclusion, what is extremely important, in the case of serum TWEAK and urinary RANTES it was possible to determine the optimal cut-off values, exceeding of which may indicate impaired renal function in patients with a solitary functioning kidney. It might be useful in clinical practice in establishing the reference values of new biomarkers in patients with solitary functioning kidney.

Reached results indicate that the tumor necrosis factor inducer, TWEAK, and the cytokine RANTES may serve as potential biomarkers of early renal impairment and suggest possible relationship between TWEAK and uRANTES levels and the degree of renal impairment. However, more studies on a larger group of patients are needed to confirm these preliminary data.

Author Contributions: H.N. and K.T.-J. designed the study, and wrote the manuscript. K.K., K.B. and A.W. contributed to collection and interpretation of data, and assisted in the preparation of the manuscript. D.J. performed statistical analysis and assisted in the preparation of the manuscript. All authors approved the final version of the manuscript. All authors have read and agreed to the published version of the manuscript.

Funding: This work has been financed by grant from the Medical University of Bialystok, Poland (grant number: SUB/1/DN/18/006/1141).

Institutional Review Board Statement: The study was conducted according to the guidelines of the Declaration of Helsinki and approved by the Institutional Review Board of the Medical University of Bialystok (R-I-002/137/2018).

Informed Consent Statement: Informed consent was obtained from all subjects involved in the study.

Conflicts of Interest: All the authors declared no competing interest.

References

1. Westland, R.; Schreuder, M.F.; Bökenkamp, A.; Spreeuwenberg, M.D.; van Wijk, J.A. Renal injury in children with a solitary func-tioning kidney—the KIMONO study. *Nephrol. Dial. Transplant.* **2011**, *26*, 1533–1541. [CrossRef] [PubMed]
2. Schreuder, M.F. Life with one kidney. *Pediatr. Nephrol.* **2018**, *33*, 595–604. [CrossRef] [PubMed]
3. Brenner, B.M.; Lawler, E.V.; Mackenzie, H.S. The hyperfiltration theory: A paradigm shift in nephrology. *Kidney Int.* **1996**, *49*, 1774–1777. [CrossRef] [PubMed]
4. Chicheportiche, Y.; Bourdon, P.R.; Xu, H.; Hsu, Y.-M.; Scott, H.S.; Hession, C.; Garcia, I.; Browning, J.L. TWEAK, a New Secreted Ligand in the Tumor Necrosis Factor Family That Weakly Induces Apoptosis. *J. Biol. Chem.* **1997**, *272*, 32401–32410. [CrossRef] [PubMed]
5. Sanz, A.B.; Justo, P.; Sanchez-Niño, M.D.; Blanco-Colio, L.; Winkles, J.A.; Kreztler, M.; Jakubowski, A.; Blanco, J.; Egido, J.; Ruiz-Ortega, M.; et al. The Cytokine TWEAK Modulates Renal Tubulointerstitial Inflammation. *J. Am. Soc. Nephrol.* **2008**, *19*, 695–703. [CrossRef] [PubMed]
6. Sanz, A.B.; Sanchez-Niño, M.D.; Izquierdo, M.C.; Jakubowski, A.; Justo, P.; Blanco-Colio, L.; Ruiz-Ortega, M.; Egido, J.; Ortiz, A. Tweak induces proliferation in renal tubular epithelium: A role in uninephrectomy induced renal hyperplasia. *J. Cell. Mol. Med.* **2009**, *13*, 3329–3342. [CrossRef] [PubMed]
7. Kułaga, Z.; Litwin, M.; Grajda, A.; Kułaga, K.; Gurzkowska, B.; Góźdź, M.; Pan, H. Oscillometric blood pressure percentiles for Polish normal-weight school-aged children and adolescents. *J. Hypertens.* **2012**, *30*, 1942–1954. [CrossRef]
8. Schwartz, G.J.; Muñoz, A.; Schneider, M.F.; Mak, R.H.; Kaskel, F.; Warady, B.A.; Furth, S.L. New Equations to Estimate GFR in Children with CKD. *J. Am. Soc. Nephrol.* **2009**, *20*, 629–637. [CrossRef]
9. Goldfarb, D.A.; Matin, S.F.; Braun, W.E.; Schreiber, M.J.; Mastroianni, B.; Papajcik, D.; Rolin, H.A.; Flechner, S.; Goormastic, M.; Novick, A.C. Renal outcome 25 years after donor nephrectomy. *J. Urol.* **2001**, *166*, 2043–2047. [CrossRef]
10. Gai, M.; Giunti, S.; Lanfranco, G.; Segoloni, G.P. Potential risks of living kidney donation a review. *Nephrol. Dial. Transplant.* **2007**, *22*, 3122–3127. [CrossRef]
11. Seeman, T.; Patzer, L.; John, U.; Dušek, J.; Vondrák, K.; Janda, J.; Misselwitz, J. Blood Pressure, Renal Function, and Proteinuria in Children with Unilateral Renal Agenesis. *Kidney Blood Press. Res.* **2006**, *29*, 210–215. [CrossRef] [PubMed]
12. Dursun, H.; Bayazit, A.K.; Cengiz, N.; Seydaoglu, G.; Buyukcelik, M.; Soran, M.; Noyan, A.; Anarat, A. Ambulatory blood pressure monitoring and renal functions in children with a solitary kidney. *Pediatr. Nephrol.* **2007**, *22*, 559–564. [CrossRef] [PubMed]

13. Schnaper, H.W. Remnant nephron physiology and the progression of chronic kidney disease. *Pediatr. Nephrol.* **2014**, *29*, 193–202. [CrossRef] [PubMed]
14. Cochat, P.; Febvey, O.; Bacchetta, J.; Bérard, E.; Cabrera, N.; Dubourg, L. Towards adulthood with a solitary kidney. *Pediatr. Nephrol.* **2018**, *34*, 2311–2323. [CrossRef] [PubMed]
15. Sanz, A.B.; Moreno, J.A.; Sanchez-Nino, M.D.; Ucero, A.C.; Benito, A.; Santamaria, B.; Justo, P.; Izquierdo, M.C.; Egido, J.; Blanco-Colio, L.M. TWEAKing renal injury. *Front. Biosci.* **2008**, *13*, 580–589. [CrossRef] [PubMed]
16. Burkly, L.C.; Michaelson, J.S.; Zheng, T.S. TWEAK/Fn14 pathway: An immunological switch for shaping tissue responses. *Immunol. Rev.* **2011**, *244*, 99–114. [CrossRef]
17. Schreuder, M.F.; E Langemeijer, M.; Bokenkamp, A.; Waal, H.A.D.-V.D.; Van Wijk, J.A. Hypertension and microalbuminuria in children with congenital solitary kidneys. *J. Paediatr. Child Health* **2008**, *44*, 363–368. [CrossRef]
18. Radhakrishna, V.; Govindarajan, K.K.; Sambandan, K.; Jindal, B.; Naredi, B. Solitary functioning kidney in children: Clinical implications. *J. Bras Nefrol.* **2018**, *40*, 261–265. [CrossRef]
19. Sanna-Cherchi, S.; Ravani, P.; Corbani, V.; Parodi, S.; Haupt, R.; Piaggio, G.; Degli Innocenti, M.L.; Somenzi, D.; Trivelli, A.; Caridi, G.; et al. Renal outcome in patients with congenital anomalies of the kidney and urinary tract. *Kidney Int.* **2009**, *76*, 528–533. [CrossRef]
20. Akl, K. The anomalies associated with congenital solitary functioning kidney in children. *Saudi J. Kidney Dis. Transplant.* **2011**, *22*, 67–71.
21. Westland, R.; Kurvers, R.A.J.; Van Wijk, J.A.; Schreuder, M.F. Risk Factors for Renal Injury in Children With a Solitary Functioning Kidney. *Pediatrics* **2013**, *131*, 478–485. [CrossRef] [PubMed]
22. Schwartz, N.; Michaelson, J.S.; Putterman, C. Lipocalin-2, TWEAK, and other cytokines as urinary biomarkers for lupus nephritis. *Ann. N. Y. Acad. Sci.* **2007**, *1109*, 265–274. [CrossRef] [PubMed]
23. Schwartz, N.; Rubinstein, T.; Burkly, L.C.; E Collins, C.; Blanco, I.; Su, L.; Hojaili, B.; Mackay, M.; Aranow, C.; Stohl, W.; et al. Urinary TWEAK as a biomarker of lupus nephritis: A multicenter cohort study. *Arthritis Res. Ther.* **2009**, *11*, R143. [CrossRef] [PubMed]
24. El-Shehaby, A.; Darweesh, H.; El-Khatib, M.; Momtaz, M.; Marzouk, S.; El-Shaarawy, N.; Emad, Y. Correlations of Urinary Biomarkers, TNF-Like Weak Inducer of Apoptosis (TWEAK), Osteoprotegerin (OPG), Monocyte Chemoattractant Protein-1 (MCP-1), and IL-8 with Lupus Nephritis. *J. Clin. Immunol.* **2011**, *31*, 848–856. [CrossRef] [PubMed]
25. Xuejing, Z.; Jiazhen, T.; Jun, L.; Xiangqing, X.; Shuguang, Y.; Fuyou, L. Urinary TWEAK level as a marker of lupus nephritis activ-ity in 46 cases. *J. Biomed. Biotechnol.* **2012**, *2012*, 359647. [CrossRef]
26. Schwartz, N.; Goilav, B.; Putterman, C. The pathogenesis, diagnosis and treatment of lupus nephritis. *Curr. Opin. Rheumatol.* **2014**, *26*, 502–509. [CrossRef]
27. Campbell, S.; Burkly, L.C.; Gao, H.X.; Berman, J.W.; Su, L.; Browning, B.; Zheng, T.; Schiffer, L.; Michaelson, J.S.; Putterman, C. Proin-flammatory effects of TWEAK/Fn14 interactions in glomerular mesangial cells. *J. Immunol.* **2006**, *176*, 1889–1898. [CrossRef]
28. Wang, X.; Lieske, J.C.; Alexander, M.P.; Jayachandran, M.; Denic, A.; Mathew, J.; Lerman, L.O.; Kremers, W.K.; Larson, J.J.; Rule, A.D. Tu-buloinersttial Fibrosis of Living Donor Kidneys Associates with Urinary Monocyte Chemoattractant Protein 1. *Am. J. Nephrol.* **2016**, *43*, 454–459. [CrossRef]
29. Pastore, V.; Calè, I.; Aceto, G.; Campanella, V.; Lasalandra, C.; Magaldi, S.; Niglio, F.; Basile, A.; Cocomazzi, R.; Bartoli, F. Prospective Study on Several Urinary Biomarkers as Indicators of Renal Damage in Children with CAKUT. *Eur. J. Pediatr. Surg.* **2018**, *29*, 215–222. [CrossRef]
30. Chan, R.W.; Lai, F.M.; Li, E.K.; Tam, L.S.; Chow, K.M.; Li, P.K.; Szeto, C.C. Messenger RNA expression of RANTES in the urinary sedi-ment of patients with lupus nephritis. *Nephrology (Carlton)* **2006**, *11*, 219–225. [CrossRef]
31. Tian, S.; Li, J.; Wang, L.; Liu, T.; Liu, H.; Cheng, G.; Liu, D.; Deng, Y.; Gou, R.; Wan, Y.; et al. Urinary levels of RANTES and M-CSF are predictors of lupus nephritis flare. *Inflamm. Res.* **2007**, *56*, 304–310. [CrossRef] [PubMed]

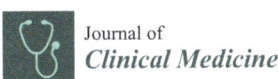

Review

The Use of Artificial Intelligence Algorithms in the Diagnosis of Urinary Tract Infections—A Literature Review

Natalia Goździkiewicz [1,*], Danuta Zwolińska [2] and Dorota Polak-Jonkisz [2]

[1] Department of Pediatric Nephrology, University Hospital in Wroclaw, 50-556 Wrocław, Poland
[2] Department of Pediatric Nephrology, Wroclaw Medical Univeristy, 50-556 Wrocław, Poland; danuta.zwolinska@umed.wroc.pl (D.Z.); dorota.polak-jonkisz@umed.wroc.pl (D.P.-J.)
* Correspondence: natalia.gozdzikiewicz@gmail.com; Tel.: +48-717-364-400

Abstract: Urinary tract infections (UTIs) are among the most common infections occurring across all age groups. UTIs are a well-known cause of acute morbidity and chronic medical conditions. The current diagnostic methods of UTIs remain sub-optimal. The development of better diagnostic tools for UTIs is essential for improving treatment and reducing morbidity. Artificial intelligence (AI) is defined as the science of computers where they have the ability to perform tasks commonly associated with intelligent beings. The objective of this study was to analyze current views regarding attempts to apply artificial intelligence techniques in everyday practice, as well as find promising methods to diagnose urinary tract infections in the most efficient ways. We included six research works comparing various AI models to predict UTI. The literature examined here confirms the relevance of AI models in UTI diagnosis, while it has not yet been established which model is preferable for infection prediction in adult patients. AI models achieve a high performance in retrospective studies, but further studies are required.

Keywords: urinary tract infections; artificial intelligence; machine learning; medical decision support system

1. Introduction

Urinary tract infections (UTIs) are among the most common bacterial infections, affecting 150 million people each year [1]. UTI is a collective term describing infections that involve the colonization of pathogens found anywhere in the urinary system, comprising cystitis, pyelonephritis, renal abscess, urethritis, and prostatitis. In clinical practice, UTIs are categorized as uncomplicated or complicated. Uncomplicated UTIs include acute uncomplicated cystitis (AUC)—infection of the bladder or lower urinary tract—and acute uncomplicated pyelonephritis (AUP)—infection of the kidney or upper urinary tract—which occur in patients who have a regular, unobstructed urinary tract with no history of recent instrumentation. Complicated urinary tract infections can arise in a urinary tract that has metabolic, functional, or structural abnormalities. Complex UTIs may involve any part of the urinary tract. The main consequence of UTIs is that they critically increase the possibility of a failure of therapy.

UTIs are caused by both Gram-negative and Gram-positive bacteria, as well as by certain types of fungi. The dominant infectious microorganism for both uncomplicated and complicated UTIs is uropathogenic *Escherichia coli* (UPEC), although the distribution of pathogens causing UTIs varies [2].

The diagnostic process of a UTI is usually carried out based on a combination of clinical symptoms of infection and a positive urine analysis or culture [3]. Some of these features have been combined into clinical predictors, but the predictive values remain sub-optimal. Although the culture of the urine remains the gold standard for diagnosing and treating UTIs, technical considerations including the methods of collection of the urine as well as the

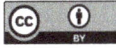

time necessary for obtaining culture results remain problematic. Urine culture examination has the disadvantage of taking at least 48 h to produce an outcome. Rapid, cost-effective methods for UTI diagnosis are required as an alternative form of scanning. Moreover, the diagnosis of UTIs using clinical criteria alone has an error rate of approximately 33% [4]. Therefore, the development of better diagnostic tools for UTIs is essential for improving antimicrobial stewardship and to reduce the morbidity associated with this condition.

The choice of management options for UTIs depends on whether they are uncomplicated or complicated. Most guidelines for non-complex UTIs recommend treatment with empirical antibiotics; however, this accounts for a considerable percentage of antibiotic prescriptions. Anti-microbial drugs should not be prescribed excessively, as they may result in antibiotic overuse and contribute to the development of antimicrobial resistance. In the management of pyelonephritis, clinicians need to correctly differentiate between acute uncomplicated forms and complicated, often obstructive, forms of UTIs that require early appropriate imaging. Quick and proper treatment can prevent urosepsis.

As UTIs are a major issue in all age groups and are thus significant in clinical practice, a high level of diagnostic accuracy is crucial.

Digitalization in Medical Field

Making sense of human language has been a goal of artificial intelligence researchers since the 1950s. Technological development in the health industry has increased significantly over the last 10–15 years. In most industrialized countries, a shortage of medical professionals has stimulated the need for technology, especially new and inventive implementations of artificial intelligence models and algorithms. Applying this kind of software in order to solve medical problems can prove to be highly beneficial, especially in terms of cutting costs, lowering the amount of required time and the need for human knowledge and resources, and reducing the number of medical errors.

Artificial intelligence, as an advanced science technology, has been widely used in medical fields to promote medical development, mainly considering the early detection [5], diagnosis [6], and management of diseases [7]. For instance, Secinaro et al. [7] in their research extensively described the impact and potential use of AI in healthcare. They pointed out that AI helps in diagnostic accuracy and has the potential to analyze health data by comparing thousands of medical records, thus providing efficient management of health services and places of care.

AI models can be used not only to identify UTIs, but also to recognize patients at highest risk for serious complications such as sepsis. The systematic review presented by Choudhury, A., and Asan, O. [5] indicates that AI-enabled decision support systems, when implemented correctly, can aid in enhancing patient safety by improving error detection, patient stratification, and drug management.

The objective of this study was to analyze current views regarding attempts at applying AI techniques in clinical practice, as well as to find promising methods to diagnose UTIs in more efficient ways. We also compared the currently used AI models and identified the most effective one.

2. Methods

Our narrative review contains a critical and objective analysis of the current knowledge on the use of AI in UTI diagnostics. This study was reported according to the Preferred Reporting Items for Systematic Reviews and Meta-Analysis (PRISMA) guidelines. We followed the PRISMA Checklist. Our protocol was registered with the Open Science Framework on 3 April 2022.

We searched for publications in the Pub Med, ProQuest, and Cochrane databases from January 2006 to August 2021.

The search strategy included randomized controlled trials, clinical trials, and observational studies. The reference lists of articles were examined for additional relevant studies.

The keywords used in the search were initially determined by a preliminary review of the literature.

The final search query for PubMed was as follows: ("artificial intelligence" [MeSH] OR "artificial intelligence" OR "machine learning" [MeSH] OR "machine learning" OR "deep learning" [MeSH] OR "deep learning" OR "natural language processing" [MeSH] OR "natural language processing") AND ("urinary tract infection*" [MeSH] OR "urinary tract infection*" OR "bacteriuria" [MeSH] OR "bacteriuria"). The search was restricted only to English-language literature.

We excluded any study if the data were insufficient for outcome assessment, when recurrent UTIs were analyzed, opinion/review papers, and studies involving the pediatric population. Six trials met the required criteria (Figure 1). The collected data from the chosen trials are summarized in Table 1.

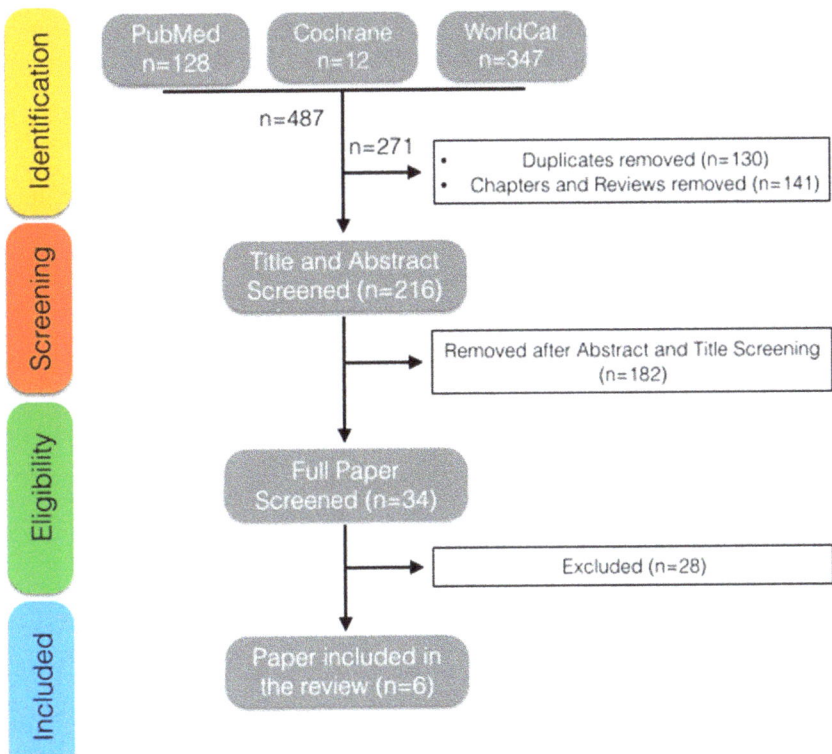

Figure 1. Search strategy.

3. Overview of AI Applications in UTI Diagnosis

AI is defined as the science and engineering of creating intelligent machines that behave in a way that could be considered intelligent if it was done by a human being [8]. One of the major branches of AI is machine learning, which is defined as the study of algorithms and statistical models that computer systems use to learn from sample data and past experience, without being explicitly programmed to perform specific tasks [9–11].

With the capacity to identify hidden patterns in the data, machine learning can be used to solve various problems, such as finding the associations between two variables, classifying subjects by certain criteria, making predictions based on baseline characteristics, and recognizing objects with similar patterns. Popular machine learning algorithms include support vector machine (SVM), random forest (RF), gradient boosting decision tree (GBDT), and artificial neural network (ANN) [12].

SVM is a well-known method, especially for classification where sample sizes are small. In a multidimensional environment, SVM is the linear separator between data samples that classify them by creating an optimal hyperplane.

RF is a technique that produces multiple classification and regression (CART) trees. Each tree is trained on a bootstrap sample of the original training data and searches a random subset of variables; thus, every tree is "voting". Classification is a result of the average vote of all of the trees.

ANN is a common method that consists of single or multiple layers, and it is made up of processing units that are called nodes/neurons. Signals travel though the network via nodes that are interconnected. There are three types of neurons: input (receives information), hidden (main task is extracting patterns), and output (responsible for final network result).

Boosting algorithms are becoming more and more popular because of their high interpretability, ease of implementation, and high prediction accuracy. There are several types of boosting algorithms, such as the AdaBoost algorithm, gradient boosting algorithm, and XG boost algorithm. Boosting algorithms produce a decision tree based on a sample of the training data. The main goal of the algorithm is to build a basic weak classifier, and then the algorithm uses it for continuous learning.

Taylor et al. [13] performed a single-center, multi-site, retrospective cohort analysis of 80,387 adults who visited the emergency department considering urine culture results and UTI manifestation. These authors tried to answer the question of which currently known AI algorithm has the highest specificity and sensitivity in UTI diagnosis using clinical symptoms, blood, and urine samples. They developed models for UTI prediction with six machine learning algorithms: RF, extreme gradient boosting, adaptive boosting, SVM, elastic net, and ANN using both laboratory and clinical data. Models were developed with both the full set of 211 factors and a reduced set of 10 variables (age, gender, UA nitrites, UA WBC, UA bacteria, UA blood, UA epithelial cells, history of UTI, and dysuria). UTI predictions were compared with the previous documentation of UTI diagnosis and antibiotic administration. Taylor RA et al. found that the top performing algorithm for both the full and reduced models was extreme gradient boosting (XGBoost), which had an area under the curve of 0.904 [8]. The XGBoost full and reduced models demonstrated greatly improved specificity in comparison with the provider judgment proxy of UTI diagnosis or antibiotic administration, while also demonstrating superior sensitivity when compared with the documentation of UTI diagnosis. The study concluded that the application of the algorithm in real life would allow approximately 1 in 4 patients to be re-categorized from false positive to true negative, and 1 in 11 patients to be re-categorized from false negative to true positive.

The literature suggests that approximately two-thirds of urine samples typically yield negative culture results [14]. Burton and colleagues [14] in their study tried to use artificial intelligence to reduce diagnostic workload without compromising the detection of UTIs. The researchers' aim was to identify which markers in the urine samples were the most sensitive and specific in order to help diagnose UTIs without the need to culture. They retrospectively analyzed 212,554 urine reports. They used two methods of classification, a heuristic model and a machine learning approach, testing three algorithms (random forest, neural network, and extreme gradient boosting). The study concluded that, in a heuristic model, the combination of the white blood cell count and bacteria count showed the strongest correlation with the probability of significant bacterial growth on the culture. The optimum minimum thresholds for WBC and bacterial counts were found to be 30 μL and 100 μL, respectively. They found that, with the application of these criteria, there would be a 39.1% reduction in the number of samples needing culture and a sensitivity of 96% for the positive bacterial culture. For the machine learning algorithms, models were developed using the set of 16 factors. All of the machine learning algorithms outperformed the heuristic model. After further analysis, the authors concluded that the samples from pregnant patients and children (age 11 or younger) required independent evaluation [14]. It turned out that the best overall solution was to combine three extreme gradient boosting algorithms, trained independently for the classification of pregnant patients, children, and then all other patients. When combined, this system granted a relative workload reduction of 41% and a sensitivity of 95% for each of the stratified patient groups.

In their research, the Advanced Analytics Group of Pediatric Urology and ORC Personalized Medicine Group tried to create a model that could identify children with an initial UTI who were at the highest risk for both recurrent UTIs (rUTI) and vesicoureteral reflux (VUR), in order to allow for targeted voiding cystourethrogram (VCUG), while children at low risk could be observed [15]. The authors enrolled 500 subjects (305 RIVUR and 195 CUTIE) in their study. The mean age was 21 ± 19 months. In this study, 72 patients developed rUTI, out of which 53 also had VUR (10.6% of the total). The final model was developed with a set of variables including age, gender, race, weight, systolic blood pressure percentile, dysuria, urine albumin/creatinine ratio, prior antibiotics exposure, and current medication. Compared with children without rUTI-associated VUR, patients with rUTI-associated VUR were significantly more likely to be white (91% vs. 72%), taking over-the-counter or prescription medication (74% vs. 49), and have a higher index UTI temperature (mean 39.8 vs. 39.4 °C). The final model had an area under the curve of 0.761. The study concluded that the predictive model provides a promising performance to facilitate the individualized management of children with initial UTIs [15].

The research conducted by Ozkan et al. [16] aimed to identify if an AI model could predict the probability of cystitis and non-specific urethritis diseases with similar symptoms from the urinary tract and, if so, to identify which one performed the best. For this purpose, the results of routine examination, urinalysis, and diagnostic medical sonography of 59 patients were collected and composed as a UTI dataset. Four different artificial intelligence methods, i.e., decision tree (DT), SVM, random forest (RF), and ANN, which are widely used in medical diagnosis systems, were used to create classification structures. Accuracy, specificity, and sensitivity statistical measurements were used to determine the performance of the created models. The comparison of individual AI methods showed that ANN had the highest accuracy result of 98.3% for UTI diagnosis. Unlike clinical-based diagnosis, this ANN model only needs the variables of pollakiuria, suprapubic pain, and erythrocyturia to receive a proper diagnosis with similar accuracy. The conclusion of this study indicated that the possibility of making a decision about complicated UTIs using factors of suprapubic pain, pollakiuria, and urinalysis result, assisted by AI methods, is very much real and applicable in the modern world. It was shown that the ANN-based model structure could classify UTIs without the need for expensive laboratory tests and ultrasounds, and thus has a a lower diagnostic cost, shorter decision time, and no need for invasive methods. Additionally, different types of data augmentation can be used to increase the accuracy of the model.

The cohort study from 2019 performed by Gadalla et al. [17] was the first attempt to use cloudiness and immunological biomarkers in urine samples as key factors in machine learning algorithms (RF and SVM) for UTI prediction. The authors investigated whether it was possible to use clinical and urinary immunological biomarkers to predict UTIs. In their study, the researchers included female patients who presented in primary care with at least one of following symptoms: dysuria, urgency, or frequency. Patients with signs of complicated UTIs, current use of antibiotics, and functional or anatomical genitourinary tract abnormalities, as well as pregnant women, were excluded from further research. General practitioners (GPs) collected the information and evaluated the symptoms on a scale from 0 = no symptoms to 6 = severe to measure its intensity. In uncomplicated UTIs, white blood cells, red blood cells, epithelial cells, and microorganisms can cause the urine to become cloudy. Urine cloudiness was also reported by GPs following sample examination and emerged to be particularly helpful in ruling out uncomplicated UTI cases. During this study, 17 clinical and 42 immunological potential predictors for bacterial culture were found using RF or SVM coupled with recursive feature elimination. Urine cloudiness was the best performing clinical predictor to rule out (negative likelihood ratio [LR−] = 0.4) and rule in (LR+ = 2.6) UTIs. Using a more discriminatory scale to assess cloudiness (turbidity) further increased the accuracy of UTI prediction (LR+ = 4.4). Urinary levels of MMP9, NGAL, CXCL8, and IL-1β together had a higher LR+ (6.1) and similar LR−(0.4) compared with cloudiness. Clinical and urinary immunological biomarkers for UTI diagnosis are important predictors and could be used to develop a point-of-care test for UTIs, but require further validation.

Heckerling and colleagues [18] used ANN coupled with genetic algorithms to determine combinations of clinical variables optimized for predicting UTIs. The ANN examined 212 women enrolled in the study aged between 19 and 84 with symptoms of UTIs. Confirmation of infections in the urinary tract was defined based on different criteria in separate models, as uropathogen counts of $\geq 10^5$ colony-forming units (CFU) per milliliter and uropathogen counts of $\geq 10^2$ CFU per milliliter. Five-variable sets were created that classified cases of urinary tract infection and non-infection with receiver operating characteristic (ROC) curve areas that ranged from 0.853 (95% CI, 0.796–0.909) for uropathogen counts of ≥ 105 CFU per milliliter to 0.792 (95% CI, 0.726–0.858) for uropathogen counts of ≥ 102 CFU per milliliter. Network influence analyses revealed that some factors predicted urine infection in unexpected ways, and interacted with other variables when making predictions. While they found that cloudiness was associated with an increased LR+, their genetic algorithm did not retain it for the creation of the neural network. It is possible that this reflects the differences between neural networks and RF models [18].

Table 1. An overview of the current knowledge regarding various AI models in UTI diagnostics.

Authors	Cohort Size	Research Type	Top Performing Algorithm	Sensitivity (%)	Specificity (%)	Predictors Used in Developing of AI Models
Taylor et al. [13]	80.387	Retrospective cohort study	XGBoost	61,7 (60.0–63.3)	94.9 (94.5–95.3)	Age, gender, UA WBC (white blood cells), UA nitrates, UA leukocytes, UA bacteria, UA blood, UA epithelial cells, history of previous UTI, and dysuria
Burton et al. [14]	212.554	Retrospective cohort study	XGBoost (combined)	95.2 [+/−0.22]	60.93 [+/−0.62]	Demographics, historical urine culture results, and clinical details
Ozkan et al. [16]	59	Retrospective study	ANN	97.77	100	Pollacuria, suprapubic pain, and erythrocyturia
Advanced Analytics Group of Pediatric Urology et al. [15]	500 (children)	Observational cohort study	NA	NA	NA	Age, gender, race, weight, SBP (percentile), dysuria, ACR, and current and prior antibiotics
Gadalla et al. [17]	183	Retrospective cohort study	RF/SVM	NA	NA	Urine cloudness and urinary levels of MMP9, NGAL, CXC8, and IL-β
Heckerling et al. [18]	212	Retrospective cohort study	ANN + genetic algorithm	82.1 (69.2–90.7)	74.4 (66.6–80.9)	Urinary frequency; dysuria; foul urine odor; symptom duration; history of diabetes; leukocyte esterase on a urine dipstick; and red blood, cells, epithelial cells, and bacteria upon urinalysis

ACR—urine: albumin/creatine ratio; AI—artificial intelligence; ANN—artificial neutral networks; NA—not available; RF—random forest; SBP—systolic blood pressure; SVM—support vector machine; UA—urinalysis.

4. Conclusions and Future Directions

AI algorithms can reveal parsimonious variable sets that are accurate at predicting urinary tract infections, as well as novel relationships between symptoms, urinalysis findings, and inflammatory processes in the urinary tract. Accurate and rapid decision making can assist physicians in daily practice, especially considering children and infants. The literature examined here confirms the relevance of AI models in UTI diagnosis, whereas it has not yet been established which model is preferable for infection prediction in adult patients and in pediatric populations. The challenge is that a tremendous amount of big data are needed in order to construct a base for the application of a machine learning algorithm. Using new techniques in medicine could decrease the amount of time required for proper UTI diagnosis, which benefits from quick and proper treatment. Hopefully deep learning methods will prevent the overuse of anti-microbial drugs, which is particularly important in children. Artificial intelligence models have achieved a high performance in retrospective studies, but further studies are required in order to introduce advanced technology into everyday healthcare, nephrology, and urology, which could be beneficial, especially in children with recurrent urinary tract infections.

Author Contributions: Conceptualization N.G. and D.P.-J.; methodology, N.G.; validation, N.G., D.P.-J. and D.Z.; formal analysis, N.G.; investigation, N.G.; resources N.G. and D.P.-J.; data curation, N.G. and D.P.-J.; writing—original draft preparation, N.G.; writing—review and editing, N.G. and D.P.-J.; visualization, N.G.; supervision, D.P.-J. and D.Z.; project administration, N.G. and D.P.-J. All authors have read and agreed to the published version of the manuscript.

Funding: This research received no external funding.

Institutional Review Board Statement: Not applicable.

Informed Consent Statement: Not applicable.

Conflicts of Interest: The authors declare no conflict of interest.

References

1. Stamm, W.E.; Norrby, S.R. Urinary Tract Infections: Disease Panorama and Challenges. *J. Infect. Dis.* **2001**, *183*, S1–S4. [CrossRef] [PubMed]
2. Flores-Mireles, A.L.; Walker, J.N.; Caparon, M.; Hultgren, S.J. Urinary Tract Infections: Epidemiology, Mechanisms of Infection and Treatment Options, Nature Reviews. *Microbiology* **2015**, *13*, 269–284. [CrossRef] [PubMed]
3. Wilson, M.L.; Gaido, L. Laboratory Diagnosis of Urinary Tract Infections in Adult Patients. *Clin. Infect. Dis.* **2004**, *38*, 1150–1158. [CrossRef] [PubMed]
4. Schmiemann, G.; Kniehl, E.; Gebhardt, K.; Matejczyk, M.M.; Hummers-Pradier, E. The Diagnosis of Urinary Tract Infection: A Systematic Review. *Dtsch. Arztebl. Int.* **2010**, *107*, 361–367. [CrossRef] [PubMed]
5. Choudhury, A.; Asan, O. Role of artificial intelligence in patient safety outcomes: Systematic literature review. *JMIR Med. Inform.* **2020**, *8*, e18599. [CrossRef] [PubMed]
6. Choudhury, A.; Renjilian, E.; Asan, O. Use of machine learning in geriatric clinical care for chronic diseases: A systematic literature review. *JAMIA Open* **2020**, *3*, 459–471. [CrossRef] [PubMed]
7. Secinaro, S.; Calandra, D.; Secinaro, A.; Muthurangu, V.; Biancone, P. The role of artificial intelligence in healthcare: A structured literature review. *BMC Med. Inform. Decis. Mak.* **2021**, *21*, 125. [CrossRef] [PubMed]
8. McCarthy, J. What Is Artificial Intelligence? Stanford University, Computer Science Department. 2007. Available online: http://www-formal.stanford.edu/jmc/whatisai/whatisai (accessed on 28 November 2019).
9. FDA. Proposed Regulatory Framework for Modifications to Artificial Intelligence/Machine Learning (AI/ML)-Based Software as a Medical Device (SaMD). Available online: https://www.fda.gov/files/medical%20devices/published/US-FDA-Artificial-Intelligence-and-Machine-Learning-Discussion-Paper.pdf (accessed on 5 April 2022).
10. Asan, O.; Bayrak, A.E.; Choudhury, A. Artificial intelligence and human trust in healthcare: Focus on clinicians. *J. Med. Internet Res.* **2020**, *22*, e15154. [CrossRef] [PubMed]
11. FDA. What Are Examples of Software as a Medical Device? 2017. Available online: https://www.fda.gov/medical-devices/software-medical-device-samd/what-are-examples-software-medical-device (accessed on 5 April 2022).
12. Xie, G.; Chen, T.; Li, Y.; Chen, T.; Li, X.; Liu, Z. Artificial Intelligence in Nephrology: How Can Artificial Intelligence Augment Nephrologists' Intelligence? *Kidney Dis.* **2020**, *6*, 1–6. [CrossRef] [PubMed]
13. Taylor, R.A.; Moore, C.L.; Cheung, K.H.; Brandt, C. Predicting urinary tract infections in the emergency department with machine learning. *PLoS ONE* **2018**, *13*, e0194085. [CrossRef] [PubMed]

14. Burton, R.J.; Albur, M.; Eberl, M.; Cuff, S.M. Using Artificial Intelligence to Reduce Diagnostic Workload without Compromising Detection of Urinary Tract Infections. *BMC Med. Inform. Decis. Mak.* **2019**, *19*, 171. [CrossRef] [PubMed]
15. Advanced Analytics Group of Pediatric Urology and ORC Personalized Medicine Group. Targeted Workup after Initial Febrile Urinary Tract Infection: Using a Novel Machine Learning Model to Identify Children Most Likely to Benefit from Voiding Cystourethrogram. *J. Urol.* **2019**, *202*, 144–152. [CrossRef] [PubMed]
16. Ozkan, I.A.; Koklu, M.; Sert, I.U. Diagnosis of Urinary Tract Infection Based on Artificial Intelligence Methods. *Comput. Methods Programs Biomed.* **2018**, *166*, 51–59. [CrossRef] [PubMed]
17. Gadalla, A.A.H.; Friberg, I.M.; Kift-Morgan, A.; Zhang, J.; Eberl, M.; Topley, N.; Weeks, I.; Cuff, S.; Wootton, M.; Gal, M.; et al. Identification of clinical and urine biomarkers for uncomplicated urinary tract infection using machine learning algorithms. *Sci. Rep.* **2019**, *9*, 19694. [CrossRef] [PubMed]
18. Heckerling, P.S.; Canaris, G.J.; Flach, S.D.; Tape, T.G.; Wigton, R.S.; Gerber, B.S. Predictors of Urinary Tract Infection Based on Artificial Neural Networks and Genetic Algorithms. *Int. J. Med. Inform.* **2007**, *76*, 289–296. [CrossRef] [PubMed]

Review

Current Concepts of Pediatric Acute Kidney Injury—Are We Ready to Translate Them into Everyday Practice?

Kinga Musiał

Department of Pediatric Nephrology, Wrocław Medical University, Borowska 213, 50-556 Wrocław, Poland; kinga.musial@umed.wroc.pl

Abstract: Pediatric acute kidney injury (AKI) is a major cause of morbidity and mortality in children undergoing interventional procedures. The review summarizes current classifications of AKI and acute kidney disease (AKD), as well as systematizes the knowledge on pathophysiology of kidney injury, with a special focus on renal functional reserve and tubuloglomerular feedback. The aim of this review is also to show the state-of-the-art in methods assessing risk and prognosis by discussing the potential role of risk stratification strategies, taking into account both glomerular function and clinical settings conditioned by fluid overload, urine output, or drug nephrotoxicity. The last task is to suggest careful assessment of eGFR as a surrogate marker of renal functional reserve and implementation of point-of-care testing, available in the case of biomarkers like NGAL and [IGFBP-7] × [TIMP-2] product, into everyday practice in patients at risk of AKI due to planned invasive procedures or treatment.

Keywords: furosemide stress test; hyperfiltration; [IGFBP-7] × [TIMP-2]; NGAL; renal angina index; renal functional reserve; tubular damage; tubuloglomerular feedback

1. Introduction

Pediatric acute kidney injury (AKI) is a serious clinical condition, associated with increased morbidity and mortality, as reported in large observational studies like AWARE (Assessment of Worldwide Acute Kidney Injury, Renal Angina, and Epidemiology) or AWAKEN (Assessment of Worldwide Acute Kidney Injury Epidemiology in Neonates) [1–3]. Yet, defining an efficient and reliable tool for kidney injury assessment in children is still a challenge. Despite longitudinal efforts and a wide range of methods tested in adults, the results seem difficult to be transferred directly into the pediatric background, where the results and their interpretation are age-dependent. While methods of evaluating renal function in stable milieu are established, the real task is how to predict the kidney ability to preserve function despite injury under stress conditions. Thus, we should search for static and dynamic markers of kidney function, as well as parameters of functional flexibility, predicting recovery after injury.

The history of progress in diagnosing kidney injury and predicting prognosis screens through various classifications, identification of risk factors, discovery and increasing role of damage biomarkers, evaluation of renal functional reserve and usage of stress tests, and finally search for predictors of progression from AKI to CKD or of recovery. The major task for the future is how to translate the adult experience into the pediatric clinical setting in order to prevent kidney injury or provide recovery from it.

2. Classical AKI Definitions

Defining acute kidney injury was a milestone towards understanding the nature of renal damage. The goal behind subsequently developed criteria (RIFLE, pRIFLE, AKIN) was to find the most accurate tool for early diagnosis and efficient treatment of AKI [4–6]. Finally, the KDIGO AKI definition was developed as a unified classification for children and adults and is now recommended for pediatric AKI [7–9] (Table 1).

Table 1. KDIGO acute kidney injury (AKI) and acute kidney disease (AKD) definitions [7,8]. eGFR, estimated glomerular filtration rate.

Stages of AKI	Serum Creatinine	eGFR	Urine Output (UOP)
Stage 1	1.5-fold increase of baseline creatinine in 7 days or increase by ≥0.3 mg/dL within 48 h	-	<0.5 mL/kg b.w./h in 6–12 h
Stage 2	2-fold increase	-	<0.5 mL/kg b.w./h in ≥12 h
Stage 3	3-fold increase or increase by ≥0.5 mg/dL within 48 h or serum creatinine ≥4.0 mg/dL	decrease to <35 mL/min/1.73 m^2 in patients <18 years or receipt of renal replacement therapy	<0.3 mL/kg b.w./h in ≥24 h or anuria in ≥12 h
AKD	Serum creatinine	eGFR	Markers of damage
For ≤3 months	increase by >50%	decrease by ≥35%	present

However, all these classifications still depend mainly on serum creatinine, an imperfect kidney function evaluation tool. Indeed, creatinine clearance may reflect eGFR in steady conditions, but stress modifies its value owing to creatinine excretion by proximal tubules. Moreover, creatinine concentration is biased with multiple modifiers (muscle mass, metabolism, hydration status, use of diuretics) and delayed toward actual time of injury. Thus, further research has concentrated on finding markers that would precede creatinine rising. The whole domain of injury biomarkers has evolved from a new understanding of AKI, according to which functional loss and damage may follow each other or exist concurrently [10].

3. Expanded AKI Definition

Recommendations given by the 10th Acute Dialysis Quality Initiative (ADQI) have combined functional and damage markers and created four categories in the AKI field [10]. The classification distinguishes between loss of glomerular function and presence of tubular damage, showing that they may appear separately, subsequently, or concomitantly [10]. This new classification underlines the idea of transition between categories and assessment of the kidney status over time. The term of "functional AKI", where glomerular filtration rate is decreased, but markers of damage are absent, covers all cases of volume-dependent, time-sensitive, and potentially reversible alterations in kidney function preceding damage. Such transient elevation of serum creatinine could be observed in the early phases of "pre-renal azotemia" resulting from dehydration or "post-renal AKI" with urinary tract obstruction without signs of damage. The idea of "subclinical AKI" is new, stressing the fact that damage may precede functional loss, like in the case of drugs with nephrotoxic potential (Figure 1). Therefore, damage markers may become promising early predictors of incipient AKI. The "combined AKI" category unified the two former conditions, whereas "no AKI" was complementary to normal renal function without signs of damage (Figure 1). Moreover, the authors proposed a hypothesis that all options may turn into one another, thus defining various types of AKI-associated injury as potentially reversible processes [10].

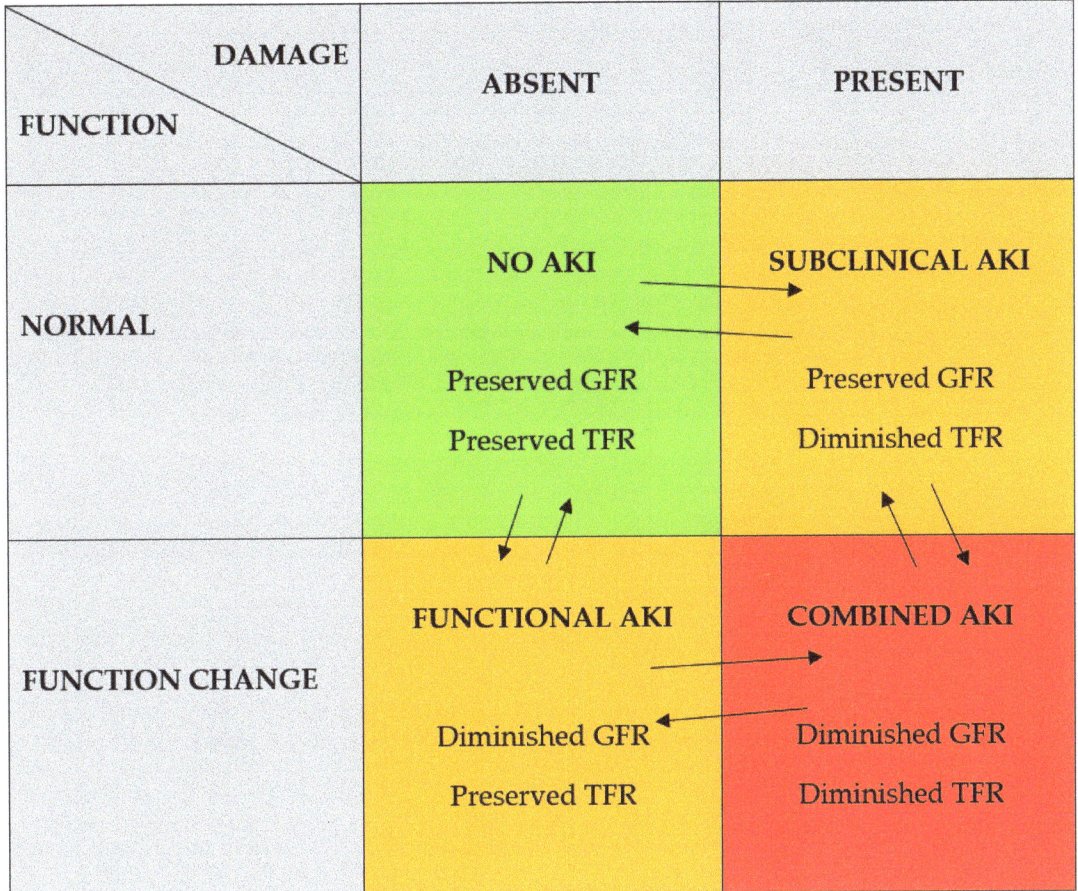

Figure 1. Expanded acute kidney injury (AKI) criteria combining function and damage biomarkers, glomerular functional reserve (GFR), and tubular functional reserve (TFR) (according to [10], modified).

4. Markers of Injury

The spectrum of AKI biomarkers in the pediatric population has been reviewed extensively elsewhere [11–14]. However, their implementation is restricted to small groups of patients and the results, rather of scientific than diagnostic value, could not modify the strategy of improvement for pediatric AKI [15]. Thus, despite the robustness of markers tested in the AKI conditions, only a few proved their usefulness in the prediction of AKI or prediction of recovery and found their place in everyday practice. Out of a wide range of candidates, only NGAL and [IGFBP7] × [TIMP-2] product were put into the form of point-of-care testing, thus serving as diagnostic tools.

4.1. Neutrophil Gelatinase-Associated Lipocalin (NGAL)

NGAL is a low molecular weight protein (25 kDa), filtered freely by glomeruli and reabsorbed by the proximal tubules. The distal tubular epithelial cells are the main source of NGAL, but its urinary increase is a sign of proximal tubule injury, especially due to ischemia. AKI triggers the release of a monomeric form into the urine. Serum, plasma, and urine NGAL are useful in predicting AKI, although recent meta-analysis has confirmed the superiority of urine NGAL over serum/plasma measurements (area under the curve

(AUC) = 0.92 for urine NGAL, AUC = 0.87 for serum NGAL, and AUC = 0.84 for plasma NGAL) in patients with sepsis [16]. Urine NGAL also performed well in the pediatric population. It could predict 30-day and 3-month mortality in children with AKI [17], and its concentration could distinguish between patients at risk of developing AKI as a consequence of nephrotoxicity [18]. Most recently, uNGAL has shown its usefulness, together with CT-scan, in the assessment of AKI in patients suffering from SARS-CoV 2 infection [19].

4.2. Insulin-Like Growth Factor-Binding Protein (IGFBP)-7

IGFBP-7 is another low molecular weight (30 kDa) protein freely filtered by glomeruli and reabsorbed by proximal tubules. Renal injury results in its increased tubular expression and tubular cell cycle arrest in the G1 phase. The consequence is decreased energy consumption in the course of a self-protective mechanism. Increased IGFBP-7 urinary concentrations were noticed in children and neonates from intensive care units. They predicted renal outcome and distinguished between patients with and without AKI, or between those with early recovery from AKI and late or non-recovery [20,21].

4.3. Tissue Inhibitor of Metalloproteinase (TIMP)-2

TIMP-2 (21 kDa), similarly to IGFBP-7, is another marker of cell cycle arrest. It proved its superiority over damage markers, like urinary NGAL, KIM-1, or L-FABP, in AKI prediction among critically ill patients. The assessment of [IGFBP-7] × [TIMP-2] product gave even better results in the prediction of progression to mild/severe AKI and of 30-day and 3-month mortality due to AKI [20–22]. Moreover, similarly to NGAL, [IGFBP-7] × [TIMP-2] is now available in the form of a point-of-care test, Nephrocheck. Nalesso et al. [23] have analyzed the usefulness of Nephrocheck based on the literature analysis. The authors concluded that the use of this test should be considered in the case of any large surgery or when invasive procedure is planned. The major restriction is the fact that the predictive value of [IGFBP-7] × [TIMP-2] product increases with the severity of patient condition. In practice, the marker distinguishes quite precisely between those who develop severe AKI and no AKI, but copes rather poorly with the prediction of mild forms of AKI [23].

The above-mentioned examples clearly show that the biomarker universum is still under construction. Additionally, the ongoing discussion shows large discrepancies among scientists and clinicians regarding their accuracy and predictive value [24–26]. Yet, their diagnostic value is restricted to the short period between pre-AKI and AKI time points.

5. From AKI into Acute Kidney Disease (AKD)

Adding markers of injury to the current understanding of AKI has expanded diagnostic possibilities [10]. However, AKI milieu according to KDIGO criteria is restricted to one week from the set point of injury, concentrating on the dynamics and progression of damage. The current concept of kidney dysfunction takes into account both pre-injury and post-injury conditions, putting stress on factors predicting damage and assessing a chance for recovery. The latter seems of paramount prognostic value, distinguishing between potentially reversible acute injury and irreversible chronic kidney disease (CKD).

The consensus report of the Acute Disease Quality Initiative (ADQI) has aimed at describing conditions of ongoing pathophysiological process in the kidney after AKI [27]. According to ADQI, acute kidney disease (AKD) encompasses all episodes of kidney injury persisting for more than 7 days, but less than 90 days [27].

The current KDIGO definition of AKD takes into account the exclusive or concurrent persistence of serum creatinine rise/eGFR decrease/damage marker presence [8] (Table 1). ADQI consensus has divided AKD into stages, congruent with AKI stages 1–3 (Table 2). Additionally, "subacute AKD", called stage zero, was added and subdivided into three categories, depending on the unchanged/increased serum creatinine or absence/presence of damage markers (Table 2).

Table 2. Stages of AKD according to Acute Disease Quality Initiative (ADQI) consensus [10].

Stages of AKD	Serum Creatinine	Markers of Damage
Stage 0A	Return to baseline values	No evidence of injury Risk of long-term events
Stage 0B	Return to baseline values	Ongoing kidney damage/injury Loss of renal reserve
Stage 0C	Increase less than 1.5-fold	Ongoing kidney damage/injury
Stage 1	1.5-fold increase	Ongoing kidney damage/injury
Stage 2	2-fold increase	Ongoing kidney damage/injury
Stage 3	3-fold increase	Ongoing kidney damage/injury
Ongoing RRT	Receipt of renal replacement therapy (RRT)	

As the AKI definition requires strict time limits that do not fit every patient with kidney damage, AKD seems to have a chance to classify those who did not fulfill the criteria of AKI, but demonstrate persistent features of renal injury. Moreover, an extended observation period is essential in establishing the future direction of changes—to recovery or toward irreversible damage.

Indeed, ADQI has proposed several hypothetical trajectories of AKD sequelae from day 0 (injury) to day 28. Their range was from rapid reversal of normal kidney function within 48 h to systematic progression from subacute AKI towards AKD stage 3 within 28 days [27]. Of note, those who developed AKI stage 3 within the first 48 h could partially improve within 7 days to AKI stage 2, then to AKD stage 2, and finally to stage 1. However full recovery was not possible [27].

6. AKI–AKD–CKD Continuum

The above-mentioned hypothetical models aimed to show the idea of the continuum between AKI, AKD, and CKD, where AKD is a link between AKI and CKD [27]. However, AKD in this concept should be understood as an AKI sequel, with an ongoing recovery or damage and possibility of either favorable or adverse consequences. Treating AKD like a CKD prequel may trigger an unexpected bias, because, among all definitions of kidney injury, only CKD bears the burden of irreversibility.

AKI in the Presence of Pre-Existing CKD

All AKI definitions concentrate on the actual kidney dysfunction without considering potential previous episodes of injury. Such conjecture is justified in the situation when the focus is on the proportional change in serum creatinine or estimated glomerular filtration rate, rather than on their absolute post-exposure values. The latter may be biased with different threshold values when current injury develops on the basis of chronic kidney disease. Moreover, the ability of the kidney to use its functional reserve may maintain apparently normal eGFR values despite ongoing kidney function decline. Silent loss of nephrons during the AKI–AKD–CKD continuum may be difficult to perceive, but current knowledge provides tools to diagnose this process.

7. Renal Functional Reserve

The term renal functional reserve (RFR) was established in the 1980s to describe the difference between the baseline eGFR value and its increase after stimulation by protein intake [28]. The concept of discrepancy between kidney function in stable versus stress conditions originates from the observation that baseline kidney capacity is at approximately 75% of its maximal filtration [28,29]. Such reserve secures quick adaptation to physiological demands, like protein intake or excessive/insufficient fluid supplementation. A similar ability allows to compensate transient decrease in functioning renal mass during pathological conditions. The value of basal eGFR and the extent to which it can increase in stress conditions both depend on the intact renal mass. In consequence, return to the baseline eGFR value after a temporary decline in the course of a single episode of AKI can be achieved, although it is reached at the cost of reduced RFR [30]. Repeat AKI episodes may lead to continuous mobilization of RFR to maintain eGFR. Such worsening of kidney function would pass unnoticed until RFR becomes exhausted with subsequent injuries. It is assumed that the loss of functioning nephrons may remain undiagnosed, owing to unchanged eGFR values, as long as the intact renal mass is reduced by no more than 50%. Beyond this threshold, the rate of kidney damage may grow exponentially [29].

The Mechanism of eGFR Increase

The mechanism by which eGFR increases is triggered depending on the presence/absence of underlying renal injury. Physiologically, stress conditions evoke additional recruitment of intact nephron units and subsequent increased filtration, as observed during pregnancy, in patients with solitary kidney or in those who became living related donors. This apparently normal eGFR is maintained at the cost of RFR stimulation. Under pathological conditions, the reduced mass of functioning nephrons can only respond by augmented filtration of a single nephron, resulting in hyperfiltration [29]. Such a scenario accompanies obesity, diabetic nephropathy, or primary glomerulopathies. Yet, it is also based on persistent stimulation of RFR. In consequence, decompensation of regulatory mechanisms may follow.

Indeed, large observational studies concluded that, even in health, the presence of hyperfiltration signifies further eGFR decline and risk of CKD development [31,32]. The Japanese study revealed that basic eGFR values in people with hyperfiltration were significantly higher (although within normal range) than in those who did not develop hyperfiltration [31]. Moreover, those increased values persisted for 3.3 ± 1.9 years before they reached the threshold of hyperfiltration. Then, the eGFR decline followed, and it was accelerated in patients with hyperfiltration when compared with those without it [31]. The Korean experience proved that hyperfiltration was connected with the increased risk of incident proteinuria and 30% eGFR decline [32]. The authors concluded that hyperfiltration may be treated as an indicator of increased risk of developing CKD in an apparently healthy population. The study held in Singapore has strengthened the above conclusions by showing that the risk of renal decline was even higher in patients with hyperfiltration caused by diabetes [33]. Summing up, the expense of hyperfiltration is costly even in the healthy population, although those with comorbidities pay more.

These observations urge to describe the phenomenon of hyperfiltration. The hypothetical process has been analyzed in detail in the case of oral protein load or amino acid infusion [30,34]. The major force triggering hyperfiltration in this case is tubuloglomerular feedback.

8. Tubuloglomerular Feedback

Tubuloglomerular feedback (TGF) is an autoregulatory mechanism to control glomerular filtration at a single nephron level. The major goal for TGF is to maintain glomerular capillary pressure within a safe range. The control of vascular tone within the afferent arteriole is adjusted to water and salt delivery to the distal tubule sensing site—macula densa. When distal tubular delivery of NaCl aggravates, macula densa triggers vasoconstriction of the above mentioned artery, glomerular capillary pressure decreases, and eGFR value declines.

Diabetes is the most spectacular example of interactions between tubules and glomeruli, with subsequent hyperfiltration and diabetic kidney disease [35]. When the increased content of filtered glucose reaches proximal tubules, sodium-glucose cotransporters 2 and 1 (SGLT2 and SGLT1) are responsible for enhanced reabsorption of glucose, together with sodium, chloride, and fluid [35]. This phenomenon is aggravated by tubular hypertrophy, resulting from hyperglycemia, and subsequent increased expression of high-capacity transporter SGLT2 in the early proximal tubule. Decreased delivery of Na, Cl, and fluid to macula densa triggers tubuloglomerular feedback with hyperfiltration. Additionally, reduced fluid content, reaching distal tubule, decreases hydrostatic back pressure in the Bowman's capsule, thus enhancing glomerular filtration and physical stress on the filtration barrier [35].

Oral protein intake or amino acid infusion result in the increased filtered load of amino acids and their aggravated reabsorption, together with NaCl, by proximal tubules [30]. In consequence, diminished delivery of NaCl to distal tubules senses macula densa to inhibit the activity of tubuloglomerular feedback and evoke hyperfiltration through vasodilatation of the afferent artery. Preglomerular vessel dilatation provokes increase in renal plasma flow (RPF), without changing filtration fraction. Among factors responsible for this phenomenon, paracrine and endocrine stimuli seem of paramount importance. One of the major regulators in TGF is nitric oxide (NO).

Amino acid infusion increases the intrarenal synthesis of nitric oxide (NO). Experimental data have proven the direct impact of neuronal nitric oxide synthase β (NOS1 β) from macula densa on TGF and subsequent change in eGFR [36]. Wild-type mice on a 4-week high-protein diet demonstrated kidney hypertrophy, glomerular hyperfiltration, increased blood flow, decreased renal vascular resistance, as well as upregulated expression and activity of macula densa NOS1 β, in comparison with mice fed a low-protein diet. Meanwhile, the TGF response was blunted both in vivo (measurement by micropuncture) and in vitro (measurement of diameters of the afferent artery), but to a greater extent in mice on the high-protein diet. Macula densa NOS1 β knockout mice demonstrated attenuation of all these reactions despite high-protein diet intake [36].

Although TGF is most efficient in response to short-term stimuli, the above mentioned results suggest that chronic TGF stimulation may establish a new set point of distal tubular flow. In practice, TGF becomes less sensitive to increased NaCl load and single nephron eGFR remains increased. Such a concept would explain the tight connections between tubules and glomeruli, not only in acute conditions, but also as a consequence of chronic kidney injury, leading, e.g., to diabetic kidney disease.

9. Tubular Function Testing

Renal functional reserve provides the information on maximal capacity of glomerular filtration in stress conditions. The major challenge in everyday practice is the fact that no routine test for clinical assessment of RFR exists. Once TGF was revealed, it became clear that eGFR value is tightly connected with proximal tubule function. Having said that, is it worth testing tubular function as an equivalent of renal capacity to adapt to unfavorable conditions? The concept of the tubular stress test is parallel to the glomerular stress test after protein/amino acid load—tubular secretion of creatinine is assessed after protein meal and confronted with the baseline secretion value [37]. Although available in clinical practice, this test still requires standardization.

Furosemide Stress Test

Contrary to the tubular stress test, the furosemide stress test is used routinely to assess tubular damage in patients with AKI. Recent evidence shows that its result can be interpreted as a predictive tool in assessing the risk of progression into AKI stage 3 and need for renal replacement therapy. The concept is based on loop diuretic pharmacodynamics. Furosemide is secreted by proximal tubules and acts at the intraluminal side of the ascending limb of the loop of Henle, where it inhibits the Na K Cl2 cotransporter and induces natriuresis [37]. In practice, 1–1.5 mg/kg b.w. of Furosemide is given and urine output is assessed after 2 h [37]. Volume exceeding 200 mL is a predictor of good prognosis.

The above-mentioned tests should open the discussion about introducing tubular functional reserve into the future panel of renal injury/recovery markers. Glomerular functional reserve and tubular functional reserve, analyzed together with damage markers, may complete the picture of kidney dysfunction (Figure 1).

10. Risk Stratification Strategy

Combined glomerular and tubular function assessment in static and dynamic conditions does not provide a complete evaluation of the patient's current status or prognosis. Clinical perspective is essential and cannot be neglected. The complex analysis of biomarker/stress test/functional reserve interrelations, together with the clinical context, has evolved into various evaluating systems able to stratify the risk of AKI development/progression to AKI stage 3/progression to CKD/recovery. The above-mentioned complex analysis is best illustrated by two systems of risk evaluation: renal angina index (RAI) and fluid overload kidney injury score (FOKIS).

10.1. Renal Angina Index (RAI)

RAI was created in order to recognize patients at risk of developing AKI within 72 h [38]. The classification categorizes patients according to two major features: risk and injury. Within the risk category, scoring encompasses moderate (one point), high (three points), and very high (five points) risk. Moderate risk is connected with admission to pediatric intensive care unit, high risk encompasses patients after stem cell transplantation, whereas very high risk patients are on ventilation. The category of injury identifies changes in creatinine clearance and fluid overload [38]. One point is dedicated to patients with unchanged kidney function and moderate (<5%) fluid overload (FO). The two-point evaluation is given to those whose eGFR has decreased by no more than 25%, while FO has exceeded 5%. Four points describe patients with 25–50% eGFR decrease and >5% FO. Finally, eight points means >50% eGFR decrease and >5% FO. The risk score is multiplied by the injury score, thus the range of points is from 1 to 40. Anyone obtaining more than eight points in the final assessment will most probably develop AKI within 72 h. The values below eight have a strong negative predictive value toward developing AKI in the next 3 days [38].

10.2. Fluid Overload Kidney Injury Score (FOKIS)

Fluid overload seriously worsens the prognosis in AKI. Pathologic accumulation of interstitial fluid in the kidney may additionally impair perfusion by the obstruction of capillary blood flow. Calculation of FO is based on multiple equations taking into account fluid balance or patient weight [39]. It is assumed that 10% FO is a threshold value for intervention.

FOKIS is a newly developed four-dimentional score putting together different categories: urine output (UOP), fluid overload (FO), serum creatinine, and nephrotoxin use [39]. Both UOP and changes in kidney function (eGFR decrease) are classified according to the pRIFLE categories and gain points from 0 to 3. The FO criteria range from <15% (1 point) to >35% (5 points). The category of nephrotoxins scores a patient treated with less than three nephrotoxic drugs (0 points), with three nephrotoxic medications (1 point), and allows to give another point (+1 point) for every additional nephrotoxic agent [39].

11. How to Prevent Kidney Injury in Children?

The above-mentioned tools stratify the risk of developing AKI based on clinical data and glomerular function. Yet, none of the classifications dedicated to children encompasses the use of biomarkers.

Relying on the values of estimated GFR while assessing kidney function in children may give discrepant results. AKI provides dynamic conditions and highly changeable concentrations of serum creatinine, delayed in their dynamics toward the time of injury. Age-dependent variability of its values increases potential bias. Therefore, an efficient future strategy facing current demands should be implemented based on available tools.

The first attempt should be to properly evaluate renal function and functional reserve, taking into account the fact that these two strongly depend on one another. A patient with hyperfiltration has a decreased renal functional reserve, and thus is potentially at risk of developing AKI in unfavorable conditions. Thus, increased eGFR values cannot diminish the vigilance, whereas "normal" records should urge the search for past injuries and factors forcing mobilization of renal functional reserve.

One of the examples is the recently published data on renal function and AKI incidence in children undergoing hematopoietic stem cell transplantation (HSCT), who are classified by RAI as those at high risk of developing AKI. Most of the pediatric patients presented with hyperfiltration even before the procedure and its presence was correlated with previous chemotherapy [40]. Of note, the percentage of children with increased eGFR values was the highest among those who have undergone HSCT for oncological reasons. Moreover, urinary concentrations of tubular damage markers in these patients were significantly higher than in the age-matched healthy controls, even before HSCT, and rose after the procedure [41]. These observations suggested that children undergoing HSCT most probably approach this procedure with already diminished renal functional reserve. Such suggestions should urge to establish the next goal in AKI prevention among children. This task should be to implement the already available point-of-care tests, like urinary NGAL or [IGFBP-7] × [TIMP-2] product, in the risk groups prepared for planned interventions or procedures like stem cell transplantation or surgery.

The next move should be toward expanding the diagnostic abilities by forming "AKI panels", allowing sequential assessment of various markers adjusted to the time after injury. Recent data show that combining serum creatinine, cystatin C, and urinary NGAL identifies better those children undergoing HSCT who are at risk of adverse outcomes [42]. This strategy would require establishment of reference ranges of damage markers for the pediatric population. Fortunately, first attempts have already been made, giving a chance for reliable results in the assessment of urinary NGAL, KIM-1, or L-FABP [43].

12. Conclusions

Current concepts of the nature of AKI show the complexity of interrelations between glomerular and tubular function, as well as the paramount role of cell damage in the early phase of AKI or even before it. The state-of-the-art in AKI gives multiple tools to complex assessment of actual kidney function, renal functional reserve, and stage of cellular damage in the context of clinical background. This combined analysis allows to grade the patients depending on the risk of AKI development, progression into serious AKI, CKD development, or recovery. However, serum creatinine remains the major index of AKI and the only biomarker put into everyday practice. Facing the future in prevention of pediatric AKI should mean identifying the patients at risk before the injury is fulfilled, preferably by assessing kidney functional reserve and using point-of-care testing before planned interventions. Coping with AKI diagnostics should concentrate on creation of sequential "AKI panels", where various markers are evaluated according to the sequence of their appearance in serum/urine.

Funding: This research received no external funding.

Institutional Review Board Statement: Not applicable.

Informed Consent Statement: Not applicable.

Data Availability Statement: Not applicable.

Conflicts of Interest: The author declares no conflict of interest regarding the publication of this manuscript.

References

1. Basu, R.K.; Kaddourah, A.; Terrell, T.; Mottes, T.; Arnold, P.; Jacobs, J.; Andringa, J.; Goldstein, S.L. Assessment of worldwide acute kidney injury, renal angina and epidemiology in critically ill children (AWARE): Study protocol for a prospective observational study. *BMC Nephrol.* **2015**, *16*, 24. [CrossRef]
2. Kaddourah, A.; Basu, R.K.; Goldstein, S.L.; Sutherland, S.M.; AWARE Investigators. Oliguria and acute kidney injury in critically ill children: Implications for diagnosis and outcomes. *Pediatr. Crit. Care Med.* **2019**, *20*, 332–339. [CrossRef]
3. Jetton, J.; Boohaker, L.J.; Sethi, S.K.; Wazir, S.; Rohatgi, S.; E Soranno, D.; Chishti, A.S.; Woroniecki, R.; Mammen, C.; Swanson, J.R.; et al. Incidence and outcomes of neonatal acute kidney injury (AWAKEN): A multicentre, multinational, observational cohort study. *Lancet Child. Adolesc. Health* **2017**, *1*, 184–194. [CrossRef]

4. Bellomo, R.; Ronco, C.; Kellum, J.A.; Mehta, R.L.; Palevsky, P. Acute Dialysis Quality Initiative workgroup: Acute renal failure—Definition, outcome measures, animal models, fluid therapy and information technology needs: The Second International Consensus Conference of the Acute Dialysis Quality Initiative (ADQI) Group. *Crit. Care* **2004**, *8*, R204–R212.
5. Akcan-Arikan, A.; Zappitelli, M.; Loftis, L.L.; Washburn, K.K.; Jefferson, L.S.; Goldstein, S.L. Modified RIFLE criteria in critically ill children with acute kidney injury. *Kidney Int.* **2007**, *71*, 1028–1035. [CrossRef]
6. Mehta, R.L.; Kellum, J.A.; Shah, S.V.; Molitoris, B.A.; Ronco, C.; Warnock, D.G.; Levin, A. Acute Kidney Injury Network: Acute kidney injury network: Report of an initiative to improve outcomes in acute kidney injury. *Crit. Care* **2007**, *11*, R31. [CrossRef]
7. Kidney Disease: Improving Global Outcomes (KDIGO) Acute Kidney Injury Work Group. KDIGO Clinical Practice Guideline for Acute Kidney Injury. *Kidney Int. Suppl.* **2012**, *2*, 1–138.
8. Levey, A.S.; Eckardt, K.U.; Dorman, N.M.; Christiansen, S.L.; Hoorn, E.J.; Ingelfinger, J.R.; Inker, L.A.; Levin, A.; Mehrotra, R.; Palevsky, P.M.; et al. Nomenclature for kidney function and disease: Report of a Kidney Disease: Improving Global Outcomes (KDIGO) Consensus Conference. *Kidney Int.* **2020**, *97*, 1117–1129. [CrossRef]
9. Sethi, S.K.; Bunchman, T.; Chakraborty, R.; Raina, R. Pediatric acute kidney injury: New advances in the last decade. *Kidney Res. Clin. Pract.* **2021**, *40*, 40–51. [CrossRef]
10. Murray, P.T.; Mehta, R.L.; Shaw, A.; Ronco, C.; Endre, Z.H.; Kellum, J.A.; Chawla, L.S.; Cruz, D.N.; Ince, C.; Okusa, M.D.; et al. Potential use of biomarkers in acute kidney injury: Report and summary of recommendations from the 10th Acute Dialysis Quality Initiative consensus conference. *Kidney Int.* **2014**, *85*, 513–521. [CrossRef]
11. McCaffrey, J.; Dhakal, A.K.; Milford, D.V.; Webb, N.J.A.; Lennon, R. Recent developments in the detection and management of acute kidney injury. *Arch. Dis. Child.* **2017**, *102*, 91–96. [CrossRef]
12. van Donge, T.; Welzel, T.; Atkinson, A.; van den Anker, J.; Pfister, M. Age-dependent changes in kidney injury biomarkers in pediatrics. *J. Clin. Pharmacol.* **2019**, *59*, S21–S32.
13. Musiał, K.; Zwolińska, D. New markers of acute kidney injury in children undergoing hematopoietic stem cell transplantation. In *Advances in Critical Care Pediatric Nephrology*; Sethi, S.K., Raina, R., McCulloch, M., Bunchman, T.E., Eds.; Springer: Singapore, 2021; Chapter 14, pp. 133–140.
14. Morgans, H.A.; Warady, B.A. CKD management post-AKI: The role of biomarkers. In *Advances in Critical Care Pediatric Nephrology*; Sethi, S.K., Raina, R., McCulloch, M., Bunchman, T.E., Eds.; Springer: Singapore, 2021; Chapter 17, pp. 167–176. [CrossRef]
15. Selewski, D.T.; Askenazi, D.J.; Kashani, K.; Basu, R.K.; Gist, K.M.; Harer, M.W.; Jetton, J.G.; Sutherland, S.M.; Zappitelli, M.; Ronco, C.; et al. Quality improvement goals for pediatric acute kidney injury: Pediatric applications of the 22nd Acute Disease Quality Initiative (ADQI) conference. *Pediatr. Nephrol.* **2021**, *36*, 733–746. [CrossRef]
16. Zhou, H.; Cui, J.; Lu, Y.; Sun, J.; Liu, J. Meta-analysis of the diagnostic value of serum, plasma and urine neutrophil gelatinase-associated lipocalin for the detection of acute kidney injury in patients with sepsis. *Exp. Ther. Med.* **2021**, *21*, 836. [CrossRef]
17. Westhoff, J.H.; Seibert, F.S.; Waldherr, S.; Bauer, F.; Tönshoff, B.; Fichtner, A.; Westhoff, T.H. Urinary calprotectin, kidney injury molecule-1, and neutrophil gelatinase-associated lipocalin for the prediction of adverse outcome in pediatric acute kidney injury. *Eur. J. Pediatr.* **2017**, *176*, 745–755. [CrossRef]
18. Goldstein, S.L.; Krallman, K.A.; Schmerge, A.; Dill, L.; Gerhardt, B.; Chodaparavu, P.; Radomsky, A.; Kirby, C.; Askenazi, D.J. Urinary neutrophil gelatinase-associated lipocalin rules out nephrotoxic acute kidney injury in children. *Pediatr. Nephrol.* **2021**, *36*, 1915–1921. [CrossRef]
19. He, L.; Zhang, Q.; Li, Z.; Shen, L.; Zhang, J.; Wang, P.; Wu, S.; Zhou, T.; Xu, Q.; Chen, X.; et al. Incorporation of urinary neutrophil gelatinase-associated lipocalin and computed tomography quantification to predict acute kidney injury and in-hospital death in COVID-19 patients. *Kidney Dis.* **2021**, *7*, 120–130. [CrossRef]
20. Bai, Z.; Fang, F.; Xu, Z.; Lu, C.; Wang, X.; Chen, J.; Pan, J.; Wang, J.; Li, Y. Serum and urine FGF23 and IGFBP-7 for the prediction of acute kidney injury in critically ill children. *BMC Pediatr.* **2018**, *18*, 192. [CrossRef]
21. Chen, J.; Sun, Y.; Wang, S.; Dai, X.; Huang, H.; Bai, Z.; Li, X.; Wang, J.; Li, Y. The effectiveness of urinary TIMP-2 and IGFBP-7 in predicting acute kidney injury in critically ill neonates. *Pediatr. Res.* **2020**, *87*, 1052–1059. [CrossRef]
22. Westhoff, J.H.; Tönshoff, B.; Waldherr, S.; Pöschl, J.; Teufel, E.; Westhoff, T.H.; Fichtner, A. Urinary tissue inhibitor of metalloproteinase-2 (TIMP-2)x insulin-like growth factor-binding protein 7 (IGFBP-7) predicts adverse outcome in pediatric acute kidney injury. *PLoS ONE* **2015**, *10*, e0143628. [CrossRef]
23. Nalesso, F.; Cattarin, L.; Gobbi, L.; Fragasso, A.; Garzotto, F.; Calo, L.A. Evaluating Nephrocheck as a predictive tool for acute kidney injury. *Int. J. Nephrol. Renovasc. Dis.* **2020**, *13*, 85–96. [CrossRef]
24. Vanmassenhove, J.; Kielstein, J.T.; Ostermann, M. Have renal biomarkers failed in acute kidney injury? Yes. *Intensive Care Med.* **2017**, *43*, 883–886. [CrossRef]
25. McMahon, B.; Koyner, J.L. Have renal biomarkers failed in acute kidney injury? No. *Intensive Care Med.* **2017**, *43*, 887–889. [CrossRef]
26. Prowle, J.R.; Rosner, M.H. Have renal biomarkers failed in acute kidney injury? We are not sure. *Intensive Care Med.* **2017**, *43*, 890–892. [CrossRef]
27. Chawla, L.; Bellomo, R.; Bihorac, A.; Goldstein, S.L.; Siew, E.D.; Bagshaw, S.M.; Fitzgerald, D.B.R.L.; Fitzgerald, D.B.R.L.; Mehta, D.C.E.M.R.; Mehta, D.C.E.M.R.; et al. Acute kidney disease and renal recovery: Consensus report of the Acute Disease Quality Initiative (ADQI) 16 workgroup. *Nat. Rev. Nephrol.* **2017**, *13*, 241–257. [CrossRef]

28. Bosch, J.P.; Saccaggi, A.; Lauer, A.; Ronco, C.; Belledonne, M.; Glabman, S. Renal functional reserve in humans. Effect of protein intake on glomerular filtration rate. *Am. J. Med.* **1983**, *75*, 943–950. [CrossRef]
29. Ronco, C.; Bellomo, R.; Kellum, J. Understanding renal functional reserve. *Intensive Care Med.* **2017**, *43*, 917–920. [CrossRef]
30. Jufar, A.H.; Lankadeva, Y.R.; May, C.N.; Cochrane, A.D.; Bellomo, R.; Evans, R.G. Renal functional reserve: From physiological phenomenon to clinical biomarker and beyond. *Am. J. Physiol. Regul. Integr. Comp. Physiol.* **2020**, *319*, R690–R702. [CrossRef]
31. Shimada, Y.; Nakasone, Y.; Hirabayashi, K.; Sakuma, T.; Koike, H.; Oguchi, T.; Yamashita, K.; Uchimido, R.; Moriya, T.; Komatsu, M.; et al. Development of glomerular hyperfiltration, a multiphasic phenomenon. *Am. J. Physiol. Renal. Physiol.* **2020**, *319*, F1037–F1041. [CrossRef]
32. Oh, S.W.; Yang, J.H.; Kim, M.-G.; Cho, W.Y.; Jo, S.K. Renal hyperfiltration as a risk factor for chronic kidney disease: A health checkup cohort study. *PLoS ONE* **2020**, *15*, e0238177. [CrossRef]
33. Low, S.; Zhang, X.; Wang, J.; Yeoh, L.Y.; Liu, Y.L.; Ang, K.K.L.; Tang, W.E.; Kwan, P.Y.; Tavintharan, S.; Sum, C.F.; et al. Long-term prospective observation suggests that glomerular hyperfiltration is associated with rapid decline in renal filtration function: A multiethnic study. *Diab. Vasc. Dis. Res.* **2018**, *15*, 417–423. [CrossRef]
34. Fuhrman, D.Y. The role of renal functional reserve in predicting acute kidney injury. *Crit. Care Clin.* **2020**. [CrossRef]
35. Vallon, V.; Thomson, S.C. The tubular hypothesis of nephron filtration and diabetic kidney disease. *Nat. Rev. Nephrol.* **2020**, *16*, 317–336. [CrossRef]
36. Wei, J.; Zhang, J.; Jiang, S.; Wang, L.; Persson, E.G.; Liu, R. High protein diet-induced glomerular hyperfiltration is dependent on NOS1β in the macula densa via tubuloglomerular feedback response. *Hypertension* **2019**, *74*, 864–871. [CrossRef]
37. Mittal, A.; Sethi, S.K. Functional renal reserve and furosemide stress test. In *Advances in Critical Care Pediatric Nephrology*; Sethi, S.K., Raina, R., McCulloch, M., Bunchman, T.E., Eds.; Springer: Singapore, 2021. [CrossRef]
38. Basu, R.K.; Wang, Y.; Wong, H.R.; Chawla, L.S.; Wheeler, D.S.; Goldstein, S.L. Incorporation of biomarkers with the renal angina index for prediction of severe AKI in critically ill children. *Clin. J. Am. Soc. Nephrol.* **2014**, *9*, 654–662. [CrossRef]
39. Plaud, A.; Siddiqui, S.; Arikan, A.A. Fluid overload and kidney injury score. In *Advances in Critical Care Pediatric Nephrology*; Sethi, S.K., Raina, R., McCulloch, M., Bunchman, T.E., Eds.; Springer: Singapore, 2021; Chapter 10, pp. 93–102. [CrossRef]
40. Musiał, K.; Kałwak, K.; Zwolińska, D. The impact of allogeneic hematopoietic stem cell transplantation on kidney function in children—A single center experience. *J. Clin. Med.* **2021**, *10*, 1113. [CrossRef]
41. Musiał, K.; Augustynowicz, M.; Miśkiewicz-Migoń, I.; Kałwak, K.; Ussowicz, M.; Zwolińska, D. Clusterin as a new marker of kidney injury in children undergoing allogeneic hematopoietic stem cell transplantation—A pilot study. *J. Clin. Med.* **2020**, *9*, 2599. [CrossRef]
42. Benoit, S.W.; Dixon, B.P.; Goldstein, S.L.; Bennett, M.R.; Lane, A.; Lounder, D.T.; Rotz, S.J.; Gloude, N.J.; Lake, K.E.; Litts, B.; et al. A novel strategy for identifying early acute kidney injury in pediatric hematopoietic stem cell transplantation. *Bone Marrow Transplant.* **2019**, *54*, 1453–1461. [CrossRef]
43. Bennett, M.R.; Nehus, E.; Haffner, C.; Ma, Q.; Devarajan, P. Pediatric reference ranges for acute kidney injury biomarkers. *Pediatr. Nephrol.* **2015**, *30*, 677–685. [CrossRef]

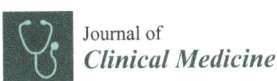

Review

Bacterial Colonization as a Possible Source of Overactive Bladder Symptoms in Pediatric Patients: A Literature Review

Katarzyna Kilis-Pstrusinska [1,*], Artur Rogowski [2,3] and Przemysław Bienkowski [4]

1. Department of Pediatric Nephrology, Wroclaw Medical University, Borowska 213, 50-556 Wroclaw, Poland
2. Faculty of Medicine, Cardinal Stefan Wyszyński University in Warsaw, Collegium Medicum, Kazimierza Wóycickiego 1/3, 01-938 Warsaw, Poland; arogowski@op.pl
3. Department of Obstetrics and Gynecology, Mother and Child Institute, 01-211 Warsaw, Poland
4. Department of Psychiatry, Medical University of Warsaw, Nowowiejska 27, 00-665 Warsaw, Poland; pbienko@yahoo.com
* Correspondence: katarzyna.kilis-pstrusinska@umed.wroc.pl; Tel.: +48-71-7364400; Fax: +48-71-7364409

Abstract: Overactive Bladder (OAB) is a common condition that is known to have a significant impact on daily activities and quality of life. The pathophysiology of OAB is not completely understood. One of the new hypothetical causative factors of OAB is dysbiosis of an individual urinary microbiome. The major aim of the present review was to identify data supporting the role of bacterial colonization in overactive bladder symptoms in children and adolescents. The second aim of our study was to identify the major gaps in current knowledge and possible areas for future clinical research. There is a growing body of evidence indicating some relationship between qualitative and quantitative characteristics of individual urinary microbiome and OAB symptoms in adult patients. There are no papers directly addressing this issue in children or adolescents. After a detailed analysis of papers relating urinary microbiome to OAB, the authors propose a set of future preclinical and clinical studies which could help to validate the concept in the pediatric population.

Keywords: overactive bladder; urinary microbiome; children; adolescents

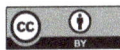

1. Introduction

Overactive Bladder (OAB) is a common condition that is known to have a significant impact on daily activities and quality of life [1–4]. In the pediatric population, OAB may not only burden child development but also have a negative impact on the family situation [5,6]. OAB is a form of lower urinary tract dysfunction caused by involuntary detrusor contractions during the filling phase. It is characterized by urgency and increased voiding frequency with or without incontinence in the absence of urinary tract infection [7]. OAB is not associated with neurological and anatomical alterations of the lower urinary tract. The recent International Children's Continence Society (ICCS) document proposes using the term daytime lower urinary tract (LUT) conditions to group all functional bladder problems in children [8]. OAB is the second most common bladder dysfunction following nocturnal enuresis [9]. Comorbid conditions associated with bladder dysfunction include urinary tract infections, vesicoureteral reflux, constipation, and encopresis [1,9–11]. In addition, there appears to be an increased frequency of behavioral and neurodevelopmental issues [5,6]. One should bear in mind that the course and clinical picture of OAB in children differ substantially from that observed in adult patients. On a theoretical ground, there are several unique factors to consider in the context of pediatric OAB, including the role of general child development, mode of delivery, mother microbiome, maturation of the nervous and endocrine systems, and development of the urinary tract [12–16].

The overall OAB prevalence in the pediatric population ranges from 1.5% to 36.4% [17–19]. It is known that the peak incidence occurs between 5 and 7 years of age, with a higher prevalence in males [1,12,20]. Overactive bladder decreases with age [13,21]. Results of a cross-sectional survey of 19,240 Korean schoolchildren identified the overall incidence of OAB, defined as urgency with or without incontinence, was 17%. The highest incidence of 23% was noted in five-year-old children and the lowest (12%) in 13-year-old patients [17]. Although OAB can resolve itself spontaneously, urinary symptoms can persist into adulthood [14,22]. The prevalence estimates for urge UI ranged from 1.8% to 30.5% in the European population, from 1.7% to 36.4% in the US population, and from 1.5% to 15.2% in the Asian population [2].

The pathophysiology of OAB is not completely understood and is believed to be multifactorial [15,23–26]. One proposed hypothesis is that dysbiosis of an individual urinary microbiome could induce or potentiate OAB symptoms [16,27–30]. The major aim of the present review was to identify data supporting the role of bacterial colonization in overactive bladder symptoms in children and adolescents. The second aim of our study was to identify major gaps in current knowledge and possible areas for future clinical research.

2. Methods

The present work was not intended to directly answer a well-defined clinically meaningful question or to modify current practice and thus could hardly fulfill the definition of a systematic review. The paucity of clinical data and lack of randomized clinical trials on the role of the microbiome in overactive bladder symptoms in children precluded a meaningful scoping review approach [31]. Hence, the present review was designed as a narrative mini-review with an assumption that an increase in the number of full-text papers may allow us to use a scoping or systematic review approach in the future [32].

Full-text papers focused on the association between the microbiome and overactive bladder symptoms were identified by searching MEDLINE and Google Scholar from inception to December 2020. Keywords included the following terms: "bacterial colonization" OR "microbiome" OR "urobiome" OR "dysbiosis" AND "overactive bladder" OR "urgency" OR "urge incontinence". A manual search of reference lists of relevant papers was also performed. One hundred and fifty-six papers were identified and screened for eligibility. Twelve original studies on microbiome and OAB were finally included in the review process. All efforts were made to identify studies on the pediatric population through manual search of abstracts and method sections for the age of recruited subjects.

Three independent reviewers screened abstracts for eligibility. Clinical studies on human subjects written in English with an available full text were included. Book chapters and conference abstracts were checked but excluded if not followed by a full-text publication.

3. Theoretical and Clinical Background

3.1. OAB

The pathophysiology of OAB is not completely understood and is believed to be multifactorial [24,25,29,33]. One theory is that the urgency and related symptoms stem from a cortical immaturity of the centers responsible for controlling urination [15,34]. Voluntary and coordinated urination is developed over time. In the first year of life, voiding is mainly controlled by the brainstem [35]. Then, cortical inhibitory pathways and the pontine micturition center along with periaqueductal grey matter, anterior cingulate gyrus, and the autonomic, somatic, and sensorial autonomic nervous systems are developed, and urination becomes voluntary [36]. The prefrontal cortex starts to maintain top-down control over more primitive afferent pathways of the brain, such as the limbic and paralimbic systems [24].

Another concept, the so-called "bladder-brain dialogue", suggests a mutual interaction between the brain and the bladder rather than unidirectional control by the brain [26,33,36]. The role of inflammation in OAB is also under investigation [25,37]. Bladder biopsies from patients with OAB without urinary tract infection (UTI) showed inflammatory changes [38]. Ghoniem et al. demonstrated upregulation of a selective subset of proinflammatory cytokines and chemokines in patients with OAB [39]. Urgency is attributed to abnormal neuromuscular signaling resulting from the stimulation of cholinergic receptors, which causes involuntary bladder muscle contractions [40,41]. However, in urodynamic studies, detrusor overactivity was only observed in approximately 58% of women with urge UI [42]. Therapy with anticholinergic drugs which mainly inhibit the function of efferent neurons in the detrusor muscle is ineffective for approximately half of patients that use them [43]. Comparable observations have been made concerning children. In case series of children with voiding dysfunction symptoms, detrusor overactivity detected by urodynamic testing was present in 52% to 58% of patients compared with 5% to 18% of asymptomatic children [44,45]. Moreover, a prospective multicenter study reported a poor correlation between symptoms and urodynamic testing in children with incontinence [46]. In a study by Bael et al., 60 of 91 children with urgency did not have evidence of an overactive bladder during bladder filling when urodynamic testing. In addition, there was a poor correlation between urodynamic findings and the response to the treatment [46].

An active exploration of etiological factors and pathophysiological mechanisms standing behind OAB symptoms in children is a prerequisite for developing safe and efficacious treatment strategies.

3.2. Microbiome

The term microbiome refers to the bacterial milieu present within various environment niches. Each individual's microbiome is unique and adapts during life as a result of environmental and genetic influences [47,48]. The maternal microbiome is a dominant factor in the development of the neonatal skin, oral mucosa, and nasopharyngeal microbiome, regardless of the delivery mode [49,50]. In the next period of life, the maternal microbiome further affects the child's microbiome through multiple transmission routes. What is interesting is a metatranscriptomic analysis of bacterial strains specific to mother-infant pairs suggests that gastrointestinal bacteria were not only transferred from the maternal gut to the infant gut environment but that the bacteria adapted effectively to the infant gut [50].

The microbiome can assist in maintaining healthy states in the human body including homeostasis and immune defense [48]. On the other hand, alterations to the microbial community structure may be also implicated in disease [51,52].

3.3. Urinary Microbiome

In the past, the urinary tract (without urethra) was considered to be sterile under normal conditions. The advances in bacterial assessment in the past decade, particularly 16S rRNA gene sequencing and expanded quantitative urine culture (EQUC), have shown that the urinary tract is not sterile [27,28,38,52–55]. Up to 80% of bacteria can be isolated using modified culture techniques for a sample that has been classified as having no growth according to the standard method [54]. According to an analysis of the literature performed by Morand et al., the urinary tract bacterial microbiome contains 21.4% of the known prokaryotic diversity associated with human beings (464 species in common), and it shares 23.6% of species with the human gut microbiota (350 species in common, 62.3% of the urine species) [56]. Females have predominantly *Lactobacillus* and *Gardnerella* species, while males carry *Corynebacterium*, *Staphylococcus*, and *Streptococcus* as dominant species [38,55]. In addition, females tend to have a more heterogeneous urinary microbiome. The species found in urine can be pathogenic or commensal. At least 60.0% of the urine microbiota is not reported in the literature as causing human UTI [56].

The characteristics and role of urinary microbiota are currently debated [33,51,52]. Urinary tract microbiota influences UTI [16,57,58]. Modification of bacterial components in urine has been associated with kidney stones, bladder cancer, and urinary incontinence [16,27,51,59]. In the context of the urinary microbiome, the gut and vaginal microbiome are also of interest, since there is evidence that implies that there is some degree of cross-talk between the bacterial flora of these organs [60–63].

The majority of urinary microbiome studies focus on adult subjects and papers concerning children are scarce. The pediatric studies on the urinary microbiome are collected in Table 1. The natural history of the urinary microbiome remains mostly unexplored.

However, to understand the role of the urinary microbiome in disease states, both in children and adults, it is necessary to know what may constitute a healthy urinary microbiome and how it develops in early childhood.

Table 1. Pediatric studies of the urinary microbiome.

	Study Group: Age, n	Key Results
Lucas et al. [64]	60 female children divided into four developmental groups: 0–3 m/o (n = 15), 4–10 m/o (n = 15), 2–6 y/o (n = 15), 7–12 y/o premenstrual girls (n = 15)	Significant shifts in the perianal and periurethral/perivaginal (PUPV) microbiome compositions during childhood, corresponding to important developmental milestones. Significant differences in the PUPV microbiome of girls with a history of UTI, likely influenced by both the UTI and the antibiotic exposure.
Curley et al. [58]	Review	Review of the literature on the role of the microbiome in recurrent UTIs, focusing on female pediatric patients when able.
Forster at al. [65]	34 children with neuropathic bladders with UTI (n = 11, mean age 11 y/o), ASB (n = 19, mean age 8.8 y/o), and with negative urine culture (n = 4, mean age 15 y/o)	The most predominant bacteria in the urine microbiomes are from the *Enterobacteriaceae* family. No difference in the urine microbiome between children with UTI, ASB, and negative urine cultures. Route of catheterization may affect the composition of the urine microbiome.
Kinneman et al. [57]	85 children < 48 months of age (72 less than 24 months)	Urinary microbiome was identified in every child, even in 3 subjects less than 30 days of age. Changes in microbiome diversity and composition were observed in subjects with a standard culture-positive UTI.
Kassiri et al. [66]	Prepubertal boys (n = 20, ages 3 months–8 years; median age 15 months)	The first characterizations of the urinary microbiome in prepubertal males. Defining the baseline healthy microbiome in children may lay the foundation for understanding the long-term impact of factors such as antibiotic use in the development of a healthy microbiome as well as the development of future diseases.
Kispal et al. [67]	12 children, 6–17 years (median age at the time of surgery 11 years)	After bladder augmentation, the native urinary bladder and augmented intestinal segments host similar microbiota despite their distinct differences of originating mucosal anatomy. Age at sampling had a statistically significant influence on β-diversity at the genus level.
Gerber et al. [16]	Review	Review of the literature on the effects of the microbiome on urologic diseases that affect the pediatric patient, including UTI, urge urinary incontinence/overactive bladder, and urolithiasis.
Ollberding et al. [68]	49 cases (delivery < 37 weeks gestation) and 48 controls (delivery ≥ 37 weeks gestation)	No difference in taxa richness, evenness, or community composition between cases and controls or for gestational age modeled as a continuous variable.

UTI-urinary tract infection; ASB-asymptomatic bacteriuria.

The relation between the urinary microbiome of parents and their children is largely unknown because to date no study has directly addressed this topic. Given the anatomic relationship between the vagina and the urinary tract, the vaginal microbiome may be relevant to the urinary microbiome. However, Hickey et al. stated that the vaginal microbiome of adolescent girls was not compatible with that of their mothers [60]. This suggests, as was the case with the gut microbiome, that the acquisition of the female "adult-form" microbiome is more of a maturation of the microbiome rather than a transition in the species representation. Currently, the data concerning the vaginal microbiome of girls are not consistent. According to a review paper by Smith and Ravel, the prepubertal vaginal microbiome is dominated by a variety of anaerobes, diphtheroid, coagulase-negative *Staphylococci*, and *E. coli*, while the postmenarcheal vaginal microbiome is most similar to adult vaginal microbiomes, dominated by *Lactobacillus* [61]. However, a prospective longitudinal study of perimenarcheal girls documented that *Lactobacillus* dominated the vaginal microbiome before the onset of menarche [60]. In addition, *Gardnerella vaginalis*, classically considered to be pathogenic, was found in up to one-third of perimenarcheal subjects. Probably, these bacteria play a commensal role in the prepubertal period.

The vaginal microbiome can be of importance in an analysis of a healthy urinary microbiome and its dysbiosis or perturbations. Urine, intestinal and vaginal microbiomes are interconnected. For example, intestinal bacteria may colonize the vaginal entrance and periurethra, and then ascend up the urethra to the bladder. The vaginal microbiome may be a natural line of defense against invading uropathogens or it may alter the urinary microbiome [62].

Kinneman et al. [57] assessed the urinary microbiome in children younger than 48 months undergoing a urinary catheterization, with and without UTI. A urinary microbiome was identified in every child. The 5 most abundant families were tissierellaceae, prevotellaeae, veillonellaceae, enterobacteriaceae, and comamonadaceae. The 5 most abundant genera were *Prevotella, Peptoniphilus, Escherichia, Veillonella*, and *Finegoldia*. Alpha diversity, which refers to the number of different species in a single site, did not differ by age, gender, antibiotic use 15 days to three months before the urine sample was obtained, maternal ethnicity, country of origin, delivery mode, or probiotic use. Decreased diversity and changes in the compositions of urinary microbiome were observed in children with standard culture-positive UTI. The authors noticed that antibiotic use affected the urinary microbiome only for a short time (up to two weeks).

Kassiri et al. [66] examined the urinary microbiome in 20 prepubertal males (aged 3 months-8 years; median age 15 months) with and without prior antibiotic exposure. The majority of patients had representation from *Staphylococcus* and *Varibaculum* species and to a lesser extent *Peptoniphilus* and *Actinobaculum*. Several of the detected genera have been previously identified in the urine of adult men. However, urinary microbial communities profiled in children were different from those described in adults. For example, *Staphylococcus* and *Corynebacterium* were present in children but were not dominant. The authors stated that the composition of the urinary microbiome in children may begin to develop early in life and evolve over time, becoming more stable in adulthood. Moreover, the study also showed differences in both the urinary and gastrointestinal microbiome in children with prior antibiotic exposure, confirming the effect of drugs on the child microbiome.

Forster et al. [65] performed a cross-sectional analysis of the urine microbiome of children with neuropathic bladders. *Enterobacteriaceae* are the most predominant bacteria in the urine microbiomes, along with *Staphylococcus, Streptococcus*, and *Enterococcus*. There was no difference in the urine microbiome between children with UTI, asymptomatic bacteriuria, and negative standard cultures. It has been observed that the route of catheterization may affect the composition of the urine microbiome. Children who catheterize their urethra have a higher proportion of *Staphylococcus*, while the urinary microbiome of patients who catheterize through a Mitrofanoff was composed of *Enterobacteriaceae* family bacteria.

In summary, the urinary microbiome in the pediatric population has just begun to be explored. Further studies that focus on the potential variables influencing the urinary microbiome are needed.

3.4. Review of Studies on Urinary Microbiome and OAB

The first studies investigating the urinary microbiome in patients with urgency concerned women suffering from urge UI who had no signs of infection [53,54]. Research studies confirmed urinary bacterial DNA and the relation of bladder polymicrobial community to certain clinical variables such as baseline urgency urinary incontinence episodes, treatment response, and post-treatment UTI risk [29]. When comparing women with and without urge UI, *Gardnerella* and *Lactobacillus gasseri* were associated with urge UI, while *Lactobacillus crispatus* was detected most frequently in controls, indicating the possibility of a protective effect of *Lactobacillus crispatus* in preventing the development of urge UI [27]. Karstens et al. revealed that the urine microbiome composition of women with normal bladder function and women with urge UI not only varies in the type of bacteria that are present but also in the number of different bacteria and abundance of these bacteria [69]. Women with more severe urge UI symptoms have decreased microbial diversity in their urinary microbiomes. Moreover, the authors noted that of the nine species found to be overrepresented in the urine of patients with urge UI, five bacteria reported as pathogens causing UTI are not routinely detected by routine cultures. This suggests that a persistent low-grade infection by such bacteria could potentially be responsible for the irritating symptoms of urge UI. In another study, it has been established that the uropathogenic bacteria *Proteus* was more commonly isolated from women with OAB. On the other hand, the genus *Lactobacillus* was present less commonly in urine from OAB patients when compared to urine taken from controls [70]. The results are in line with studies describing a significantly greater prevalence of *Lactobacillus* in controls compared to patients with bladder symptoms. The protective role of *Lactobacilli* is explained by their ability to produce bacteriocins, which have activity against uropathogenic bacteria [63].

The above-mentioned studies suggest that perturbations in the urinary microbiome, a state referred to as *dysbiosis*, may predispose to the development of OAB. However, the kind of microbiome diversity connected with OAB is not clear. Thomas-White et al. found that women with urge UI had a different and more diverse microbiome as compared to unaffected women [71]. Among patients treated with solifenacin, an anticholinergic drug, a better response was observed in women with fewer bacteria and a less diverse microbiome whereas non-responders had a community that often included bacteria not typically found in responders. However, in most studies, a decrease in species diversity was associated with urgency UI [69,70].

One should bear in mind that the above studies were cross-sectional in nature and it is not clear whether the differences in the urinary microbiome are the cause or consequences of OAB. It is possible that the urinary frequency typically associated with urgency urinary incontinence alters the microbial community. Significant new findings have highlighted the non-barrier role of the urothelium, especially its sensory functions [24,33,72,73]. As there is clear evidence of communication between the bladder and the brain, it is biologically plausible that the urinary microbiota may play some role in this communication. Therefore, the urothelial sensory signaling and its alteration may be responsible for bladder dysfunction.

4. Conclusions and Future Directions for Studies on Urinary Microbiome and Pediatric OAB

The increasing body of evidence tends to indicate some relationship between qualitative and quantitative characteristics of individual urinary microbiome and OAB symptoms in adult patients [29,69–71]. Surprisingly little is known about the possible associations between the urinary microbiome and OAB symptoms in the pediatric population. In fact, we were unable to identify papers that would specifically address this issue in children or adolescents.

Given the variety of etiopathological concepts and clinical presentations of OAB and the plethora of its somatic and psychological consequences in pediatric patients, studies on the role of the urinary microbiome in OAB could be of clear theoretical and practical importance. The following paragraphs may provide some basic ideas and impetus for research on the link between the urinary microbiome and OAB in children and adolescents.

From a theoretical point of view, future clinical studies could target specific quantitative and/or qualitative traits of the urinary microbiome as correlates of bladder physiology and pathophysiology assessed with the aid of a urine test, an ultrasound of the urinary tract, a bladder diary, dysfunctional elimination symptom questionnaires, and urodynamic methods. Microbiological and molecular approaches could help to identify bacterial species and their metabolic products directly responsible for local alterations in the urothelial milieu even in the absence of obvious symptoms of lower urinary tract infection.

From a practical point of view, it remains to be established whether qualitative and/or quantitative features of the urinary microbiome could be risk or protective factors for the development of OAB in pediatric patients. As clinicians are typically confronted with sick children rather than healthy at-risk individuals, one may also wish to know whether urinary microbiome fingerprints could provide some markers of OAB symptom severity and long-term prognosis in already diagnosed cases. For obvious reasons, it would be of value to correlate the history of lower urinary tract infections and cumulative antibiotic exposure with alterations in the urinary microbiome and OAB symptomatology.

Last but not least, future randomized clinical trials could address the role of antibiotics and probiotics in the primary or secondary prevention of OAB as well as in the treatment of OAB in children and adolescents. Gender, age, hormonal status as well as neuropsychiatric, metabolic (e.g., obesity), renal, urological, and gynecological comorbidities may pose a set of hypothetical factors modifying possible associations between the urinary microbiome and OAB in the pediatric population.

Author Contributions: K.K.-P. and P.B.: conception, study design, collection and interpretation of data, and manuscript writing; A.R.: collection and interpretation of data, revision of the manuscript. All authors have read and agreed to the published version of the manuscript.

Funding: This research received no external funding.

Institutional Review Board Statement: Not applicable.

Informed Consent Statement: Not applicable.

Data Availability Statement: Not applicable.

Conflicts of Interest: All the authors declared no conflict of interest.

References

1. Ramsay, S.; Bolduc, S. Review overactive bladder in children. *Can. Urol. Assoc. J.* **2017**, *1*, S74–S79. [CrossRef] [PubMed]
2. Milsom, I.; Coyne, K.S.; Nicholson, S.; Kvasz, M.; Chen, C.I.; Wein, A.J. Global prevalence and economic burden of urgency urinary incontinence: A systematic review. *Eur. Urol.* **2014**, *65*, 79–95. [CrossRef] [PubMed]
3. Bartoli, S.; Aguzzi, G.; Tarricone, R. Impact on quality of life of urinary incontinence and overactive bladder: A systematic literature review. *Urology* **2010**, *75*, 491–500. [CrossRef] [PubMed]
4. Reynolds, W.S.; Fowke, J.; Dmochowski, R. The burden of overactive bladder on US public health. *Curr. Bladder Dysfunct. Rep.* **2016**, *11*, 8–13. [CrossRef]
5. Landgraf, J.M.; Abidari, J.; Cilento, B.G., Jr.; Cooper, C.S.; Schulman, S.L.; Ortenberg, J. Coping, commitment, and attitude: Quantifying the everyday burden of enuresis on children and their families. *Pediatrics* **2004**, *113*, 334–344. [CrossRef] [PubMed]
6. Franco, I. Overactive bladder in children. *Nat. Rev. Urol.* **2016**, *13*, 520–532. [CrossRef] [PubMed]
7. Austin, P.F.; Bauer, S.B.; Bower, W.; Chase, J.; Franco, I.; Hoebeke, P.; Rittig, S.; Walle, J.V.; Von Gontard, A.; Wright, A.; et al. The standardization of terminology of lower urinary tract function in children and adolescents: Update report from the standardization committee of the International Children's Continence Society. *Neurol. Urodynamics* **2016**, *35*, 471–481. [CrossRef]
8. Tekgul, S.; Stein, R.; Bogaert, G.; Undre, S.; Nijman, R.J.M.; Quaedackers, J.; 't Hoen, L.; Kocvara, R.; Silay, M.S.; Radmayr, C.; et al. EAU-ESPU guidelines recommendations for daytime lower urinary tract conditions in children. *Eur. J. Pediatrics* **2020**, *179*, 1069–1077. [CrossRef] [PubMed]
9. Hellerstein, S.; Zguta, A.A. Outcome of overactive bladder in children. *Clin. Pediatrics* **2003**, *42*, 553–556. [CrossRef] [PubMed]
10. Ural, Z.; Ulman, I.; Avanoglu, A. Bladder dynamics and vesicoureteral reflux: Factors associated with idiopathic lower urinary tract dysfunction in children. *J. Urol.* **2008**, *179*, 1564–1567. [CrossRef]
11. Koff, S.A.; Wagner, T.T.; Jayanthi, V.R. The relationship among dysfunctional elimination syndromes, primary vesicoureteral reflux and urinary tract infections in children. *J. Urol.* **1998**, *160*, 1019–1022. [CrossRef]
12. UpToDate. Etiology and Clinical Features of Bladder Dysfunction in Children. Available online: www-1uptodate-1com-12 h8moszo02a5.han.bg.umed.wroc.pl/contents/etiology-and-clinical-features-of-bladder-dysfunction-in-children (accessed on 2 March 2021).
13. Hellström, A.; Hanson, E.; Hansson, S.; Hjalmas, K.; Jodal, U. Micturition habits and incontinence at age 17—Reinvestigation of a cohort studied at age 7. *Br. J. Urol.* **1995**, *76*, 231–234. [CrossRef] [PubMed]

14. Fitzgerald, M.P.; Thom, D.H.; Wassel-Fyr, C.; Subak, L.; Brubaker, L.; Van den Eeden, S.K.; Brown, J.S. Reproductive risks for incontinence study at Kaiser research group. Childhood urinary symptoms predict adult overactive bladder symptoms. *J. Urol.* **2006**, *175*, 989–993. [CrossRef]
15. Oliveira, R.G.; Baross, U., Jr. Overactive bladder in children. *Eur. Med. J.* **2018**, *3*, 70–77.
16. Gerber, D.; Forster, C.S.; Hsieh, M. The role of the genitourinary microbiome in pediatric urology: A Review. *Curr. Urol. Rep.* **2018**, *19*, 13. [CrossRef]
17. Chung, J.M.; Lee, S.D.; Kang, D.I.; Kwon, D.D.; Kim, K.S.; Kim, S.Y.; Kim, H.G.; Moon, D.G.; Park, K.H.; Park, Y.H.; et al. Korean enuresis association. prevalence and associated factors of overactive bladder in Korean children 5–13 years old: A nationwide multicenter study. *Urology* **2009**, *73*, 63–67. [CrossRef]
18. Kajiwara, M.; Inoue, K.; Kato, M.; Usui, A.; Kurihara, M.; Usui, T. Nocturnal enuresis and overactive bladder in children: An epidemiologic study. *Int. J. Urol.* **2006**, *13*, 36–41. [CrossRef]
19. Middleton, T.; Ellsworth, P. Pharmacologic therapies for the management of non-neurogenic urinary incontinence in children. *Expert. Opin. Pharmacother.* **2019**, *20*, 2335–2352. [CrossRef]
20. Wall, D.L.L.; Heesakkers, J.P. Effectiveness of percutaneous tibial nerve stimulation in the treatment of overactive bladder syndrome. *Res. Rep. Urol.* **2017**, *9*, 145–157. [PubMed]
21. Hellström, A.; Hanson, E.; Hansson, S.; Hjalmas, K.; Jodal, U. Micturition habits and incontinence in 7-year-old Swedish school entrants. *Eur. J. Pediatrics* **1990**, *149*, 434–437. [CrossRef]
22. Sampaio, A.S.; Fraga, L.G.A.; Salomão, B.A.; Oliveira, J.B.; Seixas, C.L.; Veiga, M.L.; Netto, J.M.B.; Barroso, U. Are lower urinary tract symptoms in children associated with urinary symptoms in their mothers? *J. Pediatric Urol.* **2017**, *13*, e1–e269. [CrossRef] [PubMed]
23. Vrijens, D.; Drossaerts, J.; Van Koeveringe, G.; Van Kerrebroeck, P.; Van Os, J.; Leue, C. Affective symptoms and the overactive bladder—A systematic review. *J. Psychosom. Res.* **2015**, *78*, 95–108. [CrossRef]
24. Kim, J.W.; Kim, S.J.; Park, J.M.; Na, Y.G.; Kim, K.H. Past, present, and future in the study of neural control of the lower urinary tract. *Int. Neurol. J.* **2020**, *24*, 191–199. [CrossRef] [PubMed]
25. Farhan, B.; Chang, H.; Ahmed, A.; Zaldivar, F.; Ghoniem, G. Characterisation of urinary monocyte chemoattractant protein 1: Potential biomarker for patients with overactive bladder. *Arab. J. Urol.* **2019**, *17*, 58–60. [CrossRef]
26. Zuo, L.; Zhou, Y.; Wang, S.; Wang, B.; Gu, H.; Chen, J. Abnormal brain functional connectivity strength in the overactive bladder syndrome: A Resting-state fMRI study. *Urology* **2019**, *131*, 64–70. [CrossRef]
27. Pearce, M.M.; Hilt, E.E.; Rosenfeld, A.B.; Zilliox, M.J.; Thomas-White, K.; Fok, C.; Kliethermes, S.; Schreckenberger, P.C.; Brubaker, L.; Gai, X.; et al. The female urinary microbiome: A comparison of women with and without urgency urinary incontinence. *MBio* **2014**, *5*, e01283-14. [CrossRef]
28. Magistro, G.; Stief, C.G. The urinary tract microbiome: The answer to all our open questions? *Eur. Urol. Focus* **2019**, *5*, 36–38. [CrossRef]
29. Pearce, M.M.; Zilliox, M.J.; Rosenfeld, A.B.; Thomas-White, K.J.; Richter, H.E.; Nager, C.W.; Visco, A.G.; Nygaard, I.E.; Barber, M.D.; Schaffer, J.; et al. Pelvic floor disorders network. The female urinary microbiome in urgency urinary incontinence. *Am. J. Obstet. Gynecol.* **2015**, *213*, e1–e11. [CrossRef] [PubMed]
30. Antunes-Lopes, T.; Vale, L.; Coelho, A.M.; Silva, C.; Rieken, M.; Geavlete, B.; Rashid, T.; Rahnama'i, S.M.; Cornu, J.N.; Marcelissen, T. The role of urinary microbiota in lower urinary tract dysfunction: A systematic review. *Eur. Urol. Focus* **2020**, *6*, 361–369. [CrossRef]
31. Baethge, C.; Goldbeck-Wood, S.; Stephan Mertens, S. SANRA—A scale for the quality assessment of narrative review articles. *Res. Integr. Peer Rev.* **2019**, *4*, 5. [CrossRef]
32. Ferrari, R. Writing narrative style literature reviews. *Med. Writing* **2015**, *24*, 230–235. [CrossRef]
33. Smith, A.L. Understanding overactive bladder and urgency incontinence: What does the brain have to do with it? *F1000Res.* **2018**, *7*, F1000 Faculty Rev-1869. [CrossRef]
34. Bauer, S.B.; Yeung, C.K.; Sihoe, J.D. Voiding Dysfunction in Children: Neurogenic and Non-Neurogenic. In *Campbell's Urology*, 9th ed.; Kavoussi, L.R., Novick, A.C., Partin, A.W., Peters, C.A., Wein, A.J., Eds.; WB Saunders Co.: Philadelphia, PA, USA, 2007; pp. 3604–3655.
35. Sillén, U. Bladder function in healthy neonates and its development during infancy. *J. Urol.* **2001**, *166*, 2376–2381. [CrossRef]
36. Griffiths, D.; Derbyshire, S.; Stenger, A.; Resnick, N. Brain control of normal and overactive bladder. *J. Urol.* **2005**, *174*, 1862–1867. [CrossRef] [PubMed]
37. Tyagi, P.; Barclay, D.; Zamora, R.; Yoshimura, N.; Peters, K.; Vodovotz, Y.; Chancellor, M. Urine cytokines suggest an inflammatory response in the overactive bladder: A pilot study. *Int. Urol. Nephrol.* **2010**, *42*, 629–635. [CrossRef] [PubMed]
38. Lewis, D.A.; Brown, R.; Williams, J.; White, P.; Jacobson, S.K.; Marchesi, J.R.; Drake, M.J. The human urinary microbiome; bacterial DNA in voided urine of asymptomatic adults. *Front. Cell. Infect. Microbiol.* **2013**, *3*, 41. [CrossRef] [PubMed]
39. Ghoniem, G.; Faruqui, N.; Elmissiry, M.; Mahdy, A.; Abdelwahab, H.; Oommen, M.; Abdel-Mageed, A.B. Differential profile analysis of urinary cytokines in patients with overactive bladder. *Int. Urogynecol. J.* **2011**, *22*, 953–961. [CrossRef] [PubMed]
40. Al-Ghazo, M.A.; Ghalayini, I.F.; Al-Azab, R.; Hani, O.B.; Matani, Y.S.; Haddad, Y. Urodynamic detrusor overactivity in patients with overactive bladder symptoms. *Int. Neurol. J.* **2011**, *15*, 48–54. [CrossRef] [PubMed]

41. Ptashnyk, T.; Hatzinger, M.; Zeller, F.L.; Kirschner-Hermanns, R. Overactive bladder syndrome—Focus onto detrusor overactivity. *Scand. J. Urol.* **2020**, *55*, 56–60. [CrossRef]
42. Hashim, H.; Abrams, P. Is the bladder a reliable witness for predicting detrusor overactivity? *J. Urol.* **2006**, *175*, 191–194. [CrossRef]
43. Nitti, V.W.; Kopp, Z.; Lin, A.T.L.; Moore, K.H.; Oefelein, M.; Mills, I.W. Can we predict which patient will fail drug treatment for overactive bladder? At think tank discussion. *Neurourol. Urodyn.* **2010**, *29*, 652–657. [CrossRef] [PubMed]
44. Schulman, S.L.; Quinn, C.K.; Plachter, N.; Kodman-Jones, C. Comprehensive management of dysfunctional voiding. *Pediatrics* **1999**, *103*, E31. [CrossRef] [PubMed]
45. Hoebeke, P.; Van Laecke, E.; Van Camp, C.; Raes, A.; Van De Walle, J. One thousand video-urodynamic studies in children with non-neurogenic bladder sphincter dysfunction. *BJU Int.* **2001**, *87*, 575–580. [CrossRef]
46. Bael, A.; Lax, H.; Jong, D.T.P.; Hoebeke, P.; Nijman, R.J.; Sixt, R.; Verhulst, J.; Hirche, H.; Van Gool, J.D. European bladder dysfunction study (European Union BMH1-CT94-1006). The relevance of urodynamic studies for urge syndrome and dysfunctional voiding: A multicenter controlled trial in children. *J. Urol.* **2008**, *180*, 1486–1493. [CrossRef]
47. Benson, A.K.; Kelly, S.A.; Legge, R.; Ma, F.; Low, S.J.; Kim, J.; Zhang, M.; Oh, P.L.; Nehrenberg, D.; Hua, K.; et al. Individuality in gut microbiota composition is a complex polygenic trait shaped by multiple environmental and host genetic factors. *Proc. Natl. Acad. Sci. USA* **2010**, *107*, 18933–18938. [CrossRef] [PubMed]
48. Cho, I.; Blaser, M.J. The human microbiome: At the interface of health and disease. *Nat. Rev. Genet.* **2012**, *13*, 260–270. [CrossRef] [PubMed]
49. Dominguez-Bello, M.G.; Costello, E.K.; Contreras, M.; Magris, M.; Hidalgo, G.; Fierer, N.; Knight, R. Delivery mode shapes the acquisition and structure of the initial microbiota across multiple body habitats in newborns. *Proc. Natl. Acad. Sci. USA* **2010**, *107*, 11971–11975. [CrossRef]
50. Asnicar, F.; Manara, S.; Zolfo, M.; Truong, D.T.; Scholz, M.; Armanini, F.; Ferretti, P.; Gorfer, V.; Pedrotti, A.; Tett, A.; et al. Studying vertical microbiome transmission from mothers to infants by strain-level metagenomic profiling. *mSystems* **2017**, *2*, e00164-16. [CrossRef]
51. Aragón, I.M.; Herrera-Imbroda, B.; Queipo-Ortuño, M.I.; Castillo, E.; Del Moral, J.S.; Gómez-Millán, J.; Yucel, G.; Lara, M.F. The urinary tract microbiome in health and disease. *Eur. Urol. Focus* **2018**, *4*, 128–138. [CrossRef]
52. Ackerman, A.L.; Chai, T.C. The bladder is not sterile: An update on the urinary microbiome. *Curr. Bladder Dysfunct. Rep.* **2019**, *14*, 331–341. [CrossRef]
53. Wolfe, A.J.; Toh, E.; Shibata, N.; Rong, R.; Kenton, K.; Fitzgerald, M.P.; Mueller, E.R.; Schreckenberger, P.; Dong, Q.; Nelson, D.E.; et al. Evidence of uncultivated bacteria in the adult female bladder. *J. Clin. Microbiol.* **2012**, *50*, 1376–1383. [CrossRef] [PubMed]
54. Hilt, E.E.; McKinley, K.; Pearce, M.M.; Rosenfeld, A.B.; Zilliox, M.J.; Mueller, E.R.; Brubaker, L.; Gai, X.; Wolfe, A.J.; Schreckenberger, P.C. Urine is not sterile: Use of enhanced urine culture techniques to detect resident bacterial flora in the adult female bladder. *J. Clin. Microbiol.* **2014**, *52*, 871–876. [CrossRef] [PubMed]
55. Fouts, D.E.; Pieper, R.; Szpakowski, S.; Pohl, H.; Knoblach, S.; Suh, M.J.; Huang, S.H.; Ljungberg, I.; Sprague, B.M.; Lucas, S.K.; et al. Integrated next-generation sequencing of 16S rDNA and metaproteomics differentiate the healthy urine microbiome from asymptomatic bacteriuria in neuropathic bladder associated with spinal cord injury. *J. Transl. Med.* **2012**, *10*, 174. [CrossRef] [PubMed]
56. Morand, A.; Cornu, F.; Dufour, J.C.; Tsimaratos, M.; Lagier, J.C.; Raoult, D. Human bacterial repertoire of the urinary tract: A potential paradigm shift. *J. Clin. Microbiol.* **2019**, *57*, e00675-18. [CrossRef] [PubMed]
57. Kinneman, L.; Zhu, W.; Wong, W.S.W.; Clemency, N.; Provenzano, M.; Vilboux, T.; Jane't, K.; Seo-Mayer, P.; Levorson, R.; Kou, M.; et al. Assessment of the urinary microbiome in children younger than 48 months. *Pediatric Infect. Dis. J.* **2020**, *39*, 565–570. [CrossRef]
58. Curley, T.; Forster, C.S. Recurrent UTIs in girls: What is the role of the microbiome? *Urology* **2020**. [CrossRef] [PubMed]
59. Popović, V.B.; Šitum, M.; Chow, C.-E.T.; Chan, L.S.; Roje, B.; Terzić, J. The urinary microbiome associated with bladder cancer. *Sci. Rep.* **2018**, *8*, 12157. [CrossRef] [PubMed]
60. Hickey, R.J.; Zhou, X.; Settles, M.L.; Erb, J.; Malone, K.; Hansmann, M.A.; Shew, M.L.; Van Der Pol, B.; Fortenberry, D.J.; Forney, L.J. Vaginal microbiota of adolescent girls prior to the onset of menarche resemble those of reproductive-age women. *MBio* **2015**, *6*, e00097-15. [CrossRef]
61. Smith, S.B.; Ravel, J. The vaginal microbiota, host defence and reproductive physiology. *J. Physiol.* **2017**, *595*, 451–463. [CrossRef] [PubMed]
62. Komesu, Y.M.; Dinwiddie, D.L.; Richter, H.E.; Lukacz, E.S.; Sung, V.W.; Siddiqui, N.Y.; Zyczynski, H.M.; Ridgeway, B.; Rogers, R.G.; Arya, L.A.; et al. Pelvic floor disorders network. Defining the relationship between vaginal and urinary microbiomes. *Am. J. Obstet. Gynecol.* **2020**, *222*, e1–e154. [CrossRef]
63. Gorbachinsky, I.; Sherertz, R.; Russell, G.; Krane, L.S.; Hodges, S.J. Altered perineal microbiome is associated with vulvovaginitis and urinary tract infection in preadolescent girls. *Ther. Adv. Urol.* **2014**, *6*, 224–229. [CrossRef]
64. Lucas, E.J.; Ching, C.B.; Saraswat, S.; Dabdoub, S.M.; Kumar, P.P.; Justice, S.S. Acquisition, divergence, and personalization of the female perineal microbiomes are driven by developmental milestones and disrupted by urinary tract infection: A pilot study. *Front. Pediatrics* **2020**, *8*, 542413. [CrossRef] [PubMed]
65. Forster, C.S.; Panchapakesan, K.; Stroud, C.; Banerjee, P.; Gordish-Dressman, H.; Hsieh, M.H. A cross-sectional analysis of the urine microbiome of children with neuropathic bladders. *J. Pediatrics Urol.* **2020**, *16*, e1–e593. [CrossRef] [PubMed]

66. Kassiri, B.; Shrestha, E.; Kasprenski, M.; Antonescu, C.; Florea, L.D.; Sfanos, K.S.; Wang, M.H. A prospective study of the urinary and gastrointestinal microbiome in prepubertal males. *Urology* **2019**, *13*, 204–210. [CrossRef]
67. Kispal, Z.F.; Vajda, P.; Kardos, D.; Klymiuk, I.; Moissl-Eichinger, C.; Castellani, C.; Singer, G.; Till, H. The local microbiome after pediatric bladder augmentation: Intestinal segments and the native urinary bladder host similar mucosal microbiota. *J. Pediatrics Urol.* **2019**, *15*, e1–e30. [CrossRef] [PubMed]
68. Ollberding, N.J.; Völgyi, E.; Macaluso, M.; Kumar, R.; Morrow, C.; Tylavsky, F.A.; Piyathilake, C.J. Urinary microbiota associated with preterm birth: Results from the conditions affecting neurocognitive development and learning in early childhood (CANDLE) study. *PLoS ONE* **2016**, *11*, e0162302. [CrossRef] [PubMed]
69. Karstens, L.; Asquith, M.; Davin, S.; Stauffer, P.; Fair, D.; Gregory, W.T.; Rosenbaum, J.T.; McWeeney, S.K.; Nardos, R. Does the urinary microbiome play a role in urgency urinary incontinence and its severity? *Front. Cell. Infect. Microbiol.* **2016**, *6*, 78. [CrossRef] [PubMed]
70. Curtiss, N.; Balachandran, A.; Krska, L.; Peppiatt-Wildman, C.; Wildman, S.; Duckett, J. A case controlled study examining the bladder microbiome in women with overactive bladder (OAB) and healthy controls. *Eur. J. Obstet. Gynecol. Reprod. Biol.* **2017**, *214*, 31–35. [CrossRef] [PubMed]
71. Thomas-White, K.J.; Hilt, E.E.; Fok, C.; Pearce, M.M.; Mueller, E.R.; Kliethermes, S.; Jacobs, K.; Zilliox, M.J.; Brincat, C.; Price, T.K.; et al. Incontinence medication response relates to the female urinary microbiota. *Int. Urogynecol. J. Pelvic Floor Dysfunct.* **2016**, *27*, 723–733. [CrossRef]
72. Dalghi, M.G.; Montalbetti, N.; Carattino, M.D.; Apodaca, G. The urothelium: Life in a liquid environment. *Physiol. Rev.* **2020**, *100*, 1621–1705. [CrossRef]
73. Roberts, M.W.G.; Sui, G.; Wu, R.; Rong, W.; Wildman, S.; Montgomery, B.; Ali, A.; Langley, S.; Ruggieri, M.R., Sr.; Wu, C. TRPV4 receptor as a functional sensory molecule in bladder urothelium: Stretch-independent, tissue-specific actions and pathological implications. *FASEB J.* **2020**, *34*, 263–286. [CrossRef] [PubMed]

MDPI
St. Alban-Anlage 66
4052 Basel
Switzerland
Tel. +41 61 683 77 34
Fax +41 61 302 89 18
www.mdpi.com

Journal of Clinical Medicine Editorial Office
E-mail: jcm@mdpi.com
www.mdpi.com/journal/jcm

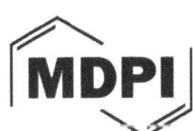